The Molecular Basis of Autism

The Molecular Basis of Autism

Editor: Gweneth Hopkins

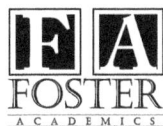

FA
FOSTER
ACADEMICS

www.fosteracademics.com

www.fosteracademics.com

FOSTER
ACADEMICS

Cataloging-in-Publication Data

The molecular basis of autism / edited by Gweneth Hopkins.
    p. cm.
Includes bibliographical references and index.
ISBN 978-1-63242-789-2
    1. Autism--Molecular aspects. 2. Hyperlexia--Molecular aspects.
3. Autism spectrum disorders--Molecular aspects. I. Hopkins, Gweneth.
RC553.A88 M65 2019
616.858 82--dc23

Foster Academics,
118-35 Queens Blvd., Suite 400,
Forest Hills, NY 11375, USA

ISBN 978-1-63242-789-2 (Hardback)

Contents

Preface

An individual with autism experiences difficulties with social interactions and communication, and exhibits restricted and repetitive behavior. The underlying cause of the disease is not entirely understood but can be ascribed to a combination of genetic and environmental factors. The genetics of autism are complex. The associated behaviors of autism may have multiple pathophysiologies. It does not have a unifying mechanism at the cellular, molecular or systems level, but it is believed that autism may be caused due to converging mutations on common molecular pathways. Autistic children experience faster growth of brain in early stages, followed by relatively slower or normal growth during childhood. This early overgrowth is hypothesized to be due to a disturbed neuronal migration during early gestation, an excess of neurons which causes local overconnectivity in specific brain areas, unbalanced excitatory-inhibitory networks, etc. This book covers in detail some existing theories and innovative concepts revolving around the pathophysiology of autism. It presents researches and studies performed by experts across the globe on the molecular basis of autism. It will help new researchers by foregrounding their knowledge in this domain.

The researches compiled throughout the book are authentic and of high quality, combining several disciplines and from very diverse regions from around the world. Drawing on the contributions of many researchers from diverse countries, the book's objective is to provide the readers with the latest achievements in the area of research. This book will surely be a source of knowledge to all interested and researching the field.

In the end, I would like to express my deep sense of gratitude to all the authors for meeting the set deadlines in completing and submitting their research chapters. I would also like to thank the publisher for the support offered to us throughout the course of the book. Finally, I extend my sincere thanks to my family for being a constant source of inspiration and encouragement.

Editor

Randomised controlled trial of simvastatin treatment for autism in young children with neurofibromatosis type 1 (SANTA)

Stavros Stivaros[1,2†], Shruti Garg[3†], Maria Tziraki[4], Ying Cai[5], Owen Thomas[6], Joseph Mellor[7], Andrew A. Morris[8], Carly Jim[9], Karolina Szumanska-Ryt[4], Laura M Parkes [4], Hamied A. Haroon[4], Daniela Montaldi[4], Nicholas Webb[10], John Keane[7], Francisco X. Castellanos[11], Alcino J. Silva[5], Sue Huson[12], Stephen Williams[2], D. Gareth Evans[12], Richard Emsley[13], Jonathan Green[3*†] [iD] and SANTA Consortium

Abstract

Background: Neurofibromatosis 1 (NF1) is a monogenic model for syndromic autism. Statins rescue the social and cognitive phenotype in animal knockout models, but translational trials with subjects > 8 years using cognition/behaviour outcomes have shown mixed results. This trial breaks new ground by studying statin effects for the first time in younger children with NF1 and co-morbid autism and by using multiparametric imaging outcomes.

Methods: A single-site triple-blind RCT of simvastatin vs. placebo was done. Assessment (baseline and 12-week endpoint) included peripheral MAPK assay, awake magnetic resonance imaging spectroscopy (MRS; GABA and glutamate+glutamine (Glx)), arterial spin labelling (ASL), apparent diffusion coefficient (ADC), resting state functional MRI, and autism behavioural outcomes (Aberrant Behaviour Checklist and Clinical Global Impression).

Results: Thirty subjects had a mean age of 8.1 years (SD 1.8). Simvastatin was well tolerated. The amount of imaging data varied by test. Simvastatin treatment was associated with (i) increased frontal white matter MRS GABA ($t(12) = -2.12$, $p = .055$), GABA/Glx ratio ($t(12) = -2.78$, $p = .016$), and reduced grey nuclei Glx (ANCOVA $p < 0.05$, Mann-Whitney $p < 0.01$); (ii) increased ASL perfusion in ventral diencephalon (Mann-Whitney $p < 0.01$); and (iii) decreased ADC in cingulate gyrus (Mann-Whitney $p < 0.01$). Machine-learning classification of imaging outcomes achieved 79% ($p < .05$) accuracy differentiating groups at endpoint against chance level (64%, $p = 0.25$) at baseline. Three of 12 (25%) simvastatin cases compared to none in placebo met 'clinical responder' criteria for behavioural outcome.

Conclusions: We show feasibility of peripheral MAPK assay and autism symptom measurement, but the study was not powered to test effectiveness. Multiparametric imaging suggests possible simvastatin effects in brain areas previously associated with NF1 pathophysiology and the social brain network.

Trial registration: EU Clinical Trial Register (EudraCT) 2012-005742-38 (www.clinicaltrialsregister.eu)

Keywords: Autism, Neurofibromatosis type 1, Neuroimaging, Randomised controlled trial, Statin, Simvastatin

* Correspondence: jonathan.green@manchester.ac.uk
†Equal contributors
[3]Division of Neuroscience and Experimental Psychology, School of Biological Sciences, Faculty of Biology, Medicine and Health, University of Manchester, Manchester Academic Health Science Centre, Manchester University NHS Foundation Trust, Greater Manchester Mental Health NHS Foundation Trust, Room 3.311, Jean McFarlane Building, Oxford Road, Manchester M13 9PL, UK
Full list of author information is available at the end of the article

Background

Neurofibromatosis 1 (NF1) is the most common autosomal dominant single-gene neurodevelopmental disorder with incidence of 1:2700, [1] caused by loss of function mutations in the NF1 gene on chromosome 17q11.2 encoding for neurofibromin. Although identified by neurocutaneous manifestations, morbidity in childhood NF1 usually relates to cognitive, social and behavioural difficulties, with moderate cognitive impairment and academic underachievement in about 80% [2] and attention-deficit/hyperactivity disorder (ADHD) in 38–50% [2, 3]. Recent evidence of autism spectrum disorder (ASD) prevalence of ~ 25% with partial traits in a further 20% [4, 5] support NF1 as a promising single-gene syndromic model for understanding ASD pathology [6].

The neurobiology of the social and learning deficits in NF1 has been studied in $Nf1^{+/-}$ mouse models and recent in-human studies [7]. Neurofibromin is a negative regulator of rat-sarcoma viral oncogene homologue (Ras); loss of neurofibromin causes disinhibition of the RasMAPK pathway with consequent GABA/glutamate disequilibrium, impairment in long-term potentiation (LTP) and synaptic plasticity [8]. Upregulation of the Ras pathway can also directly affect myelin formation and axonal integrity [9] and dysregulate nitric oxide signalling pathways in oligodendrocytes [10]. Recent diffusion tensor imaging (DTI) study in human NF1 [11] demonstrated increased apparent diffusion coefficient (ADC) values localised in the caudate and other deep grey nuclei, diencephalon and frontal white matter in NF1 children compared to controls, consistent with decreased neuronal density or myelin sheath disorganisation; the extent of these effects was associated with neurological symptoms. Other imaging studies in human NF1 have identified reduced cortical GABA [12, 13], reduced cerebral perfusion [14], alteration in diffusion-weighted imaging [15] and abnormal network connectivity on resting state fMRI [16, 17].

This emerging understanding of NF1 neural system pathophysiology from animal and human studies has provided a rationale for experimental intervention trials. Compensatory downregulation of Ras activation can be achieved by blocking its farnesylation, using 3-hydroxy-3-methylglutaryl coenzyme A (HMG-CoA) reductase inhibitors (statins). Attenuation of Ras activity in $Nf1^{+/-}$ mouse models using lovastatin [18] or, alternatively, through genetic co-deletion of the Pak1 gene ($Nf1^{+/-}, Pak1^{+/-}$) [7] rescues the biochemical, electrophysiological and behavioural deficits, including normalisation of social memory and autism-like behavioural phenotypes. Convergence in effect of these two methods supports the specificity of the target mechanism. Further, the Pak1 gene co-deletion experiment illustrated the potential of such studies to illuminate causal pathogenic

pathways, by suggesting functional localisation of the primary Ras-related pathology in the amygdala and other parts of the social brain network, and causal involvement of specific synaptic proteins [7].

Translational statin intervention studies in human NF1, based on the Ras downregulation hypothesis, have had mixed results. Improvements in verbal and nonverbal memory were reported within a 12-week phase 1 single-arm study examining the safety and tolerability of lovastatin in 23 children aged 10–17 years [19] and in a 14-week randomised controlled trial (RCT) of lovastatin in 44 10–50-year-olds [20]. Normalisation of pseudo-resting state functional connectivity in areas of the default mode network (DMN) following lovastatin treatment was found in a case series of 7 children from the prior child cohort [21]. A case-control study of transcranial magnetic stimulation in 11 adults with NF1 showed impaired synaptic plasticity and deficits in phasic alertness at baseline compared to controls, which improved after 4 days of high-dose (200 mg) lovastatin [22]. However, larger statin trials have found little effect. A 12-week double-blind, placebo-controlled RCT of simvastatin in 62 children with NF1 aged 8–16 found no group differences on primary behavioural outcome measures and minimal improvements in cognitive aspects of visual synthesis in the simvastatin group; [23] another RCT of simvastatin (84 children aged 8–16 years) found no improvements in cognitive deficits or parent-reported behavioural problems [24]. A 16-week RCT of lovastatin in 146 8–15-year-olds with NF1 and visuospatial learning/attention deficits found no improvements on a paired associate learning task [25].

This human intervention work has been on mid-childhood or older cohorts rather than in earlier development. Trials have also not specifically targeted NF1-autism behavioural outcomes or used multiparametric imaging techniques. We report here therefore on the first experimental trial of a statin in young children with NF1 with co-occurring autism, using detailed multilevel measurements designed to assess the pathogenic pathway identified in NF1 animal models from gene disruption to cognitive and behavioural pathology. These included (i) statin effects at a cellular level on Ras activation, using peripheral MAPKinase assay; (ii) multiparametric imaging to reflect different related aspects of neural system structure, neurophysiology and in vivo function; and (iii) NF1-relevant cognitive and autism-related behavioural outcomes. By investigating statin effects on these different levels, we aim to illuminate the dynamics and possible causal relationships of this pathogenic pathway in humans. Hypotheses were that (i) statin treatment in young children with NF1-autism would be feasible, safe and acceptable to families; (ii) peripheral MAPKinase assay and awake multiparametric imaging could be acquired; and (iii) that although the study was not powered for definitive treatment effect estimation, signals of change in MAPK and multimodal imaging parameters would be detectable, along with change in autism and other cognitive and behavioural symptoms. Specific imaging parameters for testing and hypothesised parameter changes were selected on the basis of the existing imaging literature in NF1, especially those linked to known abnormalities in idiopathic autism. Thus, we expected normalisation of the reduced GABA and perfusion metrics, and reduction in the abnormalities in DTI and connectivity metrics found in NF1 (see "Methods" section).

Methods

Design and participants

A single-site triple-blind (clinician, family, assesor) RCT of simvastatin vs. placebo in children with NF1-autism, the SimvAstatin in Neurofibromatosis Type 1-Autism (SANTA) trial, was registered with EudraCT number 2012-005742-38. Study protocol is available on http://research.bmh.manchester.ac.uk/santa. Participants were children between 4.5–10.5 years meeting diagnostic criteria for (i) NF1 (National Institutes of Health criteria) [26] (ii) autism spectrum disorder (ASD) using Collaborative Program of Excellence in Autism (CPEA) criteria, based on Autism Diagnostic Interview-Revised (ADI-R), Autism Diagnostic Observation Scale-2 and WASI (Wechsler Abbreviated Scale of Intelligence) verbal IQ, [27] after positive initial screening ($T > 60$) on parent-rated Social Responsiveness Scale (SRS). They were recruited via local and regional UK NF1 clinics (Manchester, Leeds, Newcastle, Edinburgh, Wirral, Warrington and Edinburgh, UK) and through NF charities' newsletters, websites and social media pages. Exclusion criteria were (i) severe learning disability (WASI verbal IQ < 50); (ii) in active treatment for another NF1 complication (e.g., chemotherapy for optic pathway or other low-grade glioma, Ilizarov frame for pseudarthrosis) or clinically significant unrelated illness; (iii) abnormal liver function or creatinine kinase at baseline (iv) parents of participants with insufficient English to complete the ASD screening assessments; (v) use of psychotropic medication other than stimulants, current simvastatin use or any investigational drug within 4 months of screening; (vi) participants with planned surgery within 16 weeks of potential enrolment. Participants on a stable dose of stimulants for at least 3 months prior to screening were permitted to participate.

Measures

MAPK assay (baseline, 12-week endpoint) in peripheral lymphocytes was used as a marker of the effectiveness of statin-induced downregulation of the intracellular Ras pathway. In animal models, peripheral estimation of this kind has shown consistency with neural Ras activity, and in humans, has been associated with cognitive function in Alzheimer's disease and cognitive impairment [28, 29]. Details of methodology and assay are given in Additional file 1.

Brain imaging (baseline, 12-week endpoint) on a Philips 3T Achieva scanner (Eindhoven, The Netherlands) was implemented using a 32-channel head coil for signal reception and body coil for transmission with no contrast or sedation. Imaging parameters were purposefully selected on the basis of prior hypotheses relating to existing imaging findings in NF1 on cortical GABA spectroscopy [12, 13], MR cerebral perfusion [14], alteration in diffusion-weighted imaging [15] and abnormal network connectivity on resting state fMRI [16, 17]. Additional file 1: Table S1 outlines the imaging protocol, along with our patient preparation protocol to facilitate awake scanning in this challenging imaging cohort. No visual stimulation was allowed for the initial resting state fMRI acquisition, but following this, the children were allowed to watch a projected film of their choice or listen to music if they preferred. Imaging data were acquired at week 0 and then again following either exposure to placebo or simvastatin for 12 weeks. In four cases, where the initial imaging dataset was incomplete, a week 4 scan was performed which acquired only the missing week 0 imaging datasets (T1 volume and diffusion data).

Autism symptoms (baseline, 4 weeks, 12-week endpoint) were quantified using standard measures of proven specificity and sensitivity to treatment effect over short periods and widely used in autism psychopharmacology trials [30, 31]. Parent-rated *Aberrant Behaviour Checklist* (ABC) [32] has 58-items on 1–4 Likert scale with five subscales: irritability, hyperactivity, lethargy/withdrawal, stereotypy and inappropriate speech. *Parent-defined target symptoms* [33] was based on blinded researcher interview. One or two problems of greatest concern to parents at baseline, rated on frequency, duration, intensity and functional impairment, were assessed on a 9-point scale as 1 = normal, 2 = markedly improved, 3 = definitely improved, 4 = equivocally better, 5 = no change, 6 = equivocally worse, 7 = definitely worse, 8 = markedly worse, and 9 = disastrously worse. Ratings across the two target symptoms were averaged. *Clinical Global Impression Scale* (CGI-S) [34] was used in measuring severity of psychopathology on a 7-point scale, change from the initiation of treatment on a similar 7-point scale and the drug efficacy index. Over three decades of research the CGI correlates well with standard research drug efficacy scales [34]. *Overactivity symptoms* were assessed using the standard parent-rated Conners questionnaire [35]. Following standard practice in autism medication trials [36], *clinical responders* were defined as children with 25% reduction in the parent-rated ABC irritability score plus a rating of 'much improved' or 'very much improved' on the clinician-rated CGI scale.

Acceptability

Telephone interviews were conducted at 16 weeks (4 weeks after the end of the trial) by researchers independent of the trial research team, and blind to treatment arm, to assess parent acceptability of the trial protocol. This 19-item interview was rated on a 5-point Likert scale from strongly disagree to strongly agree for each stem statement.

Procedures

Eligible participants were randomised on a 1:1 ratio by the clinical trial pharmacy at Manchester University NHS Foundation Trust using web-based randomisation with blocks of 2 and 4. The results of the randomisation were not communicated outside the pharmacy, which delivered the appropriate masked drug bottles to the research team. All investigators, participants and their parents were kept masked to treatment allocation.

Simvastatin is an HMG-CoA reductase inhibitor. It has a UK and US licence for use in age 10 and above, and there is extensive off-label clinical experience of its use in younger children with other disorders such as familial hypercholesterolaemia and Smith Lemli Opitz Syndrome. The bioavailability of simvastatin is 42.5% ± 42.5. The only other available statin which crosses the blood brain barrier (lovastatin) is not licenced for use in children in Europe.

Assessments were carried out at the NIHR/Wellcome Trust Clinical Research Facility, Manchester University NHS Foundation Trust at baseline and weeks 4 and 12. After baseline and randomisation, participants were treated with simvastatin or placebo in liquid preparation at 0.5 mg/kg in a single daily dose. At week 4, in the absence of any reported adverse effects, or abnormalities of plasma biochemistry (LFTs and CK), simvastatin dose was increased to 1 mg/kg/day to a maximum of 30 mg/day. This dosing regime was similar to those used in other studies of simvastatin in young children [37] and was selected for known safety and indirectly for known efficacy in such other contexts.

Consent and ethics

We obtained informed oral and written consent from parents and assent from children where developmentally appropriate. The local ethics committee approved the study (REC Reference 13/NW/0111). The trial was conducted in agreement with the Declaration of Helsinki and Good Clinical Practice Guidelines.

Statistical analysis
Behavioural measures

Statistical analysis was performed in Stata version 14, based on an intention-to-treat approach using all randomised patients and followed the CONSORT statement and trial protocol. The only protocol measure not presented in this report is the Judgement of Line Orientation Test, for which insufficient analysable data were available (details in Additional file 1). The primary analysis was based on tabulated and associated graphical summaries of feasibility indicators: patient recruitment, checks for the absence of selective recruitment of participants; baseline balance of summary statistics and patient flow. The study was not powered for formal analysis of between-group treatment effect on clinical and behavioural outcomes; the presented results focus on point estimates and associated 95% confidence intervals rather than statistical significance. Analysis was performed using linear regression models to estimate the effect of random allocation on autism and behavioural symptom outcomes at 12 weeks, adjusting for baseline values of the relevant outcome as a linear covariate. Bootstrapping with 500 replications was used to estimate standard errors for all models.

Imaging analysis (further details in Additional file 1)

GABA spectroscopy GABA measurements were taken from (i) frontal white matter (FWM) and (ii) deep grey nuclei (DGN) using the localised spectroscopy sequence MEGA-PRESS, using the unsuppressed water signal as a reference. GABA measurement is defined as 'GABA+', due to macromolecular signal contribution [38]. The sum of glutamate and glutamine (Glx) was measured via the same acquisition, giving a peak centred at 3.75 ppm. A non-water-suppressed acquisition from the same locations was acquired to act as reference. Statistical analyses in SPSS 22.0 considered the absolute and between-group change from baseline to endpoint, with and without adjustment for baseline variation. Parametric (*t* test) and non-parametric (Mann-Whitney test with covariate adjustment) [39] tests were used for comparison, based on normality of the data. No correction was made for testing across multiple regions.

Perfusion imaging Pulsed arterial spin labelling images were acquired using a modified 'STAR' technique [40], together with co-aligned proton density images. Perfusion images were obtained by subtracting control images from labelled images and fitting to a single blood-compartment model using an in-house code provided by LP (see Additional file 1: Table S1). The median regional CBF values were calculated following CBF map registration to the corresponding structural T1 images.

Diffusion imaging We applied a diffusion-weighted multislice spin echo single-shot echo planar imaging sequence transaxially: slices 55 contiguous, $b = 1000$ s/mm^2 (Δ/δ 36.4/22.7 ms) in 6 non-collinear directions. One volume (b0 image) was also acquired without a diffusion gradient; $b = 0$ s/mm^2. The median regional ADC values were calculated following ADC map registration to the corresponding structural T1 images.

Resting state fMRI Single-shot, whole brain coverage, echo planar imaging was used to acquire resting state data (Additional file 1: Table S1). Spatial networks demonstrating strong temporal co-activation in the resting BOLD fMRI responses were defined using probabilistic independent component analysis (ICA). The analysis for differences between groups was performed using a dual regression technique, which allowed for voxel-by-voxel comparisons of functional connectivity.

Machine learning The whole imaging dataset was analysed for stratification into simvastatin or placebo groups with a Random Forest machine learning classifier. Cross-validation was performed, such that each fold contained at least one example of each group. The significance of the resulting area under the curve (AUC) score was assessed using a test where the group labels were permuted (Python scikit-learn library) [41].

Results

Trial flow
Additional file 1: Figure S4 shows the CONSORT flow chart for the study. Ninety-one completed parent-reported SRS questionnaires were received between October 2013 and June 2015. Of these, 71 met eligibility criteria and were invited for in-depth assessment; 53 were seen for baseline ASD assessments, from which 30 met CPEA criteria for ASD and were randomised (placebo, 16; simvastatin, 14); 26 completed endpoint assessment at 12 weeks. All analyses were by assigned groups.

Demographics and baseline status
Additional file 1: Tables S2 and S3 shows baseline demographic and clinical data for the two groups. The mean age of the sample was 8.10 years. Two participants in the simvastatin arm and two in the placebo arm had a pre-existing diagnosis of ADHD and were on stimulant medication. Baseline measures including ADI-R, ADOS, Verbal IQ and SRS scores were generally well matched across the groups, and the screening and diagnostic autism measures all showed values well within the standardised autism range (Additional file 1: Table S2). In the simvastatin group, 21.4% had inherited the NF1 mutations as opposed to 62.5% in the placebo group, but we have no evidence of any differential effect from familial or sporadic cases on

any baseline or outcome variable from our previous studies [4, 42]. Genotype data on the cohort is presented in Additional file 1: Table S7 where it is also compared to a large recently published genotyped cohort from our group [43]. There are no obvious differences in mutation type between the SANTA cohort and the larger cohort, suggesting representativeness of the SANTA cohort. There was no SPRED1 and only one microdeletion in the cohort. Patient defined target symptoms included hyperactivity, aggression, social inappropriateness, difficulties with communication, inflexibility/obsessionality and learning problems. In four cases (three in simvastatin, one in placebo), there was movement artefact on the T1 volume and diffusion sequences, and these parameters were then re-acquired at week 4 visit.

Acceptability
Sixteen-week telephone interview data was available for 25 participants. The scanning protocol was acceptable for all of these families, 21/25 families felt that the habituation CD helped with the scanning process.

Adverse events
Adverse events (AEs) recorded are set out in Additional file 1: Table S4. These were all minor and not specific to the simvastatin arm; none resulted in drug discontinuation or dose reduction. There were no severe adverse events or suspected unexpected serious adverse reactions.

Outcome estimation
Peripheral MAPK activity
Completed assay was achieved in 27/30 cases (12/14 simvastatin, 15/16 placebo) at baseline and 22/26 (9/11 simvastatin, 13/15 placebo) at endpoint. Missing data is related to inadequate venesection volumes and the need to prioritise adverse event monitoring. Representative Western blot assays are shown in Fig. 1 and quantification of outcomes in Additional file 1: Figure S6. Assay results showed wide variance; robust estimation using a linear method gave a moderate between-group treatment effect size point estimate of 0.60 reduction of pMAPK in favour of intervention, but with 95% CI – .34 to 1.54, ranging from small increase to large reduction (Fig. 2).

Imaging
MR spectroscopy MRS data was acquired for frontal white matter (FWM) in 27/30 cases at baseline and 19/26 at endpoint. Within this, endpoint voxel assessment of GABA+ data was possible in 5/11 simvastatin and 9/15 placebo and showed a trend towards between-group increase in the simvastatin group compared to placebo (mean 1.82 placebo vs. 2.39 simvastatin ($t(12) = -2.12$, $p = .055$, two-

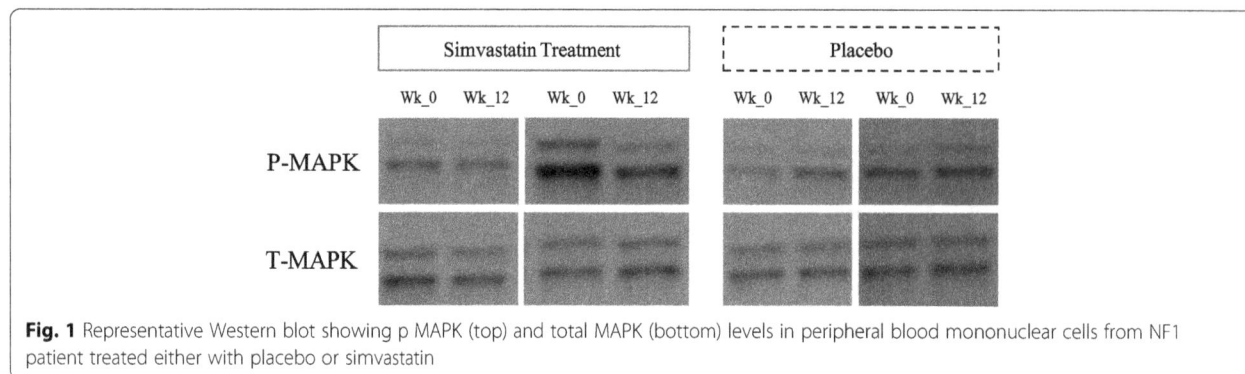

Fig. 1 Representative Western blot showing p MAPK (top) and total MAPK (bottom) levels in peripheral blood mononuclear cells from NF1 patient treated either with placebo or simvastatin

tailed uncorrected), although this was not present when adjusted for baseline values (ANCOVA $p = 0.188$, Mann-Whitney $p = 0.66$; Fig. 3a). Glx showed no effect, but GABA/Glx ratio showed significant endpoint difference $(t(12) = -2.78, p = .016$ two-tailed, uncorrected). MRS data for deep grey nuclei (DGN) was acquired in 24/30 at baseline and 23/26 at endpoint. Pre-post analysis was possible on 13 simvastatin and 12 placebo; it showed no change in GABA+ value but a significant post-treatment reduction in Glx compared to placebo (ANCOVA $p < 0.05$, Mann-Whitney $p < 0.01$; Fig. 3b), although uncorrected for a significantly lower Glx in the treatment group at baseline $(t(18) = -3.08, p = .006)$.

Perfusion and diffusivity assessment Validated data for diffusion analysis were acquired on 20/30 cases at baseline (10/14 simvastatin, 10/16 placebo) and 16/26 at endpoint (8/11 simvastatin, 8/15 placebo). Perfusion data analysis was available on 28/30 cases at baseline (12/14 simvastatin cases and 14/16 placebo) and 23/30 cases post treatment (10/14 simvastatin and 13/16 placebo). Analysis of available paired pre-post data (7 simvastatin and 13 placebo) showed significant increase in perfusion within the ventral diencephalon associated with statin treatment (ANCOVA $p < 0.01$ and Mann-

Whitney $p < 0.01$, uncorrected; Fig. 4a). Analysis of available paired pre-post data (5 simvastatin and 6 placebo) showed decrease in ADC within the cingulate gyrus associated with statin treatment (ANCOVA $p = 0.01$, Mann-Whitney $p < 0.01$, uncorrected; Fig. 4b).

Resting state fMRI Probabilistic ICA identified the default mode network (DMN) separately in both baseline (10/14 simvastatin, 11/16 placebo) and week 12 (6/11 simvastatin, 11/15 placebo) rsfMRI acquisitions. Dual regression did not identify any significant differences between simvastatin and placebo groups in the DMN spatial maps when tested at the 5% significance level (corrected for multiple comparisons). However, at the 10% significance level foci of decreased co-activation in the simvastatin group compared to placebo were seen within the right occipital lobe and left perirolandic region ($p = 0.093$ and 0.092, respectively, corrected, voxel counts 11 and 3; Fig. 5). No significant differences were seen at the 10% level in the DMN at week zero nor in the sensorimotor or medial visual networks at either time point.

Machine learning The whole imaging dataset was entered for analysis. Baseline classification accuracy was 64% ($p = 0.25$) compatible with stratification into groups on the basis of chance alone. Following treatment, the features with best statistical power for group allocation were the ADC values in the occipital cortex, the occipital white matter and the parietal white matter. We compared changes in the left- and right-sided ADC metric in these regions between both groups and found classification accuracy rose from baseline to 79% ($p < 0.05$; Fig. 6), suggesting a simvastatin treatment effect.

Behavioural outcomes
Behavioural symptom endpoint outcomes are shown in Table 1 (and week 4 intermediate outcomes in Additional file 1: Table S5). The trial was not powered to show significant between-group behaviour effects, and

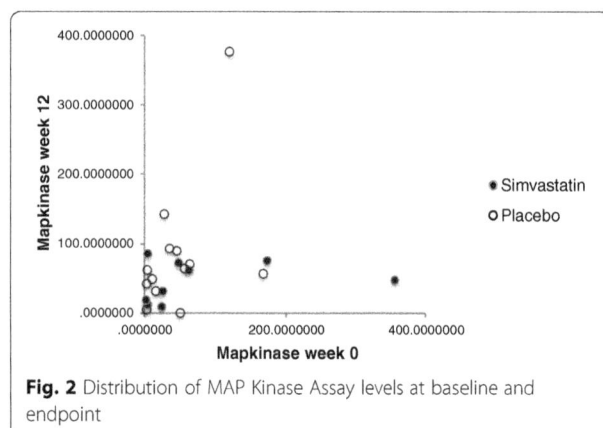

Fig. 2 Distribution of MAP Kinase Assay levels at baseline and endpoint

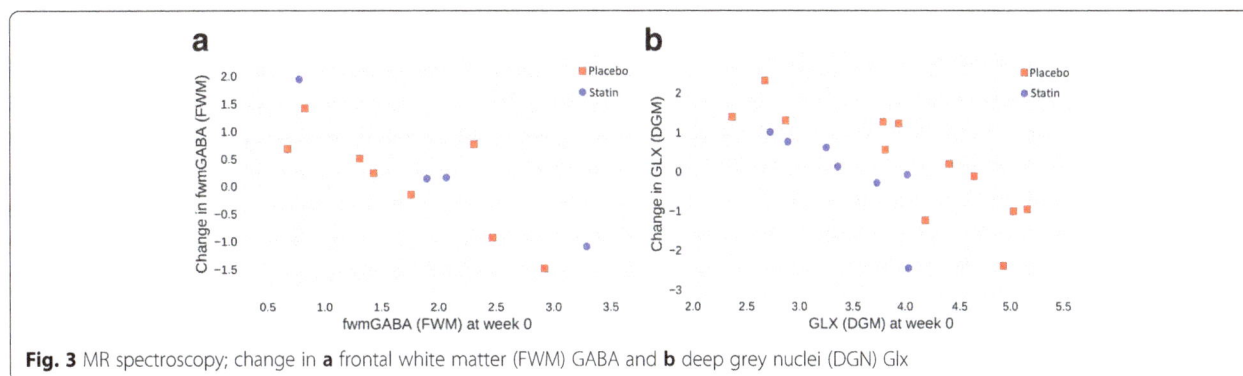

Fig. 3 MR spectroscopy; change in **a** frontal white matter (FWM) GABA and **b** deep grey nuclei (DGN) Glx

none were seen. At endpoint, 3/12 (25%) of the statin treatment cases were classified as clinical responders using standard RUPP (Research Units of Paediatric Psychopharmacology) criteria [26] compared to 0/14 (0%) in the placebo group. Each of these responders also met subsidiary standards for response on the patient-defined target symptoms (PDTS < 3). Two further cases in the statin group and 2/14 in the placebo group met PDTS responder criteria only. The responder group (*n* = 3) was characterised clinically by being male, with the mean age of 9.29 years (SD 0.77), with a relatively high-baseline ADOS total score of 17.0 (SD 1.73) but other metrics similar to group means (baseline SRS total score = 87.6 (SD 2.08), ADI-R social interaction 20.66 (SD 1.52), communication 15 (SD1.73) and RRBs 5.33 (1.55).

Discussion

Previous statin trials in older children and adults have shown mixed effects, but most used lovastatin and measured outcomes at just cognitive or behavioural levels. This trial used simvastatin, considered the most effective neuroprotective statin [44]. It is also the first trial that has looked in detail at statin effects on 'upstream' process at cell and neural system levels, reflecting a pathogenic pathway between gene disruption and the autism-related behavioural psychopathological outcomes known in NF1. We interpret the outcomes therefore in relation to each of these levels, while acknowledging that

the restricted sample size in this data-rich trial, and the variable amounts of data available for different analyses, limits precision of estimation.

At the *cellular level*, the moderate between-group point estimate showing peripheral lymphocyte reduction of MAPK function was in the hypothesised direction, consistent with a statin effect at the cell level on the Ras pathway activation; the wide 95% CI values ranged from a large decrease to a small increase. Preparation, international transport and storage of the samples may have introduced increased variance in the assay results.

At a *neural system level*, neuroimaging shows evidence of specific statin effects in regions of interest of the brain including frontal white matter, deep grey nuclei (lentiform, caudate and thalamic nuclei), cingulate gyrus, ventral diencephalon and occipital/occipito-parietal cortex. Detection of GABA in white matter has been reported in other studies, albeit at lower levels than in grey matter [45]. The effects of the statin on the multiparametric data are in a direction consistent with normalising many aspects of the underlying NF1-related neuropathology identified in previous studies. Thus, the suggested increased absolute GABA levels in frontal white matter is consistent with reversing the reduced cortical GABA found in previous studies in children and young adults with NF1 [12, 13] (a contrast to the increase found in animal experiments [7, 18]). The variation in GABA findings by brain region in our study is echoed in a

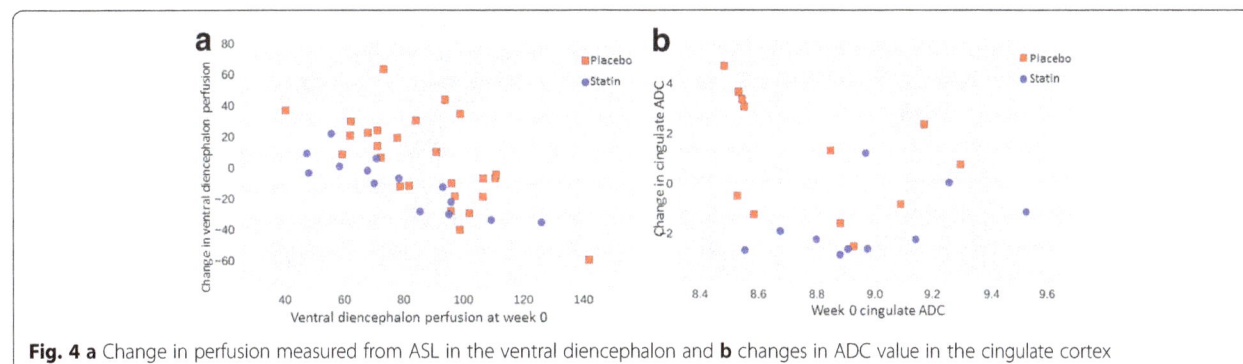

Fig. 4 a Change in perfusion measured from ASL in the ventral diencephalon and **b** changes in ADC value in the cingulate cortex

Table 1 Endpoint behavioural outcomes

Week 12 outcomes	Summary statistics			Mean difference			
	Sample	Placebo	Simvastatin	Adjusted mean difference (95% CI)	Bootstrap SE	Effect size (95% CI)	Number analysed
ABC	$N = 28$	$N = 15$	$N = 13$				
Irritability	19.14 (11.62)	16.40 (10.82)	22.31 (12.14)	1.66 (− 4.61, 7.93)	3.20	0.14 (− 0.40, 0.68)	28
Lethargy[*]	12.63 (10.01)	10.53 (9.61)	15.25 (10.30)[*]	3.60 (− 4.09, 11.28)	3.92	0.29 (− 0.41, 1.13)	26
Stereotypy	5.71 (5.08)	3.93 (3.63)	7.77 (5.83)	1.61 (− 0.98, 4.20)	1.32	0.32 (− 0.19, 0.83)	28
Hyperactivity	23.61 (13.68)	19.13 (13.17)	28.77(12.83)	3.87 (− 3.28, 11.01)	3.65	0.28 (− 0.24, 0.80)	28
Inappropriate speech	5.89 (3.11)	4.80 (2.54)	7.15 (3.31)	1.77 (− 0.10, 3.63)	0.95	0.57 (− 0.03, 1.17)	28
25% reduction irritability subscale	$N = 11$	$N = 5$	$N = 6$				
Conners	$N = 28$	$N = 15$	$N = 13$				
Inattention	77.25 (12.57)	74.53 (14.16)	80.38 (10.08)	5.33 (− 0.96, 11.61)	3.21	0.42 (− 0.08, 0.92)	27
Hyperactivity	73.54 (15.92)	69.40 (17.12)	78.31 (13.51)	−0.98 (− 8.09, 6.13)	3.63	−0.06 (− 0.51, 0.39)	27
Learning problems	69.25 (14.62)	65.40 (12.91)	73.69 (15.71)	1.59 (− 2.13, 5.30)	1.89	0.11 (− 0.15, 0.36)	27
Executive function	71.82 (14.59)	68.20 (16.24)	76.00 (11.66)	4.04 (− 2.51, 10.59)	3.34	0.28 (− 0.17, 0.73)	27
Aggression	70.43 (18.98)	68.40 (20.86)	72.77 (17.09)	− 0.05 (− 11.05,10.96)	5.61	− 0.00 (− 0.58, 0.58)	27
Peer relations	83.89 (11.53)	82.00 (13.51)	86.08 (8.73)	1.38 (− 4.45, 7.21)	2.97	0.12 (− 0.39, 0.63)	27
Parent-defined target symptoms (PDTS)	$N = 26$	$N = 14$	$N = 12$				
Mean (SD)	3.52 (1.77)	3.75 (1.86)	3.25 (1.68)				
Responders (PDTS score < 3)	7	2	5				
CGI[*]	$N = 26$	$N = 14$	$N = 12$				
Global improvement Mean (SD)	3.31 (0.84)	3.57 (0.85)	3.00 (0.74)				
Treatment responder+	$N = 3$	$N = 0$	$N = 3$				

[*]1 additional observation missing. +Treatment responder defined as > 25% reduction in ABC irritability subscale and a score of improved or much improved on CGI

Higher scores on ABC, Conners and CGI are indicative of higher levels of impairment

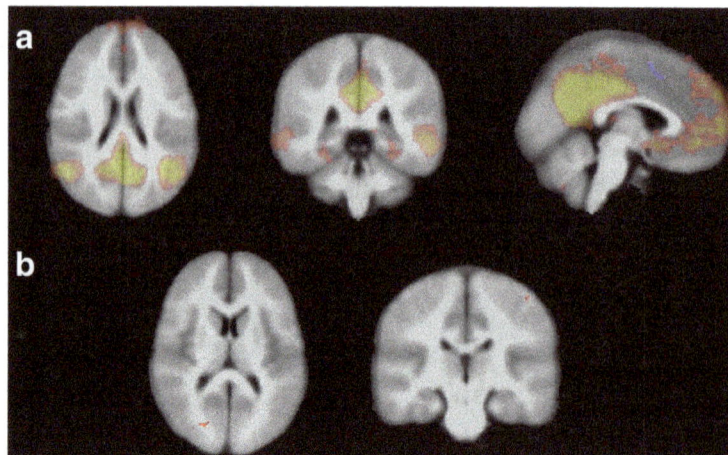

Fig. 5 rsfMRI **a** default mode network (DMN) demonstrated by probabilistic group ICA of week 12 acquisitions (axial, coronal, sagittal). **b** At week 12, foci of decreased DMN co-activation were identified at the 10% level within the right occipital and left perirolandic regions. No significant differences in the DMN were identified at the 5% level, corrected

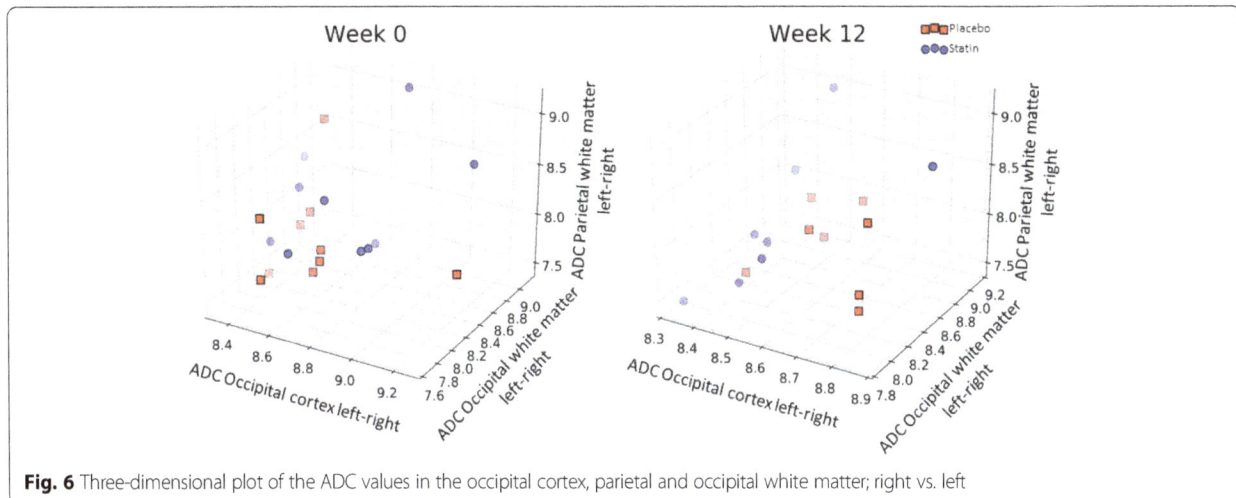

Fig. 6 Three-dimensional plot of the ADC values in the occipital cortex, parietal and occipital white matter; right vs. left

recent NF1 animal study, [46] reporting differential localization of GABA between prefrontal cortex and hippocampus and speculating that this may relate to differential effects on pre- and post-synaptic receptors. In the future, it would be possible to study this important variability further in humans by measuring GABA type A receptor binding using $[^{11}C]$-flumazenil PET alongside GABA concentration with MRS, as in [12].

Interpretation of our evidence suggesting reduced Glx concentration in deep grey nuclei in relation to the existing NF1 literature is uncertain since findings on Glx concentration in NF1 have been previously conflicting. However, in young children with idiopathic autism, elevated deep brain Glx has been found in the anterior cingulate cortex in one large sample study [47] and reported to correlate with quality of social interaction in another [48]. The finding in this current study therefore can be interpreted within this context as positive in relation to autism symptoms.

The reduction in ADC found within the cingulate gyrus, and the significant ADC finding within the machine learning analysis, needs to be interpreted in the context of other work, which has shown increased ADC and decreased FA values in NF1 including in the cingulate [15]. Such findings suggest reduction in cellular packing and intra-myelinic oedema and have been associated with NF1 neurological symptom status [11]. The effects found in this current study therefore are consistent with reduced extra-cellular water free diffusion in NF1, and a positive simvastatin effect to reduce intra-myelinic oedema and improve cellular packing. The presence of microstructural abnormalities, reflected in increased ADC values, have also been described beyond NF1 in idiopathic autism [49–51] and potentially give these findings wider relevance in relation to this NF1-autism cohort.

The increased perfusion in the ventral diencephalon can be understood in the context of diminished perfusion in cingulate gyrus, medial frontal cortex, centrum semiovale, thalamus and temporo-occipital cortex found in NF1 children ($n = 14$, mean age = 10.2 years) [14] and related hypo-metabolism predominantly within the thalamus in FDG PET studies [52–54]. Statins may increase cerebral blood flow by improving cerebral vasomotor reactivity through increased NO bioavailability, promotion of microvascular reperfusion, and enhanced eNOS in the thalamus, as well as cerebellum, visual cortex and posterior cingulate [55].

No statistically robust difference in the DMN was identified between treatment and placebo groups, but findings at the 10% level raise the possibility of a trend that might be detected in a larger study. Diminished functional connectivity has been found in the posterior cingulate in human NF1 [16], and there is evidence from a small case series with children that statin treatment can induce improvements in functional connectivity in posterior cingulate cortex [21]. Here, simvastatin could potentially be acting in a focal manner on microstructural and vascular changes resulting in better regulation of function through a regional improvement in myelination and resultant neuronal function.

For *behavioural outcomes*, while the sample was too small for definitive estimation, we found that 25% of the simvastatin sample, compared to none of the placebo group, showed a clinical response using standard criteria measured using independently triangulated parent-report with clinician judgement.

Limitations

Dosing of simvastatin in this study was based on safety and efficacy evidence from use of statins in other human disease contexts; we do not know how appropriate it might be for effectiveness in this context. Animal work showed phenotypic rescue [12] with lovastatin at doses equivalent to those commonly prescribed for children (AJS, data not shown); however, differences in mode of delivery (intraperitoneal in animal studies) and the relative brain penetration of the statins (much higher in simvastatin) make direct comparison between the animal and human studies not meaningful. A valuable next step in this context would be further pre-clinical dose-finding studies in animal models using both statins with a mode of administration comparable to that in humans. Our treatment study was relatively short term, and we cannot generalise in relation to any longer term effects. There is no controlled data as yet to confirm a specific link between peripheral pMAPK assay and neural Ras function in human NF1 (although links have been found in cognitive impairment and Alzheimer's disease); further work will be necessary to confirm its value as a biomarker. Due to the technical challenges of imaging children with developmental disability at this age, the amount of analysable data varied for each imaging parameter. The study was not powered for a formal test of effectiveness; inferences on statin effects are preliminary and serve to indicate hypotheses and outcomes of interest for future larger scale work.

Conclusions

This study demonstrates the acceptability and safety of simvastatin treatment for young children with NF1 and autism; feasibility of awake scanning, data acquisition and peripheral biomarker assay in such children given the right preparation; and the value of such a multiparametric approach in capturing the likely complexity of pathogenic mechanisms.

The trial findings are suggestive of specific simvastatin effects in brain areas that have been shown to be part of NF1 neural pathology in previous studies. Furthermore, many of these areas have functional significance as part of the 'social brain network', highly associated with social impairment and autism psychopathology [56]. This functional localisation may thus be relevant both to the high autism prevalence in NF1 and to how simvastatin could have specific remedial effects on NF1-autism at the level of brain structure and function.

In terms of pathophysiological mechanism, the initial rationale for statin intervention was its action in NF1 animal models to downregulate the Ras pathway with consequent effect to reduce GABA, improve synaptic long-term potentiation and rescue the behavioural phenotype [7, 8, 18]. This trial in young children gives evidence consistent with that model operating in humans through its evidence of a simvastatin treatment effect (albeit with wide CI) towards reduced cellular pMAPK activation on peripheral assay, and associated

biologically plausible effects found on GABA/glutamate balance in FWM and DGN. However, the results also suggest simvastatin action through additional mechanisms, such as direct effects on myelin formation and regional axonal and astrocyte integrity in NF1. Pleiotropic effects of this kind from statins in the CNS are well recognised [57–59]. Our findings further suggest that treatment may affect such mechanisms in relevant functional brain areas in NF1 autism. This has future potential for insights into causal pathogenesis in autism and NF1 as well as suggesting more focused treatment targets. Larger studies will be necessary to further test these possibilities and to link them to any confirmed effect on behavioural symptom outcomes. While the initial results are encouraging and suggest specific hypotheses for further testing, this preliminary study was not powered to provide evidence to support clinical use of simvastatin in the disorder in children at this time.

In a wider context, the SANTA trial is, to our knowledge, the first RCT in syndromic autism, or indeed in clinical neuroscience generally, to have successfully tested effects simultaneously on relevant cellular activity markers, neural system multiparametric imaging and behavioural outcomes. As such, it provides a model of a new cohort of experimental intervention designs to link brain process and behavioural outcomes in the context of an experimental intervention trial. This has the eventual goal of treatment discovery in autism, plus the illumination of pathogenic pathways from gene effect to behavioural outcome in neuropsychiatric disorder; in terms of both regional brain localization and underlying pathogenic mechanisms.

Additional file

Additional file 1: Supplementary Materials. Table S1. MRI sequence parameters and scan time duration for a complete imaging acquisition lasting approximately 45 min (including scout sequences and planning time). Table S2. Baseline descriptive data. Table S3. Baseline clinical findings. Table S4. Adverse events. Table S5. Week 4 intermediate outcomes. Table S6. Quantification of MAPK outcomes at baseline and endpoint. Table S7. A comparison of the mutation data in the SANTA sample to previously reported data from a clinic referred NF1 sample (see text). Figure S1. a) Spectrum obtained from 3 × 3 × 3 voxel placed in deep grey matter of a 5-year-old child using MEGA-PRESS suppression scheme at 3T (top, non-edited subspectrum; bottom, GABA-edited spectrum) showing signals from amino-acid protons (AA), choline-containing compounds (cho), creatine + phosphocreatine (cr), N-acetylaspartate (NAA), GABA and glutamate + glutamine (Glx). b) Figure depicting example output of AMARES Model fitting in jMRUI. Figure S2. Example locations of VOI (3 × 3 × 3 cm³) acquired from a) left fontal white matter and b) deep grey matter (including caudate, lentiform nucleus, thalamus and putamen). Figure S3. Example illustrating in sagittal view the position of the perfusion-imaging slices, which were planed above the ventricles and the labelling slab (150 mm) that was set 10 mm below the imaging slices. Figure S4. SANTA CONSORT flow diagram. (DOCX 914 kb)

Abbreviations
ABC: Aberrant Behaviour Checklist; ADC: Apparent Diffusion Coefficient; ADI-R: Autism Diagnostic Interview Revised; ADOS: Autism Diagnostic Observation Schedule; ASD: Autism spectrum disorder; CGI: Clinical Global Impression; DMN: Default mode network; DTI: Diffusion tensor imaging; MRS: Magnetic resonance spectroscopy; NF1: Neurofibromatosis 1; PDTS: Parent-defined target symptoms; SRS: Social Responsiveness Scale; WASI: Wechsler Abbreviated Scale of Intelligence

Acknowledgements
We gratefully acknowledge the collaboration of Rosemont Pharmaceuticals (https://www.rosemontpharma.com/), who supplied the study drug and placebo formulation. Neither funder nor drug supplier had any involvement in the design or conduct of the trial, analysis or interpretation of the data. The study was conducted with the support of the NIHR Manchester Clinical Research Facility, and we gratefully acknowledge the staff and services of this facility and Dr. R. A. Edden (Johns Hopkins, Baltimore, MD USA) for providing the MEGA-PRESS sequence supported by tools developed under NIH R01 EB016089 and P41 EB015909.
Santa consortium Santa Team: Suzanne Campbell, Ruth Ellicott, Emma Harrison, Akhtar Kapasi, Giangiacomo Mercatali, Rachel Moon, Hannah Tobin, Srilaxmi Velandy, Rose Wagstaffe. *NF1 Clinical consortium Manchester NF1 service*: Emma Burkitt-Wright, Grace Vassallo, Siobhan West, Judith Eelloo, Eileen Hupton, Sonia Patel, Elizabeth Howard, Karen Tricker, Lauren Lewis *Yorkshire Regional NF1 service*: Angus Dobbie, Ruth Drimer, Saghira Malik Sharif. *Alder Hey NF1 clinic*: Zahabiyah Bassi, Jamuna Acharya *Edinburgh Genetic Service*: Wayne Lam. *Sheffield NF1 clinic*: Neil Harrower, Oliver Quarrell, Alyson Bradbury. *Newcastle NF1 service*: Miranda Splitt, Susan Musson, Rachel Jones, Helen Bethell, Catherine Prem. *Sunderland NF1 clinic*: Karen Horridge. *Warrington NF1 clinic*: Shaheena Anjum. *Wirral University Hospitals NF1 clinic*: Christine Steiger.

Funding
DGE is an NIHR Senior investigator and is supported by the NIHR All Manchester Biomedical Research Centre. SS was an NIHR Clinician Scientist and was supported by the NIHR during this study. The trial was funded by a Research and Innovation Award from Manchester University NHS Foundation Trust, who also sponsored the trial. It was conducted within the Manchester Academic Health Sciences Centre. The views expressed are those of the authors and not necessarily those of the Manchester University NHS Foundation Trust, the NIHR or the Department of Health.

Authors' contributions
The trial was initiated by JG, SG, SH, and SS and designed by JG, SG, SH, SS, RE, DGE, NW, AM, MT, JK, SW, AS, YC, FC, and CJ. Additional consultation on imaging analysis was provided by OT, DM, LP, HH. RE, SS, and MT, and JK led the data analysis. RW, JM, and GM contributed to the data analysis. All authors reviewed the final manuscript. JG, SG, SS, and RE had access to the trial data and decided on submission.

Competing interests
D. Gareth Evans had a travel for a trial meeting paid for by the Amgen and declared no other conflicts of interest. All other authors declare that they have no competing interests.

Author details
[1]Academic Unit of Paediatric Radiology, Royal Manchester Children's Hospital, Central Manchester University Hospitals NHS Foundation Trust, Manchester Academic Health Sciences Centre, Manchester, UK. [2]Division of Informatics, Imaging and Data Sciences, School of Health Sciences, Faculty of Biology, Medicine and Health, University of Manchester, Manchester Academic Health Science Centre, Manchester, UK. [3]Division of Neuroscience and Experimental Psychology, School of Biological Sciences, Faculty of Biology, Medicine and Health, University of Manchester, Manchester Academic Health Science Centre, Manchester University NHS Foundation Trust, Greater Manchester Mental Health NHS Foundation Trust, Room 3.311, Jean McFarlane Building, Oxford Road, Manchester M13 9PL, UK. [4]Division of Neuroscience and Experimental Psychology, School of Biological Sciences, Faculty of Biology, Medicine and Health, University of Manchester, Manchester Academic Health Science Centre, Manchester, UK. [5]Departments of Neurobiology, Psychiatry and Biobehavioral Sciences and Psychology, Integrative Center for Learning and Memory, Brain Research Institute, Brain Research Institute, University of California, California, LA 90095, USA. [6]Academic Unit of Radiology, Salford Royal Foundation NHS Trust, Manchester Academic Health Sciences Centre, Manchester, UK. [7]Computer Science, University of Manchester, Manchester, UK. [8]Manchester University NHS Foundation Trust, Manchester Academic Health Sciences Centre, Manchester, UK. [9]Manchester Metropolitan University, Manchester, UK. [10]Department of Paediatric Nephrology, Royal Manchester Children's Hospital, Manchester University NHS Foundation Trust, Academic Health Sciences Centre, Manchester, UK. [11]Hassenfeld Children's Hospital at NYU Langone, Nathan S. Kline Institute for Psychiatric Research, New York, USA. [12]Manchester Centre for Genomic Medicine, St Mary's Hospital, Manchester University NHS Foundation Trust, Academic Health Sciences Centre, Manchester, UK. [13]Centre for Biostatistics, School of Health Sciences, Faculty of Biology, Medicine and Health, University of Manchester, Manchester, UK.

References
1. Evans D, Howard E, Giblin C, Clancy T, Spencer H, Huson S, et al. Birth incidence and prevalence of tumor-prone syndromes: estimates from a UK family genetic register service. Am J Med Genet. 2010;152A:327–32.
2. Hyman S, Shores A, North K. The nature and frequency of cognitive deficits in children with neurofibromatosis type 1. Dev Med Child Neurol. 2007; 4812:973–7. 2005;65(7):1037-44
3. Mautner V, Kluwe L, Thakker S, Leark R. Treatment of ADHD in neurofibromatosis type 1. Dev Med Child Neurol. 2002;44(3):164–70.
4. Garg S, Green J, Leadbitter K, Emsley R, Lehtonen A, Evans DG, et al. Neurofibromatosis type 1 and autism spectrum disorder. Pediatrics. 2013; 132(6):e1642–8.
5. Plasschaert E, Descheemaeker MJ, Van Eylen L, Noens I, Steyaert J, Legius E. Prevalence of autism spectrum disorder symptoms in children with neurofibromatosis type 1. Am J Med Genet B Neuropsychiatr Genet. 2014;
6. Morris SM, Acosta MT, Garg S, Green J, Huson S, Legius E, et al. Disease burden and symptom structure of autism in neurofibromatosis type 1: a study of the International NF1-ASD Consortium Team (INFACT). JAMA Psychiatry. 2016;73(12):1276–84.
7. Molosh AI, Johnson PL, Spence JP, Arendt D, Federici LM, Bernabe C, et al. Social learning and amygdala disruptions in Nf1 mice are rescued by blocking p21-activated kinase. Nat Neurosci. 2014;17(11):1583–90.
8. Cui Y, Costa RM, Murphy GG, Elgersma Y, Zhu Y, Gutmann DH, et al. Neurofibromin regulation of ERK signaling modulates GABA release and learning. Cell. 2008;135(3):549–60.
9. Ishii A, Furusho M, Dupree JL, Bansal R. Strength of ERK1/2 MAPK activation determines its effect on myelin and axonal integrity in the adult CNS. J Neurosci. 2016;36(24):6471–87.
10. Mayes DA, Rizvi TA, Titus-Mitchell H, Oberst R, Ciraolo GM, Vorhees CV, et al. Nf1 loss and Ras hyperactivation in oligodendrocytes induce NOS-driven defects in myelin and vasculature. Cell Rep. 2013;4(6):1197–212.
11. Ertan G, Zan E, Yousem DM, Ceritoglu C, Tekes A, Poretti A, et al. Diffusion tensor imaging of neurofibromatosis bright objects in children with neurofibromatosis type 1. Neuroradiol J. 2014;27(5):616–26.
12. Violante IR, Patricio M, Bernardino I, Rebola J, Abrunhosa AJ, Ferreira N, et al. GABA deficiency in NF1: a multimodal [11C]-flumazenil and spectroscopy study. Neurology. 2016;87(9):897–904.
13. Violante IR, Ribeiro MJ, Edden RA, Guimaraes P, Bernardino I, Rebola J, et al. GABA deficit in the visual cortex of patients with neurofibromatosis type 1: genotype-phenotype correlations and functional impact. Brain. 2013;136(Pt 3):918–25.

14. Yeom KW, Lober RM, Barnes PD, Campen CJ. Reduced cerebral arterial spin-labeled perfusion in children with neurofibromatosis type 1. AJNR Am J Neuroradiol. 2013;34(9):1823–8.

15. Karlsgodt KH, Rosser T, Lutkenhoff ES, Cannon TD, Silva A, Bearden CE. Alterations in white matter microstructure in neurofibromatosis-1. PLoS One. 2012;7(10):e47854.

16. Tomson SN, Schreiner MJ, Narayan M, Rosser T, Enrique N, Silva AJ, et al. Resting state functional MRI reveals abnormal network connectivity in neurofibromatosis 1. Hum Brain Mapp. 2015;36(11):4566–81.

17. Loitfelder M, Huijbregts SC, Veer IM, Swaab HS, Van Buchem MA, Schmidt R, et al. Functional connectivity changes and executive and social problems in neurofibromatosis type I. Brain Connectivity. 2015;5(5):312–20.

18. Li W, Cui Y, Kushner SA, Brown RA, Jentsch JD, Frankland PW, et al. The HMG-CoA reductase inhibitor lovastatin reverses the learning and attention deficits in a mouse model of neurofibromatosis type 1. Curr Biol. 2005; 15(21):1961–7.

19. Acosta M, Kardel P, Walsh K, Rosenbaum K, Gioia G, Packer R. Lovastatin as treatment for neurocognitive deficits in neurofibromatosis type 1: phase 1 study. Pediatr Neurol. 2011;45:241–5.

20. Bearden CE, Hellemann GS, Rosser T, Montojo C, Jonas R, Enrique N, et al. A randomized placebo-controlled lovastatin trial for neurobehavioral function in neurofibromatosis I. Ann Clin Transl Neurol. 2016;3(4):266–79.

21. Chabernaud C, Mennes M, Kardel P, Gaillard W, Kalbfleisch L, VanMeter J, et al. Lovastatin regulates brain spontaneous low-frequency brain activity in neurofibromatosis type 1. Neurosci Lett. 2012;515:28–33.

22. Mainberger F, Jung NH, Zenker M, Wahllander U, Freudenberg L, Langer S, et al. Lovastatin improves impaired synaptic plasticity and phasic alertness in patients with neurofibromatosis type 1. BMC Neurol. 2013;13:131.

23. Krab L, de Goede-Bolde RA, Aarsen F, Pluijm S, Bouman M, van der Geest J, et al. Effect of simvastatin on cognitive functioning in children with neurofibromatosis type 1: a randomized controlled trial. JAMA. 2008;300(3):287–94.

24. van der Vaart T, Plasschaert E, Rietman AB, Renard M, Oostenbrink R, Vogels A, et al. Simvastatin for cognitive deficits and behavioural problems in patients with neurofibromatosis type 1 (NF1-SIMCODA): a randomised, placebo-controlled trial. Lancet Neurol. 2013;12(11):1076–83.

25. Payne JM, Barton B, Ullrich NJ, Cantor A, Hearps SJ, Cutter G, et al. Randomized placebo-controlled study of lovastatin in children with neurofibromatosis type 1. Neurology. 2016;87(24):2575–84.

26. National Institutes of Health Consensus Development Conference. Neurofibromatosis conference statement. Arch Neurol. 1988;45:575–8.

27. Lainhart JE, Bigler ED, Bocian M, Coon H, Dinh E, Dawson G, et al. Head circumference and height in autism: a study by the Collaborative Program of Excellence in Autism. Am J Med Genet A. 2006;140(21):2257–74.

28. Kayano M, Higaki S, Satoh JI, Matsumoto K, Matsubara E, Takikawa O, et al. Plasma microRNA biomarker detection for mild cognitive impairment using differential correlation analysis. Biomarker Res. 2016;4:22.

29. Kiddle SJ, Steves CJ, Mehta M, Simmons A, Xu X, Newhouse S, et al. Plasma protein biomarkers of Alzheimer's disease endophenotypes in asymptomatic older twins: early cognitive decline and regional brain volumes. Transl Psychiatry. 2015;5:e584.

30. Sandler A, Sutton K, DeWeese J, Girardi M, Sheppard V, Bodfish J. Lack of benefit of a single dose of synthetic human secretin in the treatment of autism and pervasive developmental disorders. N Engl J Med. 1999;341(24):1801–6.

31. Berry-Kravis E, Sumis A, Hervey C, Nelson M, Porges S, Weng N, et al. Open-label treatment trial of lithium to target the underlying defect in fragile X syndrome. J Dev Behav Pediatr. 2008;29:293–302.

32. Aman M. Aberrant behaviour checklist––community. East Aurora, NY: Slosson Educational Publications; 1994.

33. Arnold LE, Vitiello B, McDougle C, Scahill L, Shah B, Gonzalez NM, et al. Parent-defined target symptoms respond to risperidone in RUPP autism study: customer approach to clinical trials. J Am Acad Child Adolesc Psychiatry. 2003;42(12):1443–50.

34. Leucht S, Engel RR. The relative sensitivity of the Clinical Global Impressions Scale and the Brief Psychiatric Rating Scale in antipsychotic drug trials. Neuropsychopharmacology. 2006;31(2):406–12.

35. Conners K, Sitarenios G, Parker J, Epstein J. The revised Conners' parent rating scale (CPRS-R): factor structure, reliability, and criterion validity. J Abnorm Child Psychol. 1998;26(4):257–68.

36. McCracken JT, McGough J, Shah B, Cronin P, Hong D, Aman MG, et al. Risperidone in children with autism and serious behavioral problems. N Engl J Med. 2002;347(5):314–21.

37. Haas D, Garbade SF, Vohwinkel C, Muschol N, Trefz FK, Penzien JM, et al. Effects of cholesterol and simvastatin treatment in patients with Smith-Lemli-Opitz syndrome (SLOS). J Inherit Metab Dis. 2007;30(3): 375–87.

38. Mullins PG, McGonigle DJ, O'Gorman RL, Puts NA, Vidyasagar R, Evans CJ, et al. Current practice in the use of MEGA-PRESS spectroscopy for the detection of GABA. NeuroImage. 2014;86:43–52.

39. Vermeulen K, Thas O, Vansteelandt S. Increasing the power of the Mann-Whitney test in randomized experiments through flexible covariate adjustment. Stat Med. 2015;34(6):1012–30.

40. Petersen ET, Lim T, Golay X. Model-free arterial spin labeling quantification approach for perfusion MRI. Magn Reson Med. 2006;55(2):219–32.

41. Pedregosa F, Varoquaux G, Gramfort A, Michel V, Thirion B, Grisel O, et al. Scikit-learn: machine learning in python. J Mach Learn Res. 2011;12:2825–30.

42. Garg S, Lehtonen A, Huson SM, Emsley R, Trump D, Evans DG, et al. Autism and other psychiatric comorbidity in neurofibromatosis type 1: evidence from a population-based study. Dev Med Child Neurol. 2013; 55(2):139–45.

43. Evans DG, Bowers N, Burkitt-Wright E, Miles E, Garg S, Scott-Kitching V, et al. Comprehensive RNA analysis of the NF1 gene in classically affected NF1 affected individuals meeting NIH criteria has high sensitivity and mutation negative testing is reassuring in isolated cases with pigmentary features only. EBioMed. 2016;7:212–20.

44. Sierra S, Ramos MC, Molina P, Esteo C, Vazquez JA, Burgos JS. Statins as neuroprotectants: a comparative in vitro study of lipophilicity, blood-brain-barrier penetration, lowering of brain cholesterol, and decrease of neuron cell death. J Alzheimers Dis. 2011;23(2):307–18.

45. Mikkelsen M, Singh KD, Brealy JA, Linden DE, Evans CJ. Quantification of gamma-aminobutyric acid (GABA) in 1H MRS volumes composed heterogeneously of grey and white matter. NMR Biomed. 2016;29(11): 1644–55.

46. Goncalves J, Violante IR, Sereno J, Leitao RA, Cai Y, Abrunhosa A, et al. Testing the excitation/inhibition imbalance hypothesis in a mouse model of the autism spectrum disorder: in vivo neurospectroscopy and molecular evidence for regional phenotypes. Mol Autism. 2017;8:47.

47. Ito H, Mori K, Harada M, Hisaoka S, Toda Y, Mori T, et al. A proton magnetic resonance spectroscopic study in autism spectrum disorder using a 3-tesla clinical magnetic resonance imaging (MRI) system: the anterior cingulate cortex and the left cerebellum. J Child Neurol. 2017;32(8):731–9.

48. Doyle-Thomas KA, Card D, Soorya LV, Wang AT, Fan J, Anagnostou E. Metabolic mapping of deep brain structures and associations with symptomatology in autism spectrum disorders. Res Autism Spectr Disord. 2014;8(1):44–51.

49. Sundaram SK, Kumar A, Makki MI, Behen ME, Chugani HT, Chugani DC. Diffusion tensor imaging of frontal lobe in autism spectrum disorder. Cereb Cortex. 2008;18(11):2659–65.

50. Ben Bashat D, Kronfeld-Duenias V, Zachor DA, Ekstein PM, Hendler T, Tarrasch R, et al. Accelerated maturation of white matter in young children with autism: a high b value DWI study. NeuroImage. 2007; 37(1):40–7.

51. Mengotti P, D'Agostini S, Terlevic R, De Colle C, Biasizzo E, Londero D, et al. Altered white matter integrity and development in children with autism: a combined voxel-based morphometry and diffusion imaging study. Brain Res Bull. 2011;84(3):189–95.

52. Kaplan AM, Chen K, Lawson MA, Wodrich DL, Bonstelle CT, Reiman EM. Positron emission tomography in children with neurofibromatosis-1. J Child Neurol. 1997;12(8):499–506.

53. Balestri P, Lucignani G, Fois A, Magliani L, Calistri L, Grana C, et al. Cerebral glucose metabolism in neurofibromatosis type 1 assessed with [18F]-2-fluoro-2-deoxy-D-glucose and PET. J Neurol Neurosurg Psychiatry. 1994; 57(12):1479–83.

54. Buchert R, von Borczyskowski D, Wilke F, Gronowsky M, Friedrich RE, Brenner W, et al. Reduced thalamic 18F-flurodeoxyglucose retention in adults with neurofibromatosis type 1. Nucl Med Commun. 2008; 29(1):17–26.

55. Beason-Held L, Thambisetty M, Kraut M, Ferrucci L, Elkins W, Zonderman A, et al. Longitudinal changes in brain function related to statin use. Alzheimers Dement. 2012;8(4):701.

56. Johnson MH, Griffin R, Csibra G, Halit H, Farroni T, de Haan M, et al. The emergence of the social brain network: evidence from typical and atypical development. Dev Psychopathol. 2005;17(3):599–619.

2

A behavioral test battery for mouse models of Angelman syndrome: a powerful tool for testing drugs and novel *Ube3a* mutants

Monica Sonzogni[1,2†], Ilse Wallaard[1,2†], Sara Silva Santos[1,2†], Jenina Kingma[1,2], Dorine du Mee[1,2], Geeske M. van Woerden[1,2] and Ype Elgersma[1,2*] [iD]

Abstract

Background: Angelman syndrome (AS) is a neurodevelopmental disorder caused by mutations affecting UBE3A function. AS is characterized by intellectual disability, impaired motor coordination, epilepsy, and behavioral abnormalities including autism spectrum disorder features. The development of treatments for AS heavily relies on the ability to test the efficacy of drugs in mouse models that show reliable, and preferably clinically relevant, phenotypes. We previously described a number of behavioral paradigms that assess phenotypes in the domains of motor performance, repetitive behavior, anxiety, and seizure susceptibility. Here, we set out to evaluate the robustness of these phenotypes when tested in a standardized test battery. We then used this behavioral test battery to assess the efficacy of minocycline and levodopa, which were recently tested in clinical trials of AS.

Methods: We combined data of eight independent experiments involving 111 *Ube3a* mice and 120 wild-type littermate control mice. Using a meta-analysis, we determined the statistical power of the subtests and the effect of putative confounding factors, such as the effect of sex and of animal weight on rotarod performance. We further assessed the robustness of these phenotypes by comparing *Ube3a* mutants in different genetic backgrounds and by comparing the behavioral phenotypes of independently derived *Ube3a*-mutant lines. In addition, we investigated if the test battery allowed re-testing the same animals, which would allow a within-subject testing design.

Results: We find that the test battery is robust across different *Ube3a*-mutant lines, but confirm and extend earlier studies that several phenotypes are very sensitive to genetic background. We further found that the audiogenic seizure susceptibility phenotype is fully reversible upon pharmacological treatment and highly suitable for dose-finding studies. In agreement with the clinical trial results, we found that minocycline and levodopa treatment of *Ube3a* mice did not show any sign of improved performance in our test battery.

Conclusions: Our study provides a useful tool for preclinical drug testing to identify treatments for Angelman syndrome. Since the phenotypes are observed in several independently derived *Ube3a* lines, the test battery can also be employed to investigate the effect of specific *Ube3a* mutations on these phenotypes.

Keywords: Angelman syndrome, UBE3A, Mouse model, behavior, drug screening

* Correspondence: y.elgersma@erasmusmc.nl
†Monica Sonzogni, Ilse Wallaard and Sara Silva Santos contributed equally to this work.
[1]Department of Neuroscience, Erasmus Medical Center, Rotterdam, Netherlands
[2]ENCORE Expertise Center for Neurodevelopmental Disorders, Erasmus Medical Center, Rotterdam, Netherlands

Background

Angelman syndrome (AS) is a neurodevelopmental disorder first described in 1965 by Harry Angelman, with a birth incidence of approximately 1:20,000 [1]. AS is caused by the functional loss of the maternal allele encoding an E3 ubiquitin-protein ligase (UBE3A) [2]. Loss of functional UBE3A results in the core phenotypes of severe intellectual disability, motor coordination deficits, absence of speech, and abnormal EEG, as well as in high comorbidity of sleep abnormalities, epilepsy, and phenotypes related to autism spectrum [3].

Currently, only symptomatic treatments are available for AS, primarily aimed at reducing seizures and improving sleep [4]. The development of targeted treatments for AS heavily relies on the ability to test the efficacy of treatments in mouse models of the disorder. The success of such translational studies depends on three critical factors [5]: (1) high construct validity, (2) high face validity, and (3) robustness of the behavioral phenotypes. First, the construct validity (shared underlying etiology between mouse models and patients) of the AS mouse model is very good, since AS mouse models recapitulate the patient genetics by carrying a mutated $Ube3a$ gene specifically at the maternal allele. However, it should be noted that the majority of the AS patients carry a large deletion (15q11-15q13) which encompasses also other genes besides the $UBE3A$ gene, and which may contribute to a more severe phenotype [6]. Second, with respect to face validity (i.e., similarity of phenotypes between patient and the mouse model), the AS mouse model captures many neurological key features of the disorder really well (e.g., epilepsy, motor deficits, abnormal EEG), as well as some of the behavioral abnormalities (abnormal sleep patterns, increased anxiety, repetitive behavior) [7–12]. Robustness of the behavioral phenotypes is the third important aspect to identify novel treatments, as it allows experiments to be sufficiently powered to detect the effect of the treatment, and meanwhile minimizes a type I error in which a drug is declared effective whereas it is not. Robustness, as well as face validity, also takes into account the sensitivity to genetic background and the extent in which a phenotype is also observed in independently derived mouse models. Notably, almost all behavioral testing described in literature has been performed using the original $Ube3a^{tm1Alb}$ mouse strain generated in the Beaudet lab [7–9]; hence, it is unknown to what extent the reported phenotypes are actually specific to this mouse line.

We previously developed a series of behavioral paradigms in the domains of motor performance, anxiety, repetitive behavior, and seizure susceptibility, for testing the effect of $Ube3a$ gene reinstatement in the inducible $Ube3a^{mSTOP/p+}$ ($Ube3a^{tm1Yelg}$) mice [13]. Here, we used these paradigms in a highly standardized way, to assess phenotypes in the independently derived $Ube3a^{tm1Alb}$ and $Ube3a^{mE113X/p+}$ ($Ube3a^{tm2Yelg}$) maternal knockout strains. We combined data of eight independent experiments across five experimenters involving 111 $Ube3a^{tm1Alb}$ and 120 wild-type littermate control mice. Using a meta-analysis, we determined the statistical power of the different behavioral tests and the effect of putative confounding factors, such as the effect of sex differences. We further assessed the robustness of these phenotypes by comparing $Ube3a$ mutants in different genetic backgrounds. Finally, we employed this behavioral test battery to reassess the efficacy of minocycline and levodopa in the AS mouse model. Minocycline is a matrix metalloproteinase-9 inhibitor (MMP9), a tetracycline derivative which possesses antibiotic as well as neuroprotective activity [14, 15]. Its antibiotic properties against both gram-positive and gram-negative bacteria are related to its ability to bind to the bacterial 30S ribosomal subunit, thereby inhibiting protein synthesis [14].

Levodopa is the precursor of dopamine and was shown to be effective in treating Parkinsonism in two adults with Angelman syndrome [16]. Moreover, it is able to reduce CAMK2 phosphorylation [17], which was shown to be increased in a mouse model for Angelman syndrome [18, 19]. Minocycline and levodopa were previously tested in the AS mouse model and based on the favorable outcome of these preclinical experiments, three clinical trials were performed [20–22]. Unfortunately, none of these drugs showed a significant improvement in AS patients.

Methods

Mouse husbandry and breeding

For this study, we used $Ube3a^{m-/p+}$ mice ($Ube3a^{tm1Alb}$; MGI 2181811) [7] and $Ube3a^{mE113X/p+}$ mutants ($Ube3a^{tm2Yelg}$; MGI5911277) as previously described [23]. $Ube3a^{tm1Alb}$ mice were maintained (> 40 generations) in the 129S2 background (full name: 129S2/SvPasCrl) by crossing male $Ube3a^{m+/p-}$ mice with female 129S2 wild-type mice. $Ube3a^{tm2Yelg}$ mice were maintained (> 20 generations) in the C57BL/6J (Charles River) background by crossing male $Ube3a^{m+/pE113X}$ mice with female C57BL/6J wild-type mice. For the seizure susceptibility experiments with $Ube3a^{mE113X/p+}$ animals, this line was backcrossed eight times in 129S2 by crossing $Ube3a^{pE113X/m+}$ males with 129S2 wild-type females.

For behavioral experiments, female $Ube3a^{tm1Alb}$ ($Ube3a^{m+/p-}$) mice were bred to yield $Ube3a^{m-/p+}$ mice in two different backgrounds: $Ube3a^{m-/p+}$ (AS) mice and their WT littermates in the F1 hybrid 129S2-C57BL/6J background (WT = 120, AS = 111) and in the 129S2 background (WT = 11, AS = 16). $Ube3a^{mE113X/p+}$ mice and their WT littermates were generated in the same manner in the F1 hybrid 129S2-C57BL/6J background

(WT = 10, $Ube3a^{mE113X/p+}$ = 10) and in C57BL/6J background (WT = 15, $Ube3a^{mE113X/p+}$ = 16).

For the seizure susceptibility test, we used $Ube3a^{m-/p+}$ (WT = 45, AS = 114) and $Ube3a^{mE113X/p+}$ mice (WT = 4, AS = 8) in the 129S2 background.

Mice were housed in individually ventilated cages (IVC; 1145T cages from Techniplast) in a barrier facility. Mice were genotyped when they were 4–7 days old and re-genotyped at the completion of the experiments. All animals were kept at 22 ± 2 °C with a 12-h dark and light cycle and were tested in the light period, provided with mouse chow (801727CRM(P) from Special Dietary Service) and water ad libitum. During behavioral testing, mice were group-housed with two to four animals of the same sex per cage. Fighting between males was observed a few times, and in these rare cases, mice were separated and single housed. This was not a reason for exclusion. All mice were single housed during nest building and for the subsequent forced swim test. All animal experiments were conducted in accordance with the European Commission Council Directive 2010/63/EU (CCD approval AVD101002016791).

Behavioral analysis

The weight of the animals was determined a few days before the start of the behavioral analysis. Prior to each test, mice were acclimatized to the testing room for 30 min.

All behavioral experiments were performed during the light period of the light/dark cycle. Both male and female mice at the age of 8–12 weeks were used for the experiments. Moreover, we tried to obtain a similar ratio of females/males between the WT and AS groups. Only in the experiments described in Fig. 4 ($Ube3a^{E113X}$ mice in F1 background) and in the epilepsy experiment using $Ube3a^{E113X}$ mice (Fig. 6c), the female/male ratio between the groups was significantly different ($p < 0.05$; chi-square test).

All behavioral testing and scoring was performed by experimenters who were blind to genotype and treatment. Behavioral tests were always run in the following order and with a minimal number of days between tests: (1) accelerating rotarod test for 5 consecutive days performed at the same hour every day; (2) 2 days of pause; (3) open field test; (4) 1 day of pause; (5) marble burying test; (6) between 5 and 7 days of pause to allow adaptation to being single caged; (7) nest building test for 5 consecutive days, in which the weight of the nest was assessed at the same hour every day; (8) 2 days of pause; and (9) forced swim test.

Accelerating rotarod

Motor function was tested using the accelerating rotarod (4–40 rpm, in 5 min; model 7650, Ugo Basile Biological Research Apparatus, Varese, Italy). Mice were given two trials per day with a 45–60-min inter-trial interval for 5 consecutive days (same hour every day). For each day, the average time spent on the rotarod was calculated, or the time until the mouse made three consecutive wrapping/passive rotations on the rotarod (latency in seconds). These passive rotations were observed rarely (1–2%) in 129S2 or F1 hybrid 129S2-C57BL/6J mice but rather common in (30%) C57BL/6J mice. Maximum duration of a trial was 5 min.

Open field test

To test locomotor activity and anxiety, mice were individually placed in a 110-cm-diameter circular open field and allowed to explore for 10 min. The light intensity was approximately 25–30 lx measured in the center of the arena. The total distance moved by each mouse in the open arena was recorded by an infrared camera (Noldus® Wageningen, NL) connected to the EthoVision® software (Noldus® Wageningen, NL), and the final outcome is indicated as distance moved in meters. For some groups, we also analyzed the time spent in the inner zone (IZ), middle zone (MZ), and outer zone (OZ) (IZ r = 25 cm, MZ r = 40, OZ r = 55 cm).

Marble burying test

Open Makrolon (polycarbonate) cages (50 × 26 × 18 cm) were filled with 4 cm of bedding material (Lignocel® Hygenic Animal Bedding, JRS). On top of the bedding material, 20 blue glass marbles were arranged in an equidistant 5 × 4 grid and the animals were given access to the marbles for 30 min. After the test, the mice were gently removed from the cage. Marbles covered for more than 50% by bedding were scored as buried, and the outcome measured is the number of buried marbles.

Nest building test

To measure nest building, mice were single housed for a period of 5 to 7 days before the start of the experiment. Subsequently, used nesting material was replaced and 11 g (11 ± 1) of compressed extra-thick blot filter paper (Bio-rad©) was added to the cage. The amount of the unused nest material was weighed and noted every day for a consecutive of 5 days, each day at the same hour.

Forced swim test

Mice were placed for 6 min in a cylindrical transparent tank (27 cm high and 18 cm diameter), filled with water (kept at 26 ± 1 °Celsius) 15 cm deep. The mouse was first left in the cylinder for 2 min to habituate. Immobility during the forced swim test was scored manually (stop-watch) by timing the amount of time the mouse was floating in the water (defined by lack of any movement) and was assessed during the last 4 min of the test.

The mouse was considered to be immobile when he ceased to move altogether, making only movements necessary to keep its head above water. The outcome measured is the time in seconds in which the mouse was immobile.

Susceptibility to audiogenic seizures

Because of the different genetic background requirements, an independent cohort of mice was used to test susceptibility to audiogenic seizures. Mice were placed in Makrolon (polycarbonate) cages ($50 \times 26 \times 18$ cm), and audiogenic seizures were induced by vigorously scraping scissors across the metal grating of the cage lid (which creates approximately a 100-dB sound). This noise was generated for 20 s, or less if a tonic-clonic seizure developed before that time. Susceptible mice responded with wild running and leaping followed by a tonic-clonic seizure, which typically lasted 10–20 s.

Within-subject testing

For the experiment described in Fig. 3, $Ube3a^{tm1Alb}$ mice in F1 hybrid 129S2-C57BL/6J background were subjected to the behavioral test battery for a second time. Once the first battery was completed, female mice that had been single housed for the nest building test were placed back together with the original cage mates, while male mice remained separated for the entire second set of behavioral tasks. The second test started 4 weeks after the first testing was completed.

Drug administration

Vehicle treatment

All animals used for the meta-analysis were treated with vehicle either by IP injection (max volume 10 ul/g, hypodermic-needle 25G × 16 mm (Sterican®/B-Braun)), by oral gavage (max 10 ul/g, stainless steel animal feeding tubes 20G × 38 mm (Instech Laboratories)), or by adding to the drinking water.

Minocycline treatment

The adult-treated group consisted of 8–10-week-old $Ube3a^{m-/p+}$ ($n = 11$ saline; 11 minocycline) and WT ($n = 9$ saline; 10 minocycline) littermate control mice in F1 hybrid 129S2-C57BL/6J background. Due to space limitations, only six animals per group were used for nest building. Mice were assigned to two treatment groups in such a way that both groups had a comparable distribution of males and females and mutant and wild-type mice. Mice were subjected to daily minocycline or vehicle IP injections (minocycline hydrochloride, Sigma-Aldrich 45 mg/kg in saline solution), starting 3 weeks prior to commencing behavioral testing, as previously described [20, 24]. Behavioral testing was started 1.5 h post-injection, based on the half-life of minocycline (~ 2 h in plasma), and the

peak brain levels are reached about 2 h after injection [25].

For the postnatal-treated group, cages with $Ube3a^{m-/p+}$ and WT pups in F1 hybrid 129S2-C57BL/6J background were split in two treatment groups in such a way that both groups had a comparable distribution of males and females and mutant and wild-type mice. The treatment group received minocycline via the lactating dam, which received minocycline through the drinking water (0.2 mg minocycline/ml, supplemented with 1 mg/ml aspartame to counteract the bitter taste and shielded for light) [26]. This method of administration was shown to yield detectable concentration of minocycline in the blood of adult mice [27] and in the breast milk of lactating dams [28, 29]. Once the mice were weaned, they were supplied with the same concentration of minocycline in their drinking water. Assuming a water intake of 1.5 ml/10 g body weight/day [30], and assuming an average weight of 25 g/mouse, the average amount of minocycline these mice received is approximately 30 mg/kg/day. The drinking water was refreshed every other day. Treatment continued until all behavioral experiments were completed. The control group received water with aspartame.

Levodopa/carbidopa treatment

Cages containing $Ube3a^{m-/p+}$ and wild-type littermate control mice (8–12 weeks old) in the F1 hybrid 129S2-C57BL/6J background were assigned to two treatment groups in such a way that both groups had 15 wild type and 15 mutants and a comparable distribution of males and females. Mice in the treatment group received 15 mg/kg levodopa and 3.75 mg/kg carbidopa dissolved in saline (levodopa, Sigma-Aldrich; carbidopa, Sigma-Aldrich) by IP injection with an injection volume of 10 ul/g. The untreated group received vehicle injection by IP as described by Tan et al. [21]. The mice were injected 1 h prior to carrying out the behavioral tasks, during the entire period while partaking in these tests.

Levetiracetam treatment

$Ube3a^{m-/p+}$ mice in the 129S2 background were first tested for audiogenic seizure susceptibility at baseline. Minimally 24 h later, the mice were again tested for audiogenic seizure susceptibility, this time precisely 1 h following a single IP injection of levetiracetam (0–0.5–1–2–10–15 mg/kg; Sigma-Aldrich). The injection volume used is 5 ml/kg, and the drug was dissolved in 1% Tween-80 (Sigma-Aldrich) in milliQ water as previously described [31].

Data analysis

Data was analyzed using Excel 2010 (Microsoft) and IBM SPSS software (NY, USA). The open field, marble burying, and forced swim test data were analyzed using an unpaired T test in the untreated experimental groups and a two-way ANOVA in minocycline- and levodopa-treated animals (in which we assessed a genotype-treatment interaction). Rotarod and nest building were measured with a repeated measures ANOVA in the untreated experimental groups, or with a multivariate repeated measures ANOVA (assessing significance of interaction of time, genotype, and treatment) in the minocycline and levodopa experimental groups. We used a *Bonferroni's* post hoc *test* to detect significant differences in male and female groups. For the within-subject experiment, we used a paired T test for open field, marble burying, and forced swim tests, while we used a repeated measures factorial ANOVA when analyzing the rotarod and the nest building test. For the audiogenic seizure analysis, a Fisher's exact test was used. The correlation between body weight and maximal performance on the rotarod test was assessed with a Pearson's correlation test. For the power calculation, we performed a priori analysis using G*Power 3.1 software [32] with $\alpha = 0.05$ and power $(1 - \beta) = 0.95$, 0.90, or 0.80. Data is presented as mean$\pm$ SEM in all figures. For all tests, statistical significance was denoted by $p \leq 0.05$ (*), $p < 0.01$ (**), and $p < 0.001$ (***).

A chi-square test was performed to test if there were any significant differences in the ratio of females/males between the WT and AS groups.

Results
Robust behavioral phenotypes in $Ube3a^{m-/p+}$ mice in the F1 hybrid 129S2-C57BL/6J background

We recently developed a number of behavioral tests for testing the effect of gene reinstatement in inducible $Ube3a^{mSTOP/p+}$ ($Ube3a^{tm1Yelg}$) mice [13]. These tests can be applied in successive order to assess phenotypes in the domains of motor performance, anxiety, and repetitive behavior. Here, we set out to assess the robustness of these phenotypes in an independently derived mouse model of AS, by using F1 hybrid 129S2-C57BL/6J $Ube3a^{m-/p+}$ ($Ube3a^{tm1Alb}$) mice [7], which is the $Ube3a$ mouse mutant used for nearly all behavioral studies. We have frequently used this strain to test the efficacy of novel treatments and combined all data obtained from vehicle-treated $Ube3a^{m-/p+}$ and wild-type littermate controls in the F1 hybrid 129S2-C57BL/6J background to perform a meta-analysis. In total, this constitutes the combined data of eight experiments, carried out by five experimenters and totaling 111 $Ube3a^{m-/p+}$ and 120 wild-type littermate controls (Table 1; Fig. 1).

Individuals with Angelman syndrome show clear motor impairments, and impaired performance on the accelerating rotarod is the most frequently described phenotype in $Ube3a$ mice. Indeed, our meta-analysis shows a very robust significant difference between the two genotypes ($p < 0.001$; Fig. 1a). A power analysis with

Table 1 Overview of experiments used for the meta-analysis

Exp. #	Person	WT/MUT (n)	Sex WT f/m MUT f/m (n)	Rotarod (time(s)) WT mean (SD) Mut mean (SD)	Open field (distance(m)) WT mean (SD) Mut mean (SD)	Marble burying (# marbles buried) WT mean (SD) Mut mean (SD)	Nest building (% material used) WT mean (SD) Mut mean (SD)	Forced swim test (% floating) WT mean (SD) Mut mean (SD)
1	A	15/13	8/7 6/7	128 (42) 96 (32)	41 (14) 22 (11)	11 (4) 4 (3)	14 (25) 79 (18)	53 (23) 83 (7)
2	A	15/13	5/10 3/10	142 (43) 80 (32)	49 (10) 32 (12)	8 (4) 2 (3)	36 (23) 79 (14)	44 (24) 81 (7)
3	A	15/13	5/10 3/10	133 (42) 92 (46)	40 (12) 29 (8)	11 (3) 2 (2)	27 (18) 70 (18)	41 (19) 73 (14)
4	B	21/17[1]	10/11 7/10	159 (60) 102 (36)	31 (12) 19 (11)	14(4) 4(5)	10 (11) 48 (25)	24 (22) 63 (18)
5	C	9/11[2]	5/4 6/5	163 (49) 91 (37)	25 (6) 10 (7)	12 (5) 4(5)	48 (27) 69 (12)	28 (24) 76 (8)
6	D	15/14[3]	4/11 6/8	107 (44) 74 (26)	44 (7) 29 (13)	12 (3) 3 (3)	40 (18) 79 (12)	14 (20) 60(31)
7	E	15/15	8/7 7/8	196 (57) 126(52)	45(10) 35 (7)	11 (5) 6 (3)	63 (20) 74 (14)	47 (20) 67 (14)
8	A	15/15[4]	7/8 8/7	162 (49) 95 (35)	49 (9) 33 (13)	10 (3) 2 (3)	N/A	47 (20) 88 (9)

All experiments were performed using $Ube3a^{tm1Alb}$ mice in F1 hybrid 129S2-C57BL/6J background. For all tests shown in this table, we found a significant effect of genotype ($p < 0.05$), except for the nest building test of experiment 8, which was not performed. The table indicates the individual that performed the test battery, the number of wild-type and mutant mice used for each test, the number of females and males used for each experimental group, and the mean and standard deviation of the outcomes obtained. For the rotarod, we indicated the average performance over the 5 days, while for the nest building we provided the data as measured at day 5. Note that for some of the tests, we used a different number of mice (mice were not properly tracked, or a smaller cohort was used for nest building because of space limitations). The adapted n for these experiments is as follows: [1]nest building 13/12, forced swim test 20/17; [2]nest building 6/7; [3]open field 13/14; [4]open field 10/10, nest building not performed

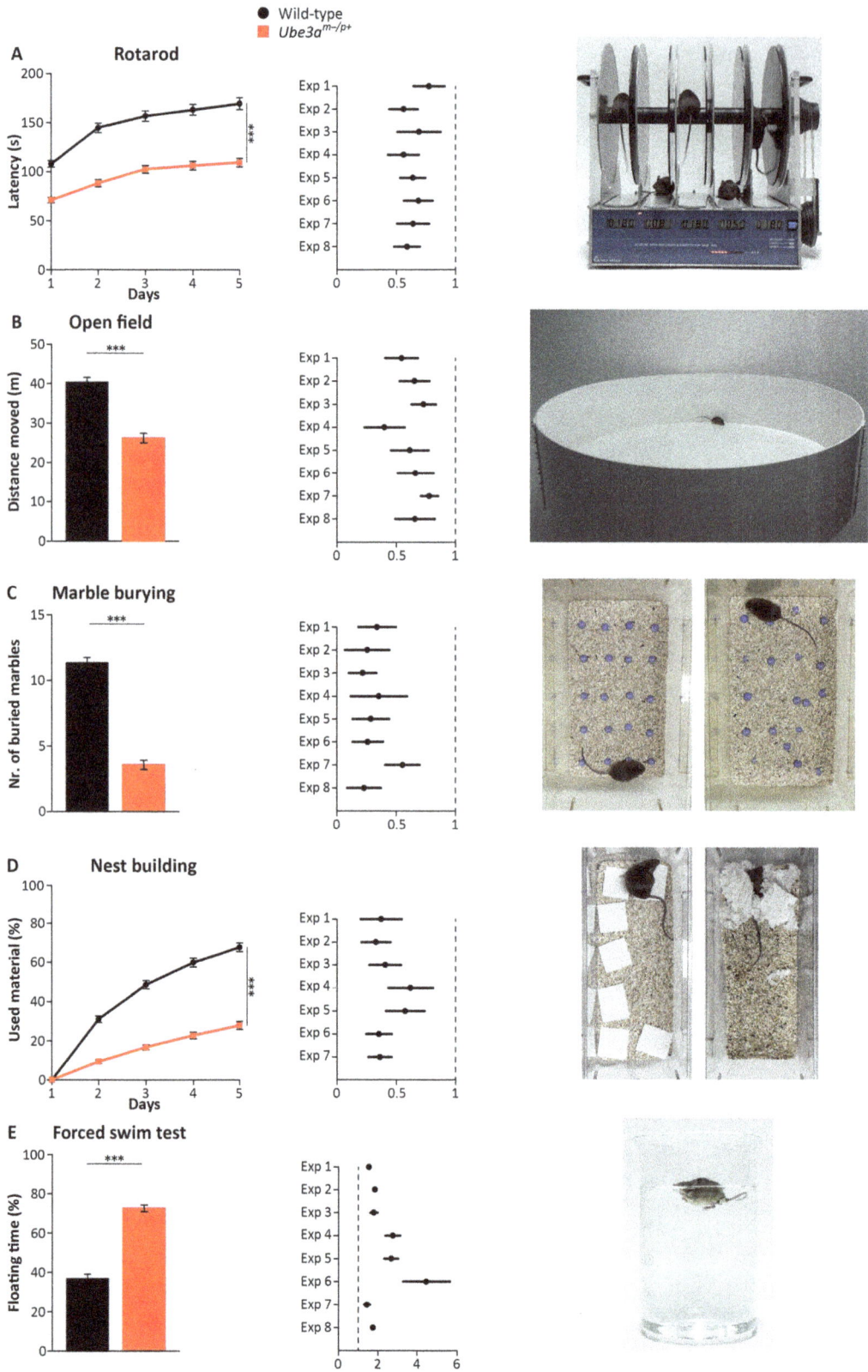

Fig. 1 (See legend on next page.)

Fig. 1 Behavioral testing of *Ube3a^{tm1Alb}* mice in F1 hybrid 129S2-C57BL/6J background. For each behavioral paradigm, the pooled (raw) data of all experiments is presented on the left panel, whereas the Forrest plots in the middle panel show the normalized data of the individual experiments (in which the data of each experiment is normalized against wild type; represented by a dashed line), as well as the 95% confidence interval. The picture on the right panel shows the behavioral set-up used for our experiments. For the marble burying test and nest building test, the picture shows the onset and finish of a behavioral experiment. **a** Accelerating rotarod in wild-type (WT) and *Ube3a$^{m-/p+}$* mice (*n* = 120, 111). **b** Open field test in WT and *Ube3a$^{m-/p+}$* mice (*n* = 113, 106). **c** Marble burying test in WT and *Ube3a$^{m-/p+}$* mice (*n* = 120, 111). **d** Nest building test in WT and *Ube3a$^{m-/p+}$* mice (*n* = 94, 86). **e** Forced swim test in WT and *Ube3a$^{m-/p+}$* mice (*n* = 120, 111). All data represent mean ± SEM. A repeated measures ANOVA or *T* test was used for statistical comparison of the non-normalized data. All tests show a significance effect of genotype (***$p < 0.001$)

$\alpha = 0.05$; $(1 - \beta) = 0.95$ showed that this task requires 14 animals per genotype (Table 2).

Following 2 days of rest, the same mice were then tested in the open field test. This paradigm is commonly used to assess anxiety in mice. Increased anxiety is commonly observed in individuals with AS [33], as well as individuals with autism spectrum disorder. In this test, we place the mice in an open arena situated in a brightly lit room and record the distance the mice travel during a 10-min time span. The measurements of the distance moved in the open arena indicated that AS mice moved significantly less (WT 40.3 ± 1.2 m; AS 26.2 ± 1.2 m; $p < 0.001$; Fig. 1b). A power analysis ($\alpha = 0.05$; $(1 - \beta) = 0.95$) showed that this task requires a minimum number of 21 mice per genotype, which makes this test a relative weak test (Table 2). Previous studies reported no significant difference observed between genotypes in the time spent in the [8, 9] inner zone of the open field, which is another measure of anxiety. Our meta-analysis revealed a significant difference between genotypes ($p < 0.005$), but this difference was small (WT 1.1% versus mutant 0.7% time in inner zone), and a significant effect was only observed in four out of the eight individual experiments (data not shown).

After 1 day of rest, the same mice were then analyzed in the marble burying test, a test used to assess repetitive and perseverative behavior as well as anxiety [34, 35]. When exposed to marbles, AS mice show a strongly impaired marble burying behavior compared to WT mice (WT 11.3 ± 0.4; AS 3.6 ± 0.3; $p < 0.001$; Fig. 1c). A power analysis ($\alpha = 0.05$; $(1 - \beta) = 0.95$) showed that seven animals/group are sufficient for this test, indicating a very robust phenotype (Table 2).

After the marble burying task, all mice were single housed for 5–7 days and then analyzed for 5 consecutive days while performing the nest building test. The nest building test assesses the innate behavior of mice to create a nest to maintain body temperature and to find shelter [36]. AS mice showed a clear phenotype compared to their WT control littermates ($p < 0.001$; Fig. 1d). As indicated in Table 2, the nest building phenotype is quite robust, since it only requires 8 mice ($\alpha = 0.05$; $(1 - \beta) = 0.95$) per group if analyzed over the last day.

Following 2 days of pause, the animals were finally subjected to the forced swim test, in which the mouse is placed in a beaker filled with water, from which the mouse will try to escape by swimming. This test is typically used to test depressive-like behavior in mice [37]. AS mice showed significant more time floating (instead

Table 2 Achieved power for each behavioral test of the behavioral test battery

	Wild type (mean ± SD)	Ube3a (mean ± SD)	Test	Achieved effect size	Sample size per group $(1-\beta) = 0.95$	Sample size per group $(1-\beta) = 0.90$	Sample size per group $(1-\beta) = 0.80$
Rotarod Time on machine (s)	149 ± 55	95 ± 40	ANOVA	0.56	14	11	9
Open field Distance moved (m)	40 ± 13	26 ± 13	*T* test	1.17	21	17	13
Marble burying (# marbles buried)	11 ± 4	4 ± 4	*T* test	2.26	7	6	5
Nest building (% used nesting material)	68 ± 23	28 ± 19	*T* test	1.95	8	7	6
Forced swim test (% floating time)	37 ± 25	73 ± 18	*T* test	1.73	10	9	7
Susceptibility to audiogenic seizure (% of animals)	7	98	*T* test	4.55	3	3	3

Data provided is based on the experiments using *Ube3a^{tm1Alb}* mice in F1 hybrid 129S2-C57BL/6J background. The table provides the obtained effect size, number of mice needed per genotype for each behavioral test (with power equal to 0.95, 0.90, 0.80), and statistical test used. For rotarod calculations, we used the average performance over the 5 days, while for the nest building we used the data of the last test day of swimming) compared to WT mice (WT 36.8 ± 2.3; AS 72.6 ± 1.7; $p < 0.001$; Fig. 1e). The power analysis test showed that this task requires a minimum of 10 mice ($\alpha = 0.05$; $(1 - \beta) = 0.95$).

Taken together, the data indicates that this test battery yields a series of robust behavioral phenotypes that can be obtained in a relative quick manner using a single cohort of mice.

The dependence of sex on the behavioral phenotypes

Angelman syndrome affects both males and females, with no known differences between the sexes. To assess if this is also the case for the *Ube3a* mouse phenotypes described above, we analyzed if there were any significant sex differences. An effect of sex was noted on the rotarod, in which female wild-type and *Ube3a* mice performed significantly better than male wild-type and *Ube3a* mice ($p < 0.001$; Fig. 2a). Since male mice are heavier than female mice and since $Ube3a^{m-/p+}$ mutants show increased weight (Fig. 2f) [8, 38], we investigated if the impaired rotarod performance as seen in $Ube3a^{m-/p+}$ mutants could be attributed to their increased weight. Hence, we performed a correlation analysis between body weight and time on the rotarod (as measured on the last training day). As shown in Fig. 2g, no meaningful correlation is observed between body weight and latency to fall in both WT mice and AS mice (WT males Pearson $r = 0.08$, AS males Pearson $r = -0.21$, WT females Pearson $r = 0.35$, AS females Pearson $r = 0.02$), although the correlation observed in WT female mice was just statistically significant ($p < 0.05$), indicating that increased bodyweight actually improves (rather than impairs) rotarod performance. Overall, we conclude that the impaired motor performance of $Ube3a^{m-/p+}$ mutants on the rotarod is not caused by the increased body weight observed in these mice, but truly reflects differences in motor performance.

We also observed a small effect of sex for the nest building task in which female $Ube3a^{m-/p+}$ mutants outperformed the male $Ube3a^{m-/p+}$ mutants ($p < 0.05$). A similar tendency was also observed in wild-type mice, but this effect was not significant (Fig. 2b). Despite the slightly better performance of female $Ube3a^{m-/p+}$ mutants, female $Ube3a^{m-/p+}$ mutants were still significantly different from wild-type mice ($p < 0.001$).

We observed no significant effect of sex in the open field test ($p = 0.25$), marble burying test ($p = 0.06$), and forced swim test ($p = 0.27$; Fig. 2c–e). Overall, these data suggest that the set of behavioral phenotypes observed in AS mice are robust and are not markedly influenced by the sex of the animal. However, given the decreased performance of male mice on the rotarod, mixed cohorts used for rotarod testing should be well balanced with respect to sex to obtain a reliable phenotype.

The behavioral test battery is suitable for within-subject testing design

A within-subject testing design is a powerful design for drug testing purposes, as it allows assessing the efficacy of a drug with considerable fewer animals. Therefore, we investigated whether the behavioral test battery allowed re-testing the same animals while maintaining a similar phenotype, which is a prerequisite for applying a within-subject design. We subjected 15 $Ube3a^{m-/p+}$ mice ($Ube3a^{tm1Alb}$) and 15 WT littermates in the F1 hybrid 129S2-C57BL/6 background to the behavioral test battery and repeated the test battery after a pause of 4 weeks. As shown in Fig. 3, performance on the rotarod test, nest building test, and forced swim test was highly similar when the initial test data were compared to the re-testing data. However, performance in the open field test as well as marble burying test was significantly different when this test was performed for the second time (open field: wild type initial vs retest $p < 0.001$, $Ube3a^{m-/p+}$ initial vs retest $p < 0.001$; marble burying: wild type initial vs retest $p < 0.001$, $Ube3a^{m-/p+}$ initial vs retest $p < 0.001$; paired T test). These differences upon re-testing are likely due to the decreased anxiety levels and or habituation of the mice upon re-testing in these paradigms. Importantly, $Ube3a^{m-/p+}$ mice remained significantly different from wild-type littermates when tested for a second time, with the exception of the marble burying test, which no longer yielded a phenotype upon re-testing ($p = 0.13$). Hence, we conclude that most tests of the behavioral test battery are suitable for a within-subject design to test the efficacy of a drug.

Behavioral phenotypes are also observed in the $Ube3a^{E113X}$ mouse model

The results above indicate that the behavioral test battery gives robust phenotypes in the $Ube3a^{tm1Alb}$ line as well as in the previously published $Ube3a^{mSTOP/p+}$ ($Ube3a^{tm1Yelg}$) line. In order to test the robustness of the battery in a third independently derived *Ube3a*-mutant strain, we used the $Ube3a^{mE113X/p+}$ ($Ube3a^{tm2Yelg}$) strain, which we recently described [23]. As shown in Fig. 4, the $Ube3a^{mE113X/p+}$-mutant mice in the F1 129S2-C57BL/6J background showed again clear impairments on the rotarod test ($p < 0.001$), open field test ($p < 0.001$), marble burying test ($p < 0.05$), nest building test ($p < 0.01$), and forced swim test ($p < 0.001$). Taken together, these data suggest that the identified set of behavioral phenotypes in this test battery is present in three independently derived *Ube3a*-mutant lines.

Mouse genetic background affects the identified AS phenotypes

Previous studies have indicated the importance of the genetic background for certain *Ube3a* phenotypes [8, 9].

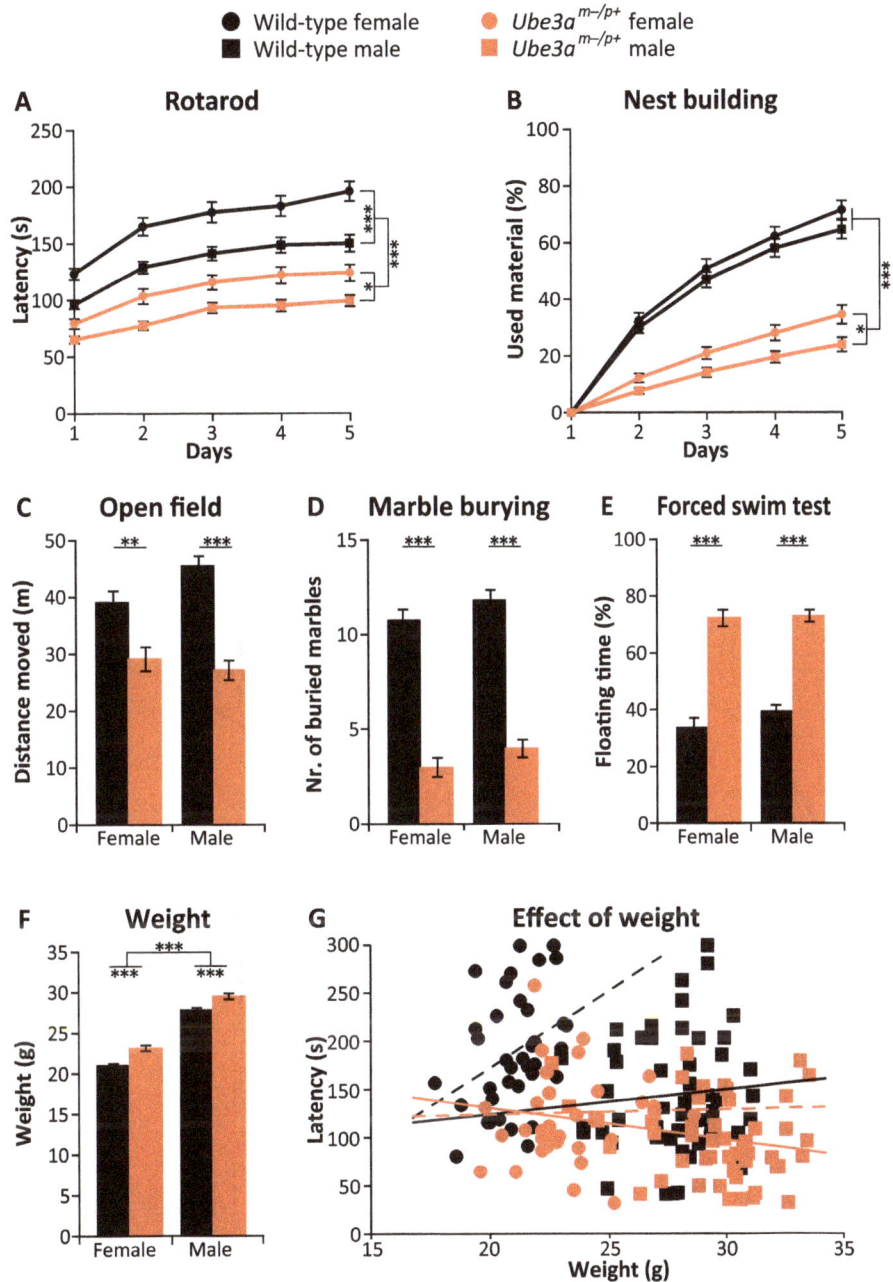

Fig. 2 Effect of sex on the behavioral phenotypes of *Ube3a^tm1Alb^* mice in F1 hybrid 129S2-C57BL/6J background. **a** Accelerating rotarod in WT and *Ube3a^m−/p+^* female mice ($n = 52, 46$) and in WT and *Ube3a^m−/p+^* male mice ($n = 68, 65$). **b** Nest building test in WT and *Ube3a^m−/p+^* female mice ($n = 42, 33$) and in WT and *Ube3a^m−/p+^* male mice ($n = 52, 53$). **c** Open field test in WT and *Ube3a^m−/p+^* female mice ($n = 47, 41$) and in WT and *Ube3a^m−/p+^* male mice ($n = 66, 65$). **d** Marble burying test in WT and *Ube3a^m−/p+^* female mice ($n = 52, 46$) and in WT and *Ube3a^m−/p+^* male mice ($n = 68, 65$). **e** Forced swim test in WT and *Ube3a^m−/p+^* female mice ($n = 52, 46$) and in WT and *Ube3a^m−/p+^* male mice ($n = 68, 65$). **f** Bodyweight in WT and *Ube3a^m−/p+^* female mice ($n = 37, 33$) and in WT and *Ube3a^m−/p+^* male mice ($n = 53, 50$). **g** Pearson correlation test between body weight and latency to fall at day 5 in WT and *Ube3a^m−/p+^* female mice ($n = 37, 33$) and in WT and *Ube3a^m−/p+^* male mice ($n = 53, 50$). Multivariate repeated ANOVA or a two-way ANOVA was used for statistical comparison. A *Bonferroni's* post hoc *test* was used to detect significant differences in behavioral phenotypes of male and female groups. All data represent mean ± SEM. Significant effects of genotype or sex are indicated as $*p < 0.05$, $**p < 0.01$, and $***p < 0.001$

To test the importance of the genetic background on the behavioral test battery, we performed the test battery on AS mice on a pure C57BL/6J (Fig. 4) and 129S2 background (Fig. 5) instead of the F1 hybrid background. *Ube3a*^mE113X/p+^ mice in C57BL/6J background showed a similar phenotype as *Ube3a*^mE113X/p+^ mutants in the F1 hybrid 129S2-C57BL/6J background with respect to the rotarod test ($p < 0.01$), marble burying test ($p < 0.001$),

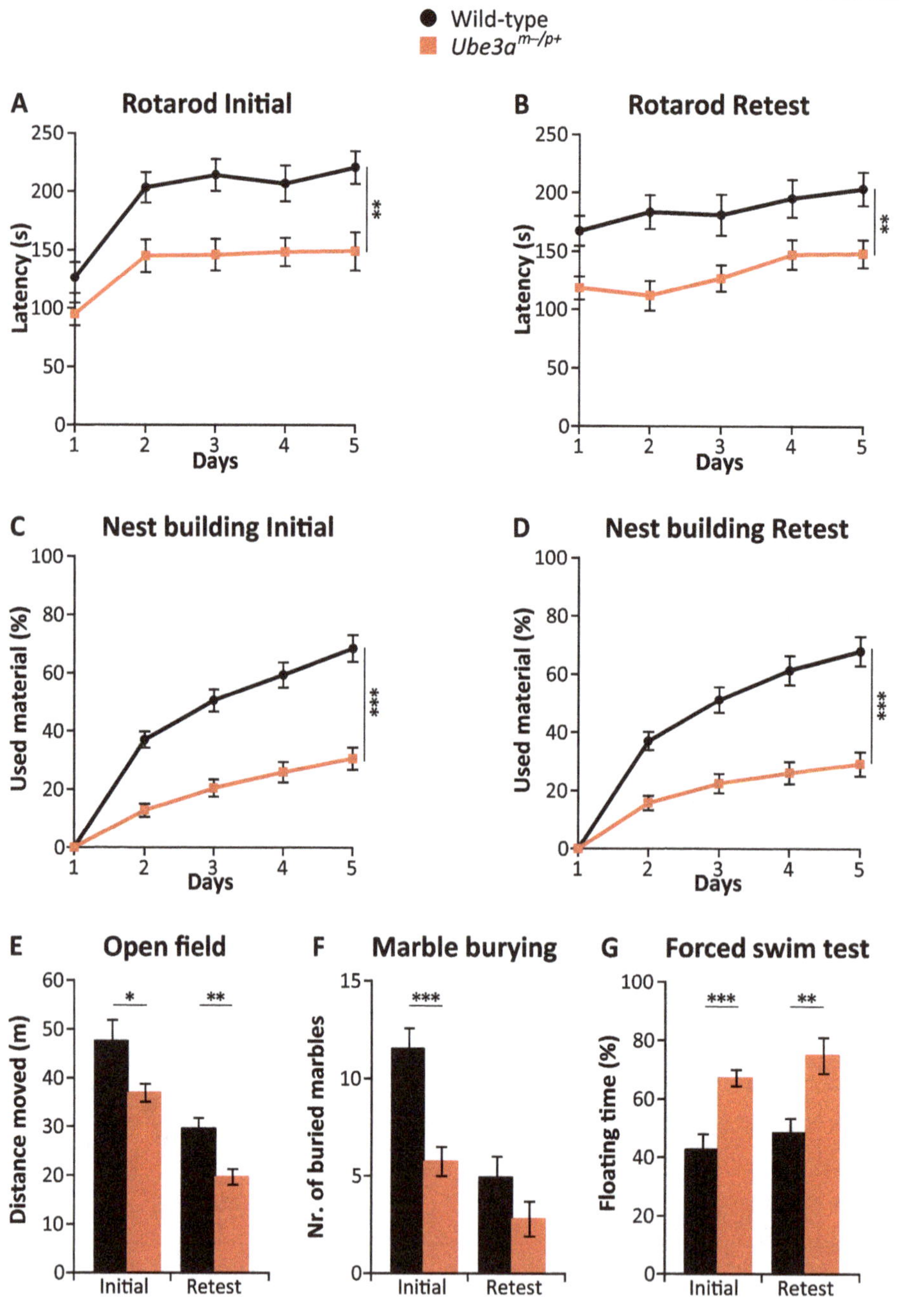

Fig. 3 Most behavioral phenotypes are stable upon re-testing $Ube3a^{tm1Alb}$ mice in F1 hybrid 129S2-C57BL/6J background. **a, c, e–g** WT and $Ube3a^{m-/p+}$ mice at initial testing and **b, d, e–g** upon re-testing. A single cohort of 15 wild-type (8 females, 7 males) and 15 $Ube3a^{tm1Alb}$ (8 females, 7 males) mice was used for all experiments. A repeated measures ANOVA or T test was used for statistical comparison of genotypes, as described in the legend of Fig. 1. All data represent mean ± SEM. Significant effects of genotype are indicated as *$p < 0.05$, **$p < 0.01$, and ***$p < 0.001$ for genotype significance

and nest building test ($p < 0.001$) (Fig. 4). No deficit was observed in the open field test ($p = 0.75$). Notably, the $Ube3a^{mE113X/p+}$ mice in C57BL/6J background showed a significant phenotype in the forced swim test ($p < 0.05$), however in the opposite direction compared to AS mice in F1 hybrid 129S2-C57BL/6J background.

The test battery was also performed using $Ube3a^{tm1Alb}$ mice in the inbred 129S2 background (Fig. 5).

$Ube3a^{tm1Alb}$ mice in the 129S2 background did not show any of the phenotypes observed in $Ube3a^{tm1Alb}$ mice in the F1 hybrid background, with the exception of the forced swim test ($p < 0.05$), which yielded a similar result as obtained in mice in the F1 hybrid background. Taken together, these data confirm and extend previous studies that most AS mouse phenotypes are strongly dependent on the genetic background.

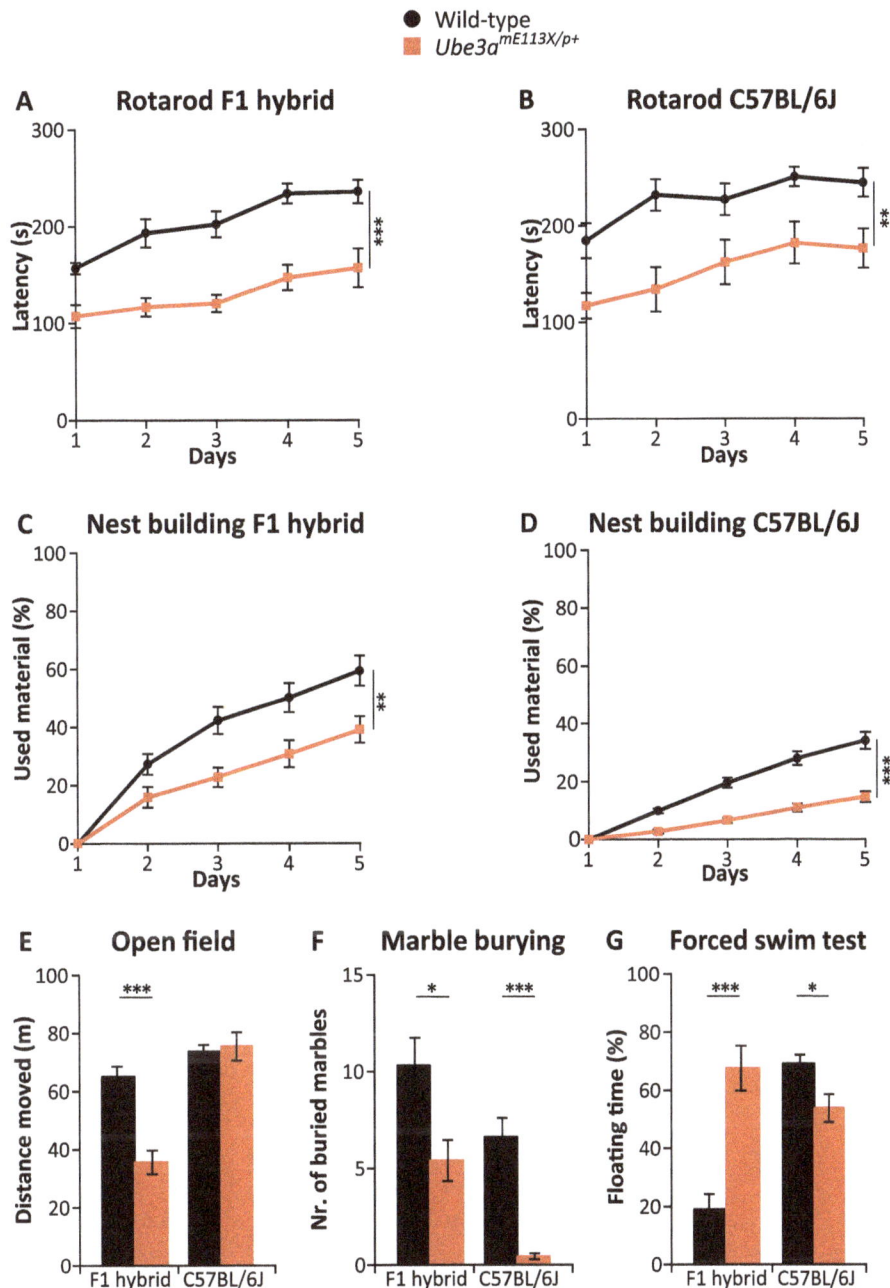

Fig. 4 Behavioral testing of $Ube3a^{mE113X/p+}$ ($Ube3a^{tm2Yelg}$) mice in the F1 hybrid 129S2-C57BL/6J and the C57BL/6J background. **a, b** Accelerating rotarod in WT and $Ube3a^{mE113X/p+}$ mice in F1 hybrid 129S2-C57BL/6J and C57BL/6J background. **c, d** Nest building test in WT and $Ube3a^{mE113X/p+}$ mice in F1 hybrid 129S2-C57BL/6J and C57BL/6J background. **e–g** Open field, marble burying, and forced swim tests in WT and $Ube3a^{mE113X/p+}$ mice in F1 hybrid 129S2-C57BL/6J and C57BL/6J background. For all behavioral tests, we used a single cohort of 10 wild-type (1 female, 9 males) and 10 $Ube3a^{mE113X/p+}$ mice (6 females, 4 males) in F1 hybrid 129S2-C57BL/6J, and 15 wild-type (11 females, 4 males) and 16 $Ube3a^{mE113X/p+}$ ($Ube3a^{tm2Yelg}$) (13 females, 4 males) mice in C57BL/6J background. All data represent mean ± SEM. A repeated measures ANOVA or T test was used for statistical comparison of genotypes, as described in the legend of Fig. 1. Significant effects of genotype are indicated as *$p < 0.05$, **$p < 0.01$, and ***$p < 0.001$

Susceptibility to audiogenic seizures

Epilepsy is a common feature of individuals with AS [39]. We previously showed that $Ube3a^{tm1Alb}$ mice as well as $Ube3a^{mSTOP/p+}$ ($Ube3a^{tm1Yelg}$) mice are highly susceptible to audiogenic seizures, a phenotype that is specifically observed in mice in the 129S2 background [7]. To investigate the strength of this test in more detail, we performed a meta-analysis of five independent experiments with a total of 114 $Ube3a^{m-/p+}$ ($Ube3a^{tm1Alb}$) mice and 45 wild-type littermates in the 129S2

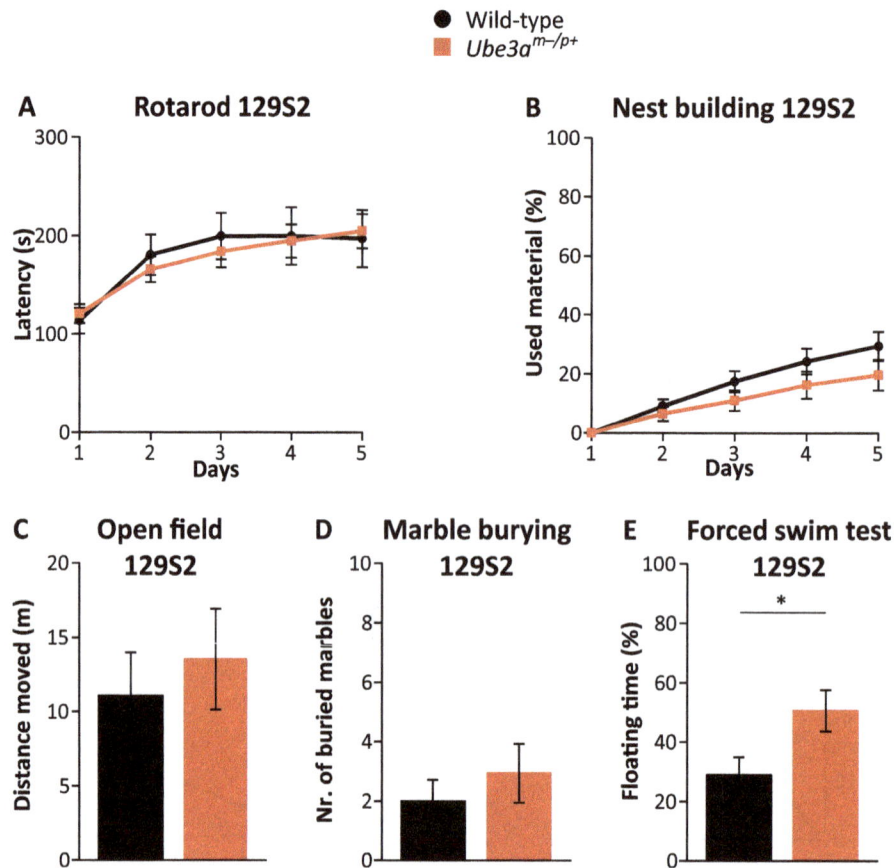

Fig. 5 Behavioral testing of Ube3a^{m−/p+} (Ube3a^{tm1Alb}) mice in the 129S2/SvPasCrl background. **a–e** Accelerating rotarod, nest building, open field, marble burying, and forced swim test in wild-type and Ube3a^{tm1Alb} mice in 129S2/SvPasCrl background (n = 11, 16) (WT = 5 females, 6 males) (Ube3a^{m−/p+} = 8 females, 8 males). A repeated measures ANOVA or T test was used for statistical comparison of genotypes, as described in the legend of Fig. 1. Significant effects of genotype are indicated as *p < 0.05

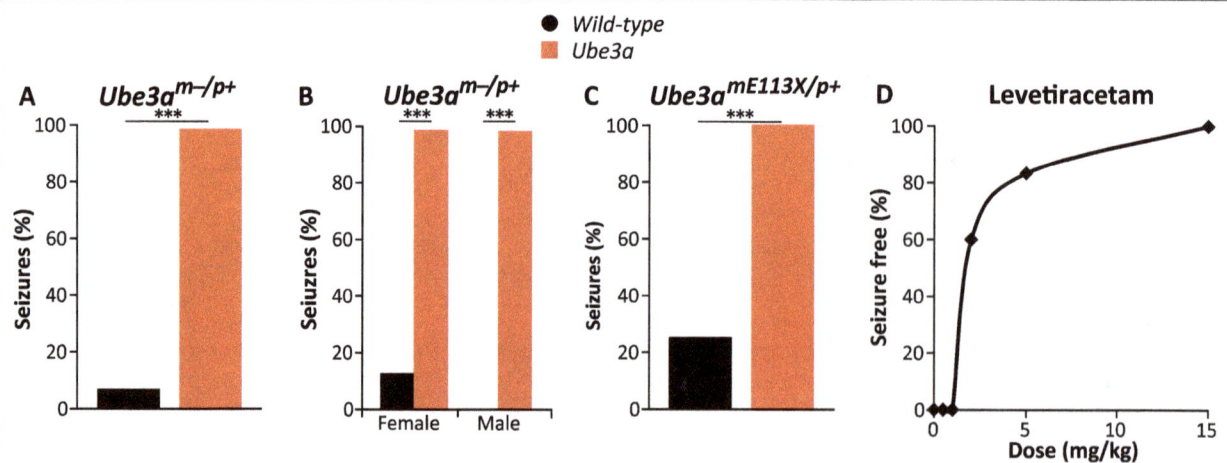

Fig. 6 Audiogenic seizure susceptibility of Ube3a^{m−/p+} and Ube3a^{mE113X/p+} mice in the 129S2/SvPasCrl background. **a** Audiogenic seizure susceptibility of WT and Ube3a^{m−/p+} mice (n = 45, 114). **b** Effect of sex on seizure susceptibility in wild-type and Ube3a^{m−/p+} mice (females n = 24, 62; males n = 21, 52). **c** Seizure susceptibility in wild-type and Ube3a^{mE113X/p+} mice (n = 4, 8) (WT = 3 females, 1 males; Ube3a^{mE113X/p+} = 1 females, 7 males). **d** Effect of increasing doses of levetiracetam on epilepsy susceptibility of Ube3a^{m−/p+} mice (0 mg/kg, n = 12; 0.5 mg/kg, n = 6; 1 mg/kg, n = 6; 2 mg/kg, n = 30; 5 mg/kg, n = 30; 15 mg/kg, n = 30). Fisher's exact test was used for statistical comparison. ***p < 0.001 for genotype significance

background. This analysis showed that this is a very robust phenotype with seizures observed in 98% of $Ube3a^{m-/p+}$ mice and in 7% of the wild-type littermates ($p < 0.001$). The robustness of this test was further confirmed by a power calculation analysis (Table 2).

We tested whether seizures were also present in the $Ube3a^{mE113X/p+}$ ($Ube3a^{tm2Yelg}$) line. To that end, we crossed $Ube3a^{pE113X/m+}$ females (backcrossed eight times in 129S2) with 129S2 males. As shown in Fig. 6, an audiogenic seizure could be provoked in all $Ube3a^{mE113X/p+}$ mutants tested ($p < 0.001$), indicating that this phenotype is observed across three independently derived $Ube3a$-mutant lines.

We previously demonstrated that the sensitivity to audiogenic seizures can be reversed upon acute treatment with anti-epileptic drugs [13]. Given the high power of this assay, we investigated if this assay is suitable to determine the effective dose of a treatment. To that end, we treated mice with levetiracetam, a compound that acts as ligand of the synaptic vesicle protein 2A, which is a commonly used anti-epileptic drug for both partial and generalized seizures and which is also often prescribed to individuals with AS [40, 41]. $Ube3a^{m-/p+}$ ($Ube3a^{tm1Alb}$) mice in 129S2 background were first assessed for their (baseline) sensitivity to audiogenically evoked seizures without treatment. After establishing that all mice were sensitive, mice received at least 1 day after baseline testing a single IP dose of levetiracetam and were tested 1 h after IP injection. As shown in Fig. 6d, a good dose-response curve could be obtained, in which 2 mg/kg levetiracetam yielded approximately 60% of mice to be resistant to audiogenic seizures. This indicates that this test is highly suitable for quickly determining the effective dose of a treatment.

Minocycline treatment does not improve behavioral phenotypes of Ube3a mice

It has previously been reported that minocycline treatment of $Ube3a$ animals improves synaptic plasticity as well as motor coordination, which was the basis for an open-label study with minocycline in individuals with AS (trial register NCT01531582 and [20]), as well as a randomized controlled trial ((NCT02056665), [22]). Unfortunately, the randomized trial showed no difference between placebo and minocycline-treated individuals [22]. To test if minocycline ameliorated the $Ube3a$-mutant phenotypes in our behavioral test battery, we subjected the animals to the same treatment protocol as used for the initial mouse study [20]. Adult-treated $Ube3a^{m-/p+}$ ($Ube3a^{tm1Alb}$) mice and littermate controls (8–12 weeks of age) in the F1 hybrid 129S2-C57BL/6J background received daily minocycline (45 mg/kg) or control saline IP injections starting 3 weeks prior to behavioral

testing. After 3 weeks of daily injections, the mice were sequentially subjected to the behavioral test battery as described above. In contrast to the previous finding (trial register NCT01531582), we did not observe a rescue on the rotarod. We also observed no effect of minocycline on any of the other tests of the behavioral battery (Fig. 7; two-way ANOVA, genotype/treatment interaction $p > 0.08$ in all tests). Notably, prolonged exposure to daily minocycline injections resulted in yellow deposits over the organs and dullness of the liver (data not shown), confirming previous studies that IP administration of minocycline is not the best choice of administration [42].

Minocycline has also been used to reverse the behavioral deficits of a mouse model of Fragile X [26, 43]. Notably, in these studies, minocycline treatment was initiated immediately after birth and provided though the drinking water. Since we previously showed that a behavioral rescue of $Ube3a$ mice may also depend on the timing of treatment initiation [13], we decided to treat $Ube3a$ animals immediately after birth, using the same protocol as described for FMRP mice [26]. However, also this prolonged postnatal treatment regimen did not yield a significant behavioral improvement, as none of these tests showed a significant interaction of genotype and treatment (two-way ANOVA, genotype/treatment interaction $p > 0.16$ in all tests) (Fig. 7).

Levodopa/carbidopa treatment does not improve behavioral phenotypes of Ube3a mice

A recent study showed that treatment of $Ube3a$ mice with levodopa resulted in improvement of their motor skills compared to untreated $Ube3a$ mice [21]. Based on this preclinical observation, a placebo-controlled trial of levodopa was initiated in 55 children between 4 and 12 years diagnosed with AS. Unfortunately, no significant improvement was observed on any of the outcomes measured following a 1-year treatment (trial register NCT01281475 and [21]). To test as to what extent levodopa ameliorated the phenotypes of $Ube3a^{m-/p+}$ ($Ube3a^{tm1Alb}$) mice in our behavioral battery, we subjected the animals to the same treatment protocol as used for the initial mouse study [21]. $Ube3a^{m-/p+}$ and wild-type littermates (8–12 weeks of age) in F1 hybrid 129S2-C57BL/6J background received daily levodopa/carbidopa (15 mg/kg levodopa and 3.75 mg/kg carbidopa) or control saline IP injections, starting 1 h prior to behavioral testing. In contrast to the earlier finding [21], we did not observe a rescue on the rotarod. We also observed no effect of levodopa treatment on any of the other tests of the behavioral battery (two-way ANOVA, genotype/treatment interaction $p > 0.17$ in all tests) (Fig. 8).

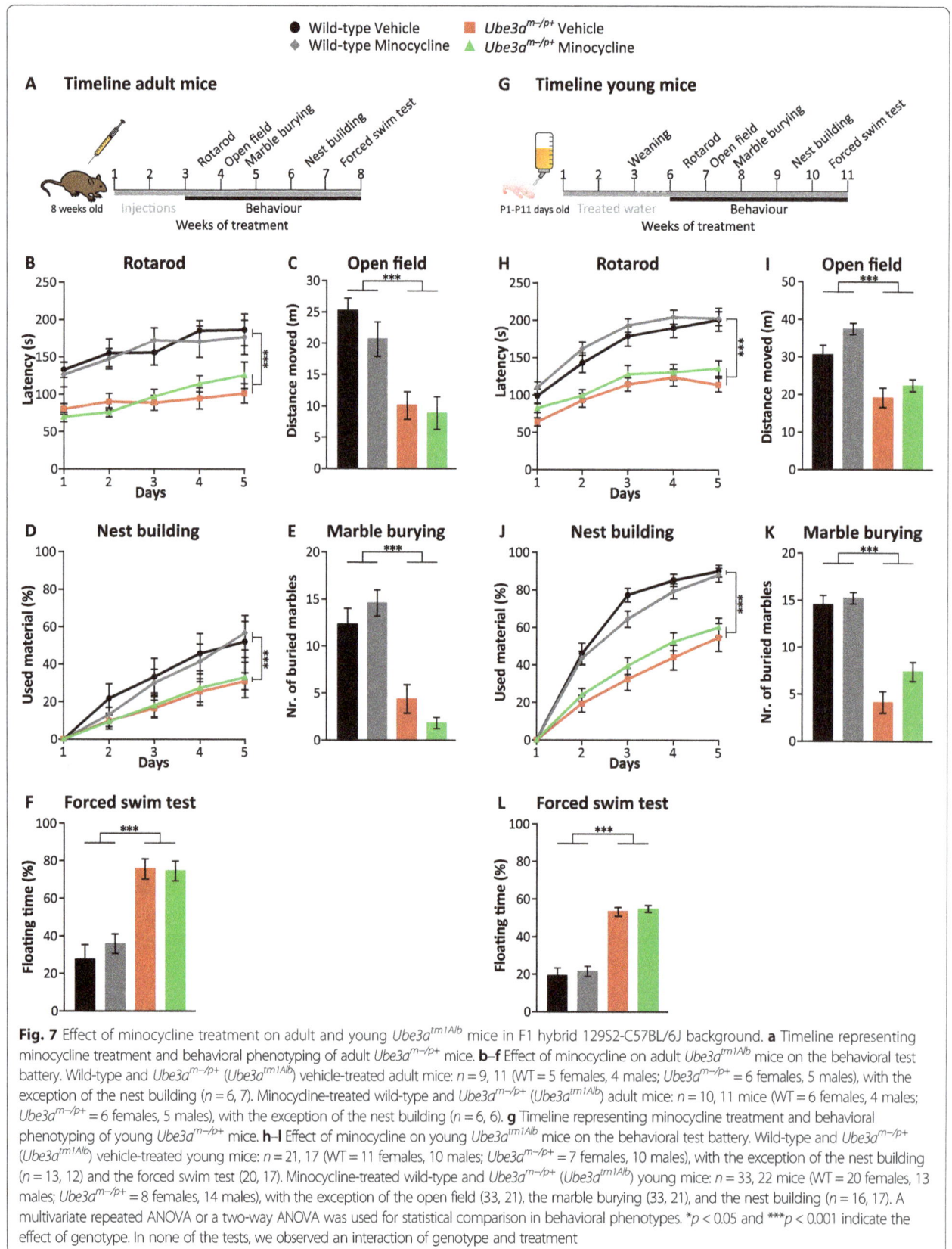

Fig. 7 Effect of minocycline treatment on adult and young *Ube3a^{tm1Alb}* mice in F1 hybrid 129S2-C57BL/6J background. **a** Timeline representing minocycline treatment and behavioral phenotyping of adult *Ube3a^{m−/p+}* mice. **b–f** Effect of minocycline on adult *Ube3a^{tm1Alb}* mice on the behavioral test battery. Wild-type and *Ube3a^{m−/p+}* (*Ube3a^{tm1Alb}*) vehicle-treated adult mice: $n = 9, 11$ (WT = 5 females, 4 males; *Ube3a^{m−/p+}* = 6 females, 5 males), with the exception of the nest building ($n = 6, 7$). Minocycline-treated wild-type and *Ube3a^{m−/p+}* (*Ube3a^{tm1Alb}*) adult mice: $n = 10, 11$ mice (WT = 6 females, 4 males; *Ube3a^{m−/p+}* = 6 females, 5 males), with the exception of the nest building ($n = 6, 6$). **g** Timeline representing minocycline treatment and behavioral phenotyping of young *Ube3a^{m−/p+}* mice. **h–l** Effect of minocycline on young *Ube3a^{tm1Alb}* mice on the behavioral test battery. Wild-type and *Ube3a^{m−/p+}* (*Ube3a^{tm1Alb}*) vehicle-treated young mice: $n = 21, 17$ (WT = 11 females, 10 males; *Ube3a^{m−/p+}* = 7 females, 10 males), with the exception of the nest building ($n = 13, 12$) and the forced swim test (20, 17). Minocycline-treated wild-type and *Ube3a^{m−/p+}* (*Ube3a^{tm1Alb}*) young mice: $n = 33, 22$ mice (WT = 20 females, 13 males; *Ube3a^{m−/p+}* = 8 females, 14 males), with the exception of the open field (33, 21), the marble burying (33, 21), and the nest building ($n = 16, 17$). A multivariate repeated ANOVA or a two-way ANOVA was used for statistical comparison in behavioral phenotypes. *$p < 0.05$ and ***$p < 0.001$ indicate the effect of genotype. In none of the tests, we observed an interaction of genotype and treatment

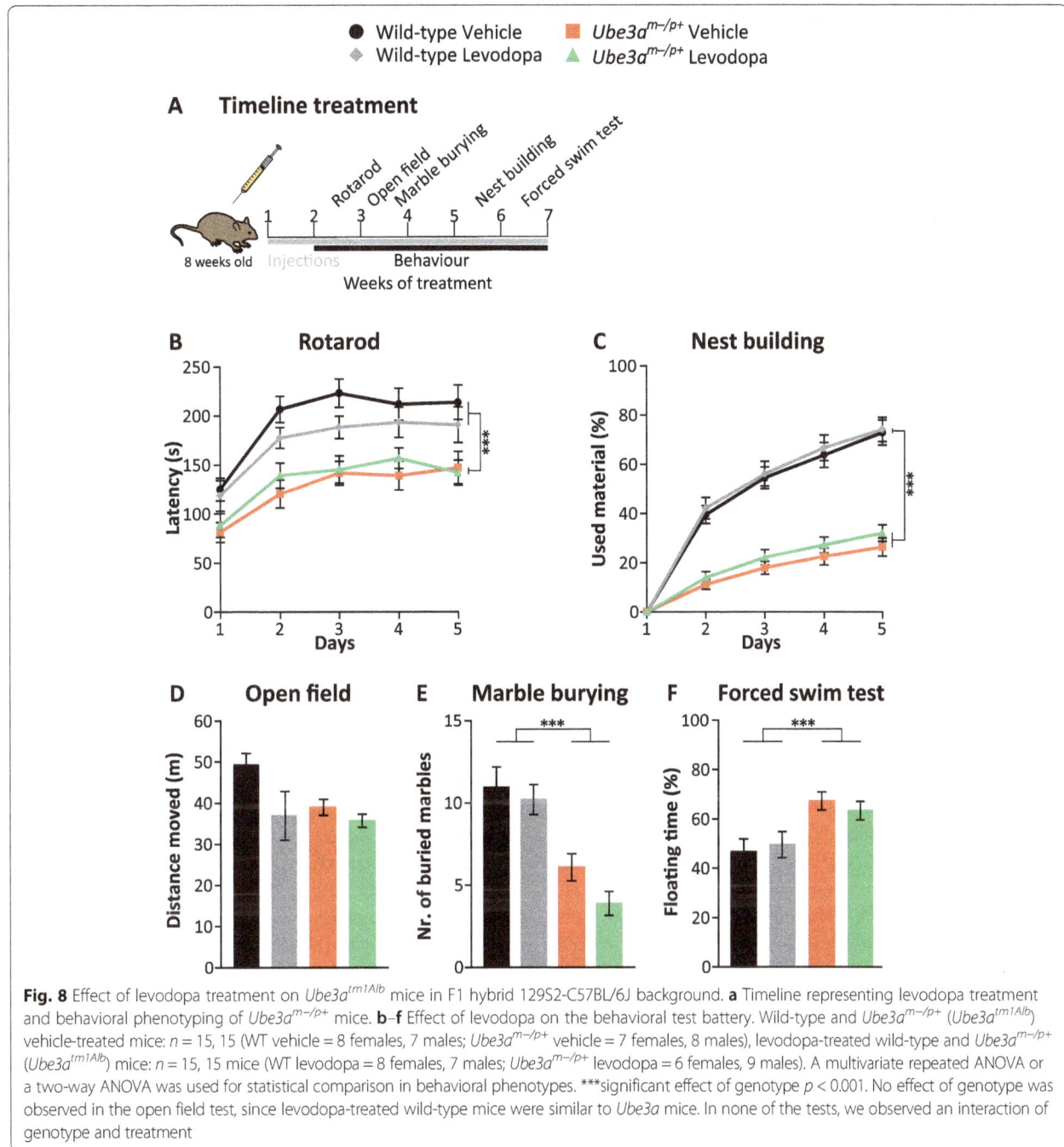

Fig. 8 Effect of levodopa treatment on $Ube3a^{tm1Alb}$ mice in F1 hybrid 129S2-C57BL/6J background. **a** Timeline representing levodopa treatment and behavioral phenotyping of $Ube3a^{m-/p+}$ mice. **b–f** Effect of levodopa on the behavioral test battery. Wild-type and $Ube3a^{m-/p+}$ ($Ube3a^{tm1Alb}$) vehicle-treated mice: $n = 15, 15$ (WT vehicle = 8 females, 7 males; $Ube3a^{m-/p+}$ vehicle = 7 females, 8 males), levodopa-treated wild-type and $Ube3a^{m-/p+}$ ($Ube3a^{tm1Alb}$) mice: $n = 15, 15$ mice (WT levodopa = 8 females, 7 males; $Ube3a^{m-/p+}$ levodopa = 6 females, 9 males). A multivariate repeated ANOVA or a two-way ANOVA was used for statistical comparison in behavioral phenotypes. ***significant effect of genotype $p < 0.001$. No effect of genotype was observed in the open field test, since levodopa-treated wild-type mice were similar to $Ube3a$ mice. In none of the tests, we observed an interaction of genotype and treatment

Discussion

Robust behavioral phenotypes with high construct and face validity in mouse models of disease are critical for the identification of novel treatments and the successful translation of these therapies to clinical trials. These pre-clinical studies may give us important information about the therapeutic dose, optimal age of treatment, and the best outcome measures to be used in a clinical trial. Given the high failure rate of clinical trials aimed at improving cognitive function [44], it is absolutely critical that the preclinical data is robust (reproducible results

across different mutant lines and different experimenters) and that the animal studies have high construct and face validity.

In this study, we investigated the robustness of a number of behavioral phenotypes, which we previously described using the inducible $Ube3a^{mSTOP/p+}$ ($Ube3a^{tm1Yelg}$) mice [13]. These phenotypes were assessed in two independently derived $Ube3a$ lines: in the commonly used $Ube3a^{tm1Alb}$ line [7] and the recently generated $Ube3a^{mE113X/p+}$ ($Ube3a^{tm2Yelg}$) line [13]. Recently, we have tested two additional novel $Ube3a$ lines in this test battery with the same results; the $Ube3a^{tm1.1Bdph}$ line (MGI:5882092) and a novel (unpublished) $Ube3a$ line ($Ube3a^{em1Yelg}$). Thus, taken together, a total of five independently derived $Ube3a$ lines show phenotypes on all the behavioral tests of the test battery described in this study. In all cases, we used heterozygous $Ube3a$ mice in which the mutation was located on the maternally inherited $Ube3a$ allele. Therefore, we conclude that construct validity is very high. However, since the majority of individuals with AS carries a large chromosomal deletion of the AS critical region (15q11-q13) which encompasses also other genes besides $Ube3a$ and which may contribute to a more severe phenotype [6], it would be of interest to test a mouse model of AS with large maternal deletion [11] in our behavioral test battery.

In terms of face validity, we used behavioral paradigms that assess domains of motor performance, anxiety, repetitive behavior, and seizure susceptibility, which are all relevant clinical phenotypes of AS. Nevertheless, the clinical translational value of some of our tests (e.g., open field, marble burying, nest building, and forced swim tests) may be limited. Although it is notable that many of our tests involve a strong motor component, we think that it is unlikely that the phenotypes observed in the open field, marble burying, nest building, and forced swim tests are solely related to deficits in the domain of motor functioning. Most notably, we have shown that the critical period for rescuing these phenotypes is distinctly different compared to rescuing the rotarod deficit [13] (and unpublished data). For instance, we found that gene reactivation in 3-week-old mice fully rescues the rotarod phenotype, but none of the other phenotypes [13]. It is further noticeable that both WT and mutant mice behave significantly different when tested for a second time in the open field and marble burying tests, whereas no significant changes were observed in rotarod performance. This further indicates that the deficits in the open field and marble burying tests are indicative of deficits in other domains than motor performance.

An important clinical feature of AS that is lacking in our behavioral test battery is a paradigm that assesses cognitive function. Despite profound cognitive impairments in individuals with AS, learning deficits in the AS mouse model are rather mild. We and others have reported learning deficits in AS mice by using the Morris water maze [8, 18, 45]. However, this paradigm is very labor intensive and hence less suitable for drug testing. Moreover, we found that a large number of mice are needed to detect significant differences and results varied strongly among experimenters (data not shown). A good learning paradigm that is highly suitable for drug testing is fear conditioning, in which animals are

subjected to a single training session in which they are trained to associate a context (training chamber) or cue (tone) with a foot shock. However, we have not been able to get consistent results across experiments and experimenters (data not shown), and varying results are published in literature, with some studies showing a specific deficit in context conditioning [7, 46] and others a specific deficit in cued conditioning [8] or both [47–49]. Notably, the two studies that investigated the behavioral deficits of $Ube3a$ mice across strains in great detail showed no context conditioning deficit in $Ube3a$ mice in the F1 hybrid 129-C57BL/6J background and C57BL/6J background, and either normal [9] or impaired [8] cued fear conditioning in $Ube3a$ mice in the C57BL/6J background. Collectively, these studies indicate that this phenotype is rather weak, and hence results, obtained with these tests should be interpreted with care.

By combining the data of eight independent experiments performed by five different experimenters, we were able to perform a meta-analysis of 111 $Ube3a^{m-/p+}$ ($Ube3a^{tm1Alb}$) and 120 WT littermate mice in the F1 hybrid 129S2-C57BL/6J background and determine the robustness of the phenotypes. In all eight experiments, we replicated $Ube3a$ phenotypes observed on the rotarod test, open field test, marble burying test, nest building test, and the forced swim test. Deficits of $Ube3a$ mice in rotarod performance, open field behavior, and marble burying have been reported by many other investigators, and hence, our results confirm the robustness of these tests. Impaired nest building behavior and impaired performance in the forced swim test of $Ube3a$ mice have not yet been reported by other laboratories, but our study shows that these deficits are also very robust. In fact, a power analysis showed that these tests are among the most robust tests of the behavioral test battery. The open field paradigm was found to have the weakest power.

Our meta-analysis further shows that there is no major effect of sex on the behavioral phenotypes, which is in line with the general notion that such differences are also not present in AS patients. We did however find that female wild-type and mutant mice outperformed male wild-type and mutant mice on the rotarod. Improved performance of female mice on the rotarod has also been reported previously [50] and emphasizes the need of using well-matched groups when groups of both sexes of $Ube3a$ mice are tested on the rotarod. Given that male mice are heavier than female mice, we investigated if the impaired performance of $Ube3a$ mice on the rotarod can be attributed to the increased weight of these mutants. However, we found no correlation between weight of the animal and performance on the rotarod. This observation is in line with other studies [50–52] and indicates that the reduced performance of

Ube3a mice on the rotarod represents a bona fide impairment in motor performance.

Besides the reproducibility of the observed phenotypes and the high face and construct validity, there are two additional features that make the behavioral test battery for *Ube3a* mice highly useful for drug testing. We show that with the exception of the epilepsy test, all behavioral experiments can be performed with a single cohort of mice, which greatly reduces costs as well as the number of mice needed. In addition, we found that with the exception of the marble burying task, the behavioral test battery can be performed twice with the same cohort while maintaining a phenotype. This makes it possible to test the efficacy of a drug using a within-subject design.

We confirmed previous studies that the audiogenic seizure phenotype is a very powerful test to investigate seizure susceptibility in *Ube3a* mice [7, 13, 18]. With this study, this phenotype is now also confirmed in three independently derived lines: the commonly used $Ube3a^{t-m1Alb}$ line [7], the $Ube3a^{mSTOP/p+}$ ($Ube3a^{tm1Yelg}$) line [13], and the recently generated $Ube3a^{mE113X/p+}$ ($Ube3a^{tm2Yelg}$) line [23]. Since nearly all *Ube3a* mice show this phenotype compared to less than 10% of wild-type animals, this test has very high power. Moreover, we showed that the phenotype is readily reversible with the anti-epileptic drug levetiracetam and that the test is highly suitable for dose finding. The only disadvantage of the audiogenic seizure test is that it cannot be performed on the same animals as used in the behavioral test battery, since the sensitivity to audiogenic seizures is exclusively observed in *Ube3a* mice in the 129S2 genetic background.

We also observed an effect of genetic background on the tests of the behavioral test battery. *Ube3a* mice in the C57BL/6J background showed a significant phenotype in the rotarod, nest building, and marble burying tests, but no effect of genotype was observed in the open field test. A significant effect of genotype was found in the forced swim test, but remarkably, this was in the opposite direction. In contrast, *Ube3a* mice in the 129S2 genetic background showed only a significant deficit in the forced swim test (in the same direction as F1 hybrid mice) and no phenotype on any of the other tests of the behavioral battery. This confirms previous reports that many of the *Ube3a* phenotypes are very sensitive to genetic background and not present in 129 lines [8, 9]. There are however several common findings as well as a few discrepancies between these studies and our study. With respect to the rotarod [8, 9] and marble burying phenotype [9], our findings that only *Ube3a*-C57BL/6J and *Ube3a*-F1 hybrid mice show a phenotype are in full agreement with each other (Huang et al. only tested *Ube3a*-C57BL/6J in the marble burying test). With respect to the open field test (distance traveled), the other

two studies also found no phenotype in *Ube3a*-129 mice, but in contrast to our findings, they both found a phenotype in *Ube3a*-C57BL/6J mice. One major difference between their and our experimental design is the time the mice were placed in the open field. Indeed, when we left the *Ube3a*-C57BL/6J mice for 30 min in the open field (instead of the 10 min we used), we found a nearly significant phenotype in *Ube3a*-C57BL/6J mice ($p = 0.06$; data not shown). With respect to percentage of time spent in the inner zone of the open field (which is another measure of anxiety), the other two studies showed no significant effect of genotype in any of the genetic backgrounds. Our meta-analysis did however reveal a significant difference between genotypes in F1 hybrid mice (WT 1.1% versus mutant 0.7% time in inner zone; $p < 0.01$), which further indicates that *Ube3a*-mutant mice are more anxious. However, we note that the observed difference was small and a significant effect was only observed in four out of the eight individual experiments. Hence, this measure is not very robust.

Taken all studies into consideration, it is clear that *Ube3a* mice in the F1 hybrid 129S2-C57BL/6J background show the most robust phenotypes, with the notable exception of the audiogenic seizure susceptibility test, which is strictly seen in *Ube3a*-129S2 mice. The question arises whether the observed differences between *Ube3a* mice in different genetic backgrounds have any translational significance. The lack of phenotypes of *Ube3a*-129S2 mice in most tests could simply reflect the passive/hypoactive phenotype of these mice, resulting in a floor effect. However, it could also be that the AS phenotype is sensitive to genetic background and that the changes that are observed between individuals with AS are in part caused by genetic modifiers, rather than the nature of the mutation. Detailed studies of individuals with recurrent or similar mutations could provide more insight in that question [53].

To test the translational value of the behavioral test battery, we decided to re-evaluate the two drugs that previously were tested in clinical trials involving individuals with AS: minocycline (trial register NCT01531582 [20] and NCT02056665 [22]) and levodopa (trial register NCT01281475 [21]). Both drugs were previously shown to rescue the rotarod impairment of *Ube3a* mice (see NCT01531582 for minocycline, and [21] for levodopa). In addition, minocycline rescued the hippocampal LTP deficit of *Ube3a* mice [20], whereas levodopa rescued the increased phosphorylation of CaMK2 observed in *Ube3a* mice [21]. We tested the effect of both drugs on all tests of our behavioral test battery, using the same drug administration protocols as used for the original studies. In addition, we also tested the effect of minocycline when administered from birth, as previously published for the Fragile X mouse model [26]. However, in line with the clinical trials, we did not observe any efficacy of these drugs when tested on *Ube3a* mice. Our finding that minocycline and levodopa are unable to improve performance on the rotarod is at odds with aforementioned previous preclinical studies. Failure of replication could be due to differences in strains or procedures, although there is full agreement between our labs with respect to performance of *Ube3a* mice on the rotarod and the effects of different genetic backgrounds on this performance [9]. We think it is more likely that the rotarod experiments used for the preclinical studies were underpowered, as our analysis showed that 14 mice per group are needed for a well-powered rotarod study using two groups. In the levodopa study, the authors used 6 different treatment groups and only 6 mice per group [21]. Such small sample sizes make the test underpowered and also very vulnerable for the sex differences that we describe here. Since the details of the rotarod experiments of the minocycline treatment were not provided (NCT01531582), we cannot comment on these discrepancies.

Conclusions

Here, we provided a behavioral test battery with a robust set of well-characterized *Ube3a* phenotypes, which allows researchers to investigate the effects of pharmacological and genetic interventions involving *Ube3a* mice. A standardized set of tests, in combination with a well-defined genetic background, will also be very useful to compare data across laboratories. Moreover, using a standardized behavioral test battery may reduce selective reporting bias [54]. Future studies should reveal how well the results of this behavioral test battery can be replicated between different laboratories in which housing and testing environment is different [55–58]. In addition, robust tests that capture phenotypes in the domain of cognitive function should be identified and added to this test battery.

Abbreviations
AS: Angelman syndrome; EEG: Electroencephalography; IP: Intraperitoneal; Mut: Mutant; UBE3A: Ubiquitin-protein ligase E3A; WT: Wild-type

Acknowledgements
We thank Linda Koene for the advice concerning statistical analysis and generating the figures. We thank Maria Smit and Mireia Bernabé Kleijn for the technical assistance with behavioral experiments, Mehrnoush Aghadavoud Jolfaei for genotyping, and Minetta Elgersma-Hooisma for the mouse colony management and editing of the manuscript.

Funding
MS was supported by grants from Associazione Angelman and FROM. SSS was supported by Fundação para a Ciência e Tecnologia and Fundação Amélia de Mello. GMW was funded by the Angelman Syndrome Foundation.

Authors' contributions
MS, IW, SSS, JK, and DM performed the behavioral experiments. MS, IW, SSS, and YE analyzed and interpreted the data. GMW generated the *Ube3a*^{tm2Yelg} mouse model and setup the tracking system. IW made the figures. YE designed the study. MS and YE wrote the manuscript. All authors contributed intellectually to this study and edited and approved the final manuscript.

Competing interests
The authors declare that they have no competing interests.

References
1. Petersen MB, Brøndum-Nielsen K, Hansen LK, Wulff K. Clinical, cytogenetic, and molecular diagnosis of Angelman syndrome: estimated prevalence rate in a Danish county. Am J Med Genet. 1995;60:261–2.
2. Kishino T, Lalande M, Wagstaff J. UBE3A/E6-AP mutations cause Angelman syndrome. Nat Genet. 1997;15:70–3.
3. Williams CA, Beaudet AL, Clayton-Smith J, Knoll JH, Kyllerman M, Laan LA, et al. Angelman syndrome 2005: updated consensus for diagnostic criteria. Am J Med Genet Part A. 2006;140A:413–8.
4. Tan W-HH, Bird LM. Angelman syndrome: current and emerging therapies in 2016. Am J Med Genet Part C Semin Med Genet. 2016;401:384–401.
5. Katz DM, Berger-Sweeney JE, Eubanks JH, Justice MJ, Neul JL, Pozzo-Miller L, et al. Preclinical research in Rett syndrome: setting the foundation for translational success. Dis Model Mech. 2012;5:733–45.
6. Gentile JK, Tan W-H, Horowitz LT, Bacino CA, Skinner SA, Barbieri-Welge R, et al. A neurodevelopmental survey of Angelman syndrome with genotype-phenotype correlations. J Dev Behav Pediatr. 2010;31:592–601.
7. Jiang YH, Armstrong D, Albrecht U, Atkins CM, Noebels JL, Eichele G, et al. Mutation of the Angelman ubiquitin ligase in mice causes increased cytoplasmic p53 and deficits of contextual learning and long-term potentiation. Neuron. 1998;21:799–811.
8. Huang HS, Burns AJ, Nonneman RJ, Baker LK, Riddick NV, Nikolova VD, et al. Behavioral deficits in an Angelman syndrome model: effects of genetic background and age. Behav Brain Res. 2013;243:79–90.
9. Born HA, Dao AT, Levine AT, Lee WL, Mehta NM, Mehra S, et al. Strain-dependence of the Angelman syndrome phenotypes in Ube3a maternal deficiency mice. Sci Rep. 2017;7:1–15.
10. Allensworth M, Saha A, Reiter LT, Heck DH. Normal social seeking behavior, hypoactivity and reduced exploratory range in a mouse model of Angelman syndrome. BMC Genet. 2011;12:7.
11. Jiang YH, Pan Y, Zhu L, Landa L, Yoo J, Spencer C, et al. Altered ultrasonic vocalization and impaired learning and memory in Angelman syndrome mouse model with a large maternal deletion from Ube3a to Gabrb3. PLoS ONE 5(8):e12278. https://doi.org/10.1371/journal.pone.0012278.
12. Miura K, Kishino T, Li E, Webber H, Dikkes P, Holmes GL, et al. Neurobehavioral and electroencephalographic abnormalities in Ube3a maternal-deficient mice. Neurobiol Dis. 2002;9:149–59.
13. Silva-santos S, Van Woerden GM, Bruinsma CF, Mientjes E, Jolfaei MA, Distel B, et al. Ube3a reinstatement identifies distinct developmental windows in a murine Angelman syndrome model. J Clin Invest. 2015;125Silva-s:1–8.
14. Garrido-Mesa N, Zarzuelo A, Gálvez J. Minocycline: far beyond an antibiotic. Br J Pharmacol. 2013;169:337–52.
15. Elewa HF, Hilali H, Hess DC, Machado LS, Fagan SC. Minocycline for short-term neuroprotection. Pharmacotherapy. 2006;26:515–21. https://doi.org/10.1592/phco.26.4.515.
16. Harbord M. Levodopa responsive Parkinsonism in adults with Angelman syndrome. J Clin Neurosci. 2001;8:421–2.
17. Brown AM, Deutch AY, Colbran RJ. Dopamine depletion alters phosphorylation of striatal proteins in a model of Parkinsonism. Eur J Neurosci. 2005;22:247–56.
18. Van Woerden GM, Harris KD, Hojjati MR, Gustin RM, Qiu S, Freire RDA, et al. Rescue of neurological deficits in a mouse model for Angelman syndrome by reduction of alphaCaMKII inhibitory phosphorylation. Nat Neurosci. 2007;10:280–2.
19. Weeber EJ, Jiang Y-H, Elgersma Y, Varga AW, Carrasquillo Y, Brown SE, et al. Derangements of hippocampal calcium/calmodulin-dependent protein kinase II in a mouse model for Angelman mental retardation syndrome. J Neurosci. 2003;23:2634 44. doi:23/7/2634

20. Grieco JC, Ciarlone SL, Gieron-Korthals M, Schoenberg MR, Smith AG, Philpot RM, et al. An open-label pilot trial of minocycline in children as a treatment for Angelman syndrome. BMC Neurol. 2014;14:232.

21. Tan WH, Bird LM, Sadhwani A, Barbieri-Welge RL, Skinner SA, Horowitz LT, et al. A randomized controlled trial of levodopa in patients with Angelman syndrome. Am J Med Genet Part A. 2018;176A:1099–107.

22. Ruiz-Antorán B, Sancho López A, Cazorla-Calleja R, López-Pájaro LF, Leiva Á, Iglesias-Escalera G, et al. A randomized placebo controlled clinical trial to evaluate the efficacy and safety of minocycline in patients with Angelman syndrome (A-MANECE study). Orphanet J Rare Dis. 2018;13:144. https://doi.org/10.1186/s13023-018-0891-6.

23. Wang T, van Woerden GM, Elgersma Y, Borst JGG. Enhanced transmission at the calyx of Held synapse in a mouse model for Angelman syndrome. Front Cell Neurosci. 2018;11:1–19.

24. Grieco J. Minocycline treatment and the necessity to develop a novel outcome measure for children with Angelman syndrome. Grad Theses Diss. 2015; http://scholarcommons.usf.edu/etd/5693.

25. Andes D, Craig WA. Animal model pharmacokinetics and pharmacodynamics: a critical review. Int J Antimicrob Agents. 2002;19:261–8.

26. Bilousova TV, Dansie L, Ngo M, Aye J, Charles JR, Ethell DW, et al. Minocycline promotes dendritic spine maturation and improves behavioural performance in the fragile X mouse model. J Med Genet. 2009;46:94–102.

27. Lee CZ, Yao JS, Huang Y, Zhai W, Liu W, Guglielmo BJ, et al. Dose–response effect of tetracyclines on cerebral matrix metalloproteinase-9 after vascular endothelial growth factor hyperstimulation. J Cereb Blood Flow Metab. 2006;26:1157–64.

28. Lin S, Wei X, Bales KR, Paul ABC, Ma Z, Yan G, et al. Minocycline blocks bilirubin neurotoxicity and prevents hyperbilirubinemia-induced cerebellar hypoplasia in the Gunn rat. Eur J Neurosci. 2005;22:21–7.

29. Luzi P, Abraham RM, Rafi MA, Curtis M, Hooper DC, Wenger DA. Effects of treatments on inflammatory and apoptotic markers in the CNS of mice with globoid cell leukodystrophy. Brain Res. 2009;1300:146–58.

30. Van Zutphen LFM, Baumans V, Beynen AC. Principles of laboratory animal science: a contribution to the humane use and care of animals and to the quality of experimental results. Amsterdam: Elsevier B.V.; 2001.

31. Florek-Luszczki M, Wlaz A, Luszczki JJ. Interactions of levetiracetam with carbamazepine, phenytoin, topiramate and vigabatrin in the mouse 6 Hz psychomotor seizure model – a type II isobolographic analysis. Eur J Pharmacol. 2014;723:410–8.

32. Kiel C, Faul F, Erdfelder E, Lang AG, Buchner A. G* Power 3: a flexible statistical power analysis program for the social, behavioral, and biomedical sciences. Behav Res Methods. 2007;39:175–91.

33. Pelc K, Cheron G, Dan B. Behavior and neuropsychiatric manifestations in Angelman syndrome. Neuropsychiatric Dis Treat. 2008;4(3):577–84.

34. Kedia S, Chattarji S. Marble burying as a test of the delayed anxiogenic effects of acute immobilisation stress in mice. J Neurosci Methods. 2014;233:150–4.

35. Angoa-Pérez M, Kane MJ, Briggs DI, Francescutti DM, Kuhn DM. Marble burying and nestlet shredding as tests of repetitive, compulsive-like behaviors in mice. J Vis Exp. 2013:1–7.

36. Jirkof P. Burrowing and nest building behavior as indicators of well-being in mice. J Neurosci Methods. 2014;234:139–46. https://doi.org/10.1016/j.jneumeth.2014.02.001.

37. Can A, Dao DT, Arad M, Terrillion CE, Piantadosi SC, Gould TD. The mouse forced swim test. J Vis Exp. 2011:4–8.

38. Meng L, Person RE, Huang W, Zhu PJ, Costa-Mattioli M, Beaudet AL. Truncation of Ube3a-ATS unsilences paternal Ube3a and ameliorates behavioral defects in the Angelman syndrome mouse model. PLoS Genet. 2013;9(12):e1004039. https://doi.org/10.1371/journal.pgen.1004039.

39. Fiumara A, Pittalà A, Cocuzza M, Sorge G. Epilepsy in patients with Angelman syndrome. Ital J Pediatr. 2010;36:31.

40. Weber P. Levetiracetam in nonconvulsive status epilepticus in a child with Angelman syndrome. J Child Neurol. 2010;25:393–6.

41. Thibert RL, Conant KD, Braun EK, Bruno P, Said RR, Nespeca MP, et al. Epilepsy in Angelman syndrome: a questionnaire-based assessment of the natural history and current treatment options. Epilepsia. 2009;50:2369–76.

42. Fagan SC, Edwards DJ, Borlongan CV, Xu L, Arora A, Feuerstein G, et al. Optimal delivery of minocycline to the brain: implication for human studies of acute neuroprotection. Exp Neurol. 2004;186:248–51.

43. Rotschafer SE, Trujillo MS, Dansie LE, Ethell IM, Razak KA. Minocycline treatment reverses ultrasonic vocalization production deficit in a mouse model of Fragile X syndrome. Brain Res. 2012;1439:7–14.

44. van der Vaart T, Overwater IE, Oostenbrink R, Moll HA, Elgersma Y. Treatment of cognitive deficits in genetic disorders. JAMA Neurol. 2015;72:1052.

45. Daily JL, Nash K, Jinwal U, Golde T, Rogers J, Peters MM, et al. Adeno-associated virus-mediated rescue of the cognitive defects in a mouse model for Angelman syndrome. PLoS One. 2011;6:e27221.

46. Hethorn WR, Ciarlone SL, Filonova I, Rogers JT, Aguirre D, Ramirez RA, et al. Reelin supplementation recovers synaptic plasticity and cognitive deficits in a mouse model for Angelman syndrome. Eur J Neurosci. 2015;41:1372–80.

47. Baudry M, Kramar E, Xu X, Zadran H, Moreno S, Lynch G, et al. Ampakines promote spine actin polymerization, long-term potentiation, and learning in a mouse model of Angelman syndrome. Neurobiol Dis. 2012;47:210–5.

48. Sun J, Zhu G, Liu Y, Standley S, Ji A, Tunguntla R, et al. UBE3A regulates synaptic plasticity and learning and memory by controlling SK2 channel endocytosis. Cell Rep. 2015;12:449–61. https://doi.org/10.1016/j.celrep.2015.06.023.

49. Sun J, Liu Y, Tran J, O'Neal P, Baudry M, Bi X. mTORC1–S6K1 inhibition or mTORC2 activation improves hippocampal synaptic plasticity and learning in Angelman syndrome mice. Cell Mol Life Sci. 2016;73:4303–14.

50. Kovács AD, Pearce DA. Location- and sex-specific differences in weight and motor coordination in two commonly used mouse strains. Sci Rep. 2013;3:1–7.

51. Cook MN, Bolivar VJ, McFadyen MP, Flaherty L. Behavioral differences among 129 substrains: implications for knockout and transgenic mice. Behav Neurosci. 2002;116:600–11.

52. McFadyen MP, Kusek G, Bolivar VJ, Flaherty L. Differences among eight inbred strains of mice in motor ability and motor learning on a rotorod. Genes, Brain Behav. 2003;2:214–9.

53. Abaied L, Trabelsi M, Chaabouni M, Kharrat M, Kraoua L, M'rad R, et al. A novel UBE3A truncating mutation in large Tunisian Angelman syndrome pedigree. Am J Med Genet Part A. 2010;152A:141–6.

54. Tsilidis KK, Panagiotou OA, Sena ES, Aretouli E, Evangelou E, Howells DW, et al. Evaluation of excess significance bias in animal studies of neurological diseases. PLoS Biol. 2013;11:e1001609.

55. Mineur YS, Crusio WE. Behavioral effects of ventilated micro-environment housing in three inbred mouse strains. Physiol Behav. 2009;97:334–40.

56. Richter SH, Garner JP, Würbel H. Environmental standardization: cure or cause of poor reproducibility in animal experiments? Nat Methods. 2009;6:257–61.

57. Flint J, Corley R, DeFries J, Fulker D, Gray J, Miller S, et al. A simple genetic basis for a complex psychological trait in laboratory mice. Science (80-). 1995;269:1432–5.

58. Mandillo S, Tucci V, Hölter SM, Meziane H, Al BM, Kallnik M, et al. Reliability, robustness, and reproducibility in mouse behavioral phenotyping: a cross-laboratory study. Physiol Genomics. 2008;34:243–55.

3

Robot-based intervention may reduce delay in the production of intransitive gestures in Chinese-speaking preschoolers with autism spectrum disorder

Wing-Chee So[*], Miranda Kit-Yi Wong, Wan-Yi Lam, Chun-Ho Cheng, Jia-Hao Yang, Ying Huang, Phoebe Ng, Wai-Leung Wong, Chiu-Lok Ho, Kit-Ling Yeung and Cheuk-Chi Lee

Abstract

Background: Past studies have shown that robot-based intervention was effective in improving gestural use in children with autism spectrum disorders (ASD). The present study examined whether children with ASD could catch up to the level of gestural production found in age-matched children with typical development and whether they showed an increase in verbal imitation after the completion of robot-based training. We also explored the cognitive and motor skills associated with gestural learning.

Methods: Children with ASD were randomly assigned to two groups. Four- to 6-year-old children with ASD in the intervention group ($N = 15$) received four 30-min robot-based gestural training sessions. In each session, a social robot, NAO, narrated five stories and gestured (e.g., both hands clapping for an awesome expression). Children with ASD were told to imitate the gestures during training. Age-matched children with ASD in the wait-list control group ($N = 15$) and age-matched children with typical development ($N = 15$) received the gestural training after the completion of research. Standardized pretests and posttests (both immediate and delayed) were administered to assess the accuracy and appropriateness of gestural production in both training and novel stories. Children's language and communication abilities, gestural recognition skills, fine motor proficiencies, and attention skills were also examined.

Results: Children with ASD in the intervention condition were more likely to produce accurate or appropriate intransitive gestures in training and novel stories than those in the wait-list control. The positive learning outcomes were maintained in the delayed posttests. The level of gestural production accuracy in children with ASD in the delayed posttest of novel stories was comparable to that in children with typical development, suggesting that children with ASD could catch up to the level of gestural production found in children with typical development. Children with ASD in the intervention condition were also more likely to produce verbal markers while gesturing than those in the wait-list control. Gestural recognition skills were found to significantly predict the learning of gestural production accuracy in the children with ASD, with such relation partially mediated via spontaneous imitation.

Conclusions: Robot-based intervention may reduce the gestural delay in children with ASD in their early childhood.

Keywords: Gesture, Autism spectrum disorder, Robot-based intervention, Early childhood

* Correspondence: wingchee@cuhk.edu.hk
Department of Educational Psychology, The Chinese University of Hong Kong, Hong Kong, Special Administrative Region of China

Background

Individuals with autism spectrum disorder (ASD) are characterized by impairments in social interaction and communication (Diagnostic and Statistical Manual of Mental Disorders, Fifth Edition, DSM-V; [1]). Approximately half of them do not attain fluent speech and a quarter of them do not have functional speech [25, 30, 59]. Therefore, alternative and augmentative communication (AAC) systems serve important means of their communication. Besides aided AAC including Picture Exchange Communication System (PECS) [8] and speech-generating devices (SGDs), unaided AAC, gesture, can supplement (i.e., augment) their existing speech or become their primary (i.e., alternative) method of expressive communication (see discussion of manual signs in [51]).

Of different kinds of gestures (e.g., body posture, facial expression, a motion of hand or head), the present study focused on hand gestures. Hand gestures are spontaneous hand movements produced for communication (e.g., waving a hand to say goodbye; swiping forehead with hand when feeling hot); we gesture when we talk. Previous research has found that young English-speaking children with ASD have delayed gestural development, in comparison to their age-matched children with typical development and those with developmental delay [9, 16, 45, 47, 79]. For example, young children with ASD have difficulties in producing "proto-declarative" pointing gestures (gestures that elicit joint attention and shared interests, e. g., a child points to a toy car in order to direct his or her mother's attention to it) [4, 14, 77, 78]. They also produce fewer markers (gestures that carry culturally specific meaning for communication, e.g., the raised thumb for hitchhiking) [16, 45, 47, 79] and iconic gestures (gestures that depict the actions or attributes of the entities in question, e.g., both hands flapping for a bird or to indicate flying) than children with typical development [16, 45, 79]. The delay in gestural use is still evident in middle and late childhood. In a study conducted by So et al. [73], 6- to 12-year-old children with ASD were found to gesture less often and use fewer types of gestures, especially markers, in comparison to their age-matched children with typical development. These children were also found to have difficulty producing iconic gestures at specified locations to identify entities [69, 73]. The severity of social and communication impairments may influence the production of communicative gestures [71].

However, some studies have not found this delay in gestural use throughout childhood and adolescence in individuals with ASD. Attwood et al. [2] reported that young children with ASD, children with Down's syndrome (DS), and children with typical development produce comparable numbers of markers. Similarly, Capps et al. [13] found that young children with ASD were as likely as children with developmental delay to enact activities with iconic gestures. de Marchena and Eigsti [20] have shown that there is no significant difference in overall gesture rate and in the number of different types of gestures produced between adolescents with ASD and their age-matched adolescents with typical development. Likewise, Medeiros and Winsler [50] reported that 7- to 18-year-old children with ASD and children with typical development produce similar numbers of iconic gestures and speech beats. Wong and So [82] even found that 6- to 12-year-old children with ASD produce more iconic gestures when narrating stories than their age-matched children with typical development.

While there are inconclusive results regarding the delay in gestural use in children and adolescents with ASD, Ham et al. [28] proposed that individuals with ASD may have selective delayed development of one type of gesture, namely, intransitive gestures (actions without objects but with symbolic meanings). These gestures convey socio-communicative intent (e.g., waving a hand to say goodbye, giving a thumbs-up for a great job, opening arms wide to welcome others). A case report by Ham et al. [28] found that an 11-year-old child with ASD has difficulties producing intransitive gestures. In their later work, they found that children with ASD had greater difficulties recognizing intransitive gestures than gestures that involve actions with objects [29]. Their results are in line with previous findings, in which young and school-aged children have specific difficulties producing markers [16, 45, 47, 73, 79]. Intervention studies designed to teach children with ASD the use of intransitive gestures are scarce. The present study aimed to teach children with ASD, specifically preschool children, intransitive gestures. Early intervention is the key for success in improving their communication skills and social competence before they enter mainstream primary schools. Additionally, it is easier to teach young children appropriate behaviors and new skills at the time when the brain is most easily developed.

In this study, we adopted a social robot as a teaching agent. Previous research has shown that individuals with ASD tend to have low levels of interest toward other humans and have a weaker understanding of the interpersonal world than of the object-related world (e.g., [36, 37, 40]). In addition to this, they find it challenging to pay attention to multiple cues during social interactions with humans [38]. Thus, they are not sensitive to other people's behaviors [41]. Individuals with ASD are therefore more responsive and respond more quickly to feedback given by a technological object than by a human (e.g., [58, 83]).

Among different technological objects, they prefer robot-like toys to non-robotic toys and human beings [18, 61]. Based on the empathizing-systemizing theory [5], robots, unlike humans, operate within predictable and lawful systems and are thereby favored by children with ASD. Social robots have been widely used in therapy for individuals with ASD in the past decade (see reviews in [11, 24, 42]). They (1) offer human-like social cues; (2) can be programmed in such a way that information can be repeated in the same format; and (3) are predictable and controllable. Therefore, social robots can provide structured and clear information. They also respond to children with ASD according to predictable rules [7]. Additionally, these children do not need to consider socio-emotional expectations when interacting with robots [68], thereby reducing their social anxiety [52].

Recently, So and colleagues conducted a first multiphase robot-based intervention study on gesture use for Chinese-speaking school-aged children with ASD [70]. School-aged children with ASD were taught to recognize, imitate, and produce 20 gestures of different types, demonstrated by the robot animation in three phases. Their results reported that children recognized and imitated more gestures, as well as producing them in appropriate social contexts after training. There were significant differences between the pretests and posttests across the three phases. The children also generalized their acquired gestural skills to a novel setting with a human researcher. In another study, they used a real social robot (as opposed to robot animation) to teach Chinese-speaking school-aged children with ASD to recognize and produce eight gestures that express feelings and needs (e.g., NOISY) [72] in two phases. Compared to the students in the wait-list control group who had not received training, students in the intervention group were more capable of recognizing and producing the eight gestures produced in the trained and non-trained scenarios. Significant differences between the pretests and posttests were found across the two phases. Even more promising, these students could recognize the same gestures produced by human experimenters. However, there was no strong evidence showing that the children in the intervention group could generalize the acquired gestural production skills to interactions with human experimenters.

At present, previous findings have shown that the gestural recognition and production of children with ASD improves after receiving robot-based training. These results are encouraging, as they provide an effective treatment of gestural communication for children with ASD in educational and clinical settings. Yet, it is *not* known whether or not children with ASD still have delayed gestural production, in comparison to their age-matched children with typical development, after the completion of robot-based training. The first objective of the present study addressed this issue. We investigated whether or not children with ASD could catch up to the level of gestural production found in age-matched children with

typical development in both trained and novel situations. If so, children with ASD would produce the target gestures as accurately as their age-matched children with typical development, suggesting that our robot-based intervention could reduce gestural delay in children with ASD. Otherwise, the children with ASD would still gesture less accurately than their children with typical development even after the completion of the robot-based intervention, suggesting that our robot-based intervention could not reduce gestural delay in children with ASD.

The second objective of the present study would examine whether an improvement in gestural production skills, if any, would be associated with increases in verbal imitation in children with ASD, even though our intervention did not directly target verbal imitation. Previous research has shown that better imitation skills were associated with language gains, which were found immediately after imitation training as well as a few years later, in children with ASD [14, 75, 76]. These findings suggested that imitation skills may play a fundamental role in shaping language skills in children with ASD. Among different kinds of imitation, a study by Ingersoll and Lalonde [32] reported that gestural imitation training (as opposed to object imitation training) yielded a gain in language use. During the training phase in the present study, children with ASD were encouraged to imitate the social robot to produce intransitive gestures while listening to the narration. Based on previous findings, we expected that gestural imitation would trigger verbal imitative behaviors, such that a child would learn to produce the intransitive gestures (e.g., come over) while saying the accompanying words ("come over"). The integration of speech and gestures is crucial when one is narrating a story.

Besides investigating the effectiveness of the robot-based intervention on gestural use and verbal imitation, we also examined whether underlying cognitive and motor skills may predict gestural learning outcomes in children with ASD, including language and communication ability, gestural recognition, fine motor skills, and attention skills. These factors have not been sufficiently studied in the past gestural intervention research and are therefore measured in the present study. Among these factors, language and communication ability may be correlated to the production of gestures in early childhood. Previous research has shown that bilingual preschoolers used more gestures (iconic and beat) with their stronger language than with their weaker language [53, 54]. Other studies have shown that adult speakers use gestures (deictics) more often with their weaker language (e.g., [27, 55, 66]).

In addition to language and communication ability, the ability to identify the meanings of gestures (gestural recognition) may also be associated with gestural imitation or production skills. It was proposed that the mirror neuron system (MNS) plays a role in observational learning and imitation in children [62, 63]. Children with ASD may have dysfunction in the MNS, leading to the poor observation of gestures [57, 81]. Poor observation would then result in an impaired understanding of gestures, thereby causing difficulties in gestural imitation. As a result of this, the extent to which children with ASD comprehend gestures influences how well they can imitate the gestures. This proposal is in line with previous findings, which have shown that individuals with ASD imitate meaningful gestures more successfully than non-meaningful ones (e.g., [17, 80]).

Moreover, dysfunction in the MNS may result in motor deficits in children with ASD [15], which may in turn influence children's ability to imitate and produce gestures. Motor deficits in autism can be subdivided into two main categories: (a) deficits in basic motor control and (b) difficulty with praxis performance. The latter is associated with the social, communicative, and behavioral impairments that are typical of autism [21, 22]. Recent research has shown that praxis skills are found to be correlated to the imitation of gestures [26], which requires the production of coordinated sequences of movements. Furthermore, attention is the key skill in learning, including gestural production. It is common for children with ASD to have attention impairments [19, 67], which may preclude them from developing effective learning strategies for producing gestures.

Methods

Participants

A total of 45 Chinese-speaking (Cantonese-speaking) participants aged 4 to 6 years old participated in this study. Of these, 30 had been diagnosed with autism or another autistic disorder when they were between the ages of 18 and 36 months ($M = 30.27$; SD = 8.17) by pediatricians at the Child Assessment Center for the Department of Health in Hong Kong. All the participants were attending various special care centers in Hong Kong. Their ASD diagnoses were further confirmed by clinical psychologists who administered Autism Diagnostic Observation Schedule (ADOS; [43]) and the Autism Diagnosis Interview-Revised (ADl-R; [44]) and by pediatricians from the Pamela Youde Child Assessment Center, Hong Kong, who followed the Diagnostic and Statistical Manual of Mental Disorders, Fifth Edition (DSM-V; [1]).

Participants with ASD were randomly assigned to two groups: an intervention group and a wait-list control group. Participants in the intervention group ($N = 15$, two females) received robot-based gestural training, while those in the wait-list control group ($N = 15$, one female) were trained after the completion of the research. The mean age of the participants in the intervention group was 5;10 (years; months) (SD = 0.83; range 4; 2–6;12) and that of the wait-list control group was 5;8 (SD = 0.35; range 5;1–6;4).

The remaining 15 participants were age-matched and had not been diagnosed with ASD, i.e., participants with typical development (six females: $M = 5;4$; SD = 0.67; range 4;5–6;4). These children did not receive robot-based gestural training. There was no significant difference in age between the participants with ASD and those with typical development, Mann-Whitney (U) = 147.50, $p < .11$. None of the participants with typical development had a family history of ASD or other diagnosed developmental disorders or impairments. Neither the participants with typical development nor the participants with ASD had any history of traumatic brain injuries, birth-related injuries, or disorders involving seizures. All of the procedures were approved by the institutional review board of the first author's university, in compliance with the Declaration of Helsinki (Reference no. 14600817). We obtained parents' informed consent prior to the study. The participants also gave their assent to participate in this study.

At the beginning of the experiment, the participants with ASD and the participants with typical development had their language and communication abilities, fine motor skills, attention skills, and gestural recognition assessed, as these skills could influence their gestural learning. The order of these assessments was counterbalanced across the participants. Table 1 shows the descriptive statistics of the performance in each assessment for both groups of participants.

The participants' language and communication abilities were measured by the Psychoeducational Profile, Third Edition (PEP-3; [65]). The PEP-3 examines the skills and behaviors of young children (aged from 6 months to 7 years) with autism and communication disabilities and charts their uneven and idiosyncratic development, emerging skills, and autistic behaviors. It has 10 subtests, which yield three composite scores in the following three aspects: language and communication, motor, and maladaptive behaviors. Our study focused on the language and communication composite, which measures a participant's ability to speak, listen, read, and write, with a higher score indicating better language and communication skills. We reported here the language and communication developmental ages that were converted from the raw and standardized scores based on the norming references published in the PEP-3 administration manual. Unsurprisingly, the participants with typical development had better language and communication abilities than the participants with ASD, $U = 55.50, p < .001$.

The participants' motor skills were assessed by the Bruininks-Oseretsky Test of Motor Proficiency, Second

Table 1 Descriptive statistics of the participants' performance in the PEP3, SCQ, BOT, ANT, and gestural recognition task

Groups	Descriptive statistics	Chronological age	Language and communication developmental age assessed by PEP-3	Standardized score in BOT	Proportion of accurate trials in ANT	Proportion of accurate trials in gestural recognition
Participants with ASD in the wait-list control	M	5.81	4.44	85.33	0.60	0.65
	SD	0.83	0.89	12.38	0.28	0.20
	Min	4.16	3.19	62.00	0.19	0.29
	Max	6.96	6.22	105.00	0.97	1.00
Participants with ASD in the intervention condition	M	5.65	4.95	105.07	0.74	0.69
	SD	0.35	0.44	20.15	0.21	0.25
	Min	5.06	4.53	49.00	0.31	0.14
	Max	6.28	5.83	130.00	1.00	1.00
Participants with typical development	M	5.31	5.41	112.13	0.83	0.85
	SD	0.67	0.46	14.19	0.10	0.11
	Min	4.43	4.72	86.00	0.69	0.64
	Max	6.35	6.22	128.00	1.00	1.00

PEP3 Psychoeducational Profile-Third Edition [65], *BOT* Bruininks-Oseretsky Test of Motor Proficiency, Second Edition (BOT™-2; [10]), Attention Network Task (ANT; [64])

Edition (BOT™-2; [10]). It assesses the fine motor as well as the gross motor proficiencies of children, ranging from those who are typically developing to those with mild to moderate motor control problems. It has eight subtests, including Fine Motor Precision, Fine Motor Integration, Manual Dexterity, Bilateral Coordination, Balance, Running Speed and Agility, Upper-Limb Coordination, and Strength, which yield six composite scores, including Fine Manual Control, Manual Coordination, Body Coordination, Strength and Agility, Gross Motor Composite, and Fine Motor Composite. We only report the Fine Motor Composite standardized score here, as fine motor skills are related to the production of the intransitive gestures taught in the present study. This composite consists of the following subtests: Fine Motor Precision, Fine Motor Integration, Manual Dexterity, and Upper-Limb Coordination. The participants with typical development received a higher fine motor composite standardized score than the participants with ASD, $U = 132.00, p < .03$.

The participants' attention skills were measured by the Attention Network Test (ANT) [23, 64]. This test lasts for half an hour and provides a nonverbal measure of the efficiency of the attentional networks involved in alerting, orienting, and executive attention across all ages in both typical and atypical populations. We focused on executive attention, which requires the participant to respond by pressing two keys indicating the direction (left or right) of a central arrow surrounded by congruent, incongruent, or neutral flankers. Thus, it evaluates one's ability to focus on the relevant stimulus while ignoring the distracting but irrelevant stimuli. For each participant, we averaged the proportions of the trials to which he or she responded correctly in the

congruent and incongruent conditions. There was no significant difference between the groups, $U = 162.00, p < .13$.

The participants' gestural recognition skills were measured by their ability to identify the meanings of intransitive gestures demonstrated by an experimenter [70, 72]. We videotaped an experimenter producing the 14 intransitive gestures that were taught in the present study. Each time, a child was shown a gesture (e.g., both hands clapping) and was asked to choose one of three options that best identified its meaning (e.g., HELLO, AWESOME, WELCOME). We reported the proportion of trials each child was able to recognize the meanings of gestures. The proportion of accurate trials in the recognition test was higher in the participants with typical development than in those with ASD, $U = 114.00, p < .007$.

Stimuli

Target gestures

A total of 14 intransitive gestures that are commonly used in daily life were taught in this intervention program. The findings of a study by Cabibihan, So, and Pramanik [12] showed that these gestures are easily recognized by speakers in the Chinese society.

Social robot

NAO (Aldebaran Robotics Company) was programmed to produce the 14 gestures (see Fig. 1). This robot has been widely used in autism therapy. It is 50 cm tall and anthropomorphic. It was deployed in the present study because it might facilitate children with ASD to generalize the acquired imitation and social skills to human-to-human interactions [11]. Besides, unlike other robots, NAO robot can produce a wide range of

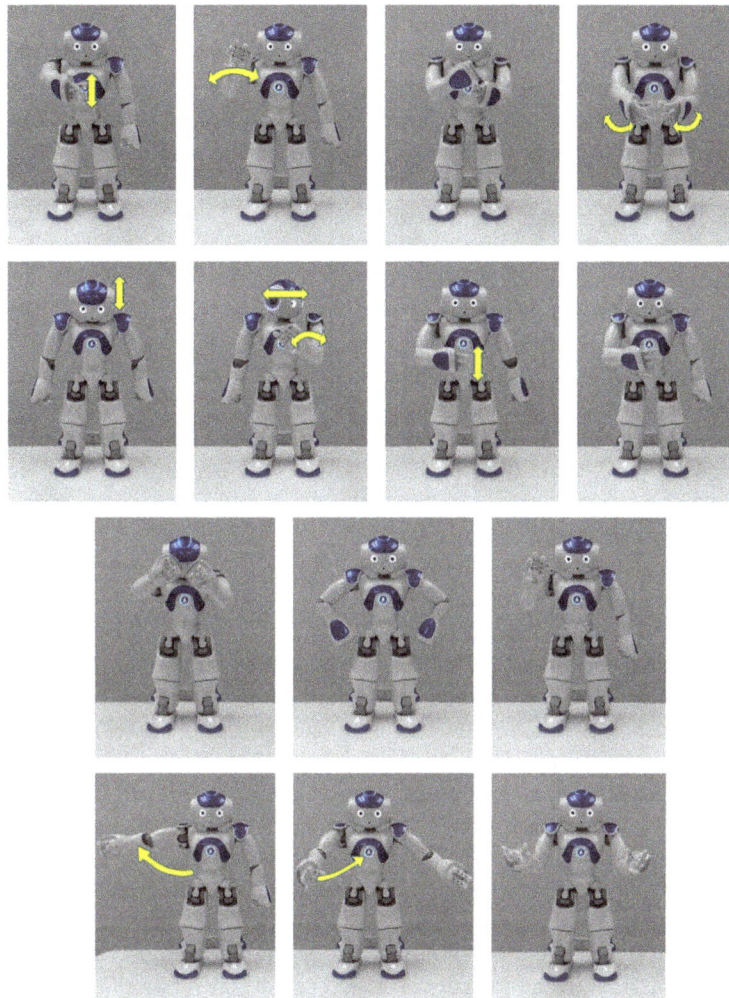

Fig. 1 Gestures performed by the NAO robot. From the upper left corner, from left to right, the following gestures are (first row) hello, bye, wrong, and awesome; (second row) yes, not allowed, hungry, and myself; (third row) annoyed, angry, and wait; and (fourth row) welcome, come, and where?

gestures. The NAO robot contains 25 degrees of freedom (DOF) from 15 joints and actuators. Our gestures were accomplished by 14 DOF from nine joints and actuators. Each of the gestural movements required two DOF in the neck, two DOF in each shoulder, two DOF on each elbow, and one DOF on each wrist. Each gesture lasted for 3–4 s.

In order to ensure that the gestures produced by the NAO robot could be recognized by the participants, we asked the participants with typical development in this study to identify the meanings of the gestures demonstrated by the robot (the robot gesture recognition task). The procedure was similar to those in the aforementioned gestural recognition task (the human gesture recognition task). The order of the human gesture recognition task and robot gesture recognition task was counterbalanced across participants. In the robot gesture recognition task, the participant was presented with one video clip each time, which showed the robot producing a gesture, and he or she was asked to choose one of three options that best described its meaning. We entered the participants' responses in both recognition tasks in the reliability analysis and found that the Cronbach's alpha was .83, suggesting that the recognition of human and robot gestures was highly correlated.

Stories

In the training sessions, the robot gestured while narrating a set of five different stories (S1, training stories). For example, one of the S1 stories was as follows: "One day, a friend visited me and she was hungry. She wanted to dine out. I asked her where we should go for lunch. She suggested eating hamburgers. I said, 'awesome'." Each story in S1 contained five sentences and two to three different gestures. Each gesture only appeared once across all stories. Five different stories thereby covered all 14 gestures. This set of stories, S1, was used for training and assessment in the standardized pretests and posttests. Another set of stories (S2, non-training stories) contained five stories that were different from those in S1. S2 was presented during the assessment (but not training) sessions in order to examine the generalization effects of the intervention in the novel context.

The stories in S1 were told by a female Cantonese speaker and her narration was recorded as audio clips. To make the recordings sound like the speech produced by a robot, robotic effects were added and the speech rate was reduced using an audio editor (Audacity, v. 2.1. 0, the Audacity Team, US state). A total of five audio clips were made, each containing one story, and these were imported to NAO. The mean length of each clip was 32.2 s (ranging from 25 to 42 s). NAO then played the audio clips and gestured during the narration. The gesture and its accompanying speech started at the same time. Thus, the participants with ASD in the intervention condition watched the gestures while listening to the stories. For example, in the aforementioned story, NAO said and gestured: "I asked her where (WHERE: two arms open wide with palms facing up) we should go for lunch". In addition to the verbal narration, the background images of the stories (e.g., a living room) were visually displayed on the laptop screen, which was placed next to NAO. One picture was shown for each story.

Procedures

The experiment was conducted in the treatment rooms at various special care centers in Hong Kong for participants with ASD and in kindergarten classrooms for the participants with typical development. The treatment rooms and classrooms were often used by the children for school activities. Each time, the room was equipped with a robot, NAO, a laptop, and a camera in front of the child (see Fig. 2). The camera videotaped the hand movements the child produced in the sessions.

The intervention program lasted for 9 weeks. It consisted of two pretests (one for each set of stories: S1 and S2), four training sessions for S1 (with two 30-min sessions per week), two immediate posttests (which were the same as the pretests), and the same follow-up posttests after 2 weeks. The posttest for S1 assessed the training effects, while that for S2 assessed the generalization effects.

For each training or assessment session, the participants were accompanied by a teacher. The training and assessment sessions were administered by a researcher, who was either the assistant or one of the authors. A small reward by way of positive reinforcement (snacks or access to toys) was offered by the teacher at the end of each pretest, posttest, and training session. All the sessions were videotaped. Each session lasted for

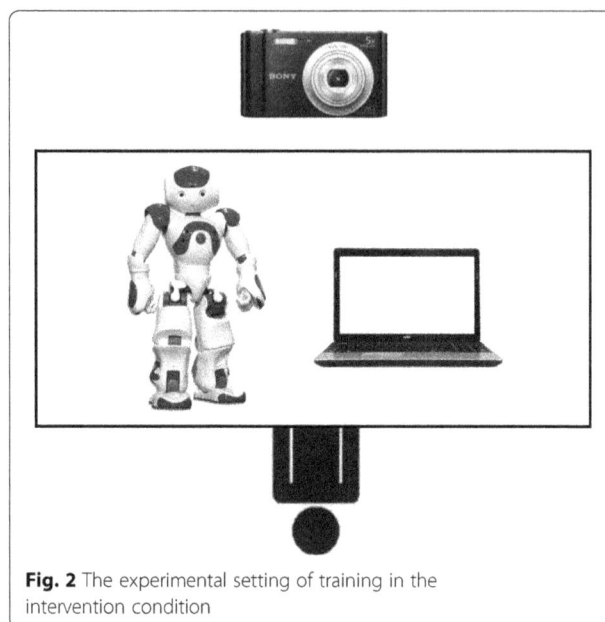

Fig. 2 The experimental setting of training in the intervention condition

approximately 30 min. Details of the intervention program are provided below.

Each pretest assessed the production of 14 intransitive gestures in different stories (S1 and S2) in the participants with ASD (both in the intervention and the waitlist control groups) and the participants with typical development. At the beginning of the pretest, the human researcher first greeted the participant then gave instructions. The researcher then asked the participant whether he or she understood the instructions. If the participant indicated that he or she did not understand the instructions, the researcher would repeat the instructions. Otherwise, the human researcher proceeded to narrate a story, with the corresponding pictures sequentially displayed on the laptop screen. After narrating a story once, the researcher repeated the sentences (e.g., "One day, a friend visited me and she was hungry."), one at a time. After finishing each sentence, the researcher asked the participant to demonstrate the corresponding gesture (e. g., "What are the hand movements for expressing the feeling of being hungry?"). The participant was given 10 s to respond. The researcher prompted the participant if he or she gave no response and gave the participant another 10 s to respond. Upon receiving the participant's response, the researcher then judged the accuracy of the gesture produced (based on the four parameters which were further elaborated in the session below) and provided feedback (correct or incorrect). The researcher then proceeded to the next sentence. After the completion of one story, the researcher moved on to the next story. The two pretests were completed after the participant had been asked to demonstrate the individual gestures in the stories in S1 and S2. Each pretest lasted for approximately 30 min. A small reward by way of positive reinforcement was provided after the pretest.

After the pretest, the participant with ASD in the intervention group proceeded to training, in which the robot narrated the stories (each one twice) while producing appropriate gestures in S1. Each time, the participant was asked to imitate the gesture. The training was completed after the five stories had been presented and the corresponding gestures had been imitated by the child in S1. The participants with ASD in the wait-list control group and the participants with typical development watched educational videos that were not relevant to gestural training (e.g., videos about animals) for 30 min.

All participants then took the posttests immediately after the training and the delayed posttests 2 weeks after the training. The human researcher administering the posttests was the same as in the pretests. The procedures in both posttests were the same as those in the pretests. All participants were able to pay attention during the training and assessments. A short break was given to the participants if requested. None of them were absent from the sessions.

Coding and scoring

We had a research assistant, who did not know the objectives of the study and was unaware of the research questions of the present study, watch the videos of the participants and counted the number of trials in which they produced the gestures correctly, according to four parameters [74]: use of hand/hands (e.g., placing the right/left hand against the head vs. using both hands), hand-shape (e.g., open palm vs. curled palm vs. fist), direction of movement (e.g., head nods vs. head shakes; moving the hand from left to right vs. moving it up and down), and placement (e.g., hand placed at the head vs. at the chest). The following gestures were considered incorrect: using only the left hand to produce the WHERE gesture (reason—incorrect use of hands); making a fist when producing the WAIT gesture (reason—incorrect hand shape); moving the right hand downward when producing the NOT ALLOWED gesture (reason—incorrect direction of movement); and covering the face when producing the MYSELF gesture (reason—incorrect placement).

For the gestures that did not follow the four parameters, we further coded whether these gestures were still appropriate. A gesture was considered appropriate if it conveyed the target meaning. For example, two index fingers formed a cross when producing the NOT ALLOWED gesture; right hand moved in a circle in the lower chest when producing the HUNGRY gesture; both hands raised up when producing the gesture AWESOME; and both hands formed a T-shape when producing the gesture WAIT.

Finally, we counted the number of trials in which the participants produced verbal imitation when they gestured (either accurately or appropriately). Verbal imitation was defined as the imitation of the robot's verbal marker during gestural production (e.g., saying, "Awesome" while producing the AWESOME gesture).

We then train a second coder, who also did not know the objectives of the study and was unaware of the research questions of the present study, to code gestures. She watched 20% of the videos. The inter-observer agreement in an evaluation of the accuracy of gesture production was .93 ($N = 756$; Cohen's kappa = .90, $p < .001$), that of appropriateness of gesture production was .96 ($N = 580$, Cohen's kappa = .92, $p < .001$), and that of verbal imitation was .92 ($N = 1336$, Cohen's kappa = .90, $p < .001$).

Results

We first report the proportion of trials in which the participants with ASD in the intervention condition and those in the wait-list control condition and the participants with typical development accurately produced gestures in the pretests and immediate and delayed posttests. All children spontaneously produced the intransitive gestures when instructed or prompted by the human researcher.

Table 2 shows the correlations among chronological age, language and communication developmental age, fine motor skills, attention skills, gestural recognition skills, and gestural production performance in the pretests and posttests (the data in both S1 and S2 were collapsed). There were significant correlations between fine motor skills, attention skills, gestural recognition skills, and gestural production performance in the pretests and/or posttests. Language and communication developmental age was marginally correlated to the gestural production performance in the pretest ($p < .07$).

Figure 3 shows the proportion of accurate trials in the gestural production pretests and immediate and delayed posttests in the participants with ASD (intervention and wait-list conditions) and in the participants with typical development. Repeated measures ANOVA, with group (participants with ASD in the intervention condition, participants with ASD in the wait-list control, participants with typical development) as the between subject factor, time (pretest, immediate posttest, delayed posttest) and story (S1, S2) as the within subject factors, and language and communication developmental age, BOT standardized score, and the proportions of correct trials in the ANT and gestural recognition tasks as covariates, was conducted. We found significant effects for group, $F(2, 38) = 24.44$, $p < .001$, $\eta p^2 = .56$, time × group interaction, $F(4, 76) = 22.39$, $p < .001$, $\eta p^2 = .54$, story × group interaction, $F(2, 38) = 30.50$, $p < .001$, $\eta p^2 = .62$, and three-way interaction, $F(4, 76) = 10.12$, $p < .001$, $\eta p^2 = .35$. All the other main and interaction effects were not significant.

Table 2 Correlations among chronological age, language and developmental ability, gestural recognition, fine motor skills, attention skills, and gestural production accuracy in pretests and immediate and delayed posttests

	Chronological age	Language and developmental ability	Gestural recognition	Fine motor skill	Attention skill	Gestural production accuracy in pretests	Gestural production accuracy in immediate posttests	Gestural production in delayed posttests
Chronological age	–							
Language and developmental ability	.65**	–						
Gestural recognition	0.02	.33*	–					
Fine motor skill	.34*	.57**	0.23	–				
Attention skill	0.10	0.25	.66**	.40*	–			
Gestural production accuracy in pretests	0.05	0.28	.63**	0.22	.64**	–		
Gestural production accuracy in immediate posttests	0.04	0.23	.33*	.44**	.36*	0.20	–	
Gestural production in delayed posttests	0.04	0.19	.41**	.33*	.50**	.36*	.68**	–

**$p < .001$, *$p < .05$

We further explored the three-way interaction by running two separate repeated measures ANOVAs for S1 and S2, respectively, after controlling for language and communication ability, fine motor skills, attention skills, and gestural recognition skills. With regard to S1, which was a set of stories presented during training, we found significant effects for group, $F(2, 38) = 37.04$, $p < .001$, $\eta p^2 = .66$, and time × group interaction effects, $F(4, 76) = 25.16$, $p < .001$, $\eta p^2 = .57$. Post hoc Tukey HSD have shown that the proportion of accurate trials in the pretest with the participants with typical development was greater than that with the participants with ASD in the intervention condition, $p < .04$, and those in the wait-list control

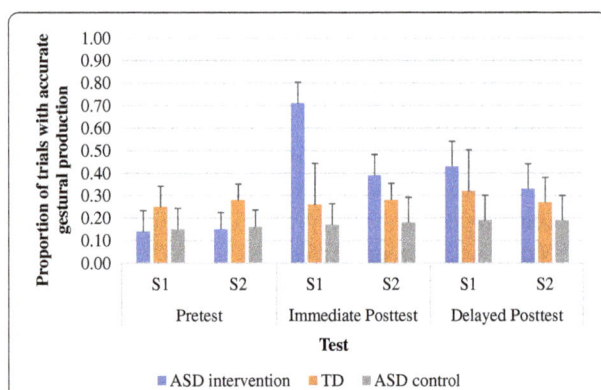

Fig. 3 The proportion of accurate trials in the pretests and immediate and delayed posttests in the ASD children (intervention and wait-list control conditions) and children with typical development (TD) in S1 and S2 narratives

condition, $p < .05$. Opposite patterns were found in the immediate posttest. The proportion of accurate trials with the participants with ASD in the intervention condition was greater than that for the participants with typical development, $p < .001$, and for the participants with ASD in the wait-list control condition, $p < .001$. Marginal significance was found between the participants with typical development and the participants with ASD in the wait-list control condition, $p < .07$. Similar findings were shown for the delayed posttest. The proportion of accurate trials with the participants with ASD in the intervention condition was greater than that for the participants with typical development, $p < .03$, and for the participants with ASD in the wait-list control condition, $p < .001$. Marginal significance was found between the participants with typical development and the participants with ASD in the wait-list control condition, $p < .08$.

Regarding S2, which was a set of stories that had not yet been taught, we found significant effects for group, $F(2, 38) = 7.24$, $p < .002$, $\eta^2 = .28$, and time × group interaction effects, $F(4, 76) = 4.47$, $p < .003$, $\eta p^2 = .19$. Post hoc Tukey HSD have shown that, similar to S1, the proportion of accurate trials in the pretest with the participants with typical development was greater than that for the participants with ASD in the intervention condition, $p < .05$, and that in the wait-list control condition, $p < .03$. Different from S1, the proportion of accurate trials in the immediate posttest with the participants with ASD in the intervention condition was comparable to that in the participants with typical development, $p < .27$, but greater than that in the participants with ASD in the wait-list control condition, $p < .001$. Significant difference was found between the participants with typical development and the participants with ASD in the wait-list control condition, $p < .04$. Likewise, the proportion of accurate trials in the delayed posttest in the participants with ASD in the intervention condition was comparable to that in the participants with typical development, $p < .16$, but greater than that in the participants with ASD in the wait-list control condition, $p < .005$. Marginal significance was found between the participants with typical development and the participants with ASD in the wait-list control condition, $p < .06$. Overall, the participants with ASD in the intervention condition were able to produce gestures as accurately as the participants with typical development in the non-training stories in the delayed posttest, suggesting that robot-based gestural intervention may reduce gestural production delay.

Interestingly, the proportions of gestures accurately produced in the participants with typical development were relatively low (below 30% for most of the assessments across all time points). Note that we coded the gestural production accuracy according to the four parameters (use of hands, hand shape, directionality of movement, and placement). It was possible that these participants produced appropriate gestures even though they did not follow the four parameters. In other words, their gestures might still convey the target meaning. We thus looked at their performance of gestural production by investigating their proportions of trials in which the gestures were accurately produced according to the four parameters as well as the proportions of trials in which the gestures were appropriate. Both proportions were then summed up.

In this analysis, we only looked at gestural production in the pretests and delayed posttest. Figure 4 shows the proportion of trials in which the participants with ASD (intervention and wait-list conditions) and the participants with typical development produced gestures accurately or produce appropriate gestures. Repeated measures ANOVA, with group (participants with ASD in the intervention condition, participants with ASD in the wait-list control, participants with typical development) as the between subject factor, time (pretest and delayed posttest) and story (S1 and S2) as the within subject factors, and language and communication developmental age and gestural recognition tasks as covariates, was conducted. We found a significant effect for group, $F(2, 38) = 3.74$, $p < .01$, $\eta p^2 = .25$. All the other main and interaction effects were not significant. Bonferroni pairwise comparisons have shown that the proportion of trials with appropriate or accurate gestural production in the participants with typical development was higher than in those with ASD in the wait-list condition, $p < .005$. However, there was no difference between the participants with typical

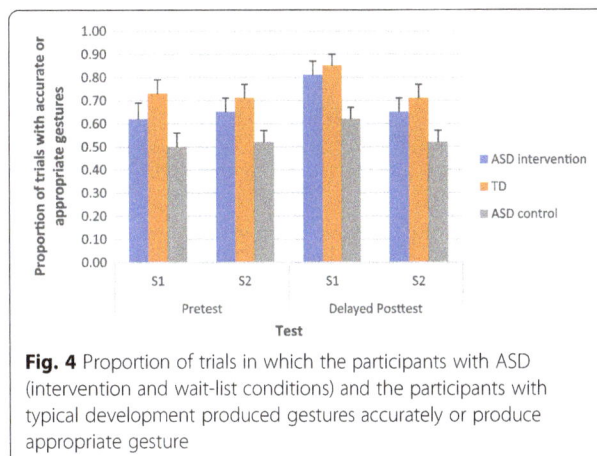

Fig. 4 Proportion of trials in which the participants with ASD (intervention and wait-list conditions) and the participants with typical development produced gestures accurately or produce appropriate gesture

development and those with ASD in the intervention condition, $p < .72$. This result supported our previous results. The participants with ASD in the intervention condition were able to produce gestures as accurately or appropriately as the participants with typical development. Additionally, the proportions of trials with appropriate or accurate gestural production in the participants with ASD in the intervention condition were higher than in those with ASD in the wait-list condition, $p < .03$, suggesting that the robot-based intervention program was effective in promoting the use of appropriate or accurate gestures.

Next, we investigated whether the participants with ASD in the intervention condition were more likely to use verbal imitation after learning target gestures. In this analysis, we compared the proportions of trials in which the participants with ASD in the intervention and wait-list control conditions used verbal imitation while producing appropriate or accurate gestures. Figure 5 shows the proportion of trials in the gestural production pretests and delayed posttests in which the participants with ASD (intervention and wait-list conditions) used verbal imitation. Repeated measures ANOVA, with group (participants with ASD in the intervention condition, participants with ASD in the wait-list control) as the between subject factor, time (pretest and delayed posttest) and story (S1 and S2) as the within subject factors, and language and communication developmental age and gestural recognition tasks as covariates, was conducted. All the main effects were not significant. Time × group interaction was significant, $F(1, 26) = 4.56$, $p < .04$, $\eta p^2 = .15$. All the other interaction effects were not significant. We further explored the time × group interaction by running two separate repeated measures ANOVAs for the participants with ASD in the intervention condition and those in the wait-list control condition, respectively, after controlling for language and communication ability and gestural recognition skills. For the participants in the intervention condition,

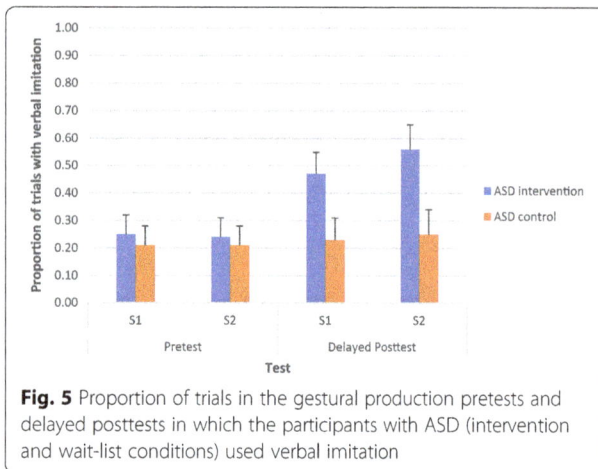

Fig. 5 Proportion of trials in the gestural production pretests and delayed posttests in which the participants with ASD (intervention and wait-list conditions) used verbal imitation

we found a significant effect for time, $F(1, 12) = 7.87$, $p < .02$, $\eta p^2 = .40$. All the other main and interaction effects were not significant. Bonferroni pairwise comparisons have shown that the proportions of trials with verbal imitation in the delayed posttests were higher than in the pretests, $p < .005$. This finding was not reported in the participants in the wait-list condition. All the main and interaction effects were not significant. These results suggested that the robot-based intervention improved the gestural production accuracy and verbal imitation in the participants with ASD in the intervention condition.

Finally, we examined whether or not language and communication ability, fine motor skills, attention skills, and gestural recognition skills would influence gestural learning in the participants with ASD in the intervention condition. In order to address this issue, we focused on their accuracy of gestural production in the delayed posttests while controlling for their performance in the pretests. We ran a generalized linear mixed model analysis with individual gestures and subjects considered as the random effects, language and communication ability, fine motor skills, attention skills, gestural recognition skills, and performance in the pretests as the fixed effects, and the participants' performance in the delayed posttest as the binomial dependent variable. The statistical analysis tools R [60] and lme4 [6] were used to perform the analyses. We collapsed the data in S1 and S2 in this analysis. We found that only gestural recognition was a significant predictor of gestural learning, $\beta = .64$, SE = $.32$, $p < .04$. Other factors were non-significant: language and communication ability, $\beta = .05$, $SE = .01$, $p < .21$; fine motor skills, $\beta = .01$, $SE = .09$, $p < .13$; and attention skills, $\beta = .87$, $SE = .82$, $p < .29$. These results suggest that a fundamental understanding of gestural meaning influences the learning of gestural production.

We ran a further analysis to explore how gestural recognition aids the learning of gestural production. Previous research has shown that imitating meaningful actions (from the perspectives of children with ASD) increases children's natural motivation to complete the actions [31]. Previous findings have also shown that individuals with ASD imitate meaningful gestures better than non-meaningful ones (e.g., [17, 80]). Based on these views, recognition of gestures might lead to spontaneous imitation during training, which in turn would promote gestural production. Therefore, we watched the videos of the training sessions and recorded whether or not the participants with ASD in the intervention condition spontaneously imitated the gestures produced by NAO.

We expected spontaneous imitation during training to act as a mediator, which would influence the effects of gestural recognition skills on gestural learning among the participants with ASD in the intervention group. Therefore, a series of linear regression analyses were conducted to investigate how gestural recognition skills predicted gestural learning via the mediation of spontaneous imitation among participants with ASD in the intervention group. Gestural learning was measured by the residual scores of gestural production performance in the delayed posttest, after controlling for the effects of gestural production performance in the pretest.

We followed four steps in establishing mediation using regression [3, 33, 35]. Table 3 shows the statistics of the four regression analyses. In the first regression analysis, we found a significant effect of gestural recognition skills on gestural learning. In the second regression analysis, we found a significant effect of gestural recognition skills on spontaneous imitation. In the third regression analysis, we found a significant effect of spontaneous imitation on gestural learning. In the fourth regression analysis, gestural recognition skills still significantly predicted gestural learning after controlling for spontaneous imitation. These findings suggest that the effect of gestural recognition skills on gestural learning was partially mediated by spontaneous imitation during training.

Discussion

To summarize, participants with ASD who received robot-based gestural training produced intransitive gestures more accurately in training stories than those who did not receive training. Similar patterns were found in non-training stories, suggesting that the acquired gestural production skills could be generalized to novel stories. Additionally, the positive learning outcomes were maintained for 2 weeks when no training was provided. Even more promising, the level of gestural production accuracy in participants with ASD in the delayed posttest of non-training stories was comparable to that in participants with typical development, suggesting

Table 3 Statistics of four regression analyses showing the effects of gestural recognition skills on gestural learning via the mediation of spontaneous imitation among the children with ASD in the intervention group

Regression analyses	β	t	R^2	ΔR^2	F
Step 1 ($N = 414$)					
DV: gestural learning					
IV: gestural recognition skills	.15	3.01**	.02	.02**	9.08**
Step 2 ($N = 402$)					
DV: spontaneous imitation					
IV: gestural recognition skills	.22	4.55***	.05	.05***	20.70
Step 3 ($N = 402$)					
DV: gestural learning					
IV: spontaneous imitation	.12	2.44*	.02	.02*	5.97*
Step 4 ($N = 402$)					
DV: gestural learning					
Block 1 IV: gestural recognition skills	.15	2.94**	.02	.02**	8.65**
Block 2 IVs: gestural recognition skills	.13	2.47*	.03	.01†	6.06**
Spontaneous imitation	.09	1.85†			

Note: $^\dagger p < .1$; $^* p < .05$; $^{**} p < .01$; $^{***} p < .001$

that participants with ASD could catch up to the level of gestural production found in participants with typical development. This finding was consistent when we also considered appropriateness of gestures. Additionally, these participants with ASD were more likely to imitate the verbal markers paired with the taught intransitive gestures in the delayed posttests of both stories than in the pretests. Gestural recognition skills were found to significantly predict the learning of gestural production in the participants with ASD, with this relation being partially mediated by spontaneous imitation.

Previous findings have shown that robot-based gestural training is effective in teaching school-aged children with ASD [70, 72]. The present study represents significant steps forward in the development and therapeutic use of robot-based intervention. First, our results document that this intervention protocol works in preschool children, thus providing an effective early intervention for nonverbal communication skills. Additionally, the findings show that robot-based intervention may reduce the delay in gestural production in participants with ASD. Previous intervention studies have not included age-matched children with typical development [70, 72], thereby leaving open the question of whether or not participants with ASD who receive robot-based gestural training could catch up to the level of gestural production found in their age-matched participants with typical development peers. We found that the participants with ASD in the intervention condition had comparable performances to the participants with typical development in the immediate as well as in the delayed posttests in regard to non-training stories. This finding is intriguing given that, in comparison to their age-

matched participants with typical development, participants with ASD have poorer language and communication abilities and fine motor proficiencies, which might influence gestural learning (see our discussion below). It also suggests that the delay in gestural production found in early childhood can be prevented by 2 weeks of robot-based gestural training.

It is interesting to observe that the participants with ASD in the intervention condition significantly outperformed the participants with typical development in the immediate posttest of the training stories. Specifically, their proportion of trials with accurate gestures increased from .15 in the pretest to .70 in the immediate posttest (while that of the participants with typical development remained at approximately .25 in both pre- and posttests). This result may be explained by the fact that the target intransitive gestures were visually presented to the participants with ASD in the intervention condition and individuals with ASD in general process information using a visually oriented approach [39]. Previous research has also shown that individuals with ASD may have superior short-term visual memory (e.g., [34, 56]). As a result of this, participants with ASD might benefit from the visual presentation of gestures and efficiently learn and memorize the gestures. Yet, their level of accuracy of gestural production declined in the delayed posttest of the same stories (.41), although it was still significantly higher than that of the participants with typical development. We did not observe superiority in the gestural production in the immediate and delayed posttests in non-training stories in the participants with ASD in the intervention condition, in comparison to the participants with typical development. This further strengthens our argument that short-term visual memory plays a significant role in learning and memorizing gestures incorporated in training stories. Despite this, the participants with ASD in the intervention condition could still generalize the acquired gestural production skills to the non-training stories, such that their accuracy of gestural production was greater than that of the participants with ASD in the wait-list control condition and was on par with that of the participants with typical development.

We also observed that the proportions of gestures accurately produced in the participants with typical development were below 30% for most of the assessments across all time points. It might be attributed to the fact that we coded the gestural production accuracy according to the four parameters (use of hands, hand shape, directionality of movement, and placement; [74]). Gestures do not contain standardized forms [48], and different forms of gestures may convey the same meaning (e.g., both hands forming a T-shape or right/left palm facing outward can request somebody else to stop from moving). Thus, the gestures produced by the participants should still be considered appropriate if they could convey the target meanings. After taking appropriateness of gestures into account, the proportions of accurate or appropriate gestures reached 70% or above in the participants with typical development across all time points. On the other hand, these proportions were comparable to those of children with ASD in the intervention condition. Taken together, the participants with ASD in the intervention condition were as capable as the participants with typical development in producing accurate gestures (i.e., those demonstrated by the robot) and appropriate gestures (i.e., those not demonstrated by the robot but were appropriate in conveying the intended meanings). In future studies, we should code the gestures in terms of their accuracy based on the four parameters as well as their appropriateness.

Previous research has shown that gestural imitation training can enhance language use [32]. In line with these findings, our study reported that participants with ASD in the intervention condition were more likely to produce the verbal markers that were co-occurring with the taught gestures in the delayed posttests than in the pretests. Such result was not found in the participants in the wait-list control condition. This was possibly because the demonstration of intransitive gestures by the robot drew the attention of the participants with ASD in the intervention condition to the verbal markers. Therefore, they noticed the gestures and verbal markers as a joint communicative art [48, 49] and produced the verbal markers while gesturing in the assessment. In this sense, gestural imitation would trigger verbal imitative behaviors. Teaching children with ASD who are non-verbal or

having relatively low verbal abilities gesture would facilitate their speech production. Future studies on gestural training in children with ASD should evaluate the learning outcomes on gestural production as well as the development of speech and gesture integration.

The other major finding in the present study was that the learning of gestural production is influenced by gestural recognition skills. After controlling for the gestural production performance in the pretests of both training and non-training stories, the proportion of trials in which the participants with ASD recognized gestures significantly predicted the proportion of trials in which they produced gestures accurately in the delayed posttests. Language and communication abilities, fine motor proficiencies, and attention skills were found to be nonsignificant. We further established that gestural recognition would influence participants' ability to produce gestures accurately, with this relation being partially mediated by the spontaneous imitation that occurred during training. These findings suggest that participants with ASD who better understand the meanings of gestures are more likely to spontaneously imitate the gestures demonstrated by the robot, which results in an enhancement in gestural production skills. These results are in line with previous research, which has shown that children with ASD have stronger motivations to imitate the gestures they understand [31]. This motivation may be reflected in the spontaneity in gestural imitation in the present study. Further intervention studies on the use of intransitive gestures should consider teaching children with ASD gestural recognition, followed by production (see [70, 72]).

Conclusions
Our study is a pioneering work showing that robot-based intervention can prevent the delay in the production of intransitive gestures in young children with ASD. Theoretically, our findings have extended the previous research, which has posited that robot-based gestural training can be considered as an effective early intervention for gestural communication. It also has strong implications for the direction in which technology-based interventions for preschoolers with ASD should proceed. Practically, our research could promote the implementation of robot-based interventions in preschool education, even for children whose language and motor skills are delayed. Note that the language and communication ages of the participants with ASD participating in this study fell behind their chronological ages, suggesting that they might have language delay. Their fine motor proficiencies were poorer than those of the age-matched participants with typical development too. However, after four robot-based gestural training sessions, they could still produce gestures as accurately as the

Robot-based intervention may reduce delay in the production of intransitive gestures in Chinese-speaking...

45

participants with typical development. Our protocol may also be useful in promoting general social competence, such as joint attention, perspective taking, and understanding others' intentions.

That said, this study has a few limitations. First, there is no evidence showing that participants with ASD who received training actually applied the acquired gestural production skills when interacting with others in their daily lives. Hence, we cannot comment on the social utility of our intervention program. In future studies, we will observe the gestural communication of the participants in schools and at home for a longer period of time. Measuring generalization and long-term maintenance effects is always challenging, because it is difficult to maintain follow-up and control confounding variables. Therefore, there are very few long-term follow-up studies [46]. Besides, one may question whether or not the robot is better than humans at being a teacher for children with ASD, which was not addressed in the present study. We are currently conducting a new study, which compares the effectiveness of robot-based intervention to that of human-based intervention on conversation skills in children with ASD. We are not proposing that either humans or robots should be the teaching agent. Rather, we propose that robots can serve as an effective agent in teaching children with ASD social and communication skills. Related to the aforementioned limitation, the present study deployed NAO, a humanoid robot, as a teacher to train children with ASD gestural communication skills. However, a recent study has reported that there may be individual variations in the preferences for different types of robots for individuals with ASD [40]. Robins et al. [61] have even shown that children with ASD were more responsive toward a theatrical robot, which has plain appearance, than a humanoid robot. Future research should be cautious with the choice of robots.

Abbreviations
AAC: Alternative and augmentative communication; ADI-R: Autism diagnosis interview-revised; ADOS: Autism diagnostic observation schedule; ANT: Attention network test; APA: American Psychiatric Association; ASD: Autism spectrum disorder; BOTTM-2: Bruininks-Oseretsky Test of Motor Proficiency, Second Edition; DOF: Degree of freedom; DS: Down's syndrome; DSM-V: Diagnostic and Statistical Manual of Mental Disorders, Fifth Edition; MNS: Mirror neuron system; PECS: Picture Exchange Communication System; PEP-3: Psychoeducational Profile, Third Edition; SCQ: Social Communication Questionnaire; SGDs: Speech-generating devices

Acknowledgements
We acknowledge the help of our research assistants, Angel Pang, Christine Cheng, and Janis Man. Special thanks to all the children and their parents for their help and dedication to education.

Funding
This research has been fully supported by the grants from the Chinese University of Hong Kong (Project no. CUHK3230211) and the Education Bureau (Project no. QEF6904338).

Authors' contributions
WCSO wrote the manuscript and designed the study. KYW wrote the manuscript and collected and coded the data. WYL programmed the robot and collected the data. CHC, JHY, YH, PN, WLW, CLH, KLY, and CCL collected and coded the data. All authors read and approved the final manuscript.

Competing interests
The authors declare that they have no competing interests.

References
1. American Psychiatric Association. Diagnostic and statistical manual of mental disorders (DSM-5). 5th ed. United State: American Psychiatric Publishing; 2013.
2. Attwood HH, Frith U, Hermelin B. The understanding and use of interpersonal gestures by autistic and Down's syndrome children. J Autism Dev Disord. 1988; https://doi.org/10.1007/BF02211950.
3. Baron RM, Kenny DA. The moderator-mediator variable distinction in social psychological research: conceptual, strategic, and statistical considerations. J Pers Soc Psychol. 1986;51(6):1173–82.
4. Baron-Cohen S. Perceptual role-taking and protodeclarative pointing in autism. Brit J Dev Psychol. 1989; https://doi.org/10.1111/j.2044-835X.1989.
5. Baron-Cohen S. Autism: the empathizing-systemizing (E-S) theory. Ann N Y Acad Sci. 2009; https://doi.org/10.1111/j.1749-6632.2009.04467.x.
6. Bates D, Maechler M, Bolker, B. lme4: Linear Mixed-Effects Models Using S4 Classes (R Package Version 0.999999-0); 2012.
7. Bolte S, Golan O, Goodwin M, Zwaigenbaum L. What can innovative technologies do for autism spectrum disorders? Autism. 2010; https://doi.org/10.1177/1362361310365028.
8. Bondy A, Frost L. PECS: the Picture Exchange Communication System training manual. Cherry Hill: Pyramid Educational Consultants; 1994.
9. Bono M, Daley T, Sigman M. Relations among joint attention, amount of intervention and language gain in autism. J Autism Dev Disord. 2004; https://doi.org/10.1007/s10803-004-2545.
10. Bruininks R, Bruininks B. Bruininks-Oseretsky test of motor proficiency. 2nd ed. Minneapolis: NCS Pearson; 2005.
11. Cabibihan JJ, Javed H, Ang M, Aljunied SM. Why robots? A survey on the roles and benefits of social robots in the therapy of children with autism. Int J Soc Robot. 2013; https://doi.org/10.1007/s12369-013-0202-2.
12. Cabibihan JJ, So WC, Pramanik S. Human-Recognizable Robotic Gestures. IEEE Trans Auton Mental Develop. 2012; https://doi.org/10.1109/TAMD.2012.2208962.
13. Capps L, Kehres J, Sigman M. Conversational abilities among children with autism and children with developmental delays. Autism. 1998; https://doi.org/10.1177/1362361398024002.
14. Carpenter M, Pennington B, Rogers S. Interrelations among social-cognitive skills in young children with autism. J Autism Dev Disord. 2002; https://doi.org/10.1023/A:1014836521114.
15. Cattaneo L, Fabbri-Destro M, Boria S, Pieraccini C, Monti A, Rizzolatti G, Cossu G. Impairment of actions chains in autism and its possible role in intention understanding. P Natl Acad Sci USA. 2007; https://doi.org/10.1073/pnas.0706273104.
16. Charman T, Drew A, Baird C, Baird G. Measuring early language development in preschool children with autism spectrum disorder using the MacArthur Communicative Development Inventory (Infant Form). J Child Lang. 2003; https://doi.org/10.1017/S0305000902005482.

17. Cossu G, Boria S, Copioli C, Bracceschi R, Giuberti V, Santelli E. Motor representation of actions in children with autism. PLoS One. 2012; https://doi.org/10.1371/journal.pone.0044779.

18. Dautenhahn K, Werry I. Towards interactive robots in autism therapy: background, motivation and challenges. Pragmat Cogn. 2004; https://doi.org/10.1075/pc.12.1.03dau.

19. Dawson G, Toth K, Abbott R, Osterling J, Munson J, Estes A, Liaw J. Early social attention impairments in autism: social orienting, joint attention, and attention to distress. Dev Psychol. 2004; https://doi.org/10.1037/0012-1649.40.2.271.

20. de Marchena A, Eigsti IM. Conversational gestures in autism spectrum disorders: asynchrony but not decreased frequency. Autism Res. 2010; https://doi.org/10.1002/aur.159.

21. Dowell LR, Mahone EM, Mostofsky SH. Associations of postural knowledge and basic motor skill with dyspraxia in autism: implications for abnormalities in distributed connectivity and motor learning. Neuropsychology. 2009; https://doi.org/10.1037/a0015640.

22. Dziuk MA, Larson JCG, Apostu A, Mahone EM, Denckla MB, Mostofsky SH. Dyspraxia in autism: association with motor, social, and communicative deficits. Dev Med Child Neurol. 2007; https://doi.org/10.1111/j.1469-8749.2007.00734.

23. Fan J, McCandliss BD, Sommer T, Raz A, Posner MI. Testing the efficiency and independence of attentional networks. J Cogn Neurosci. 2002; https://doi.org/10.1162/089892902317361886.

24. Fong I, Nourbakhsh I, Dautenhahn K. A survey of socially interactive robots. Robot Auton Syst. 2003; https://doi.org/10.1016/S0921-8890(02)00372-X.

25. Frea WD, Arnold CL, Vittimberga GL. A demonstration of the effects of augmentative communication on the extreme aggressive behavior of a child with autism within an integrated preschool setting. J Posit Behav Interv. 2001; https://doi.org/10.1177/109800700100300401.

26. Gizzonio V, Avanzini P, Campi C, Orivoli S, Piccolo B, Cantalupo G. Failure in pantomime action execution correlates with the severity of social behavior deficits in children with autism: a praxis study. J Autism Dev Disord. 2015; https://doi.org/10.1007/s10803-015-2461-2.

27. Gullberg M. Communication strategies, gestures, and grammar. Acquisition et Interaction en Langue Etrangère. 1999;8(2):61–71.

28. Ham HS, Bartolo A, Corley M. Case report: selective deficit in the production of intransitive gestures in an individual with autism. Cortex. 2010; https://doi.org/10.1016/j.cortex.2009.06.005.

29. Ham HS, Bartolo A, Corley M, Rajendran G, Szabo A, Swanson S. Exploring the relationship between gestural recognition and imitation: evidence of dyspraxia in autism spectrum disorders. J Autism Dev Disord. 2011; https://doi.org/10.1007/s10803-010-1011-1.

30. Hart SL, Banda DR. Picture exchange communication system with individuals with developmental disabilities: a meta-analysis of single subject studies. Remedial Spec Educ. 2009; https://doi.org/10.1177/0741932509338354.

31. Ingersoll B. The social role of imitation in autism: implications for the treatment of imitation deficits. Infant Young Child. 2008; https://doi.org/10.1097/01.IYC.0000314482.24087.14.

32. Ingersoll B, Lalonde K. The impact of object and gesture imitation training on language use in children with autism spectrum disorder. J Speech Lang Hear Res. 2010; https://doi.org/10.1044/1092-4388(2009/09-0043).

33. James LR, Brett JM. Mediators, moderators and tests for mediation. J Appl Psychol. 1994; https://doi.org/10.1037/0021-9010.69.2.307.

34. Jolliffe T, Baron-Cohen S. Are people with autism or Asperger syndrome faster than normal on the embedded figures task? J Child Psychol Psychiatry. 1997; https://doi.org/10.1111/j.1469-7610.1997.tb01539.x.

35. Judd CM, Kenny DA. Process analysis: estimating mediation in treatment evaluations. Eval Rev. 1981; https://doi.org/10.1177/0193841X8100500502.

36. Klin A, Jones W. Attributing social and physical meaning to ambiguous visual displays in individuals with higher-functioning autism spectrum disorders. Brain Cogn. 2006; https://doi.org/10.1016/j.bandc.2005.12.016.

37. Klin A, Lin DJ, Gorrindo P, Ramsay G, Jones W. Two-year-olds with autism orient to non-social contingencies rather than biological motion. Nature. 2009; https://doi.org/10.1038/nature07868.

38. Koegel L, Koegel R, Shoshan Y, McNerney E. Pivotal response intervention II: preliminary long-term outcome data. J Assoc Pers Severe. 1999; https://doi.org/10.2511/rpsd.24.3.186.

39. Koshino H, Kana RK, Keller TA, Cherkassky VL, Minshew NJ, Just MA. fMRI investigation of working memory for faces in autism: visual coding and underconnectivity with frontal areas. Cereb Cortex. 2008; https://doi.org/10.1093/cercor/bhm054.

40. Kumazaki H, Warren Z, Swanson A. Impressions of humanness for android robot may represent an endophenotype for autism spectrum disorders. J Autism Dev Disord. 2017; https://doi.org/10.1007/s10803-017-3365-0.

41. Lee J, Takehashi H, Nagai C, Obinata G, Stefanov D. Which robot features can stimulate better responses from children with autism in robot-assisted therapy? Int J Adv Robot Syst. 2012; https://doi.org/10.5772/51128.

42. Li H, Cabibihan JJ, Tan Y. Towards an effective design of social robots. Int J Soc Robot. 2011; https://doi.org/10.1007/s12369-011-0121-z.

43. Lord C, Risi S, Lambrecht L, Cook EH Jr, Leventhal BL, DiLavore PC, Pickles A, Rutter M. The autism diagnostic observation schedule-generic: a standard measure of social and communication deficits associated with the spectrum of autism. J Autism Dev Disord. 2000; https://doi.org/10.1023/A:1005592401947.

44. Lord C, Rutter M, Le Couteur A. Autism Diagnostic Interview-Revised: a revised version of a diagnostic interview for caregivers of individuals with possible pervasive developmental disorders. J Autism Dev Disord. 1994; https://doi.org/10.1007/BF02172145.

45. Luyster R, Lopez K, Lord C. Characterizing communicative development in children referred for autism spectrum disorder using the MacArthur-Bates Communicative Development Inventory (CDI). J Child Lang. 2007; https://doi.org/10.1017/S0305000907008094.

46. Maddox BB, Miyazaki Y, White SW. Long-term effects of CBT on social impairment in adolescents with ASD. J Autism Dev Disord. 2017; https://doi.org/10.1007/s10803-016-2779-4.

47. Mastrogiuseppe M, Capirci O, Cuva S, Venuti P. Gestural communication in children with autism spectrum disorders during mother-child interaction. Autism. 2015; https://doi.org/10.1177/1362361314528390.

48. McNeill D. Language and gesture: window into thought and action. Cambridge: Cambridge University Press; 2000.

49. McNeill D. Gesture and thought. Chicago: University of Chicago Press; 2005.

50. Medeiros K, Winsler A. Parent-child gesture use during problem solving in autism spectrum disorder. J Autism Dev Disord. 2014; https://doi.org/10.1007/s10803-014-2069-y.

51. Mirenda P. Toward functional augmentative and alternative communication for students with autism manual signs, graphic symbols, and voice output communication aids. Language, speech, and hearing services in schools; 2003. https://doi.org/10.1044/0161-1461(2003/017).

52. Mitchell P, Parsons S, Leonard A. Using virtual environments for teaching social understanding to six adolescents with autism spectrum disorders. J Autism Dev Disord. 2007; https://doi.org/10.1007/s10803-006-0189-8.

53. Nicoladis E. What's the difference between "toilet paper" and "paper toilet"? French-English bilingual children's crosslinguistic transfer in compound nouns. J Child Lang. 2002; https://doi.org/10.1017/S0305000902005366.

54. Nicoladis E, Mayberry RI, Genesee F. Gesture and early bilingual development. Dev Psychol. 1999; https://doi.org/10.1037/0012-1649.35.2.514.

55. Nicoladis E, Simone R, Yin H, Marentette M. Gesture use in story recall by Chinese-English bilinguals. Appl Psycholinguist. 2007; https://doi.org/10.1017/S0142716407070385.

56. O'Riordan MA. Superior visual search in adults with autism. Autism. 2004; https://doi.org/10.1177/1362361304045219.

57. Oberman LM, Ramachandran VS. The simulating social mind: the role of the mirror neuron system and simulation in the social and communicative deficits of autism spectrum disorders. Psychol Bull. 2007; https://doi.org/10.1037/0033-2909.133.2.310.

58. Pierno A, Mari M, Lusher D, Castiello U. Robotic movement elicits visuomotor priming in children with autism. Neuropsychologia. 2008; https://doi.org/10.1016/j.neuropsychologia.2007.08.020.

59. Ploog BO, Scharf A, Nelson D, Brooks PJ. Use of computer-assisted technologies (CAT) to enhance social, communicative, and language development in children with autism spectrum disorders. J Autism Dev Disord. 2013;43(2):301–22.

60. R Core Team. R: A Language and Environment for Statistical Computing. Vienna, Austria: R Foundation for Statistical Computing; 2012.

61. Robins B, Dautenhahn K, Dubowski J. Does appearance matter in the interaction of children with autism with a humanoid robot? Int Stud. 2006; 7(34):479–512. https://doi.org/10.1075/is.7.3.16rob.

62. Rogers S, Pennington B. A theoretical approach to the deficits in infantile autism. Dev Psychol. 1991; https://doi.org/10.1017/S0954579400000043.

63. Rogers S, Williams JH. Imitation in autism findings and controversies. In: Rogers S, Williams JH, editors. Imitation and the social mind. New York: Guilford Press; 2006. p. 277–303.

64. Rueda MR, Fan J, McCandliss BD, Halparin JD, Gruber DB, Lercari LP, Posner MI. Development of attentional networks in childhood. Neuropsychologia. 2004; https://doi.org/10.1016/j.neuropsychologia.2003.12.012.

65. Schopler E, Lansing MD, Reichler RJ, Marcus LM. Psychoeducational profile: TEACCH individualized psychoeducational assessment for children with autism spectrum disorders. 3rd ed. Austin: Pro-Ed; 2005.

66. Sherman J, Nicoladis E. Gestures by advanced Spanish-English second-language learners. Gesture. 2004; https://doi.org/10.1075/gest.4.2.03she.

67. Sigman M, Ruskin E. Continuity and change in the social competence of children with autism, Down's syndrome, and developmental delays. Monogr Soc Res Child Dev. 1999;64:256.

68. Silver M, Oakes P. Evaluation of a new computer intervention to teach people with autism or Asperger syndrome to recognize and predict emotions in others. Autism. 2001; https://doi.org/10.1177/1362361301005003007.

69. So WC, Wong MKY. I use my space not yours: use of gesture space for referential identification among children with autism spectrum disorders. Res Autism Spect Dis. 2016; https://doi.org/10.1016/j.rasd.2016.03.005.

70. So WC, Wong MKY, Cabibihan JJ, Lam KY, Chan YY, Qian HH. Using robot animation to promote gestural skills in children with autism spectrum disorders. J Comput Assist Learn. 2016; https://doi.org/10.1111/jcal.12159.

71. So WC, Wong MKY, Lam KY. Social and communication skills predict imitation abilities in children with autism. Front Educ. 2016; https://doi.org/10.3389/feduc.2016.00003.

72. So WC, Wong MKY, Lam KY, Lam WY, Chui TF, Lee TL, Ng HM, Chan CH, Fok CW. Using a social robot to teach gestural recognition and production in children with autism spectrum disorders. Disabil Rehabil. 2017; https://doi.org/10.1080/17483107.2017.1344886.

73. So WC, Wong MKY, Lui M, Yip V. The development of co-speech gesture and its semantic integration with speech in six- to 12-year-old children with autism spectrum disorders. Autism. 2015; https://doi.org/10.1177/1362361314556783.

74. Stokoe WC. Sign language structure: an outline of the visual communication systems of the American deaf. J Deaf Stud Deaf Educ. 2005; https://doi.org/10.1093/deafed/eni001.

75. Stone WL, Ousley OY, Littleford CD. Motor imitation in young children with autism: what's the object? J Abnorm Child Psychol. 1997; https://doi.org/10.1023/A:1022685731726.

76. Stone WL, Yoder PJ. Predicting spoken language level in children with autism spectrum disorders. Autism. 2001; https://doi.org/10.1177/1362361301005004002.

77. Watson LR, Crais ER, Baranek GT, Dykstra JR, Wilson KP. Communicative gesture use in infants with and without autism: a retrospective home video study. Am J Speech-Lang Pat. 2013; https://doi.org/10.1044/1058-0360(2012/11-0145.

78. Wetherby A, Prizant B. The infant toddler checklist from the communication and symbolic behavior scales. Baltimore: Brookes Publishing; 2002.

79. Wetherby AM, Woods J, Allen L, Cleary J, Dickinson H, Lord C. Early indicators of autism spectrum disorders in the second year of life. J Autism Dev Disord. 2004; https://doi.org/10.1007/s10803-004-2544-y.

80. Wild KS, Poliakoff E, Jerrison A, Gowen E. Goal-directed and goal-less imitation in autism spectrum disorder. J Autism Dev Disord. 2012; https://doi.org/10.1007/s10803-011-1417-4.

81. Williams JH, Whiten A, Suddendorf T, Perrett DI. Imitation, mirror neurons and autism. Neurosci Biobehav R. 2001; https://doi.org/10.1016/S0149-7634(01)00014-8.

82. Wong MKY, So WC. Absence of delay in spontaneous use of gestures in spoken narratives among children with autism spectrum disorders. Res Dev Disabil. 2018; https://doi.org/10.1016/j.ridd.2017.11.004.

83. Yun SS, Choi J, Park SK, Bong GY, Yoo H. Social skills training for children with autism spectrum disorder using a robotic behavioral intervention system. Autism Res. 2017; https://doi.org/10.1002/aur.1778.

4

Resveratrol ameliorates prenatal progestin exposure-induced autism-like behavior through ERβ activation

Weiguo Xie[1†], Xiaohu Ge[2†], Ling Li[3†], Athena Yao[1], Xiaoyan Wang[2], Min Li[1], Xiang Gong[1], Zhigang Chu[1], Zhe Lu[3], Xiaodong Huang[1], Yun Jiao[3], Yifei Wang[2], Meifang Xiao[3], Haijia Chen[2*], Wei Xiang[3*] and Paul Yao[1,3*] (iD)

Abstract

Background: Recent literatures indicate that maternal hormone exposure is a risk factor for autism spectrum disorder (ASD). We hypothesize that prenatal progestin exposure may counteract the neuroprotective effect of estrogen and contribute to ASD development, and we aim to develop a method to ameliorate prenatal progestin exposure-induced autism-like behavior.

Methods: Experiment 1: Prenatal progestin exposure-induced offspring are treated with resveratrol (RSV) through either prenatal or postnatal exposure and then used for autism-like behavior testing and other biomedical analyses. Experiment 2: Prenatal norethindrone (NET) exposure-induced offspring are treated with ERβ knockdown lentivirus together with RSV for further testing. Experiment 3: Pregnant dams are treated with prenatal NET exposure together with RSV, and the offspring are used for further testing.

Results: Eight kinds of clinically relevant progestins were used for prenatal exposure in pregnant dams, and the offspring showed decreased ERβ expression in the amygdala with autism-like behavior. Oral administration of either postnatal or prenatal RSV treatment significantly reversed this effect with ERβ activation and ameliorated autism-like behavior. Further investigation showed that RSV activates ERβ and its target genes by demethylation of DNA and histone on the ERβ promoter, and then minimizes progestin-induced oxidative stress as well as the dysfunction of mitochondria and lipid metabolism in the brain, subsequently ameliorating autism-like behavior.

Conclusions: We conclude that resveratrol ameliorates prenatal progestin exposure-induced autism-like behavior through ERβ activation. Our data suggest that prenatal progestin exposure is a strong risk factor for autism-like behavior. Many potential clinical progestin applications, including oral contraceptive pills, preterm birth drugs, and progestin-contaminated drinking water or seafood, may be risk factors for ASD. In addition, RSV may be a good candidate for clinically rescuing or preventing ASD symptoms in humans, while high doses of resveratrol used in the animals may be a potential limitation for human application.

Keywords: Autism spectrum disorder, Estrogen receptor β, Lipid metabolism, Mitochondria, Oxidative stress, Progestin, Resveratrol

* Correspondence: chenhaijia@saliai.com; xiangwei8@163.com; vasilis112@yahoo.com
†Weiguo Xie, Xiaohu Ge and Ling Li contributed equally to this work.
[2]SALIAI Stem Cell Institute of Guangdong, Guangzhou SALIAI Stem Cell Science and Technology Co. LTD, Guangzhou 510055, People's Republic of China
[3]Department of Pediatrics, Hainan Maternal and Child Health Hospital, Haikou 570206, People's Republic of China
[1]Institute of Rehabilitation Center, Tongren Hospital of Wuhan University, Wuhan 430060, People's Republic of China

Background

Autism spectrum disorder (ASD) is a neurological and developmental disorder that is characterized by deficits in social communication and interaction with restricted and repetitive patterns of behavior [1]. The prevalence of ASD is estimated to be 1:68 and biased towards males with a male-to-female ratio of at least 4:1 [2, 3]. Many risk factors contribute to ASD development, including genetics, sex, and environmental factors [4, 5], while the detailed mechanisms of ASD remain unclear [6].

Recent literatures have shown that dysregulation of estrogen receptor β (ERβ) is associated with ASD [7–10]. ERβ regulates the basal expression of superoxide dismutase (SOD2), which regulates oxidative stress [11], and estrogen-related receptor α (ERRα) [12], which regulates mitochondrial function and lipid metabolism [13, 14]. ERβ suppression results in oxidative stress and dysfunction of mitochondrial and lipid metabolism, subsequently triggering brain damage and autism-like behavior [9, 15]. This indicates that hormone-mediated ERβ suppression may contribute to ASD development.

It has been reported that maternal hormonal exposure is a significant risk factor for ASD [8, 16] as steroidogenic activity is elevated in some ASD patients [17] and cholesterol metabolism and various steroid abnormalities are involved in ASD development [18]. In addition, natural progesterone and synthetic progestin regulate neurogenic responses [19] and impair cognitive flexibility during development [20] as well as downregulate ERβ expression [9, 21]. We hypothesize that clinically relevant progestin may counteract estrogen-mediated neuroprotective effects via downregulation of ERβ, and contribute to ASD development [22, 23].

Resveratrol (RSV) is a natural polyphenolic compound that is present at high levels in red grapes, nuts, pomegranates, and *Polygonum cuspidatum* [24]. Resveratrol (RSV) has much therapeutic potential with its antioxidant, antitumorigenic, and cardioprotective as well as neuroprotective effects [24–28]. All of these biological activities may have potential benefits and points of interest in autism therapeutics, although very little research has been reported on its potential effect on ASD treatment [15, 29, 30].

In this study, different kinds of clinically relevant progestins were used for prenatal exposure in pregnant dams, and the offspring showed decreased ERβ expression in the brain with autism-like behavior. Oral administration of resveratrol (RSV) by either postnatal or prenatal treatment completely reversed this effect with ERβ activation and ameliorated autism-like behavior. Further investigation showed that RSV-mediated ERβ activation is due to RSV-mediated demethylation of DNA and histone on the ERβ promoter. This is the first time we have discovered the potential mechanism of ASD development due to prenatal progestin exposure-induced ERβ suppression, as well as the potential rescuing and preventive effect of RSV on autism-like behavior through ERβ activation, which may potentially be applicable in clinical treatment of ASD patients.

Methods

A detailed description can be found in Additional file 1.

Materials

17β-estradiol (E2, #E2758); progesterone (P4, #P0130); levonorgestrel (LNG, #1362602); medroxyprogesterone acetate (MPA, #1378001); nestorone (NES, # SML0550); norethindrone (NET, #1469005); norethindrone acetate (NETA, #1470004); norgestimate (NGM, # 1471914); hydroxyprogesterone caproate (OHPC, #1329006), and resveratrol (RSV, #R5010) were obtained from Sigma. Norethynodrel (NEN, #E4600–000) was obtained from Steraloids.

In vivo rat experiments

The animal protocol conformed to the US NIH guidelines (Guide for the Care and Use of Laboratory Animals, No. 85–23, revised 1996) and was reviewed and approved by the Institutional Animal Care and Use Committee from Wuhan University [9].

Protocol 1 for postnatal treatment of resveratrol

Three-month-old female Sprague Dawley rats were caged with proven males, and the verified pregnant dams were randomly assigned to either 20 mg of progestin (such as norethindrone, NET) or VEH (vehicle group that received the same volume of vehicle). Drugs were suspended in 5% ethanol in organic sesame oil and 0.1 ml was given daily through subcutaneous injection at the nape starting from day 1 until pup delivery for ~ 21 days. The male and female offspring were separated from the dams on day 21, and then at 5 weeks old, the offspring from either VEH or progestin prenatal treatment were randomly divided into two groups, a resveratrol (RSV) group and a control (CTL) group. Rats in the RSV group were orally administered (by gavage) 20 mg/kg of RVS suspended in 10 g/l carboxymethylcellulose every day for 4 weeks (28 days). Those in the CTL group were administered 10 ml/kg of 10 g/l carboxymethylcellulose during the same period. At 10 weeks old, treated offspring were used for autism-like behavior testing or were sacrificed for further experiments and biomedical analysis [9]; see schematic details in Fig. 1a.

Protocol 2 for postnatal treatment of resveratrol with infusion of shERβ lentivirus

The male offspring (8 weeks old) from the VEH and NET group in Protocol 1 were anesthetized with a mixture of ketamine (90 mg/kg) and xylazine (2.7 mg/kg) and

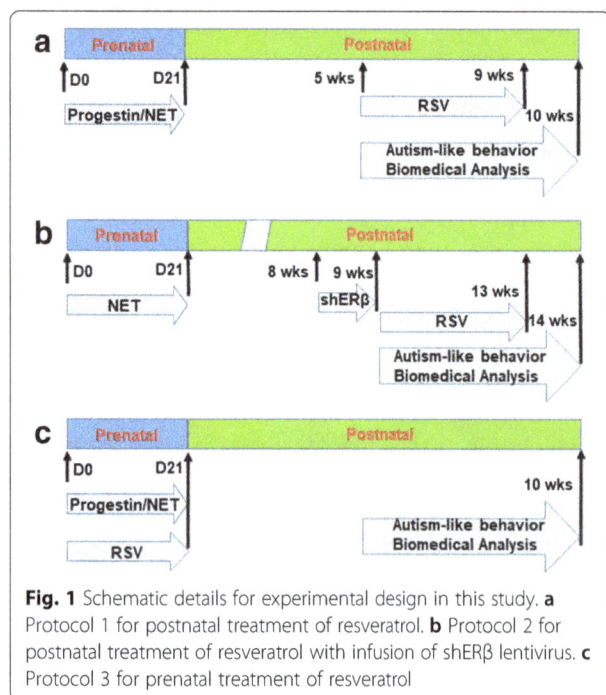

Fig. 1 Schematic details for experimental design in this study. **a** Protocol 1 for postnatal treatment of resveratrol. **b** Protocol 2 for postnatal treatment of resveratrol with infusion of shERβ lentivirus. **c** Protocol 3 for prenatal treatment of resveratrol

implanted with a guide cannula targeting the amygdala (26 gauge; Plastics One). The following coordinates were chosen for the amygdala: − 2.0 mm posterior to the bregma, ± 4.2 mm from the midline, and − 7.2 mm from the skull surface on which it was based. Cannula was attached to the skull with dental acrylic and jeweler's screws and closed with an obturator [31]. An osmotic minipump (Alzet model 2002; flow rate 0.5 µl/h; Cupertino, CA) connected to a 26-gauge internal cannula that extended 1 mm below the guide was implanted and used to deliver either ERβ knockdown (shERβ), or empty (EMP) lentivirus. Vehicle consisting of artificial cerebrospinal fluid (aCSF; 140 mM NaCl, 3 mM KCl, 1.2 mM Na$_2$HPO$_4$, 1 mM MgCl$_2$, 0.27 mM NaH$_2$PO$_4$, 1.2 mM CaCl$_2$, and 7.2 mM dextrose, pH 7.4) was used for the infusion of the lentivirus. Infusion (flow rate 0.5 µl/h) began immediately after placement of the minipump. 0.5 µl of total 2×10^3 cfu of lentivirus was infused for 1 h [9]. The experimental rats were separated into four groups (12 per group) at 9 weeks old. Group 1: VEH offspring with empty control lentivirus infusion plus oral administration of carboxymethylcellulose control treatment for 4 weeks (VEH/ EMP/CTL); Group 2: NET offspring with empty control lentivirus infusion plus oral administration of carboxymethylcellulose control treatment for 4 weeks (NET/ EMP/CTL); Group 3: NET offspring with empty control lentivirus infusion plus oral administration of resveratrol (RSV) treatment for 4 weeks (NET/EMP/RSV); Group 4: NET offspring with ERβ knockdown lentivirus infusion plus oral administration (by gavage) of RSV treatment for 4 weeks (VEH/shERβ/RSV). At 14 weeks old, the offspring

were used for behavior testing followed by biomedical analysis [9]; see schematic details in Fig. 1b.

Protocol 3 for prenatal treatment of resveratrol

Three-month-old verified pregnant dams were randomly assigned to the following four groups: Group 1: The rats received VEH (5% ethanol in organic sesame oil and 0.1 ml were given daily through subcutaneous injection at the nape) plus control (CTL) group with oral administration of 10 ml/kg of 10 g/l carboxymethylcellulose (VEH/PreCTL); Group 2: Rats received 20 µg of progestin (such as norethindrone, NET) with 5% ethanol in organic sesame oil plus) plus CTL group (NET/PreCTL); Group 3: The rats received VEH treatment plus resveratrol (RSV) group with oral administration (by gavage) of 20 mg/kg of resveratrol suspended in 10 g/l carboxymethylcellulose (VEH/PreRSV); Group 4: The rats received progestin (such as NET) group plus RSV group (NET/PreRSV). The rats received the above treatment starting from day 1 until pup delivery for ~ 21 days. Both male and female offspring were raised until 10 weeks old to be tested for autism-like behavior testing and other biomedical analysis [9], see schematic details in Fig. 1c.

Animal behavior test

The animal behavior test of offspring was carried out at 10 weeks of age. Female offspring were tested in the diestrus phase, which was confirmed by vaginal smears. Autism-like behavior was evaluated using the marble burying test (MBT) and social interaction (SI) test.

Marble burying test (MBT)

In brief, each rat is placed in a clean cage ($35 \times 23 \times 19$ cm^3) filled with wood chip bedding to a depth of 5 cm containing 20 colored glass marbles (1 cm diameter) placed in a 5×4 arrangement. The number of marbles buried (> 50% covered by bedding material) in 30 min was hand-scored by the experimenter [9, 32, 33].

Social interaction (SI) test

In short, the subjects (Test and Stranger) were separately habituated to the arena for 5 min before the test. During each test, the rats were placed into the apparatus over a period of 20 min and the time spent following, mounting, grooming, and sniffing any body parts of the other rat was taken as an indicator of social engagement, and the social interaction time was calculated and analyzed using EthoVision XT animal tracking software (Noldus, USA) [34]. The animal used as the "Stranger" was used only once and was a Sprague Dawley rat of the same gender, weight, and age, with no previous contact with the test rats [9, 32, 33].

Methods

The amygdala neurons were isolated for in vitro primary cell culture analysis [9, 35]. The DNA methylation on the rat ERβ promoter was evaluated by a real-time PCR-based methylation-specific PCR (MSP) analysis as described previously with some modifications [9, 36–38]. The lentivirus for rat ERβ shRNA and empty control (EMP) were prepared previously in our lab [9]. The mRNA was measured by real-time quantitative PCR using primers provided in Additional file 1: Table S1, and the protein was measured by western blotting [9]. The SIRT1 activity assay was evaluated in nuclear extract using a SIRT1 Fluorometric Drug Discovery Kit (Cat #: BML-AK555, Enzo Life Sciences) [39]. Oxidative stress was evaluated by in vivo superoxide anion (O_2^-) release [40] and 3-nitrotyrosine formation. DNA damage was evaluated by 8-OHdG and γH2AX formation [9]. Mitochondrial function was evaluated by mitochondrial DNA copies [9] and intracellular ATP level [40]. The histone methylation was evaluated by chromatin immunoprecipitation (ChIP) analysis [9]. Fatty acid metabolism was evaluated by in vitro lipid transport assay [41] and fatty acid oxidation assay [42, 43]. Statistical analysis was conducted using SPSS 22 software, and a P value of < 0.05 was considered significant, and the data was given as mean ± SEM [9].

Results

Postnatal resveratrol treatment reverses prenatal progestin exposure-induced ERβ suppression and autism-like behavior

We first investigated the potential effect of prenatal progestin exposure on ERβ expression in the amygdala and autism-like behavior in 10-week-old male offspring, and then evaluated whether postnatal resveratrol treatment could reverse this effect. In Table 1 (left panel of first row), several steroids, 17β-estradiol (E2), progesterone (P4), and eight different kinds of clinically relevant progestins, including levonorgestrel (LNG), medroxyprogesterone acetate (MPA), nestorone (NES), norethindrone (NET), norethindrone acetate (NETA), norethynodrel (NEN), norgestimate (NGM), and hydroxyprogesterone caproate (OHPC), were used for prenatal exposure to different 3-month-old pregnant dams for 21 days ($n = 8$). The 5-week-old male offspring were then treated by either control (CTL) or resveratrol (RSV) for 4 weeks, and the ERβ mRNA in the amygdala was evaluated by real-time PCR and the autism-like behavior was evaluated by social interaction time. Our results showed that E2 had no effect, while P4 slightly decreased ERβ expression but had no significant effect on social interaction time, and almost all the clinically relevant progestins significantly decreased ERβ expression (except the NGM), and decreased social interaction time (except the NEN) compared to the vehicle group. Furthermore, resveratrol treatment almost completely reversed the suppression effect on ERβ expression and social interaction time (partly for the NES and NGM). Our results indicate that postnatal resveratrol treatment reverses prenatal progestin exposure-induced ERβ suppression and autism-like behavior.

Prenatal resveratrol treatment prevents prenatal progestin exposure-induced ERβ suppression and autism-like behavior

We then evaluated the potential effect of prenatal resveratrol treatment on prenatal progestin exposure-induced ERβ suppression and autism-like behavior. In Table 1

Table 1 Resveratrol reverses and prevents prenatal progestin exposure-induced ERβ suppression and autism-like behavior

Rats	Postnatal treatment of RSV				Prenatal treatment of RSV			
Prenatal progestin exposure	ERβ mRNA level (%)		Social interaction time (seconds)		ERβ mRNA level (%)		Social interaction time (seconds)	
	Control	RSV	Control	RSV	Control	RSV	Control	RSV
Vehicle	100 ± 9	111 ± 10	351 ± 27	369 ± 17	100 ± 11	91 ± 11	356 ± 24	340 ± 16
E2	94 ± 12	91 ± 13	369 ± 24	343 ± 16	89 ± 13	95 ± 9	341 ± 17	336 ± 19
P4	78 ± 10*	119 ± 9	321 ± 17	339 ± 22	78 ± 8*	106 ± 8	319 ± 22	369 ± 23
LNG	54 ± 11*	89 ± 12	259 ± 19*	321 ± 19	61 ± 9*	109 ± 11	263 ± 12*	335 ± 17
MPA	72 ± 13*	115 ± 7	261 ± 24*	351 ± 28	66 ± 12*	92 ± 8	245 ± 11*	361 ± 22
NES	81 ± 11	91 ± 9	249 ± 20*	298 ± 23*	75 ± 8*	111 ± 12	266 ± 18*	350 ± 18
NET	49 ± 8*	106 ± 11	237 ± 16*	326 ± 20	55 ± 10*	106 ± 9	220 ± 25*	348 ± 20
NETA	67 ± 9*	90 ± 9	286 ± 19*	378 ± 14	72 ± 13*	113 ± 11	301 ± 17*	356 ± 25
NEN	75 ± 8*	113 ± 12	336 ± 26	361 ± 15	69 ± 14*	78 ± 9*	321 ± 25	336 ± 21
NGM	85 ± 12	90 ± 8	279 ± 22*	306 ± 22*	78 ± 9*	135 ± 11*	291 ± 23*	343 ± 24
OHPC	59 ± 10	109 ± 11	268 ± 19*	322 ± 21	63 ± 11*	106 ± 12*	287 ± 19*	326 ± 22

$n = 8$, results are expressed as mean ± SEM

Note: E2, 17β-estradiol; P4, progesterone; LNG, levonorgestrel; MPA, medroxyprogesterone acetate; NES, nestorone; NET, norethindrone; NETA, norethindrone acetate; NEN, norethynodrel; NGM, norgestimate; OHPC, hydroxyprogesterone caproate; RSV, resveratrol.

*$P < 0.05$, vs vehicle group in the same column

(right panel of first row), prenatal exposure of P4 and all the eight different kinds of clinically relevant progestins significantly decreased ERβ expression and social interaction time (except the NEN), while prenatal resveratrol treatment (oral administration of 20 mg/kg RSV for 21 days) almost completely reversed prenatal progestin exposure-induced suppression effect on ERβ expression (partly for NEN) and social interaction time. Our results indicate that prenatal resveratrol treatment prevents prenatal progestin exposure-induced ERβ suppression and autism-like behavior.

Postnatal resveratrol treatment reverses prenatal norethindrone exposure-induced suppression of ERβ and its target genes in the amygdala

In Table 1, the prenatal exposure of norethindrone (NET) in pregnant dams showed the most dramatic

suppression effect on ERβ expression and social interaction time in offspring compared to other progestins. The NET was chosen for the prenatal progestin exposure in the later experiments to investigate the detailed mechanism and effect of resveratrol on autism-like behavior. The animal was treated as shown in Fig. 1b. We first measured the gene expression of ERβ, SOD2, and ERRα in the hypothalamus and hippocampus (see Additional file 1: Figure S1). We found that prenatal NET exposure showed no effect on gene expression. Also, RSV treatment showed no effect on the expression of ERβ and SIRT1, while the expression of SOD2 and ERRα was significantly increased in both the hypothalamus and hippocampus by RSV treatment compared to the control (CTL) group. We then measured the mRNA expression of ERβ (see Fig. 2a), SOD2 (see Fig. 2b), and ERRα (see Fig. 2c) in the amygdala. We

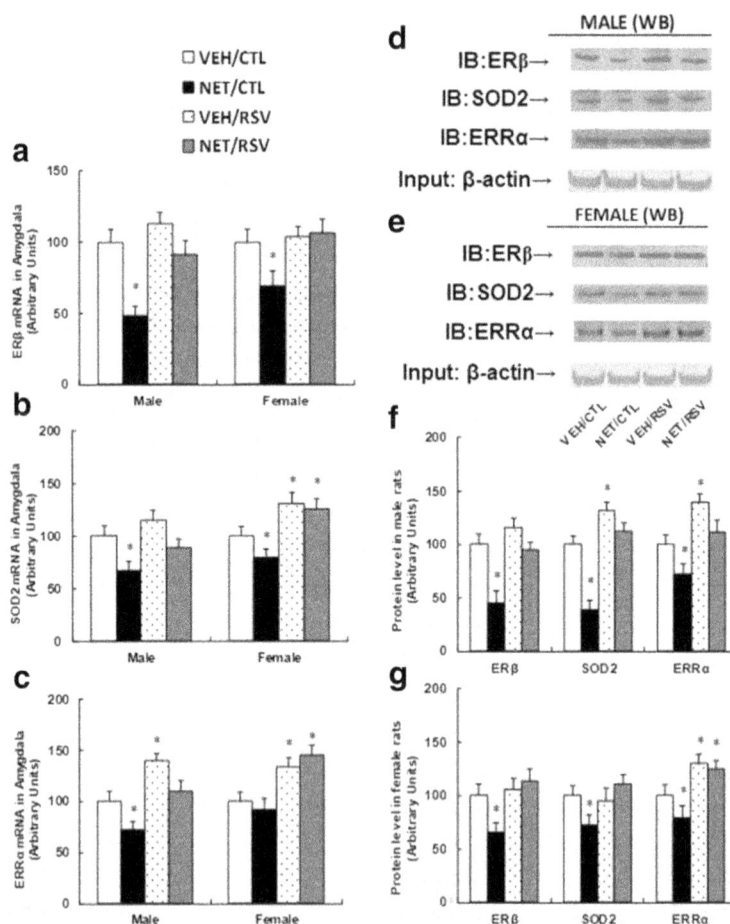

Fig. 2 Postnatal resveratrol treatment reverses prenatal norethindrone exposure-induced suppression of ERβ and its target genes. Three-month-old pregnant dams were exposed to NET (20 µg norethindrone) or VEH (vehicle, 5% ethanol in organic sesame oil) by subcutaneous daily injection of 0.1 ml for 21 days until pup delivery. Both male and female offspring were then treated with either control (CTL) or resveratrol (RSV) for 4 weeks starting from 5 weeks old. The offspring were sacrificed at 10 weeks of age to isolate the amygdala for further analysis. a–c mRNA levels in the amygdala for genes of ERβ a, SOD2 b, and ERRα c, $n = 5$. d Representative pictures of protein levels in male offspring by western blotting. e Representative pictures of protein levels in female offspring by western blotting. f Protein expression quantitation for d, $n = 5$. g Protein expression quantitation for e, $n = 5$. *, $P < 0.05$, vs VEH/CTL group; ¶, $P < 0.05$, vs NET/CTL group. Results are expressed as mean ± SEM

found that RSV treatment completely reversed prenatal NET exposure-induced suppression of ERβ, SOD2, and ERRα in both male and female offspring. Furthermore, in female offspring, RSV significantly increased expression of SOD2 and ERRα in both the VEH and NET groups, while in male offspring there was much less gene activation (see Fig. 2b, c), indicating that female offspring seem more responsive to RSV treatment compared to male offspring. We also measured the protein levels in the amygdala (see Fig. 2d–g). The results showed that RSV completely reversed the NET-mediated suppression effect on the expression of ERβ, SOD2, and ERRα. Furthermore, RSV increased ERRα expression in VEH treatment compared to the CTL group in male offspring (see Fig. 2d, f), and in female offspring, RSV significantly increased ERRα expression in both VEH and NET treatment compared to CTL group (see Fig. 2e, g). We also measured the SIRT1 mRNA expression (see Figure S2a) and SIRT1 activity (see Figure S2b), which showed no difference in any of the treatments, indicating that SIRT1 may not be involved in RSV-mediated effect (see detailed statistical information in Additional file 1: Data S1). Our results suggest that RSV reverses prenatal NET exposure-induced suppression of ERβ and its target genes, and female offspring seem more responsive than male offspring.

Postnatal resveratrol treatment diminishes prenatal norethindrone exposure-induced methylation of DNA and histone on the ERβ promoter

In Fig. 3a, b, the DNA methylation on the ERβ promoter was significantly increased by prenatal NET exposure, and RSV treatment completely diminished this effect compared to the CTL group. We then measured the histone methylation on the ERβ promoter by ChIP techniques. In male offspring (see Fig. 3c), prenatal NET exposure increased H3K9 di-methylation (H3K9me2) by 1.80-fold and H3K27 tri-methylation (H3K27me3) by 2.13-fold, while in female offspring (see Fig. 3d), it increased H3K9 di-methylation (H3K9me2) by 2.14-fold and H3K27 tri-methylation (H3K27me3) by 1.56-fold, but had no effect on H3K9 tri-methylation (H3K9me3). RSV treatment completely diminished the effect on H3K9me2, but partly diminished the effect on H3K27me3 in male offspring compared to the CTL group, while in female offspring, RSV partly diminished the effect on H3K9 di-methylation, but completely diminished the effect on H3K27 tri-methylation (see detailed statistical information in Additional file 1: Data S2). Our results indicate that postnatal RSV administration diminishes prenatal levonorgestrel exposure-induced methylation of DNA and histone on the ERβ promoter in the amygdala.

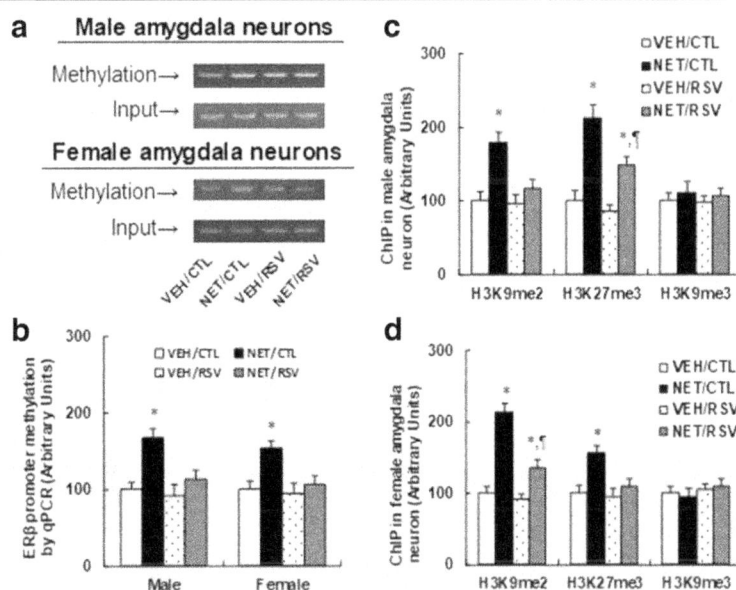

Fig. 3 Postnatal resveratrol treatment diminishes prenatal norethindrone exposure-induced methylation of DNA and histone on the ERβ promoter. The amygdala neurons were isolated from 10-week-old male/female offspring for in vitro cell culture analysis. **a** The representative bands for ERβ methylation in amygdala neurons from both male (upper panel) and female (lower panel) offspring. **b** DNA methylation on ERβ by real-time PCR-based methylation-specific PCR (MSP) analysis in amygdala neurons, n = 5. **c** ChIP analysis on the ERβ promoter in male amygdala neurons, n = 5. **d** ChIP analysis on the ERβ promoter in female amygdala neurons, n = 5. *, P < 0.05, vs VEH/CTL group; ¶, P < 0.05, vs NET/CTL group. Results are expressed as mean ± SEM

Postnatal resveratrol administration ameliorates prenatal norethindrone exposure-induced oxidative stress and dysfunction of mitochondria and lipid metabolism

We evaluated the effect of RSV treatment on prenatal NET exposure-induced ERβ suppression and the subsequent molecular consequences in the amygdala, including ROS generation, DNA damage, mitochondrial function and lipid metabolism. We found that prenatal NET exposure significantly increased superoxide anion (O_2^-) release by 2.27-fold (in male) and 1.88-fold (in female) respectively (see Fig. 4a); it increased 3-nitrotyrosine formation by 2.03-fold (in male) and 1.54-fold (in female) respectively (see Fig. 4b); it increased 8-OHdG formation by 2.65-fold (in male) and 2.27-fold (in female) respectively (see Fig. 4c); it increased γH2AX formation by 1.94-fold (in male) and 1.48-fold (in female) respectively (see Fig. 4d, e); it decreased mitochondrial DNA copies by 38% (in male) and 24% (in female) respectively (see Fig. 4f); it decreased

intracellular ATP level by 45% (in male) and 25% (in female) respectively (see Fig. 4g). Furthermore, it decreased in vivo fatty acid oxidation by 47% (in male) and 18% (in female) respectively (see Fig. 4h), and it decreased in vitro fatty acid uptake by 42% (in male) and 26% (in female) respectively (see Fig. 4i). RSV treatment partly reversed this effect in male offspring, while in female offspring, RSV completely diminished this effect. Furthermore, in VEH group, RSV treatment significantly increased mitochondrial function (see Fig. 4f, g) and in vivo fatty acid oxidation metabolism (see Fig. 4h) in both male and female offspring. On the other hand, RSV treatment increased in vitro fatty acid uptake (see Fig. 4i) in female offspring but not in male offspring from VEH group (see detailed statistical information in Additional file 1: Data S3). Our results indicate that RSV ameliorates prenatal NET exposure-induced oxidative stress and dysfunction of mitochondria and lipid metabolism, and that female

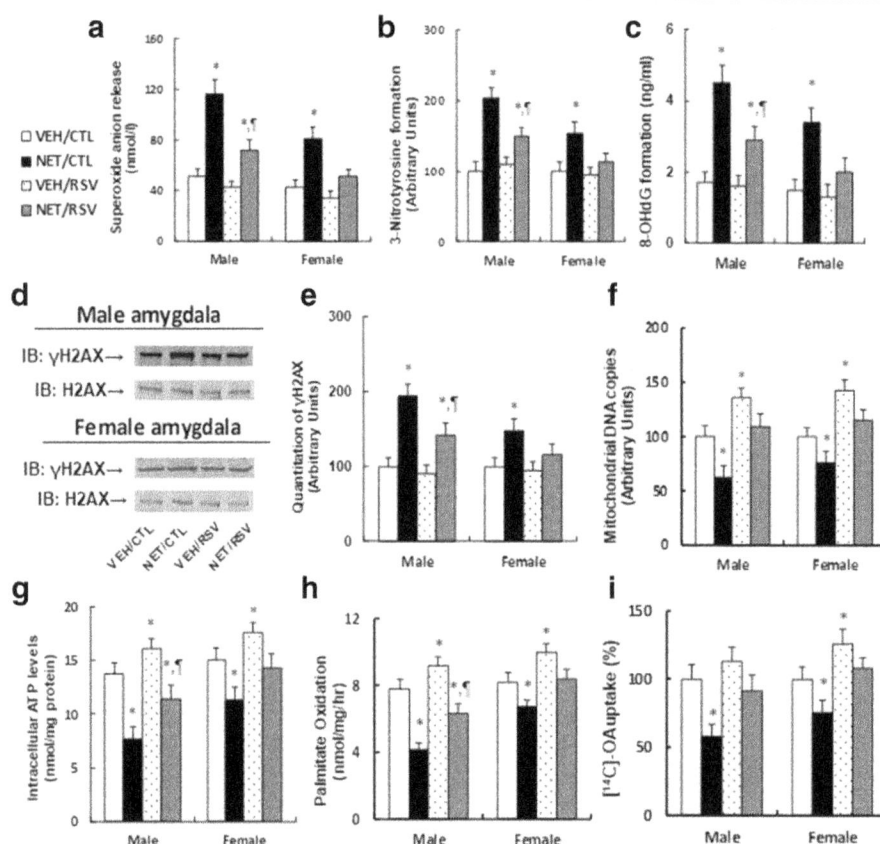

Fig. 4 Postnatal resveratrol treatment ameliorates prenatal norethindrone exposure-induced oxidative stress, dysfunction of mitochondria, and lipid metabolism. **a–h** The amygdala tissues were isolated from 10-week-old male/female offspring for further analysis. **a** In vivo superoxide anion release, $n = 5$. **b** Quantitation of 3-nitrotyrosine (3-NT) formation, $n = 5$. **c** 8-OHdG formation, $n = 5$. **d** Representative γH2AX western blotting band for both male (upper panel) and female (down panel) offspring. **e** Quantitation of γH2AX formation for **d**, $n = 5$. **f** Mitochondrial DNA copies, $n = 4$. **g** Intracellular ATP levels, $n = 5$. **h** The in vivo palmitate oxidation rate, $n = 5$. **i** The amygdala neurons were isolated from 10-week-old male/female offspring for in vitro ^{14}C-OA fatty acid uptake, $n = 5$. *, $P < 0.05$, vs VEH/CTL group; ¶, $P < 0.05$, vs NET/CTL group. Results are expressed as mean ± SEM

offspring were less responsive to NET exposure than male offspring.

Postnatal resveratrol treatment ameliorates prenatal norethindrone exposure-induced autism-like behavior

We measured the effect of RSV on prenatal NET exposure-induced autism-like behavior. In male offspring, prenatal NET exposure decreased buried marbles by 52% (see Fig. 5a), while there was no difference in female offspring. We then evaluated the social interaction time. In male offspring, the NET treatment decreased by 32% in sniffing, 48% in mounting, no difference in grooming partner, and 33% in total social interaction (see Fig. 5b), while RSV treatment completely diminished this effect. In female offspring, the NET treatment decreased by 20% in sniffing, no difference in mounting or grooming partner, and 22% in total social interaction (see Fig. 5c). Furthermore, the RSV treatment completely diminished this effect in both male and female offspring (see detailed statistical information in Additional file 1: Data S4). Our results indicate that RSV completely reverses prenatal NET exposure-induced autism-like behavior and that male offspring seem more sensitive to NET-induced effect compared to female offspring.

Postnatal resveratrol treatment ameliorates prenatal norethindrone exposure-induced autism-like behavior through ERβ activation

Prenatal NET exposure treated male offspring received lentivirus infusion of shERβ shown in Fig. 1b. We first measured the gene expression of ERβ, SOD2, and ERRα. The results showed that prenatal NET exposure significantly decreased mRNA levels (see Fig. 6a) and protein levels (see Fig. 6b, c) of those genes. We then measured prenatal NET exposure-mediated molecular consequences in the amygdala. The results showed that postnatal resveratrol treatment ameliorates prenatal NET exposure-induced oxidative stress (see Additional file 1: Figure S3a, b), DNA damage (see Additional file 1: Figure S3c, e), dysfunction of mitochondria (see Additional file 1: Figure S3f, g), and lipid metabolism (see Additional file 1: Figure S3 h, i) through ERβ activation. RSV treatment completely reversed this suppression effect, while ERβ knockdown (shERβ) significantly diminished the effect of RSV (see Additional file 1: Figure S3). Next, we investigated the potential effect of RSV treatment and ERβ expression on prenatal NET exposure-induced autism-like behavior in male offspring. We found that prenatal NET exposure (NET/EMP/CTL) decreased buried marbles by 32% (see Fig. 6d) compared to the control group. RSV treatment completely reversed prenatal NET exposure-induced

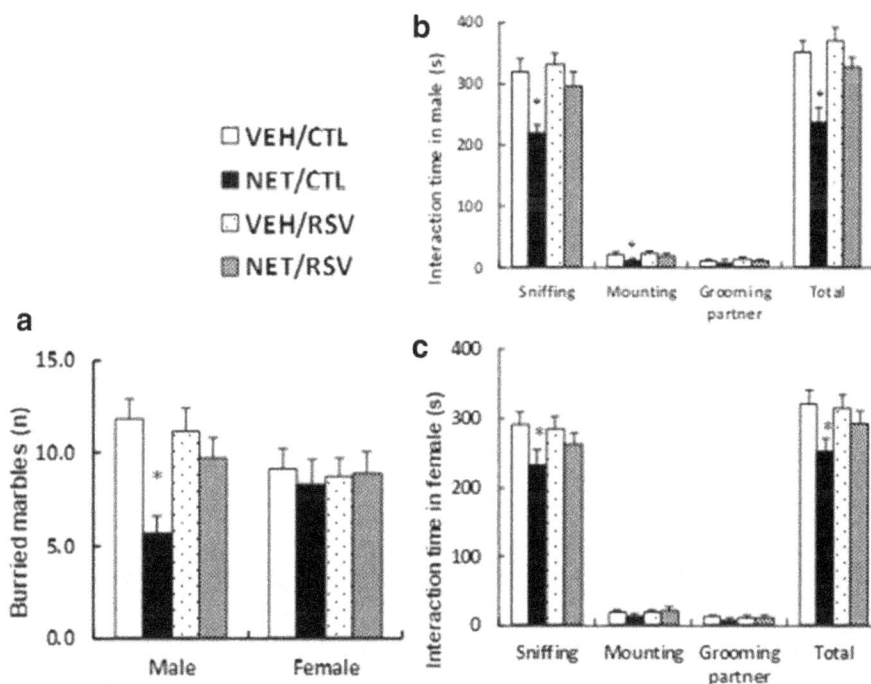

Fig. 5 Postnatal resveratrol treatment ameliorates prenatal norethindrone exposure-induced autism-like behavior. Three-month-old pregnant dams were exposed to NET (20 μg levonorgestrel) or VEH (vehicle, 5% ethanol in organic sesame oil) by subcutaneous daily injection of 0.1 ml for 21 days until pup delivery. Both male and female offspring were then treated by either control (CTL) or resveratrol (RSV) for 4 weeks starting from 5 weeks old. Both male and female offspring were used for autism-like behavior tests at 10 weeks old. **a** Buried marble tests, n = 9. **b**, **c** Social interaction time in both male (**b**) and female (**c**) offspring, n = 9. *, P < 0.05, vs VEH/CTL group; ¶, P < 0.05, vs NET/CTL group. Results are expressed as mean ± SEM

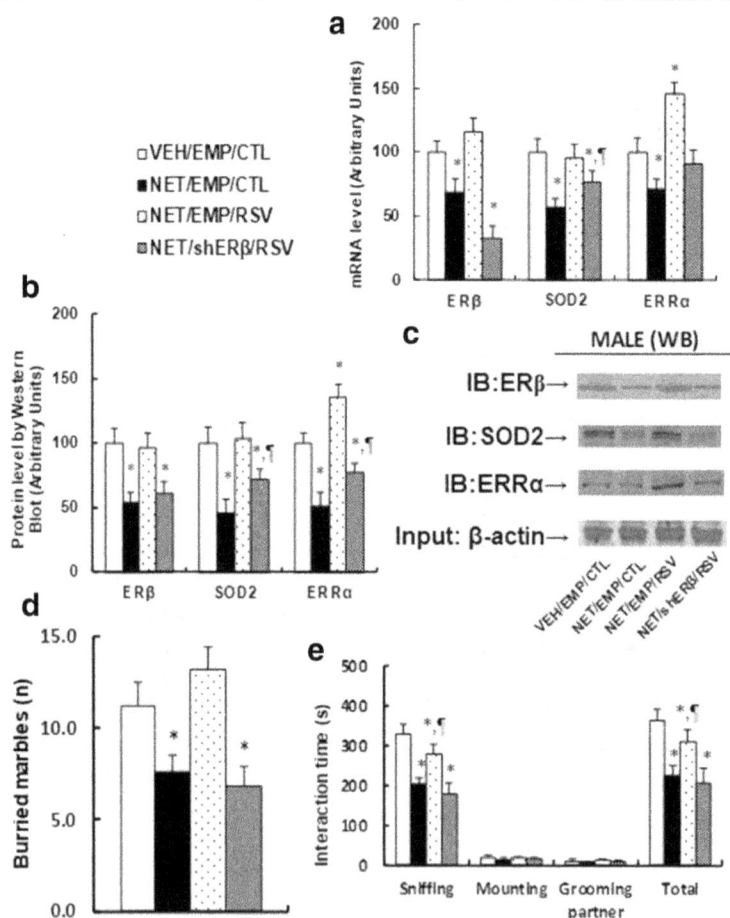

Fig. 6 Postnatal resveratrol treatment ameliorates prenatal norethindrone exposure-induced autism-like behavior through ERβ activation. The 8-week-old male offspring from VEH or NET group received either empty (EMP) or ERβ knockdown (shERβ) lentivirus infusion and were treated by either control (CTL) or resveratrol (RSV) for 4 weeks, and the offspring were sacrificed at 13 weeks of age for further analysis. **a–c** The amygdala tissues were isolated from 13-week-old treated male offspring for gene expression analysis. **a** The mRNA levels for gene expression, $n = 4$. **b** The quantitation of protein levels, $n = 5$. **c** Representative bands for western blots. **d** Buried marble tests, $n = 9$. **e** Interaction time, $n = 9$. *, $P < 0.05$, vs VEH/EMP/CTL group; ¶, $P < 0.05$, vs NET/EMP/CTL group; #, $P < 0.05$, vs NET/EMP/RSV group. Results are expressed as mean ± SEM

autism-like behavior, while ERβ knockdown (shERβ) completely diminished the effect of RSV. We also measured the social interaction time (see Fig. 6e). The results showed that prenatal NET exposure resulted in a 38% decrease in sniffing and a 37% decrease in total social interaction, while it showed no difference in mounting and grooming partner. RSV treatment partly diminished this effect, while ERβ knockdown (shERβ) completely diminished the effect of RSV (see detailed statistical information in Additional file 1: Data S5). Our results indicate that RSV ameliorates prenatal norethindrone exposure-induced autism-like behavior in offspring through ERβ activation.

Prenatal resveratrol treatment prevents prenatal norethindrone exposure-induced autism-like behavior

Three-month-old pregnant dams were exposed to either NET (20 μg norethindrone) or VEH (vehicle) for ~ 21 days during the whole pregnancy, and they also received either control (PreCTL) or resveratrol (PreRSV) prenatal treatment by oral administration. Both male and female offspring at 10 weeks of age were used for biomedical analysis and autism-like behavior testing. We first measured the ERβ gene expression (see Fig. 7a) and found that prenatal RSV treatment completely reversed prenatal NET exposure-induced ERβ suppression. We also measured the epigenetic changes with histone methylation on the ERβ promoter in both male (see Additional file 1: Figure S4a) and female offspring (see Additional file 1: Figure S4b). We found that prenatal RSV treatment completely normalized prenatal NET exposure-induced histone methylation, including H3K9me2 and H3K27me3. We also measured the oxidative stress, including superoxide anion (see Additional file 1: Figure S4c) and 8-OHdG formation (see Additional file 1: Figure S4d); mitochondria functions, including mitochondrial DNA copies (see Additional file 1: Figure S4e) and

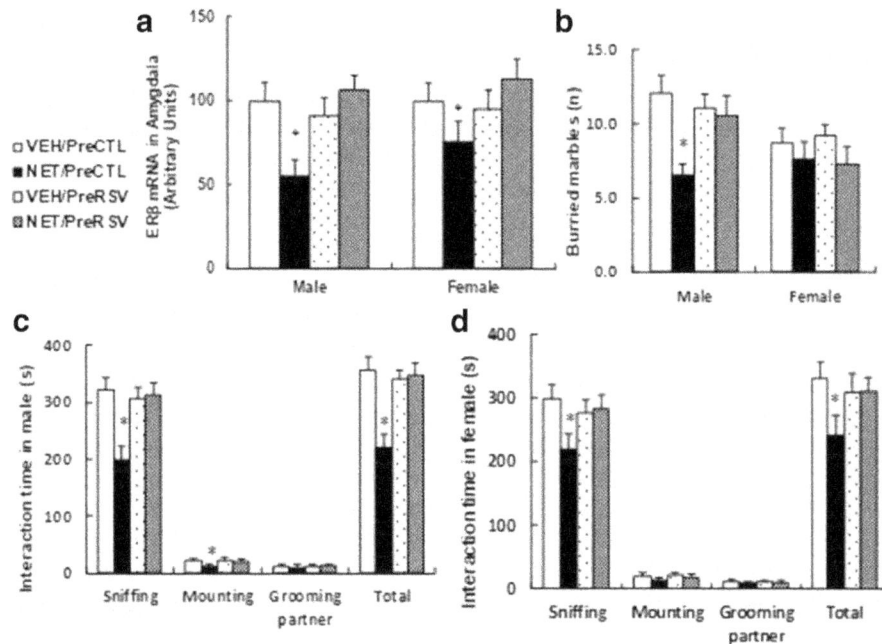

Fig. 7 Prenatal resveratrol treatment prevents prenatal norethindrone exposure-induced autism-like behavior. Three-month old pregnant dams were exposed to NET (20 μg norethindrone) or VEH (vehicle only) by subcutaneous daily injection of 0.1 ml for 21 days until pup delivery. In addition, all the dams received either control (PreCTL) or resveratrol (PreRSV) treatment by oral administration at the same time. At 10 weeks of age, both male and female offspring were used for gene expression analysis and autism-like behavior testing. **a** The ERβ mRNA level, $n = 4$. **b** Buried marble tests, $n = 9$. **c, d** Interaction time for both male (**c**) and female (**d**) offspring, $n = 9$. *, $P < 0.05$, vs VEH/CTL group. Results are expressed as mean ± SEM

intracellular ATP level (see Additional file 1: Figure S4f); as well as lipid metabolism, including palmitate oxidation (see Additional file 1: Figure S4 g) and fatty acid uptake (see Additional file 1: Figure S4 h). It showed that prenatal RSV treatment completely (in female offspring) or partly (in male offspring) reversed NET-induced effect compared to control group. Finally, we measured autism-like behavior, including buried marble testing (see Fig. 7b) and social interaction time testing for both male (see Fig. 7c) and female offspring (see Fig. 7d). We found that prenatal RSV treatment completely reversed prenatal NET exposure-induced autism-like behavior in both male and female offspring (see detailed statistical information in Additional file 1: Data S6). Our results indicate that prenatal RSV treatment prevents prenatal NET exposure-induced autism-like behavior.

Discussion

In this study, we show that prenatal progestin exposure decreases ERβ expression in the brain and induces autism-like behavior in offspring. Oral administration of RSV reverses prenatal progestin exposure-induced ERβ suppression by demethylation of DNA and histone on the ERβ promoter in the amygdala in offspring. RSV-mediated ERβ activation then upregulates the expression of SOD2 and ERRα and minimizes the

oxidative stress and dysfunction of mitochondria [6] and lipid metabolism, subsequently ameliorating prenatal progestin exposure-induced autism-like behavior. In addition, prenatal resveratrol treatment prevents prenatal progestin exposure-induced autism-like behavior in offspring.

Association of progestin and ASD development

Natural progesterone or synthetic progestins, such as hydroxyprogesterone caproate (OHPC), have been used to reduce the incidence of preterm birth [44], where there is a signal for embryo-fetal toxicity associated with OHPC in the two largest clinical trials [45]. Progestin is the major component in hormone replacement therapy (HRT) and combined oral contraceptive (COC), and taking oral contraceptives when pregnancy begins is a strong risk factor for ASD development [8]. Also, progestin concentrations found in water can suppress ERβ expression and affect brain functions [21, 46]. Our current data show that prenatal progestin exposure suppresses ERβ expression in the amygdala [47] and subsequently contributes to ASD development [9]. This consideration may potentially apply to humans, as prenatal progestin exposure may be associated with ASD development via directly or indirectly taking progestin compounds, which includes contraceptive pills, progesterone/progestin pills to prevent threatened abortion, and COC-contaminated drinking water and seafood during pregnancy [21].

Resveratrol-mediated demethylation of DNA and histone on the ERβ promoter

It has been reported that RSV inhibits DNA methyltransferases (DNMTs) [48] and subsequently decreases DNA methylation [49] and histone methylation [50, 51]. We show that RSV in vivo treatment significantly decreases both DNA methylation and histone methylation on the ERβ promoter, and subsequently increases ERβ expression. This is the first time we report the potential neuroprotective mechanism of RSV through RSV-mediated demethylation with subsequent gene activation. Furthermore, we show that RSV treatment can only demethylate prenatal NET exposure-mediated hypermethylation on both DNA and histone, while it has little effect on basal methylation in the prenatal VEH exposure group. This suggests that RSV-mediated demethylation is not only due to RSV-mediated DNMT inhibition, but rather that some other indirect factors may also be involved [52].

Resveratrol-mediated ERβ activation

We have previously reported that ERβ expression is regulated by SIRT1 through complexes of SIRT1-PPARγ/RXR-p300 on the ERβ promoter [14], and RSV has been reported to be able to activate SIRT1 either directly [53] or indirectly through AMPK activation [54]. We suppose that resveratrol treatment should be able to activate SIRT1 and subsequently upregulate ERβ expression, while our results show that RSV treatment significantly increases ERβ expression, but neither SIRT1 expression nor activity changes in the amygdala, suggesting that a SIRT1-independent ERβ activating mechanism is required for RSV-mediated ERβ activation. Our further investigation shows that RSV treatment in vivo significantly alters DNA methylation and epigenetic changes with demethylation on the ERβ promoter in the amygdala, which subsequently activates ERβ expression with ameliorated autism-like behavior. This is the first time we report the potential mechanism for RSV-mediated gene activation through demethylation of either DNA or histone in the nervous system, which sheds a light on rescuing ASD symptoms through resveratrol treatment.

Resveratrol-mediated activation of SOD2 and ERRα

Our results show that resveratrol (RSV) treatment reverses prenatal NET exposure-induced methylation of DNA and histone on the ERβ promoter and subsequently reverses prenatal NET exposure-induced ERβ suppression, but it does not change the basal DNA and histone methylation level and subsequent basal ERβ expression. On the other hand, the basal expression level of SOD2 and ERRα increases significantly in response to RSV treatment in not only the amygdala, but also in the hypothalamus and hippocampus; this kind of gene activation is not regulated by ERβ as reported previously [11, 12] since the basal ERβ expression has no change in response to RSV treatment. Also, the in vitro cell culture experiments show that RSV treatment significantly increases the expression of SOD2 and ERRα, and female offspring seem more responsive to RSV treatment compared to male offspring. This can be explained because the female offspring have higher basal ERβ expression compared to male offspring, or because RSV can directly activate SOD2 and ERRα expression through another pathway, such as PGC1α [53]. Furthermore, in female rats, RSV increased expression of both SOD2 and ERRα, even in rats that were not exposed to NET, suggesting a more general effect. Our results indicate that another factor other than ERβ may also be involved in regulating the gene activation of SOD2 and ERRα. This can be explained by RSV-mediated PGC-1α activation, as it has been reported that RSV activates PGC-1α either by SIRT1 [53] or AMPK (54)-mediated indirect activation or by direct deacetylation of PGC-1α [55], and the activated PGC-1α then upregulates the expression of ERRα [56, 57] and SOD2 [58].

Limitations

This study has several limitations. In animal behavioral tests, the marble burying test and the social interaction time were used for the evaluation of autism-like behavior, while these tests do not really reflect adequate tests of this syndrome. The marble burying test has been used to describe anxiety and repetitive behavior, but not clearly presented as a test for autism. A more common test for autism should be the social preference test and the ultrasonic vocalization test. In addition, during the animal treatment, prenatal exposure of either progestin or resveratrol was used throughout the whole pregnancy period (21 days), while this rarely happens in the human being. Usually, the first trimester during the pregnancy is considered as the most sensitive period for the prenatal exposure of risk factors; in this case, prenatal exposure of progestin or resveratrol during the first 7 days of pregnancy in dams may be more reasonable for this treatment. On the other hand, we were using higher doses of resveratrol and progestin for the treatment of pregnant dams in this study in order to achieve a significant effect in animals to mimic the long-term exposure of lower doses in humans, and this may be a potential limitation for human application.

Conclusions

Our results indicate that prenatal progestin exposure is a strong risk factor for autism-like behavior. Many potential clinical progestin applications, including oral contraceptive pills, preterm birth drugs, and progestin-contaminated drinking water or seafood, may be risk factors for potential ASD development. In addition, resveratrol may be a good candidate for rescuing and preventing ASD symptoms in humans through ERβ upregulation.

Additional file

Additional file 1: Table S1. Sequences of primers for the real time quantitative PCR (qPCR). **Figure S1.** Postnatal resveratrol treatment increases expression of SOD2 and ERRα, while it has no effect on the expression of ERβ and SIRT1 in the hypothalamus and hippocampus of prenatal norethindrone exposed offspring. **Figure S2.** Both resveratrol and norethindrone treatment do not change the expression and activity of SIRT1 in the amygdala. **Figure S3.** Postnatal resveratrol treatment ameliorates prenatal norethindrone exposure-induced oxidative stress, dysfunction of mitochondria and lipid metabolism through ERβ activation. **Figure S4.** Prenatal resveratrol treatment prevents prenatal norethindrone exposure-induced epigenetic changes, oxidative stress, and the dysfunction of mitochondria and lipid metabolism. Data S1. Statistical details for Fig. 2. Data S2. Statistical details for Fig. 3. Data S3. Statistical details for Fig. 4. Data S4. Statistical details for Fig. 5. Data S5. Statistical details for Fig. 6. Data S6. Statistical details for Fig. 7. (DOCX 402 kb)

Abbreviations

ASD: Autism spectrum disorder; ChIP: Chromatin immunoprecipitation; COC: Combined oral contraceptive; E2: 17β-estradiol; EMP: Empty control; ERRα: Estrogen-related receptor α; ERβ: Estrogen receptor β; HRT: Hormone replacement therapy; LNG: Levonorgestrel; MBT: Marbles burying test; MPA: Medroxyprogesterone acetate; NEN: Norethynodrel; NES: Nestorone; NET: Norethindrone; NETA: Norethindrone acetate; NGM: Norgestimate; OHPC: Hydroxyprogesterone caproate; P4: Progesterone; RSV: Resveratrol; SI: Social interaction; SOD2: Mitochondrial superoxide dismutase; VEH: Vehicle control

Funding

This study was financially supported by The National Natural Science Foundation of China, Project #: 81772097; Natural Science Foundation of Hubei Province of China, Project #: 2016CFB473; and Bureau of Public Health of Hainan Province, Key Project # 14A110065.

Authors' contributions

PY wrote the paper. PY, WX, and HC designed and interpreted the experiments. AY, XG, ZC, and XH performed the rat surgery and social behavior testing. XW, YW, and XG performed the virus preparation and gene analysis. ZL, YJ, and MX performed the amygdala isolation and analysis. WX, XG, and LL performed the remaining experiments. All authors read, edited, and approved the final manuscript.

Competing interests

Authors including Drs Xiaohu Ge, Xiaoyan Wang, Yifei Wang, and Haijia Chen, were employed by the company Guangzhou SALIAI Stem Cell Science and Technology Co. LTD. All other authors declare that they have no competing interests.

References

1. Abrahams BS, Geschwind DH. Advances in autism genetics: on the threshold of a new neurobiology. Nat Rev Genet. 2008;9(5):341–55.
2. Volkmar FR, Pauls D. Autism. Lancet. 2003;362(9390):1133–41.
3. Bralten J, van Hulzen KJ, Martens MB, Galesloot TE, Arias Vasquez A, Kiemeney LA, Buitelaar JK, Muntjewerff JW, Franke B, Poelmans G. Autism spectrum disorders and autistic traits share genetics and biology. Mol Psychiatry. 2018;23(5):1205–12.
4. Schaafsma SM, Pfaff DW. Etiologies underlying sex differences in autism spectrum disorders. Front Neuroendocrinol. 2014;35(3):255–71.
5. Modabbernia A, Velthorst E, Reichenberg A. Environmental risk factors for autism: an evidence-based review of systematic reviews and meta-analyses. Mol Autism. 2017;8:13.
6. Rossignol DA, Frye RE. A review of research trends in physiological abnormalities in autism spectrum disorders: immune dysregulation, inflammation, oxidative stress, mitochondrial dysfunction and environmental toxicant exposures. Mol Psychiatry. 2012;17(4):389–401.
7. Strifert K. An epigenetic basis for autism spectrum disorder risk and oral contraceptive use. Med Hypotheses. 2015;85(6):1006–11.
8. Whitaker-Azmitia PM, Lobel M, Moyer A. Low maternal progesterone may contribute to both obstetrical complications and autism. Med Hypotheses. 2014;82(3):313–8.
9. Zou Y, Lu Q, Zheng D, Chu Z, Liu Z, Chen H, Ruan Q, Ge X, Zhang Z, Wang X, et al. Prenatal levonorgestrel exposure induces autism-like behavior in offspring through ERbeta suppression in the amygdala. Mol Autism. 2017;8:46.
10. Crider A, Thakkar R, Ahmed AO, Pillai A. Dysregulation of estrogen receptor beta (ERbeta), aromatase (CYP19A1), and ER co-activators in the middle frontal gyrus of autism spectrum disorder subjects. Mol Autism. 2014;5(1):46.
11. Liu Z, Gou Y, Zhang H, Zuo H, Zhang H, Liu Z, Yao D. Estradiol improves cardiovascular function through up-regulation of SOD2 on vascular wall. Redox Biol. 2014;3(0):88–99.
12. Li H, Liu Z, Gou Y, Yu H, Siminelakis S, Wang S, Kong D, Zhou Y, Liu Z, Ding Y, et al. Estradiol mediates vasculoprotection via ERRalpha-dependent regulation of lipid and ROS metabolism in the endothelium. J Mol Cell Cardiol. 2015;87:92–101.
13. Zhan Y, Liu Z, Li M, Ding T, Zhang L, Lu Q, Liu X, Zhang Z, Vlessidis A, Aw TY, et al. ERbeta expression in the endothelium ameliorates ischemia/reperfusion-mediated oxidative burst and vascular injury. Free Radic Biol Med. 2016;96:223–33.
14. Kong D, Zhan Y, Liu Z, Ding T, Li M, Yu H, Zhang L, Li H, Luo A, Zhang D, et al. SIRT1-mediated ERbeta suppression in the endothelium contributes to vascular aging. Aging Cell. 2016;15(6):1092–102.
15. Rossignol DA, Frye RE. Evidence linking oxidative stress, mitochondrial dysfunction, and inflammation in the brain of individuals with autism. Front Physiol. 2014;5:150.
16. Mamidala MP, Polinedi A, Kumar PT, Rajesh N, Vallamkonda OR, Udani V, Singhal N, Rajesh V. Maternal hormonal interventions as a risk factor for autism spectrum disorder: an epidemiological assessment from India. J Biosci. 2013;38(5):887–92.
17. Baron-Cohen S, Auyeung B, Norgaard-Pedersen B, Hougaard DM, Abdallah MW, Melgaard L, Cohen AS, Chakrabarti B, Ruta L, Lombardo MV. Elevated fetal steroidogenic activity in autism. Mol Psychiatry. 2015;20(3):369–76.
18. Gillberg C, Fernell E, Kocovska E, Minnis H, Bourgeron T, Thompson L, Allely CS. The role of cholesterol metabolism and various steroid abnormalities in autism spectrum disorders: a hypothesis paper. Autism Res. 2017;10(6):1022–44.
19. Liu L, Zhao L, She H, Chen S, Wang JM, Wong C, McClure K, Sitruk-Ware R, Brinton RD. Clinically relevant progestins regulate neurogenic and neuroprotective responses in vitro and in vivo. Endocrinology. 2010;151(12):5782–94.
20. Willing J, Wagner CK. Exposure to the synthetic progestin, 17alpha-hydroxyprogesterone caproate during development impairs cognitive flexibility in adulthood. Endocrinology. 2016;157(1):77–82.
21. Petersen LH, Hala D, Carty D, Cantu M, Martinovic D, Huggett DB. Effects of progesterone and norethindrone on female fathead minnow (Pimephales promelas) steroidogenesis. Environ Toxicol Chem. 2015;34(2):379–90.
22. Aguirre C, Jayaraman A, Pike C, Baudry M. Progesterone inhibits estrogen-mediated neuroprotection against excitotoxicity by down-regulating estrogen receptor-beta. J Neurochem. 2010;115(5):1277–87.

23. Jayaraman A, Pike CJ. Progesterone attenuates oestrogen neuroprotection via downregulation of oestrogen receptor expression in cultured neurones. J Neuroendocrinol. 2009;21(1):77–81.

24. Dasgupta B, Milbrandt J. Resveratrol stimulates AMP kinase activity in neurons. Proc Natl Acad Sci U S A. 2007;104(17):7217–22.

25. Baur JA, Sinclair DA. Therapeutic potential of resveratrol: the in vivo evidence. Nat Rev Drug Discov. 2006;5(6):493–506.

26. Han YS, Zheng WH, Bastianetto S, Chabot JG, Quirion R. Neuroprotective effects of resveratrol against beta-amyloid-induced neurotoxicity in rat hippocampal neurons: involvement of protein kinase C. Br J Pharmacol. 2004;141(6):997–1005.

27. Valenzano DR, Terzibasi E, Genade T, Cattaneo A, Domenici L, Cellerino A. Resveratrol prolongs lifespan and retards the onset of age-related markers in a short-lived vertebrate. Curr Biol. 2006;16(3):296–300.

28. Parker JA, Arango M, Abderrahmane S, Lambert E, Tourette C, Catoire H, Neri C. Resveratrol rescues mutant polyglutamine cytotoxicity in nematode and mammalian neurons. Nat Genet. 2005;37(4):349–50.

29. Bambini-Junior V, Zanatta G, Della Flora Nunes G, Mueller de Melo G, Michels M, Fontes-Dutra M, Nogueira Freire V, Riesgo R, Gottfried C. Resveratrol prevents social deficits in animal model of autism induced by valproic acid. Neurosci Lett. 2014;583:176–81.

30. Bakheet SA, Alzahrani MZ, Nadeem A, Ansari MA, Zoheir KMA, Attia SM, Al-Ayadhi LY, Ahmad SF. Resveratrol treatment attenuates chemokine receptor expression in the BTBR T+tf/J mouse model of autism. Mol Cell Neurosci. 2016;77:1–10.

31. Hu M, Richard JE, Maliqueo M, Kokosar M, Fornes R, Benrick A, Jansson T, Ohlsson C, Wu X, Skibicka KP, et al. Maternal testosterone exposure increases anxiety-like behavior and impacts the limbic system in the offspring. Proc Natl Acad Sci U S A. 2015;112(46):14348–53.

32. Bahi A. Sustained lentiviral-mediated overexpression of microRNA124a in the dentate gyrus exacerbates anxiety- and autism-like behaviors associated with neonatal isolation in rats. Behav Brain Res. 2016;311:298–308.

33. Hippocampal BA. BDNF overexpression or microR124a silencing reduces anxiety- and autism-like behaviors in rats. Behav Brain Res. 2017;326:281–90.

34. Mufford JT, Paetkau MJ, Flood NJ, Regev-Shoshani G, Miller CC, Church JS. The development of a non-invasive behavioral model of thermal heat stress in laboratory mice (Mus musculus). J Neurosci Methods. 2016;268:189–95.

35. Hay CW, Shanley L, Davidson S, Cowie P, Lear M, McGuffin P, Riedel G, McEwan IJ, MacKenzie A. Functional effects of polymorphisms on glucocorticoid receptor modulation of human anxiogenic substance-P gene promoter activity in primary amygdala neurones. Psychoneuroendocrinology. 2014;47:43–55.

36. Ogino S, Kawasaki T, Brahmandam M, Cantor M, Kirkner GJ, Spiegelman D, Makrigiorgos GM, Weisenberger DJ, Laird PW, Loda M, et al. Precision and performance characteristics of bisulfite conversion and real-time PCR (MethyLight) for quantitative DNA methylation analysis. J Mol Diagn. 2006; 8(2):209–17.

37. Eads CA, Danenberg KD, Kawakami K, Saltz LB, Blake C, Shibata D, Danenberg PV, Laird PW. MethyLight: a high-throughput assay to measure DNA methylation. Nucleic Acids Res. 2000;28(8):E32.

38. Nosho K, Irahara N, Shima K, Kure S, Kirkner GJ, Schernhammer ES, Hazra A, Hunter DJ, Quackenbush J, Spiegelman D, et al. Comprehensive biostatistical analysis of CpG island methylator phenotype in colorectal cancer using a large population-based sample. PLoS One. 2008;3(11):e3698.

39. Hou X, Xu S, Maitland-Toolan KA, Sato K, Jiang B, Ido Y, Lan F, Walsh K, Wierzbicki M, Verbeuren TJ, et al. SIRT1 regulates hepatocyte lipid metabolism through activating AMP-activated protein kinase. J Biol Chem. 2008;283(29):20015–26.

40. Yao D, Shi W, Gou Y, Zhou X, Yee Aw T, Zhou Y, Liu Z. Fatty acid-mediated intracellular iron translocation: a synergistic mechanism of oxidative injury. Free Radic Biol Med. 2005;39(10):1385–98.

41. Hagberg CE, Falkevall A, Wang X, Larsson E, Huusko J, Nilsson I, van Meeteren LA, Samen E, Lu L, Vanwildemeersch M, et al. Vascular endothelial growth factor B controls endothelial fatty acid uptake. Nature. 2010; 464(7290):917–21.

42. Taib B, Bouyakdan K, Hryhorczuk C, Rodaros D, Fulton S, Alquier T. Glucose regulates hypothalamic long-chain fatty acid metabolism via AMP-activated kinase (AMPK) in neurons and astrocytes. J Biol Chem. 2013;288(52):37216–29.

43. Huynh FK, Green MF, Koves TR, Hirschey MD. Measurement of fatty acid oxidation rates in animal tissues and cell lines. Methods Enzymol. 2014;542: 391–405.

44. Sanchez-Ramos L, Kaunitz AM, Delke I. Progestational agents to prevent preterm birth: a meta-analysis of randomized controlled trials. Obstet Gynecol. 2005;105(2):273–9.

45. Christian MS, Brent RL, Calda P. Embryo-fetal toxicity signals for 17alpha-hydroxyprogesterone caproate in high-risk pregnancies: a review of the non-clinical literature for embryo-fetal toxicity with progestins. J Matern Fetal Neonatal Med. 2007;20(2):89–112.

46. Giatti S, Melcangi RC, Pesaresi M. The other side of progestins: effects in the brain. J Mol Endocrinol. 2016;57(2):R109–26.

47. van Wingen GA, van Broekhoven F, Verkes RJ, Petersson KM, Backstrom T, Buitelaar JK, Fernandez G. Progesterone selectively increases amygdala reactivity in women. Mol Psychiatry. 2008;13(3):325–33.

48. Hardy TM, Tollefsbol TO. Epigenetic diet: impact on the epigenome and cancer. Epigenomics. 2011;3(4):503–18.

49. Lou XD, Wang HD, Xia SJ, Skog S, Sun J. Effects of resveratrol on the expression and DNA methylation of cytokine genes in diabetic rat aortas. Arch Immunol Ther Exp. 2014;62(4):329–40.

50. Paluszczak J, Krajka-Kuzniak V, Baer-Dubowska W. The effect of dietary polyphenols on the epigenetic regulation of gene expression in MCF7 breast cancer cells. Toxicol Lett. 2010;192(2):119–25.

51. Han S, Uludag MO, Usanmaz SE, Ayaloglu-Butun F, Akcali KC, Demirel-Yilmaz E. Resveratrol affects histone 3 lysine 27 methylation of vessels and blood biomarkers in DOCA salt-induced hypertension. Mol Biol Rep. 2015;42(1):35–42.

52. Papoutsis AJ, Lamore SD, Wondrak GT, Selmin OI, Romagnolo DF. Resveratrol prevents epigenetic silencing of BRCA-1 by the aromatic hydrocarbon receptor in human breast cancer cells. J Nutr. 2010;140(9):1607–14.

53. Lagouge M, Argmann C, Gerhart-Hines Z, Meziane H, Lerin C, Daussin F, Messadeq N, Milne J, Lambert P, Elliott P, et al. Resveratrol improves mitochondrial function and protects against metabolic disease by activating SIRT1 and PGC-1alpha. Cell. 2006;127(6):1109–22.

54. Canto C, Gerhart-Hines Z, Feige JN, Lagouge M, Noriega L, Milne JC, Elliott PJ, Puigserver P, Auwerx J. AMPK regulates energy expenditure by modulating NAD+ metabolism and SIRT1 activity. Nature. 2009;458(7241):1056–60.

55. Feige JN, Lagouge M, Canto C, Strehle A, Houten SM, Milne JC, Lambert PD, Mataki C, Elliott PJ, Auwerx J. Specific SIRT1 activation mimics low energy levels and protects against diet-induced metabolic disorders by enhancing fat oxidation. Cell Metab. 2008;8(5):347–58.

56. Lin J, Handschin C, Spiegelman BM. Metabolic control through the PGC-1 family of transcription coactivators. Cell Metab. 2005;1(6):361–70.

57. Schreiber SN, Emter R, Hock MB, Knutti D, Cardenas J, Podvinec M, Oakeley EJ, Kralli A. The estrogen-related receptor alpha (ERRalpha) functions in PPARgamma coactivator 1alpha (PGC-1alpha)-induced mitochondrial biogenesis. Proc Natl Acad Sci U S A. 2004;101(17):6472–7.

58. St-Pierre J, Drori S, Uldry M, Silvaggi JM, Rhee J, Jager S, Handschin C, Zheng K, Lin J, Yang W, et al. Suppression of reactive oxygen species and neurodegeneration by the PGC-1 transcriptional coactivators. Cell. 2006; 127(2):397–408.

5

Characterization and structure-activity relationships of indenoisoquinoline-derived topoisomerase I inhibitors in unsilencing the dormant Ube3a gene associated with Angelman syndrome

Hyeong-Min Lee[1], Ellen P. Clark[1], M. Bram Kuijer[1], Mark Cushman[2], Yves Pommier[3] and Benjamin D. Philpot[1,4*] (iD)

Abstract

Background: Angelman syndrome (AS) is a severe neurodevelopmental disorder lacking effective therapies. AS is caused by mutations in ubiquitin protein ligase E3A (UBE3A), which is genomically imprinted such that only the maternally inherited copy is expressed in neurons. We previously demonstrated that topoisomerase I (Top1) inhibitors could successfully reactivate the dormant paternal allele of Ube3a in neurons of a mouse model of AS. We also previously showed that one such Top1 inhibitor, topotecan, could unsilence paternal UBE3A in induced pluripotent stem cell-derived neurons from individuals with AS. Although topotecan has been well-studied and is FDA-approved for cancer therapy, its limited CNS bioavailability will likely restrict the therapeutic use of topotecan in AS. The goal of this study was to identify additional Top1 inhibitors with similar efficacy as topotecan, with the expectation that these could be tested in the future for safety and CNS bioavailability to assess their potential as AS therapeutics.

Methods: We tested 13 indenoisoquinoline-derived Top1 inhibitors to identify compounds that unsilence the paternal allele of Ube3a in mouse neurons. Primary cortical neurons were isolated from embryonic day 14.5 (E14.5) mice with a Ube3a-YFP fluorescent tag on the paternal allele ($Ube3a^{m+/pYFP}$ mice) or mice that lack the maternal Ube3a allele and hence model AS ($Ube3a^{m-/p+}$ mice). Neurons were cultured for 7 days, treated with drug for 72 h, and examined for paternal UBE3A protein expression by Western blot or fluorescence immunostaining. Dose responses of the compounds were determined across a log range of drug treatments, and cytotoxicity was tested using a luciferase-based assay.

Results: All 13 indenoisoquinoline-derived Top1 inhibitors unsilenced paternal Ube3a. Several compounds exhibited favorable paternal Ube3a unsilencing properties, similar to topotecan, and of these, indotecan (LMP400) was the most effective based on estimated E_{max} (maximum response of unsilencing paternal Ube3a) and EC_{50} (half maximal effective concentration).

(Continued on next page)

* Correspondence: bphilpot@med.unc.edu
[1]Department of Cell Biology and Physiology, University of North Carolina School of Medicine, Neuroscience Research Building, Room 5119 115 Mason Farm Rd., Campus Box 7545, Chapel Hill, NC 27599-7545, USA
[4]UNC Neuroscience Center, Carolina Institute for Developmental Disabilities, University of North Carolina School of Medicine, Chapel Hill, NC, USA
Full list of author information is available at the end of the article

(Continued from previous page)

Conclusions: We provide pharmacological profiles of indenoisoquinoline-derived Top1 inhibitors as paternal *Ube3a* unsilencers. All 13 tested compounds were effective at unsilencing paternal *Ube3a*, although with variable efficacy and potency. Indotecan (LMP400) demonstrated a better pharmacological profile of *Ube3a* unsilencing compared to our previous lead compound, topotecan. Taken together, indotecan and its structural analogues are potential AS therapeutics whose translational potential in AS treatment should be further assessed.

Keywords: Angelman syndrome, UBE3A, Topoisomerase I, Topotecan, Indenoisoquinoline, Topoisomerase inhibitor, Indotecan

Background

Angelman syndrome (AS) is a severe neurodevelopmental disorder characterized by developmental delay, intellectual disability, speech impairment, seizures, and ataxia [1–5]. AS has a prevalence of 1:15,000 [6, 7], and these individuals need care across their full lifespan, yet no cure currently exists. Thus, it is of great importance to develop treatments for AS. AS is caused by mutation of the ubiquitin protein ligase E3A (*UBE3A*) gene, which is genomically imprinted. Only the maternally inherited copy is expressed in neurons [8], whereas *UBE3A* is biallelically expressed in most other tissues. This neuron-specific imprinting provides insight into why deletions or mutations in the maternal copy of *UBE3A* primarily impact brain function and cause AS. However, the paternal *UBE3A* allele is intact, as demonstrated by biallelic expression in other tissues, raising the possibility that AS could be treated by unsilencing the dormant paternal *UBE3A* allele in neurons.

This led us to try pharmacological approaches to identify small molecules capable of unsilencing the dormant copy of *UBE3A*. In a previous study, we developed a high-content assay to identify small molecules that could unsilence paternal *Ube3a* in mouse primary neurons. In that screen, we used knock-in mice carrying a yellow fluorescent protein (YFP)-tagged *Ube3a* reporter, allowing us to visualize maternal- or paternal-specific expression of *Ube3a-YFP* in cultured neurons. As expected, *Ube3a-YFP* was expressed in cultured neurons when inherited maternally but was not expressed (silenced) when inherited paternally. We found that topoisomerase I (Top1) inhibitors (e.g., topotecan) could effectively unsilence paternal *Ube3a* in mice [9], raising the possibility that topotecan or similar compounds [10] could become treatments for AS. The translational potential was supported by evidence that topotecan treatment biochemically rescued the function of UBE3A, unsilenced *Ube3a* in vivo in mice, and unsilenced paternal *UBE3A* in induced pluripotent stem cell-derived neurons of AS patients [11].

Topotecan is FDA-approved for the treatment of cancer and is well tolerated in adult and pediatric cancer patients [12–15]. It is also used to treat brain tumors [16, 17]. Topotecan crosses the BBB more readily than many topoisomerase inhibitors [18]. However, active pumps extrude

topotecan from the brain, which limits its functional CNS bioavailability [19, 20]. Moreover, topotecan can produce some toxicities [21, 22]. These limitations prompted us to search for novel Top1 inhibitors with better CNS bioavailability and improved safety profiles.

Indenoisoquinoline-derived Top1 inhibitors offer a promising class of compounds for paternal *Ube3a* unsilencing as many of these compounds produce particularly stable Top1 cleavage complexes [23–25], which we have shown are critical for producing paternal *Ube3a* unsilencing [26]. Over 300 indenoisoquinoline derivatives have been tested, some of which are very potent Top1 poisons and show antitumor activity in mouse models [10, 27–31]. These Top1 inhibitors work by blocking the enzymatic activity of Top1 by stabilizing cleavage complexes, which are compound-bound intermediates of Top1-DNA [10, 23–25, 32]. More importantly, when compared to topotecan, indenoisoquinoline-derived Top1 inhibitors demonstrate improved characteristics such as greater chemical stability of these cleavage complexes. In addition, they target a unique DNA sequence for cleavage (indenoisoquinolines --G$^\downarrow$C-- vs. topotecan --T$^\downarrow$G--) [23–25, 32].

The goal of this study was to establish indenoisoquinoline derivatives that could effectively unsilence paternal *Ube3a*, with the expectation that some of these compounds might prove to be safe and have favorable CNS bioavailability. All of the tested compounds showed a capacity to unsilence the paternal *Ube3a* allele, with several of the compounds exhibiting unsilencing efficacy similar to topotecan. Excitingly, two of the tested indenoisoquinoline derivatives, indotecan (LMP400) and indimitecan (LMP776), are already in clinical trials [33, 34]. The results of our study suggest additional Top1 inhibitors that should be advanced for AS preclinical testing of safety and CNS efficacy.

Methods
Animals
All animal experiments were handled with an Institutional Animal Care and Use Committee (IACUC) protocol approved by the University of North Carolina School of Medicine. AS model mice [35] (*Ube3a*$^{m-/p+}$) were

generated by crossing $Ube3a^{m+/p-}$ females with wildtype males. Paternal YFP-tagged mice [36] ($Ube3a^{m+/pYFP}$) were generated by crossing heterozygote $Ube3a$-YFP males with wildtype females. Mice were housed at 12 h:12 h LD and given ad libitum access to water and food. Both male and female mice (embryos) were used in all studies.

Chemistry

Topotecan was purchased from Cayman Chemicals. Indotecan (LMP400) and indimitecan (LMP776) were obtained from the Developmental Therapeutics Program (DTP) branch, National Cancer Institute. Eleven structural analogues of indotecan and indimitecan, all indenoisoquinoline derivatives, were provided by Dr. Mark Cushman at Purdue University. Syntheses of 12 indenoisoquinolines have been previously described: indotecan (LMP400) and indimitecan (LMP776) [33], DB-III-17, DB-IV-26, DB-IV-50, DB-IV-56, DB-IV-58, DB-V-37, DB-V-41, DB-V-46, and DB-V-47 [37], and MJ-II-66A [30]. MNR-IV-64 was synthesized by the procedure reported for the corresponding N-4′-hydroxybutyl analogue [30]. These compounds were selected because they have a wide range of cytotoxicities in cancer cell culture while maintaining some degree of Top1 inhibitory

activity. All compounds were stored at − 20 °C before being reconstituted in dimethyl sulfoxide (DMSO) prior to use.

Cell culture and drug treatment

Primary cortical neurons were isolated and cultured using previously described protocols [9]. Briefly, we isolated cortical neurons from embryos (E14.5) carrying paternal $Ube3a$-YFP ($Ube3a^{m+/pYFP}$) or maternal deletion of $Ube3a$ ($Ube3a^{m-/p+}$). Isolated cortical neurons were plated onto 384-well plates (∼ 25,000 cells/well) for high-content imaging and onto 6-well plates (∼ 1,000,000 cells/well) for Western blot analysis. Cultured neurons were initially incubated for 7 days, replacing culture medium every 3–4 days. Drugs were freshly prepared in DMSO as a 10-mM stock, unless further dilution in DMSO was necessary. On day 7 (DIV 7), the indicated compounds (topotecan, indotecan, indimitecan, DB-IV-58, and DB-V-37 in Figs. 1, 2, and 3) were directly added at 0.3 μM (final concentration in culture medium) to the neurons for 72 h to allow time for unsilencing of paternal $Ube3a$ or $Ube3a$-YFP. For dose dependence and cytotoxicity tests (Fig. 4 and Additional file 1), we used half-log molar drug concentrations, 1×10^{-10}, 3×10^{-10}, 1×10^{-9}, 3×10^{-9}, 1×10^{-8}, 3×10^{-8}, 1×10^{-7}, 3×10^{-7}, 1×10^{-6}, 3×10^{-6}, 1×10^{-5}, and 3×10^{-5} M.

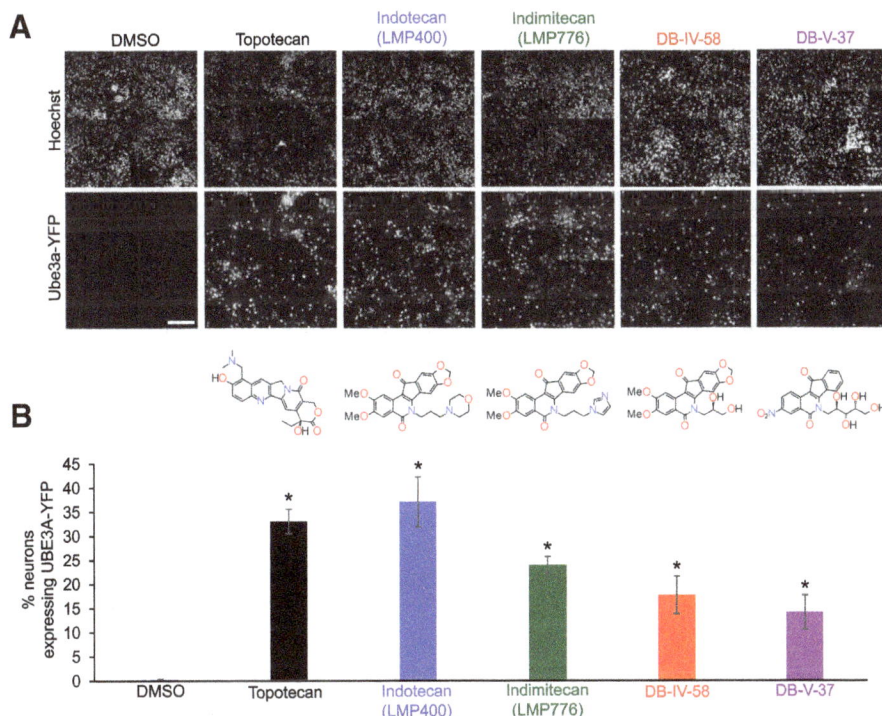

Fig. 1 Like the camptothecin-derived topotecan, indenoisoquinoline derivatives can unsilence paternal $Ube3a$-YFP in vitro. **a** Immunofluorescence images of nuclei (Hoechst stain) and paternal UBE3A-YFP in drug-treated cultured mouse cortical neurons and chemical structures of the compounds. Paternal $Ube3a$-YFP was unsilenced by the indicated drugs [topotecan (0.3 μM), indotecan (0.3 μM), indimitecan (0.3 μM), DB-IV-58 (0.3 μM), or DB-V-37 (0.3 μM)] but not by DMSO vehicle control (scale bar = 100 μm). DB-IV-58 and DB-V-37 are structural analogues of indotecan and indimitecan. **b** Quantitative analysis of neurons expressing unsilenced paternal UBE3A-YFP ($n = 4$ wells in 384-well plate/group, $*p < 0.05$)

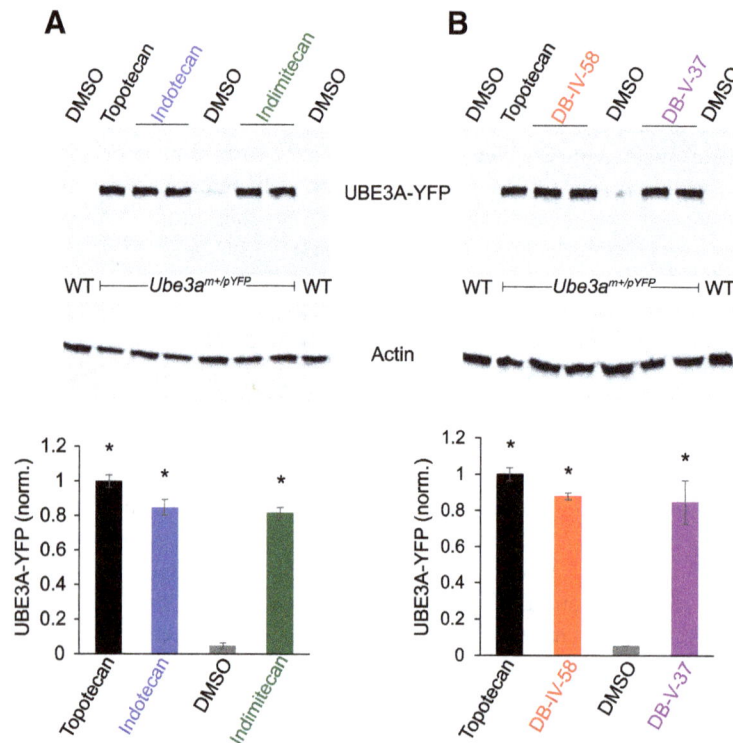

Fig. 2 Western blot analysis demonstrating the capacity of indenoisoquinoline derivatives to increase paternal UBE3A-YFP at the protein level in cultured neurons from $Ube3a^{m+/pYFP}$ mice. **a** Immunoblot and quantification of UBE3A-YFP levels normalized to actin in cultured neurons from wildtype (WT) or $Ube3a^{m+/pYFP}$ mice treated with DMSO (0.1% vehicle control), topotecan (0.3 μM), indotecan (0.3 μM), or indimitecan (0.3 μM) ($n = 3$/group, *$p < 0.05$). **b** Immunoblots and quantification of UBE3A-YFP levels normalized to actin in cultured neurons from wildtype (WT) or $Ube3a^{m+/pYFP}$ mice treated with DMSO (0.1% vehicle control), topotecan (0.3 μM), DB-IV-58 (0.3 μM), or DB-V-37 (0.3 μM) ($n = 3$/group, *$p < 0.05$)

Fluorescence immunostaining and high-content imaging

We followed the protocols for fluorescent immunostaining and high-content imaging of cortical neurons as previously described [9, 38]. Briefly, 72 h after drug treatment, the cells were fixed with 4% paraformaldehyde at room temperature for 15 min. After rinsing with phosphate-buffered saline (PBS) three times, the cells were permeabilized with 1% Triton-X 100 in PBS, followed by blocking with 5% NGS and 0.1% Triton-X 100 in PBS at room temperature for 30 min. After blocking, the cells were incubated with primary antibody, rabbit anti-GFP (1:1000, Novus Biologicals), at 4 °C overnight. The cells were then briefly rinsed with PBS followed by incubation with secondary antibody, goat anti-rabbit Alexa Fluor 488 (1:200, Thermo Fisher/Invitrogen), at room temperature. One hour after secondary antibody incubation, the cells were rinsed with PBS and fluorescent images were acquired using a BD Pathway 855 bioimager. The acquired images were processed by CellProfiler [39] to count the number of positive cells and measure fluorescent intensity (Additional file 2). To determine the percentage of neurons expressing paternal $Ube3a$-YFP, we counted the total number of cells (Hoechst) and YFP-positive cells, and the number of

YFP-positive cells was divided by the total number of cells. Fluorescence intensity was measured in neurons expressing unsilenced paternal $Ube3a$-YFP and normalized to vehicle control.

Cytotoxicity test

Toxicity of the compounds was tested in cultured cortical neurons in vitro. Using Cyto Tox-Glo assay (Promega), we followed the manufacturer's protocol to measure luminescence proportional to the number of dead vs. live cells. Briefly, 72 h after drug treatment, we directly added AAF-Glo substrates into the drug-treated (or 0.1% DMSO vehicle-treated) neurons and incubated them at room temperature for 15 min. We then measured luminescence produced by dead-cell protease activity.

Western blot analysis

We followed the same procedures of Western blot analysis as previously described [9, 38]. In brief, 72 h after drug treatment, we collected the cultured neurons from 6-well plates and extracted total protein with protein extraction buffer. Bradford assay was performed to measure protein concentration, and 30 μg of total protein was loaded for Bis-polyacrylamide gel electrophoresis

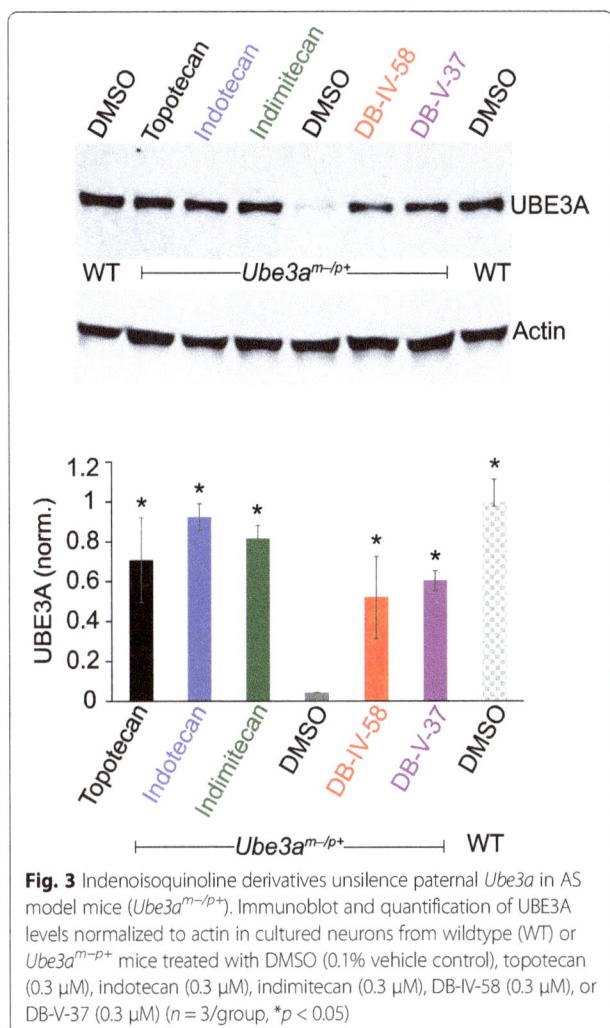

Fig. 3 Indenoisoquinoline derivatives unsilence paternal *Ube3a* in AS model mice (*Ube3a^{m−/p+}*). Immunoblot and quantification of UBE3A levels normalized to actin in cultured neurons from wildtype (WT) or *Ube3a^{m−p+}* mice treated with DMSO (0.1% vehicle control), topotecan (0.3 μM), indotecan (0.3 μM), indimitecan (0.3 μM), DB-IV-58 (0.3 μM), or DB-V-37 (0.3 μM) (n = 3/group, *p < 0.05)

Two-way ANOVA was performed to determine changes in EC_{50}, E_{max}, and LC_{50} (Table 1), with comparisons to topotecan made using a Bonferroni correction for multiple comparisons.

Results

Indenoisoquinoline-derived topoisomerase I inhibitors effectively unsilence paternal Ube3a

The goal of this study was to identify novel Top1 inhibitors as potential AS therapeutics. We chose to focus on the compounds indotecan (LMP400), indimitecan (LMP776), and their analogues because indotecan and indimitecan recently completed phase I clinical trial testing at the National Institutes of Health (ClinicalTrials.gov ID: NCT01051635). Moreover, indotecan exhibits favorable CNS penetration [40]. Thus, these drugs have already undergone a certain degree of preclinical safety testing, which could expedite clinical development if warranted.

As we anticipated, paternal *Ube3a-YFP* was not expressed at appreciable levels in cultured neurons in the presence of 0.1% DMSO (vehicle control). On the other hand, topotecan (positive control) unsilenced paternal *Ube3a-YFP* as previously reported [9] (Fig. 1a). Four indenoisoquinoline-derived compounds (indotecan, indimitecan, DB-IV-58, and DB-V-37) also successfully demonstrated unsilencing of paternal *Ube3a-YFP* in our reporter mouse (Fig. 1a). We quantified the number of Hoechst-positive cells expressing paternal *Ube3a-YFP* above a defined threshold and found that few (0.21 ± 0.17%) DMSO-treated neurons expressed *Ube3a-YFP* above threshold (Fig. 1b). In contrast, a significant (p < 0.05) number of neurons expressed paternal *Ube3a-YFP* when cultures were treated with topotecan (33.0 ± 2.56%), indotecan (37.1 ± 5.19%), indimitecan (23.9 ± 1.72%), DB-IV-58 (17.7 ± 3.87%), or DB-V-37 (14.1 ± 3.55%) (Fig. 1b). The number of cells expressing paternal *Ube3a-YFP* was similar between indotecan- and topotecan-treated neurons at a dose of 0.3 μM. At this same concentration (0.3 μM), fewer neurons treated with indimitecan, DB-IV-58, or DB-V-37 expressed paternal *Ube3a-YFP* compared to topotecan-treated neurons (p < 0.05 compared to topotecan-treated neurons).

To validate the paternal *Ube3a-YFP* unsilencing and definitively rule out the possibility of fluorescence artifacts (e.g., intrinsic fluorescence in compounds), we performed Western blot analysis using primary cultured cortical neurons. No UBE3A-YFP protein was expressed in wildtype neurons (negative control), whereas paternal UBE3A-YFP was marginally detectable in DMSO-treated cells from *Ube3a^{m+/pYFP}* mice, possibly due to contamination from glial cells that express *Ube3a* biallelically or to very modest expression of paternal *Ube3a* expressed during early stages of development. Topotecan, indotecan, indimitecan, DB-IV-58, and DB-V-37 treatments led to paternal UBE3A-YFP protein production (Fig. 2). Normalized

(Bio-Rad). Electrophoresed proteins were transferred to nitrocellulose membrane (0.45 μm, Bio-Rad). The membranes were blocked with 5% non-fat milk in TBS-T at room temperature for 30 min followed by overnight 4 °C incubation with primary antibodies (rabbit anti-GFP, 1:1000, Novus Biologicals; rabbit anti-Ube3a, 1:1000, Bethyl Lab; mouse anti-actin; 1:5000, Sigma). The next day, the membranes were rinsed with TBS-T three times and incubated with HPR-conjugated secondary antibodies for 1 h at room temperature (goat anti-rabbit, 1:1000, Vector Lab or goat anti-mouse, 1:1000, Vector Lab). Following secondary antibody incubation, the membranes were rinsed with TBS-T at room temperature for 1 h (4–5 times) and ECL substrates (Bio-Rad) were used to visualize immunostaining using an Amersham Imager 600 (AI600, GE Life Sciences).

Statistical analysis

One-way ANOVA was performed to determine significant differences in unsilencing paternal *Ube3a*-YFP or *Ube3a*, followed by Dunnett's multiple comparison test.

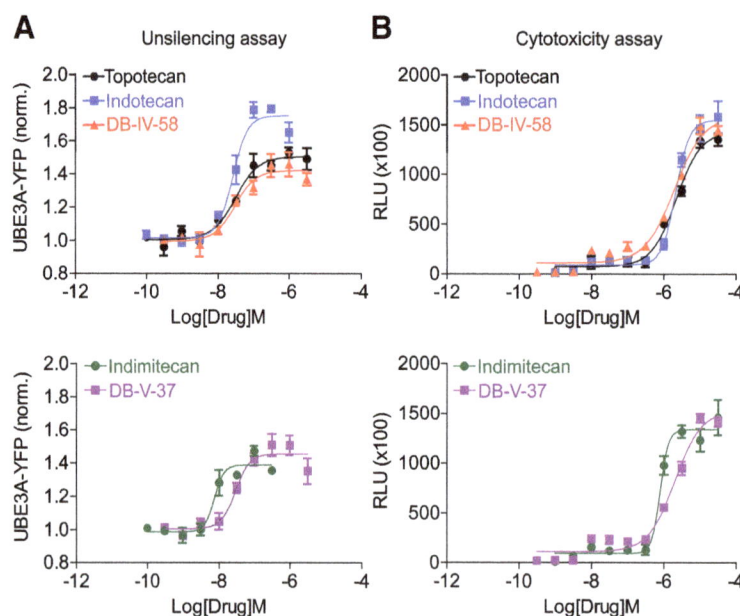

Fig. 4 Pharmacological properties of four indenoisoquinoline derivatives in unsilencing paternal *Ube3a-YFP* in vitro. **a** Dose dependence of four indenoisoquinoline derivatives and topotecan in unsilencing of paternal UBE3A-YFP ($n = 4$/group). Estimated potencies and efficacies of the drugs are summarized in Table 1. **b** Dose-dependent cytotoxicities of four indenoisoquinoline derivatives and topotecan ($n = 4$/group). Estimated LC_{50} values are summarized in Table 1

fold changes in unsilenced UBE3A-YFP were comparable in all five tested drugs (bottom panels in Fig. 2a, b).

Although unlikely, we wanted to rule out the possibility that the unsilencing was an artifact of the *Ube3a-YFP* knock-in. Thus, we tested the drug effects in AS model mice that lack the maternal *Ube3a* allele (*Ube3a*$^{m-/p+}$ mice) (Fig. 3). There was little paternal UBE3A protein in DMSO-treated *Ube3a*$^{m-/p+}$ neurons compared to *Ube3a*$^{m+/p+}$ (wildtype) neurons. Topotecan, indotecan, indimitecan, DB-IV-58, and DB-V-37 treatments result in a high level of paternal UBE3A protein compared to DMSO-treated neurons. These data confirm the ability of the tested indenoisoquinolines to unsilence paternal *Ube3a*.

Pharmacological profiling of indenoisoquinoline Top1 inhibitors in cultured cortical neurons in vitro

Once we confirmed the unsilencing effects, we performed pharmacological profiling of indotecan, indimitecan, and

their analogues for structure-activity relationships in order to identify more effective unsilencers. We performed dose-response experiments for all tested compounds (Fig. 4a and Additional file 1). These experiments identified indotecan as the most efficacious of all of drugs tested, with the potency (EC_{50}) of indotecan being significantly better than topotecan (Table 1; *$p < 0.05$). This suggests indotecan may have potential as a possible AS therapeutic. Indimitecan is less likely as a candidate therapeutic, because although it exhibited good potency in a nanomolar range and had similar efficacy as topotecan (Fig. 4a and Table 1, *$p < 0.05$), it likely has a low therapeutic index (discussed below). We also examined 11 structural analogues. Among 11 compounds, we found two of them, DB-IV-58 and DB-V-37, with similar efficacy and potency to topotecan (Fig. 4a and Table 1). However, they were less effective than indotecan.

Indenoisoquinoline derivatives were primarily designed to inhibit cancer cell growth. Because our goal is to

Table 1 Summary of efficacies and potencies of topotecan and indenoisoquinoline derivatives

Compound	EC_{50} [M]	E_{max}	LC_{50} [M]
Topotecan	3.04E−08 (± 3.40E−09)	1.51 (± 0.11)	2.30E−06 (± 2.01E−08)
Indotecan	2.56E−08 (± 1.05E−09)*	1.78 (± 0.13)*	2.01E−06 (± 1.59E−07)
Indimitecan	7.47E−09 (± 7.49E−10)*	1.47 (± 0.10)	7.89E−07 (± 3.43E−08)*
DB-IV-58	3.10E−08 (± 9.75E−09)	1.45 (± 0.12)	2.01E−06 (± 1.09E−07)
DB-V-37	2.99E−08 (± 8.29E−09)	1.48 (± 0.08)	2.02E−06 (± 1.02E−07)

EC_{50}, E_{max}, and LC_{50} are estimated from data presented in Fig. 4. Significance was tested by two-way ANOVA, followed by a Bonferroni correction for multiple comparisons to determine significant differences (*$p < 0.05$) from topotecan-treated neurons repurpose these drugs to unsilence a CNS target, it was necessary to test whether the compounds would be deleterious in neuronal cells. Toxicity testing of four indenoisoquinoline-derived compounds (indotecan, DB-IV-58, DB-V-37, and indimitecan) in the cultured neurons revealed that the cytotoxicity of the first three drugs (indotecan, DB-IV-58, and DB-V-37) was similar to that of topotecan. On the other hand, indimitecan exhibited toxicity at a significantly lower concentration than topotecan (Fig. 4b and Table 1, $*p < 0.05$), suggesting that it might have a low therapeutic index. Lastly, we also tested dose dependency of nine additional analogues (Additional file 1 and Additional file 3: Table S1). All nine compounds could unsilence paternal Ube3a-YFP to a certain degree. However, their effectiveness did not exceed that of indotecan. Three compounds (DB-IV-50, DB-IV-56, and MNR-IV-64) share similar pharmacological profiles, as their efficacy and potency were similar. However, their effectiveness of unsilencing paternal Ube3a-YFP was less than our lead compounds. Six compounds (DB-III-17, DB-IV-26, DB-V-41, DB-V-46, DB-V-47, and MJ-II-66A) unsilenced paternal Ube3a-YFP to a certain degree; however, they showed a very limited range of doses that produce Ube3a-YFP unsilencing before showing toxicities (e.g., an unfavorable therapeutic index). Because of the limited dose ranges, their EC_{50} values were not clearly determined (Additional file 3: Table S1). These data together suggest that, compared to topotecan, indotecan has a higher potency and efficacy, but similar toxicity profile, in its ability to unsilence the dormant paternal Ube3a allele in neurons.

Discussion

The goal of this study was to explore indenoisoquinoline derivatives as possible AS therapeutics by characterizing their effects on Ube3a unsilencing in mouse cortical neurons in vitro. Here, we identify indotecan (LMP400) as a potential AS therapeutic agent that warrants further examination in vivo for CNS bioavailability and safety.

The unique expression of UBE3A governed by genomic imprinting provides a therapeutic opportunity for AS by reactivating the paternal UBE3A allele [8, 9, 11]. Our research team previously reported that topoisomerase I inhibitors can reactivate the dormant UBE3A allele, providing the first proof of concept of pharmacological reactivation of paternal UBE3A as a potential therapeutic intervention for AS [9]. Because of the anticancer activity of Top1 inhibitors, many derivatives that overcome the limitations of camptothecins [10, 41, 42] have been synthesized for clinical development. Of these, topotecan, is FDA-approved for ovarian and lung cancers [43], while another, irinotecan, is approved for colon cancers [44]. However, these compounds may have limited clinical potential for treating AS. For example, topotecan has several

flaws such as decreased bioavailability due to plasma protein binding of the lactone hydrolysis product, removal from cells by drug efflux transporters, and long infusion times necessitated by relatively low stability of the ternary drug-DNA-enzyme cleavage complexes [10, 18]. These limitations prompted us to search for novel Top1 inhibitors as potential AS therapeutics, with the expectation that lead candidates could then be vetted for having improved CNS bioavailability and better safety profiles. For these studies, we focused on indenoisoquinoline-derived Top1 inhibitors that might overcome the limitations of topotecan [10]. Of many indenoisoquinoline-derived Top1 inhibitors, indotecan and indimitecan were selected to examine their unsilencing effects on paternal Ube3a because of their similar ability to effectively inhibit almost 100% of Top1 enzymatic activity [33] and recent completion of phase I clinical trials (ClinicalTrials.gov ID: NCT01051635).

Here, we demonstrate that indenoisoquinoline-derived Top1 inhibitors are potent Ube3a unsilencers, with different unsilencing properties. Of the compounds we tested in vitro, indotecan (LMP400) [10, 34] appears to have more favorable paternal Ube3a unsilencing properties than topotecan. While both topotecan and indotecan exhibit CNS penetrance [18, 40], there are not yet data available to directly compare their relative CNS bioavailability; there is a need to carefully establish the CNS bioavailability of indotecan. One potential advantage of indotecan is that it is not a substrate for the transporters ABCG2 and MDR1 [32], suggesting that it may stay longer in the CNS than topotecan because transporters extrude topotecan from the brain [19]. Moreover, although the cytotoxicity profile of indotecan is similar to that of topotecan, its efficacy and potency are better than topotecan. Indimitecan (LMP776) [10] appears to be more toxic than topotecan, while the three other indenoisoquinoline derivatives (indotecan, DB-IV-58, and DB-V-37) showed similar cytotoxicity to topotecan in our cultured cortical neurons. In addition, the efficacy of indimitecan is lower than that of topotecan. The structural differences in indenoisoquinoline-derived compounds are responsible for their different unsilencing effects. The only structural difference between indotecan and indimitecan is in the side chain which is appended to the heterocyclic system that intercalates in the DNA break generated by Top1 [10, 23]. These characteristics will be important considerations for the future design of paternal UBE3A unsilencers. Although indotecan exhibits better efficacy and potency than topotecan, the similar cytotoxicity of the two drugs must be considered for in vivo applications. Importantly, the DNA cleavage complex patterns of indotecan are different from topotecan in a manner that may confer some important advantages for clinical use. Indenoisoquinolines such as indotecan produce more stable cleavage complexes than camptothecins such as topotecan [45], which, based on the mechanism of *Ube3a* unsilencing [26], should enhance *Ube3a* unsilencing as we observed. Moreover, after drug removal, the Top1-DNA complexes induced by indenoisoquinolines persist under conditions where camptothecin-induced Top1-DNA complexes completely reverse [45]. This observation further suggests that the similar cytotoxicity of indotecan might be offset by the potential for a briefer treatment regimen in vivo, which remains to be addressed. Known off-target effects for topoisomerase inhibitors generally lead to the transient downregulation of long genes [11, 46, 47]. Genome-wide analyses are necessary to reveal all potential off-target effects for indenoisoquinolines (e.g., indotecan). Alternatively, an in silico analysis using SEA (similarity ensemble approach; http://sea.bkslab.org) enables us to predict off-targets. SEA analysis revealed that indotecan possesses 55 potential off-targets, including aurora kinase A, aurora kinase B, and acetylcholinesterase. Regardless of off-target effects, clinical trials have demonstrated that, at least at the concentrations examined, indotecan is well tolerated in a clinical population [34]. However, it still remains to be addressed whether off-target effects arise at the concentration at which indotecan is effective, as we reported that indotecan has a very low EC_{50} of ~ 26 nM to produce *Ube3a* unsilencing.

We tested 11 structural analogues of indotecan/indimitecan for their ability to unsilence paternal *Ube3a*, and these compounds could be roughly categorized based on their ability to inhibit Top1 in cell-free assays: those compounds (DB-IV-26, DB-IV-50, DB-IV-56, DB-IV-58, DB-V-37, and DB-V-41) that have 100% of the ability of camptothecin to stabilize the ternary drug-DNA-Top1 cleavage complexes [37, 48], those compounds (DB-V-46, DB-V-47, and MNR-IV-64) that inhibit between 50 and 75% of Top1 [37], and those compounds (MJ-II-66A) that inhibit between 20 and 50% of Top1 [30]. We also tested DB-III-17, as this is an intermediate compound for synthesizing or modifying the analogues. The compounds with lower Top1 inhibitory activities (DB-III-17, DB-V-46, DB-V-47, and MJ-II-66A) showed a very limited therapeutic index. Their ambiguous EC_{50} values were mainly due to limited effective dose ranges. Although we did not test their cytotoxicities in our cultured cortical neurons, we expect that they are more toxic than topotecan because we could not measure the fluorescence intensity in unsilenced UBE3A-YFP protein, possibly due to cell death produced at concentrations > 1 μM. On the other hand, we observed similar efficacy and potency of three compounds (DB-IV-50, DB-IV-56, and MNR-IV-64) with between 75 and ~ 100% Top1 inhibitory activities relative to camptothecin, but their effectiveness seems to be less than those of indotecan or topotecan. Interestingly, although DB-IV-26 and

DB-V-41 have ~ 100% Top1 inhibitory activity, their EC50 values were also ambiguous due to limited effective dose ranges. Since the cleavage complexes are critical for producing paternal *Ube3a* unsilencing [26], we suspect that their cleavage complexes may not be stable enough to produce paternal *Ube3a* unsilencing. More importantly, the various hydroxylated side chains contribute to differences in the pharmacological action in *Ube3a* unsilencing. For example, the compounds with lower Top1 inhibitory activities (DB-III-17, DB-V-46, DB-V-47, and MJ-II-66A) either lack the hydroxylated side chains that potentially serve as hydrogen-bond acceptors/donors that enable Top1 inhibitory activities and cytotoxicity at physiological pH [49] or the hydroxylated side chain is cyclic. On the other hand, other compounds possessing dimethoxy or methylenedioxy groups, and/or straight hydroxylated side chains, which appear to be the main contributors to Top1 inhibitory activity and cytotoxicity, effectively unsilence paternal *Ube3a*.

Taken together, our study suggests that clinical development of paternal *Ube3a* unsilencers will require optimization of Top1 inhibition and cytotoxicity through modulating chemical characteristics, including the length of the side chains. Although in vivo assays are necessary to further evaluate the unsilencing effects of indenoisoquinolines, this study provides a framework for developing novel AS therapies using different classes of Top1 inhibitors.

Conclusions

Angelman syndrome is a neurodevelopmental disorder without effective therapeutic interventions. However, pharmacological restoration of the epigenetically silenced copy of *UBE3A* could be one promising approach. Pharmacological inhibition of topoisomerase I (Top1) leads to re-expression of the dormant *UBE3A* allele. Here, we provided pharmacological profiles of indenoisoquinoline-derived Top1 inhibitors as *Ube3a* unsilencers in mouse neurons to identify potential AS clinical candidates. Our data suggest that a number of indenoisoquinolines, and in particular indotecan (LMP400), are potent unsilencers of the paternal *Ube3a* allele and should be further assessed in vivo for their translational potential.

Additional files

Additional file 1: Chemical structures of nine analogues of indotecan/indimitecan and their pharmacological properties in unsilencing of paternal UBE3A-YFP in vitro. A. DB-III-17, B. DB-IV-26, C. DB-IV-50, D. DB-IV-56, E. DB-V-41, F. DB-V-46, G. DB-V-47, H. MJ-II-66A, I. MNR-IV-64. Estimated potencies and efficacies of the drugs are summarized in Additional file 3: Table S1. (DOCX 13 kb)

Additional file 2: Image analysis in CellProfiler. Morphological changes in the neurons were assessed by nuclear structure of Hoechst-stained neurons. A Immunofluorescence images of Hoechst-stained neurons obtained using a BD Pathway 855 high-content imager (top). The size (between 18 and 40 pixel units) and intensity (threshold range between 0.005 and 1) of stained nuclei were used to segregate putative viable cells recognized as objects (middle, green) from clumped or dead cells (middle, red). Recognized objects were further processed based on size, intensity, and shape (round) (bottom, individual objects were assigned colors by CellProfiler to allow them to be better visualized). No objects were identified in the neurons treated with 10 μM indotecan, as no nuclei met the criteria of immunofluorescence size and intensity. B Quantitative analysis of identified objects. The average numbers of objects were comparable between neurons treated with DMSO (0.1% vehicle control) and indotecan (0.01 μM and 0.3 μM)-treated neurons. (PDF 338 kb)

Additional file 3: Table S1. Potency and efficacy of nine analogues (PDF 270 kb)

Abbreviations

AAF-Glo: Alanyl-alanyl-phenylalanyl-aminoluciferin; AS: Angelman syndrome; BBB: Blood-brain barrier; CNS: Central nervous system; DIV: Day in vitro; FBS: Fetal bovine serum; LMP: Laboratory of Molecular Pharmacology at National Cancer Institutes; NGS: Normal goat serum; PBS: Phosphate buffer saline; PBS-T: Phosphate buffer saline Triton X-100; Ube3a: Ubiquitin protein ligase E3A; $Ube3a^{m-/p+}$: Maternal deletion of ubiquitin protein ligase E3A and intact paternal Ube3a; $Ube3a^{m+/pYFP}$: Intact maternal Ube3a and paternal yellow fluorescence protein (YFP)-tagged Ube3a

Acknowledgements

We would like to thank the Developmental Therapeutics Program (DTP) branch, National Cancer Institute, for providing indotecan (LMP400) and indimitecan (LMP776). We would like to thank Erika Wittchen, PhD, for proofreading the manuscript.

Funding

The work was supported by NINDS R01NS085093 and a grant from the Angelman Syndrome Foundation to BDP. The research at Purdue was facilitated by the National Institutes of Health through support with Research Grant P30CA023168. YP's research was supported by the Center for Cancer Research, the Intramural Program of the National Cancer Institute (NIH) (Z01-BC006161).

Authors' contributions

HML designed and performed all experiments. EPC and MBK assisted and supported cell culture and neuronal isolation. MS and YP provided the compounds tested in this study. The manuscript was written by HML, MC, YP, and BDP. All authors reviewed and agreed to submit the final manuscript.

Competing interests

Not applicable to authors except MC, who is on the Board of Directors and an investor in Gibson Oncology, Inc., which has licensed indenoisoquinoline intellectual property owned by Purdue University. Neither Gibson Oncology nor any other commercial company sponsored or provided other direct financial support to the author or his laboratory for the research reported in this article.

Author details

[1]Department of Cell Biology and Physiology, University of North Carolina School of Medicine, Neuroscience Research Building, Room 5119 115 Mason Farm Rd., Campus Box 7545, Chapel Hill, NC 27599-7545, USA. [2]Department of Medicinal Chemistry and Molecular Pharmacology, Purdue University School of Pharmacy and the Purdue Center for Cancer Research, West Lafayette, IN, USA. [3]Developmental Therapeutics Branch and Laboratory of Molecular Pharmacology, Center for Cancer Research, National Cancer Institute, Bethesda, MD, USA. [4]UNC Neuroscience Center, Carolina Institute for Developmental Disabilities, University of North Carolina School of Medicine, Chapel Hill, NC, USA.

References

1. Dagli AI, Mueller J, Williams CA. Angelman syndrome. In: Adam MP, Ardinger HH, Pagon RA, Wallace SE, LJH B, Mefford HC, Stephens K, Amemiya A, Ledbetter N, editors. GeneReviews(R). Seattle (WA):University of Washington; 1993.
2. Clayton-Smith J. Angelman syndrome: a review of the clinical and genetic aspects. J Med Genet. 2003;40(2):87–95.
3. Dan B. Angelman syndrome: current understanding and research prospects. Epilepsia. 2009;50(11):2331–9.
4. Williams CA. Neurological aspects of the Angelman syndrome. Brain Dev. 2005;27(2):88–94.
5. Mabb AM, Judson MC, Zylka MJ, Philpot BD. Angelman syndrome: insights into genomic imprinting and neurodevelopmental phenotypes. Trends Neurosci. 2011;34(6):293–303.
6. Steffenburg S, Gillberg CL, Steffenburg U, Kyllerman M. Autism in Angelman syndrome: a population-based study. Pediatr Neurol. 1996;14(2):131–6.
7. Dan B. Behavior and neuropsychiatric manifestations in Angelman syndrome. Neuropsychiatr Dis Treat. 2008;4;577.
8. Vu TH, Hoffman AR. Imprinting of the Angelman syndrome gene, UBE3A, is restricted to brain. Nat Genet. 1997;17(1):12–3.
9. Huang HS, Allen JA, Mabb AM, King IF, Miriyala J, Taylor-Blake B, Sciaky N, Dutton JW Jr, Lee HM, Chen X, et al. Topoisomerase inhibitors unsilence the dormant allele of Ube3a in neurons. Nature. 2011;481(7380):185–9.
10. Pommier Y, Cushman M. The indenoisoquinoline noncamptothecin topoisomerase I inhibitors: update and perspectives. Mol Cancer Ther. 2009; 8(5):1008–14.
11. King IF, Yandava CN, Mabb AM, Hsiao JS, Huang HS, Pearson BL, Calabrese JM, Starmer J, Parker JS, Magnuson T, et al. Topoisomerases facilitate transcription of long genes linked to autism. Nature. 2013;501(7465):58–62.
12. Bomgaars L. The development of camptothecin analogs in childhood cancers. Oncologist. 2001;6(6):506–16.
13. Philpot BD, Thompson CE, Franco L, Williams CA. Angelman syndrome: advancing the research frontier of neurodevelopmental disorders. J Neurodev Disord. 2011;3(1):50–6.
14. Rodriguez-Galindo C, Poquette CA, Marina NM, Head DR, Cain A, Meyer WH, Santana VM, Pappo AS. Hematologic abnormalities and acute myeloid leukemia in children and adolescents administered intensified chemotherapy for the Ewing sarcoma family of tumors. J Pediatr Hematol Oncol. 2000;22(4):321–9.
15. Blaney SM, Phillips PC, Packer RJ, Heideman RL, Berg SL, Adamson PC, Allen JC, Sallan SE, Jakacki RI, Lange BJ, et al. Phase II evaluation of topotecan for pediatric central nervous system tumors. Cancer. 1996;78(3):527–31.
16. Feun L, Savaraj N. Topoisomerase I inhibitors for the treatment of brain tumors. Expert Rev Anticancer Ther. 2008;8(5):707–16.
17. Minturn JE, Janss AJ, Fisher PG, Allen JC, Patti R, Phillips PC, Belasco JB. A phase II study of metronomic oral topotecan for recurrent childhood brain tumors. Pediatr Blood Cancer. 2010;56(1):39–44.
18. El-Gizawy SA, Hedaya MA. Comparative brain tissue distribution of camptothecin and topotecan in the rat. Cancer Chemother Pharmacol. 1999;43(5):364–70.
19. Motl S, Zhuang Y, Waters CM, Stewart CF. Pharmacokinetic considerations in the treatment of CNS tumours. Clin Pharmacokinet. 2006;45(9):871–903.
20. Houghton PJ, Cheshire PJ, Hallman JD, Lutz L, Friedman HS, Danks MK, Houghton JA. Efficacy of topoisomerase I inhibitors, topotecan and irinotecan, administered at low dose levels in protracted schedules to mice

bearing xenografts of human tumors. Cancer Chemother Pharmacol. 1995; 36(5):393–403.

21. Stone JB, DeAngelis LM. Cancer-treatment-induced neurotoxicity--focus on newer treatments. Nat Rev Clin Oncol. 2016;13(2):92–105.

22. Soffietti R, Trevisan E, Ruda R. Neurologic complications of chemotherapy and other newer and experimental approaches. Handb Clin Neurol. 2014; 121:1199–218.

23. Ioanoviciu A, Antony S, Pommier Y, Staker BL, Stewart L, Cushman M. Synthesis and mechanism of action studies of a series of norindenoisoquinoline topoisomerase I poisons reveal an inhibitor with a flipped orientation in the ternary DNA–enzyme–inhibitor complex as determined by X-ray crystallographic analysis. J Med Chem. 2005;48(15):4803–14.

24. Marchand C, Antony S, Kohn KW, Cushman M, Ioanoviciu A, Staker BL, Burgin AB, Stewart L, Pommier Y. A novel norindenoisoquinoline structure reveals a common interfacial inhibitor paradigm for ternary trapping of the topoisomerase I-DNA covalent complex. Mol Cancer Ther. 2006;5(2):287–95.

25. Staker BL, Feese MD, Cushman M, Pommier Y, Zembower D, Stewart L, Burgin AB. Structures of three classes of anticancer agents bound to the human topoisomerase I–DNA covalent complex. J Med Chem. 2005;48(7): 2336–45.

26. Mabb AM, Simon JM, King IF, Lee HM, An LK, Philpot BD, Zylka MJ. Topoisomerase 1 regulates gene expression in neurons through cleavage complex-dependent and -independent mechanisms. PLoS One. 2016;11(5): e0156439.

27. Antony S, Kohlhagen G, Agama K, Jayaraman M, Cao S, Durrani FA, Rustum YM, Cushman M, Pommier Y. Cellular topoisomerase I inhibition and antiproliferative activity by MJ-III-65 (NSC 706744), an indenoisoquinoline topoisomerase I poison. Mol Pharmacol. 2005;67(2):523–30.

28. Cushman M, Jayaraman M, Vroman JA, Fukunaga AK, Fox BM, Kohlhagen G, Strumberg D, Pommier Y. Synthesis of new Indeno[1, 2-c]isoquinolines: cytotoxic con-camptothecin topoisomerase I inhibitors. J Med Chem. 2000; 43(20):3688–98.

29. Fox BM, Xiao X, Antony S, Kohlhagen G, Pommier Y, Staker BL, Stewart L, Cushman M. Design, synthesis, and biological evaluation of cytotoxic 11-alkenylindenoisoquinoline topoisomerase I inhibitors and indenoisoquinoline –camptothecin hybrids. J Med Chem. 2003;46(15):3275–82.

30. Strumberg D, Pommier Y, Paull K, Jayaraman M, Nagafuji P, Cushman M. Synthesis of cytotoxic indenoisoquinoline topoisomerase I poisons. J Med Chem. 1999;42(3):446–57.

31. Kinders RJ, Hollingshead M, Lawrence S, Ji J, Tabb B, Bonner WM, Pommier Y, Rubinstein L, Evrard YA, Parchment RE, et al. Development of a validated immunofluorescence assay for gammaH2AX as a pharmacodynamic marker of topoisomerase I inhibitor activity. Clinical cancer research : an official journal of the American Association for Cancer Research. 2010;16(22):5447–57.

32. Antony S, Agama KK, Miao ZH, Takagi K, Wright MH, Robles AI, Varticovski L, Nagarajan M, Morrell A, Cushman M, et al. Novel indenoisoquinolines NSC 725776 and NSC 724998 produce persistent topoisomerase I cleavage complexes and overcome multidrug resistance. Cancer Res. 2007;67(21): 10397–405.

33. Nagarajan M, Morrell A, Ioanoviciu A, Antony S, Kohlhagen G, Agama K, Hollingshead M, Pommier Y, Cushman M. Synthesis and evaluation of indenoisoquinoline topoisomerase I inhibitors substituted with nitrogen heterocycles. J Med Chem. 2006;49(21):6283–9.

34. Kummar S, Chen A, Gutierrez M, Pfister TD, Wang L, Redon C, Bonner WM, Yutzy W, Zhang Y, Kinders RJ, et al. Clinical and pharmacologic evaluation of two dosing schedules of indotecan (LMP400), a novel indenoisoquinoline, in patients with advanced solid tumors. Cancer Chemother Pharmacol. 2016;78(1):73–81.

35. Jiang YH, Armstrong D, Albrecht U, Atkins CM, Noebels JL, Eichele G, Sweatt JD, Beaudet AL. Mutation of the Angelman ubiquitin ligase in mice causes increased cytoplasmic p53 and deficits of contextual learning and long-term potentiation. Neuron. 1998;21(4):799–811.

36. Dindot SV, Antalffy BA, Bhattacharjee MB, Beaudet AL. The Angelman syndrome ubiquitin ligase localizes to the synapse and nucleus, and maternal deficiency results in abnormal dendritic spine morphology. Hum Mol Genet. 2008;17(1):111–8.

37. Beck DE, Agama K, Marchand C, Chergui A, Pommier Y, Cushman M. Synthesis and biological evaluation of new carbohydrate-substituted indenoisoquinoline topoisomerase I inhibitors and improved syntheses of the experimental anticancer agents indotecan (LMP400) and indimitecan (LMP776). J Med Chem. 2014;57(4):1495–512.

38. Kim Y, Lee HM, Xiong Y, Sciaky N, Hulbert SW, Cao X, Everitt JI, Jin J, Roth BL, Jiang YH. Targeting the histone methyltransferase G9a activates imprinted genes and improves survival of a mouse model of Prader-Willi syndrome. Nat Med. 2017;23(2):213–22.

39. Carpenter AE, Jones TR, Lamprecht MR, Clarke C, Kang IH, Friman O, Guertin DA, Chang JH, Lindquist RA, Moffat J, et al. CellProfiler: image analysis software for identifying and quantifying cell phenotypes. Genome Biol. 2006;7(10):R100.

40. Guo J, Holleran J, Schmitz JC, Czambel K, Beumer JH, Eiseman JL: Pharmacokinetics and pharmacodynamics of indenoisoquinoline LMP400 (indotecan) in BALB/c female mice bearing CT-26 colon tumors. [abstract]. Proceedings of the 106th Annual Meeting of the American Association for. Cancer Research 2015.

41. Pommier Y. Topoisomerase I inhibitors: camptothecins and beyond. Nat Rev Cancer. 2006;6(10):789–802.

42. Pommier Y, Sun Y, Huang SN, Nitiss JL. Roles of eukaryotic topoisomerases in transcription, replication and genomic stability. Nat Rev Mol Cell Biol. 2016;17(November 2016):703–21.

43. Garst J. Safety of topotecan in the treatment of recurrent small-cell lung cancer and ovarian cancer. Expert Opin Drug Saf. 2007;6(1):53–62.

44. Fuchs C, Mitchell EP, Hoff PM. Irinotecan in the treatment of colorectal cancer. Cancer Treat Rev. 2006;32(7):491–503.

45. Antony S, Jayaraman M, Laco G, Kohlhagen G, Kohn KW, Cushman M, Pommier Y. Differential induction of topoisomerase I-DNA cleavage complexes by the indenoisoquinoline MJ-III-65 (NSC 706744) and camptothecin: base sequence analysis and activity against camptothecin-resistant topoisomerases I. Cancer Res. 2003;63(21):7428–35.

46. Mabb AM, Kullmann PH, Twomey MA, Miriyala J, Philpot BD, Zylka MJ. Topoisomerase 1 inhibition reversibly impairs synaptic function. Proc Natl Acad Sci U S A. 2014;111(48):17290–5.

47. Solier S, Ryan MC, Martin SE, Varma S, Kohn KW, Liu H, Zeeberg BR, Pommier Y. Transcription poisoning by topoisomerase I is controlled by gene length, splice sites, and miR-142-3p. Cancer Res. 2013;73(15):4830–9.

48. Nagarajan M, Xiao X, Antony S, Kohlhagen G, Pommier Y, Cushman M. Design, synthesis, and biological evaluation of indenoisoquinoline topoisomerase I inhibitors featuring polyamine side chains on the lactam nitrogen. J Med Chem. 2003;46(26):5712–24.

49. Cinelli MA, Reddy PV, Lv PC, Liang JH, Chen L, Agama K, Pommier Y, van Breemen RB, Cushman M. Identification, synthesis, and biological evaluation of metabolites of the experimental cancer treatment drugs indotecan (LMP400) and indimitecan (LMP776) and investigation of isomerically hydroxylated indenoisoquinoline analogues as topoisomerase I poisons. J Med Chem. 2012;55(24):10844–62.

6

The geometric preference subtype in ASD: identifying a consistent, early-emerging phenomenon through eye tracking

Adrienne Moore*🆔, Madeline Wozniak, Andrew Yousef, Cindy Carter Barnes, Debra Cha, Eric Courchesne and Karen Pierce

Abstract

Background: The wide range of ability and disability in ASD creates a need for tools that parse the phenotypic heterogeneity into meaningful subtypes. Using eye tracking, our past studies revealed that when presented with social and geometric images, a subset of ASD toddlers preferred viewing geometric images, and these toddlers also had greater symptom severity than ASD toddlers with greater social attention. This study tests whether this "GeoPref test" effect would generalize across different social stimuli.

Methods: Two hundred and twenty-seven toddlers (76 ASD) watched a 90-s video, the Complex Social GeoPref test, of dynamic geometric images paired with social images of children interacting and moving. Proportion of visual fixation time and number of saccades per second to both images were calculated. To allow for cross-paradigm comparisons, a subset of 126 toddlers also participated in the original GeoPref test. Measures of cognitive and social functioning (MSEL, ADOS, VABS) were collected and related to eye tracking data. To examine utility as a diagnostic indicator to detect ASD toddlers, validation statistics (e.g., sensitivity, specificity, ROC, AUC) were calculated for the Complex Social GeoPref test alone and when combined with the original GeoPref test.

Results: ASD toddlers spent a significantly greater amount of time viewing geometric images than any other diagnostic group. Fixation patterns from ASD toddlers who participated in both tests revealed a significant correlation, supporting the idea that these tests identify a phenotypically meaningful ASD subgroup. Combined use of both original and Complex Social GeoPref tests identified a subgroup of about 1 in 3 ASD toddlers from the "GeoPref" subtype (sensitivity 35%, specificity 94%, AUC 0.75.) Replicating our previous studies, more time looking at geometric images was associated with significantly greater ADOS symptom severity.

Conclusions: Regardless of the complexity of the social images used (low in the original GeoPref test vs high in the new Complex Social GeoPref test), eye tracking of toddlers can accurately identify a specific ASD "GeoPref" subtype with elevated symptom severity. The GeoPref tests are predictive of ASD at the individual subject level and thus potentially useful for various clinical applications (e.g., early identification, prognosis, or development of subtype-specific treatments).

Keywords: Eye tracking, Autism spectrum disorder, Early identification, Social attention, Geometric preference

* Correspondence: armoore@ucsd.edu
Autism Center of Excellence, Department of Neurosciences, University of California San Diego, La Jolla, CA, USA

Background

Autism spectrum disorder (ASD) encompasses a heterogeneous collection of phenotypes. Some individuals with ASD are highly capable, verbally fluent individuals who view their autism as a benign difference requiring an increase in tolerance and acceptance from the neurotypical community rather than a cure [1]. Others with ASD are severely impaired with minimal ability for self-care or for communicating their perspectives or needs [2–4]. It may be possible to maximize impact of treatment for those with particularly challenging forms of ASD by intervening early in the development of symptoms [5–7]. Neurobiological differences between people who will go on to be diagnosed with ASD and those who will not have been traced back to even prenatal stages of development [8–10]. Differences in behavioral presentation at the group level between children who will and will not go on to be diagnosed with ASD have been found as early as 6 months [11–13]. However, according to recent Centers for Disease Control and Prevention reporting, most children on the autism spectrum in the USA are not diagnosed until after the age of 4 [14]. The development of effective tests that can reliably identify in their infancy which individuals will go on to be diagnosed with autism, and whether that autism will ultimately be mild or severe, is in its very early stages.

Clinician judgments of observed behavior, though vulnerable to subjective bias, remain the gold standard for ASD identification [15]. This state of affairs persists despite widespread acceptance that the origins of ASD are neurobiological and that therefore the development of highly objective tests should be achievable [16]. Eye tracking is a methodology with great potential clinical utility for screening, diagnosis, and early detection of ASD [17]. It is objective, quantitative, non-invasive, relatively inexpensive and easy to use, and appropriate for very young infants and many levels of functioning [18, 19]. Moreover, while basic oculomotor functioning has been shown not to differ in fundamental ways [19] between ASD and controls (although see [20, 21] for notable differences in spontaneous fixation durations and attentional disengagement), patterns of viewing socially relevant information reveal the phenotypic differences between ASD and typical development [22]. When paired with stimuli and tasks that have been well explored by the field of neuroscience, eye tracking may move us toward clinical approaches grounded in knowledge of the disrupted neural circuitry of ASD, with the goal of improved treatment impact [23].

Eye tracking studies of toddlers and young children with ASD have reported less time attending to biological motion [24], less attention to people's heads and more to bodies [25], less time viewing people and faces within a complex scene [13], and, when viewing faces, less time spent viewing the key feature components [26]. Young children with ASD also exhibit atypical gaze-following behavior during eye tracking paradigms [27] which is important because gaze-following is a key precursor to the development of joint attention [28]. Joint attention skills are critically associated with language acquisition in typically developing children [29] and with language and social deficits in ASD [30]. Though it has not been demonstrated, the social differences and difficulties of adults with ASD could possibly be influenced by the long-term, cumulative impact of this abnormal visual attention to what is socially meaningful during development [31–33]. Abnormal non-social attentional components (e.g., disengagement) likely add complexity to this explanation as well [34]. Intervention studies focused on improving joint attention skills have yielded promising results thus far, suggesting it may be feasible to alter this course of events as ASD unfolds across childhood [35].

Despite the many insights into ASD development stemming from eye tracking research, difficultly when comparing results from different eye tracking studies of ASD toddlers has been noted [22]. This is in part because seemingly minor changes to the stimuli presented may alter the results considerably. For example, in separate studies, Jones [31] and Chawarska [36] presented video stimuli to ASD toddlers of similar ages (mean age 2.1 years, standard deviation .65 years, and the 13- to 25-month age range, respectively). Both studies included a complex stimulus background with toys and other objects, in front of which was a centrally located female actress who looked directly into the camera while trying to attract attention with child-directed speech. However, Jones (2008) found increased looking to the mouth region and decreased looking to the eye region in ASD children compared to contrast groups. Chawarska, on the other hand, found decreased looking time to the face and specifically to the mouth region and increased looking to the hands in ASD children, yet no differences in eye region fixation per se, compared to contrast groups. There are various possible explanations for this discrepancy, and several authors have previously commented on it [22, 37]. Regardless of the cause, the sharp inconsistency of findings between such studies suggests that results when eye tracking toddlers with ASD can be very sensitive and may not generalize robustly or replicate unless many factors are controlled.

In contrast, the current eye tracking study examines whether the GeoPref test effect is robust against changes to the social images presented in a conceptual replication of the "GeoPref" subtype effect identified in our previous work (see Fig. 1). Specifically, in 2011, Pierce et al. reported eye tracking data from a preferential looking task showing that preference for viewing geometric rather than social stimuli is a risk factor for an autism diagnosis in toddlers [38]. In 2016, Pierce et al. reported that this Geometric Preference (GeoPref) test identifies

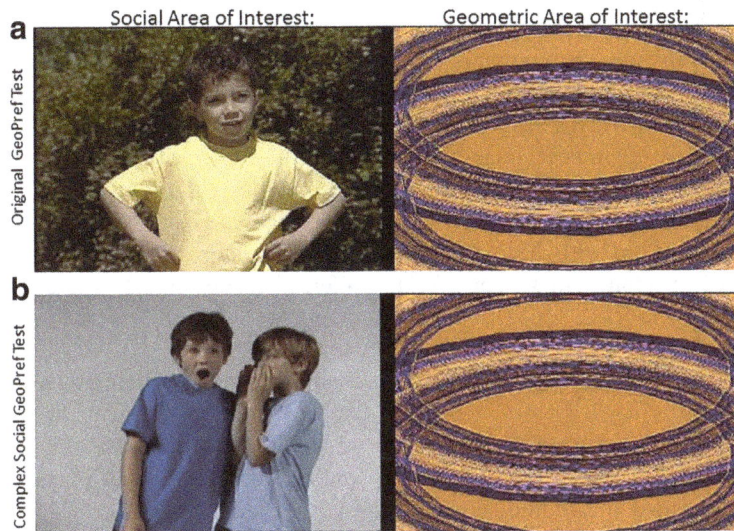

Fig. 1 Examples of stimuli. **a** Sample image from the original GeoPref test which consists of a 60-s video composed of 28 scenes, 26 of which involve one individual's movement (while the other two scenes include twins moving side by side). ©2003 Gaiam Americas, Inc., Courtesy of Gaiam Americas, Inc. As each social scene switches to a new actor, the paired geometric scene switches simultaneously to different colors and moving shapes. **b** Sample image from the Complex Social GeoPref test which consists of a 90-s video composed of nine scenes, five of which include two children interacting and four of which include one child moving enthusiastically. As each social scene changes, the paired geometric scene also switches simultaneously to a different color and moving shape, as in the original GeoPref test

an ASD subtype with increased symptom severity compared to ASD children who preferentially view social images [39]. Individuals in the GeoPref ASD subtype, who spent more than 69% of looking time viewing geometric stimuli, had higher ADOS scores, lower MSEL receptive and expressive language and visual reception scores, and lower Vineland scores for adaptive behavior.

The current study tests the Geometric Preference phenomenon identified previously by varying the social stimulus presentation's total length, scene length, and complexity of social interactions. The original study shows full body or large, dance-like movements and uniformly positive affect. The current study depicts a broader range of expressed emotions including surprise and anger, as well as happiness, and shows socially meaningful but physically more subtle actions like whispering in another's ear, hugging, and one child sticking out her tongue at another. As in the original test, these social stimuli portray biological motion and faces (though with less biological motion and more varied facial expressions), keeping the paradigm closely linked to stimuli that have been often used by cognitive neuroscience in attempts to map the social brain [40–42]. These complex social vignettes unfold more gradually than the actions in the original stimuli; therefore, the stimulus video is longer overall and composed of longer individual scenes. The geometric stimuli were not altered, other than by selecting a subset and extending the duration of presentation per scene to match the durations to the social stimuli. This was done so that by

isolating the social variables only, we could conclude that changes in the pattern of responses to viewing the stimuli were due to the social scene manipulation, thus avoiding any confounds. Because toddlers with ASD are more likely to have a reduced interest in social stimuli, we considered the fact that the sensitivity of the test (which was around 23% for the original GeoPref test) might improve if we altered the complexity of the social stimuli. That is, we predicted that a greater percentage of ASD toddlers may find the social side uninteresting (and would thus fixate on the geometric images instead) if it were made more complex. However, for typical toddlers, it may increase their interest in the social side if social interactions were depicted, which would potentially increase group differences.

In a meta-analysis of 38 articles comparing ASD and TD children using eye tracking [43], Chita-Tegmark reports that increasing the social content of stimuli by showing more than one person is the factor that best reveals the differences in social attention between ASD and TD groups. We tested the hypothesis that the original GeoPref test identifies a stable subtype of autism characterized by robust patterns of decreased social attention and increased attention to geometric repetition and therefore that the Complex Social GeoPref test should generally replicate the findings of the original GeoPref test, perhaps with amplified effects due to changes to the social stimuli used. That is, ASD children were predicted on average to have greater fixation times on geometric images than contrast groups, and above some threshold, all children with sufficiently high fixation time on geometric images were predicted to be ASD children. Further, ASD children who complete both tests within the appropriate age range were predicted to have fairly stable scores. Additionally, the ASD children with greatest fixation times on geometric images, the GeoPref ASD subtype, were predicted to also have worse cognitive, language, and social skills based on MSEL, ADOS, and VABS scores compared with ASD children with the least geometric fixation times (the ASD "SocPref" subtype).

Methods
Participant recruitment
Two hundred and seventy toddlers enrolled in and completed this study. Of the 270, 43 were excluded from data analysis for reasons detailed in Additional file 1: Figure S1 (e.g., vision abnormality, tantrum during eye tracking), leaving a final study sample of 227 toddlers. Their ages ranged from 12 to 48 months (mean 29.5 months, standard deviation 9.5). Two hundred and eleven of the 227 subjects in the present study (93%) were new and non-overlapping with our past two eye tracking papers [38, 39]. Of the 227 participants, 126 completed both the Complex Social GeoPref eye tracking test newly described herein and the original GeoPref test described in previous publications [38, 39, 44]. Sixty-eight of these 126 (54%) completed the original GeoPref test first, and 58 (46%) completed the Complex Social GeoPref test first, and no age differences were found between groups at either time point. The remaining 101 subjects completed the new Complex Social GeoPref test but not the original GeoPref test.

All diagnostic, psychometric and eye tracking tests took place at the University of California San Diego Autism Center. During data collection time periods, any child receiving an autism evaluation, regardless of referral source, was included in eye tracking testing. Fifty-four percent of the sample of 227 were referred to us by their pediatrician who participates in our general population-based screening method called the 1-Year Well-Baby Check-Up Approach [44]. This allows for the prospective study of ASD, as well as global developmental and language delay or other delays, beginning as early as 12 months, typically based on a toddler's failure of the CSBS-DP Infant-Toddler Checklist [45]. Occasionally, a child is referred by a participating pediatrician between ages 2 and 3 so the CSBS is no longer applicable, or because there is concern regarding the child's development despite a passing score on the CSBS questionnaire. The remaining 46% of subjects were not referred by their pediatricians. These participants either self-referred due to parental concern about their child's development, or participated as controls. Though they were not referred

after pediatrician screening for developmental delays, these children received identical testing to the screening referred group during their evaluations at the UCSD Autism Center. ASD children comprise 38% of the group referred through pediatrician screening and 29% of the self-referred group, and this difference falls short of statistical significance (chi-squared = 2.09, $p = .15$). Mean age at eye tracking for the pediatrician screening referred group was 29.9 months; mean age for the self-referred group was 29.0 months at eye tracking.

Diagnostic and psychometric assessments
At each visit, assessments were administered at UCSD Autism Center by PhD-level licensed clinical psychologists and included the Autism Diagnostic Observation Schedule (ADOS) module T, 1, or 2 [46], Mullen Scales of Early Learning (MSEL) [47], and Vineland Adaptive Behavior Scales (VABS) [48]; additional family and medical histories were also obtained. Toddlers who participated when younger than age 30 months were longitudinally tracked and diagnostically evaluated every 6–12 months until age 3 years when a final diagnosis was given. Any child receiving an evaluation during the data collection time period was administered eye tracking for this study, regardless of whether their visit was an intake appointment, a follow-up, or a final diagnostic appointment. Table 1 presents characteristics of the sample.

The study sample consisted of six discrete diagnostic groups of toddlers: 76 ASD, 11 ASD features, 56 DD, 51 TD, 22 Other, and 11 TypSib. The *ASD* group included toddlers who met DSM criteria for Autistic Disorder or PDD-NOS (DSM IV) or ASD (DSM V) at their final diagnostic evaluation. The *ASD features* group had significant ASD symptoms and/or elevated ADOS scores during at least one evaluation but did not meet full criteria for ASD at their final longitudinal evaluation. The *DD* group included transient and persistent language delay and global developmental delay determined by MSEL scores. The *TD* group included "type 1 errors," children who failed the CSBS screening at a pediatric visit but tested within typical levels on ADOS, MSEL, and VABS during their evaluations, as well as typically developing toddlers who both passed the CSBS and tested within the typical range on ADOS, MSEL, and VABS tests during their evaluations. In the *TypSib* group were unaffected toddlers with siblings with ASD who tested within the typical range during their evaluations. In the *Other* group were toddlers with a wide array of other conditions such as social anxiety or a tic disorder. For this study, 83% of the overall sample received a final diagnostic assessment at 30 months or older (mean age 38.3 months). The remaining 17% (*13 ASD, 18 DD, 4 TD, 2 TypSib, 1 Other*) were assigned to a diagnostic

Table 1 Participant characteristics of overall sample

	1) ASD[a]	2) ASD feat.	3) DD	4) TD	5) Other	6) Typical sibling ASD	ASD vs 2), p=	ASD vs 3), p=	ASD vs 4), p=	ASD vs 5), p=	ASD vs 6), p=
Sex, M/F	70/6	10/1	36/20	30/21	11/11	4/7	n/a	n/a	n/a	n/a	n/a
Age at eye tracking, months Mean (SD) [range]	30.0 (8.8) [12.1–47.4]	31.9 (8.9) [15.8–40.7]	26.8 (9.5) [12.4–46.0]	29.7 (9.5) [12.9–47.5]	33.6 (10.3) [13.1–47.7]	27.8 (11.2) [12.2–44.6]	NS	NS	NS	NS	NS
MSEL AE[b] scores/true age											
Visual reception	.79 (.18)	.94 (.24)	.93 (.19)	1.16 (.18)	1.05 (.20)	1.17 (.16)	NS	<.001	<.001	<.001	<.001
Fine motor	.79 (.18)	.90 (.13)	.96 (.18)	1.04 (.13)	.95 (.20)	1.04 (.16)	NS	<.001	<.001	<.01	<.001
Receptive language	.58 (.28)	.82 (.24)	.79 (.24)	1.10 (.16)	1.0 (.23)	1.03 (.15)	<.05	<.001	<.001	<.001	<.001
Expressive language	.60 (.26)	.72 (.20)	.64 (.23)	1.04 (.17)	.99 (.25)	1.04 (.13)	NS	NS	<.001	<.001	<.001
VABS[c] standard scores											
Communication	75.2 (18.8)	90.8 (17.2)	84.6 (15.4)	104.1 (9.8)	98.8 (12.0)	101.5 (5.1)	<.05	<.05	<.001	<.001	<.001
Daily living	82.4 (15.5)	99.2 (11.7)	92.2 (13.2)	101.1 (9.3)	96.7 (15.2)	98.4 (11.6)	<.005	=.001	<.001	<.001	<.005
Socialization	80.1 (16.1)	96.0 (11.3)	96.4 (11.2)	102.7 (9.2)	97.4 (13.7)	104.4 (6.6)	<.005	<.001	<.001	<.001	<.001
Motor skills	87.8 (17.3)	96.6 (10.4)	91.0 (13.4)	99.7 (9.6)	94.8 (13.3)	99.9 (6.5)	NS	NS	<.001	NS	NS
Composite score	78.8 (15.8)	94.6 (11.7)	88.6 (11.2)	102.7 (10.4)	96.1 (13.1)	100.9 (5.7)	<.005	<.001	<.001	<.001	<.001
ADOS[d] module T, 1, or 2											
SA[e]	13.2 (4.2)	6.2 (5.5)	4.3 (3.1)	2.5 (1.7)	4.3 (3.7)	3.1 (2.2)	<.001	<.001	<.001	<.001	<.001
RRB[f]	3.7 (2.0)	2.0 (1.5)	0.8 (1.8)	0.4 (0.8)	0.4 (0.6)	0.5 (0.5)	<.05	<.001	<.001	<.001	<.001
Total score	16.9 (5.2)	8.2 (6.0)	5.2 (3.8)	2.9 (2.0)	4.7 (4.0)	3.6 (2.0)	<.001	<.001	<.001	<.001	<.001

[a]See text for descriptions of diagnostic groups ASD, ASD Feat., DD, TD, Other, Typical Sibling ASD
[b]Mullen Scales of Early Learning, Age Equivalent
[c]Vineland Adaptive Behavior Scales
[d]Autism Diagnostic Observation Schedule
[e]Social Affect Score
[f]Restricted and Repetitive Behaviors Score

group based on a diagnosis given between 18 and 30 months (mean age 24.2 months).

Movie, apparatus, and eye tracking procedure

The Complex Social GeoPref test contained a 90-s movie composed of two large, rectangular areas of interest (AOIs) side by side (see Fig. 1) where one AOI displayed geometric patterns and the other social scenes. There was no audio. The geometric patterns were a subset of those of the original 60-s GeoPref test [38]; however, each geometric pattern was repeated for a longer time interval to achieve a 90-s test. Each social scene was paired with one of the moving, colorful geometric patterns, and when each social scene changed, each geometric pattern also changed. The social scenes included five scenes showing two children interacting. The interactions were dance-like twisting side by side, jumping to a high-five, whispering a secret then appearing surprised, whispering a secret then hugging, and teasing by sticking out tongues then stomping on the other's foot. To allow for cross-paradigm comparisons, a subset of 126 toddlers participated in the original GeoPref test identical to Pierce et al. [38] as well as the new Complex Social

GeoPref test on separate visits. Unlike the complex social scenes in the present design, in the original GeoPref test, all scenes similarly showed children doing rhythmic, dance-like movements all displaying a uniformly positive affect. See Fig. 1 for sample images and the movie clip "Additional file 2" for more details.

Eye tracking data were collected while toddlers, seated on a parent's lap, viewed these videos from 60 cm distance on a 17″ thin-film transistor monitor using the Tobii T-120 system set at 60 Hz. Five-point calibration was first performed with Tobii Studio software using an animated image with sound presented at known X-Y coordinates. Eye tracking data were collected only if the calibration result fell within the parameters reported by the manufacturer to yield an accuracy of 0.5° [49]. Each AOI subtended 12.9° horizontally and 9.1° vertically. This use of large, simple AOIs facilitated correct measurement of the infant/toddler population, who can yield data with accuracy below levels reported for adults under optimal conditions [50]. More information about data spatial accuracy is provided in the Additional file 1.

Fixations were classified based on gaze data averaged from both eyes using a velocity threshold Tobii Fixation

Filter set to 35 pixels/window, which interpolates to fill in data loss of less than 100 ms. For each subject, number of fixations, duration of each fixation, and sum of fixation time within the two AOIs (social and geometric) were calculated. Sum of fixation time per AOI was divided by total sum of fixation time for both AOIs to derive proportion of time spent on each AOI (i.e., "%Geo" and "%Soc") and to correct for missing data. Subjects with excessive missing data (i.e., less than 30 s of data) due to attending to neither AOI or due to inability to track eye gaze (e.g., during excessive movement) were excluded, in order to preclude inaccurate measurement of number or length of fixations and saccades. Number of fixations per AOI was divided by sum of fixation time for that AOI to derive saccade frequency as saccades per second, which was also reported in our prior publication [39]. See the Additional file 1: Figure S1 for the complete description of exclusion criteria and lab practices for assuring data accuracy and precision, and also the results regarding saccade per second differences between groups.

Statistical analyses
Percent of total fixation duration to geometric vs complex social stimuli
No age differences were found between diagnostic groups (one-way ANOVA with no overall effect of age; see Table 1). To compare percentage of total fixation time within the geometric AOI between groups, a one-way ANOVA was performed (diagnostic group (6 levels) × %Geo (1 level)). A significant main effect was followed by Bonferroni-corrected post hoc pairwise comparisons. Prior to selecting these analysis strategies, homogeneity of variance was confirmed with Levene's test. To confirm that differences in data quality between diagnostic groups were not impacting the reported results, an ANCOVA was performed as well, with six diagnostic groups as a fixed factor, %Geo as the dependent variable, and a data quality measure (percent of valid samples obtained) as a covariate. There was no significant effect of the data quality metric ($F_{5,221} = .011$, $p = .916$).

Relationships between percent of total fixation duration and clinical characteristics
All statistical values for clinical scores presented in Table 1, namely, those of ADOS, MSEL, and VABS, were calculated in the same manner: one-way ANOVAs were performed with post hoc pairwise tests and Bonferroni corrections. The relationship between Complex Social GeoPref %Geo scores and ADOS total scores was assessed with Spearman's rank-order correlations. After identifying the ASD children with the strongest preferences for geometric and for social images using %Geo and %Soc scores, within ASD analyses focused on differences in clinical characteristics between the subtypes "GeoPref" and "SocPref" followed strategies like those

described above: homogeneity of variance was assessed and no significant age difference between groups was found, so independent samples t tests were used to compare scores on ADOS, MSEL, and VABS scores. These comparisons presented in Table 2 are reported one-tailed based on a priori hypotheses from our 2016 manuscript regarding the direction of differences. Correction for multiple comparisons was performed using the Benjamini-Hochberg procedure. Cohen's d effect sizes are reported as well.

Clinical classification performance: sensitivity, specificity, PPV, NPV, and ROC curve
To assess the ability of the Complex Social GeoPref test to discriminate toddlers with ASD from other toddlers, sensitivity, specificity, positive predictive value (PPV), negative predictive value (NPV), and Receiver Operating Characteristic (ROC) area under the curve were determined. For consistency and comparison with our past publications, 69% looking time to geometric images was used as the cut-off for a positive result. Although PPV and NPV for a general population ASD screening tool would be calculated based on the 1/68 prevalence rate for ASD [14], the GeoPref tests are best suited as second

Table 2 Participant characteristics of ASD subgroups

	ASD GeoPref subtype	ASD SocPref subtype	t test, corrected p	Cohen's d
Sex, M/F	13/1	15/2	n/a	
Age at eye tracking, months Mean (SD) [range]	31.2 (9.2) [13.8–47.2]	28.7 (7.2) [16.4–45.4]	.40	.30
MSEL[a] age equivalent scores/true age				
Visual reception	.76 (.17)	.81 (.23)	.50	.25
Fine motor	.76 (.19)	.82 (.18)	.41	.32
Receptive language	.46 (.25)	.68 (.26)	.03	.86
Expressive language	.53 (.26)	.67 (.30)	.19	.50
VABS[b] standard scores				
Communication	71.0 (16.0)	81.5 (16.0)	.08	.66
Daily living	80.9 (15.2)	84.1 (15.3)	.57	.21
Socialization	77.1 (12.7)	84.8 (14.4)	.13	.57
Motor skills	84.4 (10.7)	95.7 (15.0)	.03	.87
Composite score	75.6 (12.7)	84.2 (15.9)	.11	.60
ADOS[c] module T, 1, or 2				
SA[d]	16.7 (3.2)	11.4 (4.1)	< .001	1.4
RRB[e]	4.2 (2.5)	3.1 (1.7)	.15	.51
Total score	20.9 (4.4)	14.5 (4.2)	< .001	1.5

[a]Mullen Scales of Early Learning
[b]Vineland Adaptive Behavior Scales
[c]Autism Diagnostic Observation Schedule
[d]Social affect
[e]Restricted and repetitive behaviors

tier tools, administered after a questionnaire screener which has higher sensitivity but lower specificity. Therefore, PPV and NPV were calculated here against the ASD rate in our sample (i.e., 1/3). This rate reflects a PPV and NPV that might be expected at a general ASD and developmental disorder diagnosis and evaluation clinic, where children are referred primarily due to failing a first-tier screening tool (i.e., the CSBS-DP Infant Toddler Checklist). Classification statistics are presented separately for the entire sample and for screening referred children only without including self-referred children. However, it is to be expected that in a real-world clinical setting, self-referrals will naturally occur as there are many ways outside of pediatrician screening (e.g., Google searching) that community members might become aware of the availability of evaluation services and then self-refer.

Because the greatest challenge to clinicians is distinguishing ASD toddlers from toddlers with other sorts of delays, these classification performance measures were also calculated without the inclusion of TD and TypSib groups and are presented in the Additional file 1. Because 69% was chosen in our previous work by setting the test's specificity to 99%, classification performance values are also reported for the cut-off that gives a specificity of 99% on the Complex Social GeoPref test (75% of looking time to geometric images) in the Additional file 1. Use of the Complex Social GeoPref test in order to rule out a diagnosis of ASD, where having a %Geo score below a certain threshold is considered positive, plus having any diagnosis other than ASD is considered true positive, is examined in the Additional file 1 with regard to sensitivity, specificity, PPV, NPV, and AUC.

Comparing and combining of complex social and original GeoPref tests

Differences between the Complex Social GeoPref and original GeoPref tests for the subset of children who completed both tests in the percentage of time viewing geometric stimuli (%Geo scores) were investigated in several ways. Paired samples t tests were used to compare %Geo scores for the two tests for each diagnostic group. Degree of correlation between test scores for individual children who completed both tests was assessed with Spearman's rank-order correlation. Use of both tests by a single child, where a positive score on either test (or both tests) is considered a positive result, was also examined with regard to sensitivity, specificity, PPV, NPV, and AUC. AUC for this two-test model was determined based on predicted probabilities calculated using binary logistic regression with %Geo scores for the two tests as covariates.

Results

Percent of total fixation duration of the six diagnostic groups to geometric vs complex social stimuli

In our new Complex Social GeoPref test, geometric images attracted significantly more looking time in ASD than in TD, DD, and other groups ($F_{5,221} = 9.1$, $p < .001$, partial eta-squared = .17; ASD vs TD, $p < .001$, Cohen's $d = .85$; ASD vs DD, $p < .001$, Cohen's $d = 1.0$; ASD vs other, $p < .005$, Cohen's $d = .96$). Toddlers with ASD spent an average of 48.4% of their time looking at geometric images (95% confidence interval (CI) range 43.6–53.2%); TD toddlers 31.2% of their time (95% CI 25.8–36.6%); DD toddlers 28.6% of their time (95% CI 23.8–33.4%); and other toddlers 30.0% of their time (95% CI 22.5–37.6%). Toddlers with ASD also looked more at geometric images than TypSibs (mean 32.8%, 95% CI 20.8–44.7%) and ASD features (mean 39.0%, 95% CI 28.9–49.0%), but these differences were not statistically significant, perhaps due to small sample sizes in the latter two study groups. See Fig. 2.

Within ASD: differences between the ASD GeoPref and ASD SocPref subtypes

Percent of total fixation duration per AOI and clinical characteristic comparisons

In order to compare clinical characteristics associated with ASD toddlers at either end of the fixation spectrum [39] (i.e., those who strongly preferred geometric images and those who strongly preferred social images), ASD toddlers were identified who were either the ASD GeoPref subtype (> 69% time looking at geometric images) or the ASD SocPref subtype (> 69% time looking at complex social images). The mean %Geo looking score for the ASD GeoPref subtype was 80.5% (or 19.5% social looking), and the mean %Soc looking score for the ASD SocPref subtype was 80.3% (or 19.7% geometric looking).

Clinical differences between the two ASD subtypes are shown in Table 2. Similar to our previous reports [39], as compared to the ASD SocPref subjects, the ASD GeoPref subjects had significantly increased ADOS social affect ($t_{29} = 4.0$, $p < .001$, Cohen's $d = 1.4$) and total scores ($t_{29} = 4.2$, $p < .001$, Cohen's $d = 1.5$). Further, across the entire group of 76 toddlers with ASD, %Geo scores on the Complex Social GeoPref test were significantly correlated with ADOS total scores, that is, those with greater preference for looking at the geometric stimuli had more severe autism scores (Spearman's rho = .43, $p < .001$), and this is presented in the Additional file 1. The ASD GeoPref subjects appeared to also have lower mean Mullen receptive language scores, and lower Vineland motor scores, with moderate Cohen's d effect sizes.

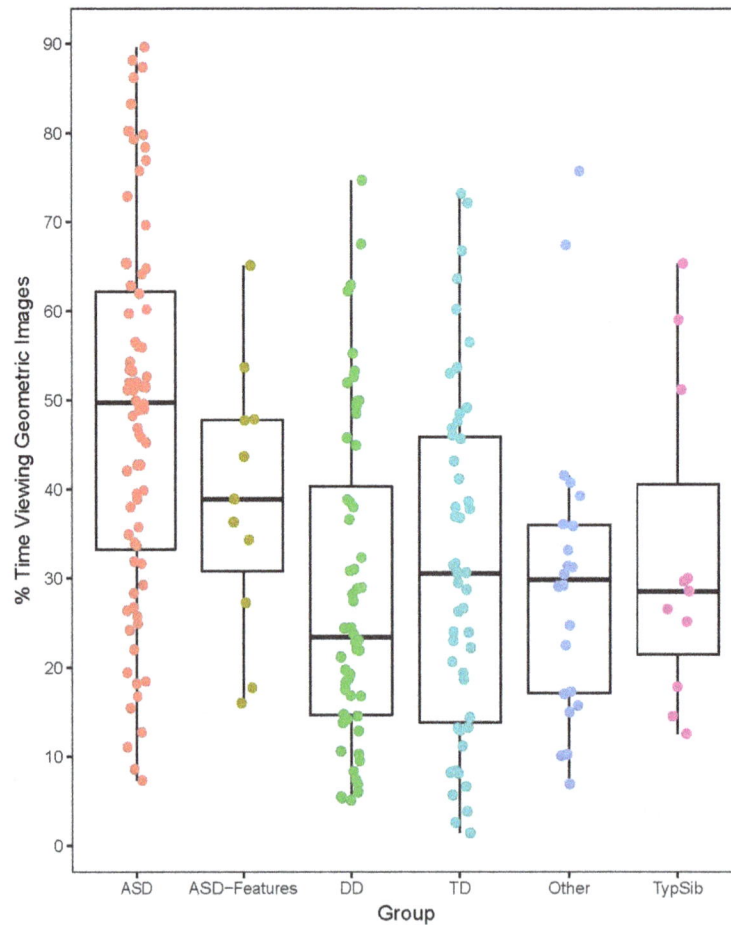

Fig. 2 Scatterplot of % time viewing geometric images (total fixation duration while viewing the dynamic geometric stimulus, divided by total fixation duration to the geometric and social stimuli combined) for all subjects who completed the Complex Social GeoPref test (n = 227) sorted by diagnostic group. Boxplots show median, range, and first and third quartiles

New Complex Social GeoPref test vs original GeoPref test
Eye tracking data were examined from 126 of the 227 study subjects (37 ASD, 10 ASD features, 30 DD, 32 TD, 7 Typ-Sibs, 10 other) who completed both the new Complex Social GeoPref test and the original GeoPref test on separate visits to the center. Sixty-seven completed the original GeoPref test first (mean age 27.3 months at original GeoPref testing) and 59 completed the Complex Social GeoPref test first (mean age 29.0 months at Complex Social GeoPref testing), and this age difference was not significant. Further, no diagnostic group differences in age at testing were found.

Across all diagnostic groups, the mean difference between the Complex Social GeoPref and original GeoPref tests in percent time looking at geometric images (%Geo) was 1.3% (%Geo = 35.4% for the Complex Social vs %Geo = 34.1% for the original GeoPref test), and this was not significant ($t_{125} = 0.6$, $p = .60$). For the ASD group, the mean %Geo score was 48.7% for the Complex Social and 44.7% for the original

GeoPref tests, which was a non-significant difference ($t_{35} = 1.0$, $p = .31$).

There was a significant within-subject correlation in %Geo of total fixation duration across the Complex Social and original GeoPref tests across all study subjects ($N = 126$; Spearman's $r = .25$, $p < .005$) and within the ASD group ($N = 37$; Spearman's $r = .47$, $p < .005$). See Fig. 3. For TD and DD groups, these scores were not significantly correlated.

ROC comparisons were all examined, with rates of specificity, sensitivity, PPV, NPV, and AUC compared between the Complex Social and original GeoPref tests in Table 3. AUC was 0.74 for the Complex Social GeoPref test. For comparison, AUC was 0.71 for the original GeoPref test in Pierce et al. (2016). Removal of typically developing children from analysis and focusing on children with some sort of delay or disorder further improved AUC to 0.75 (see Additional file 1). Removal of self-referred children and focusing on screening referred only yielded an AUC of 0.73.

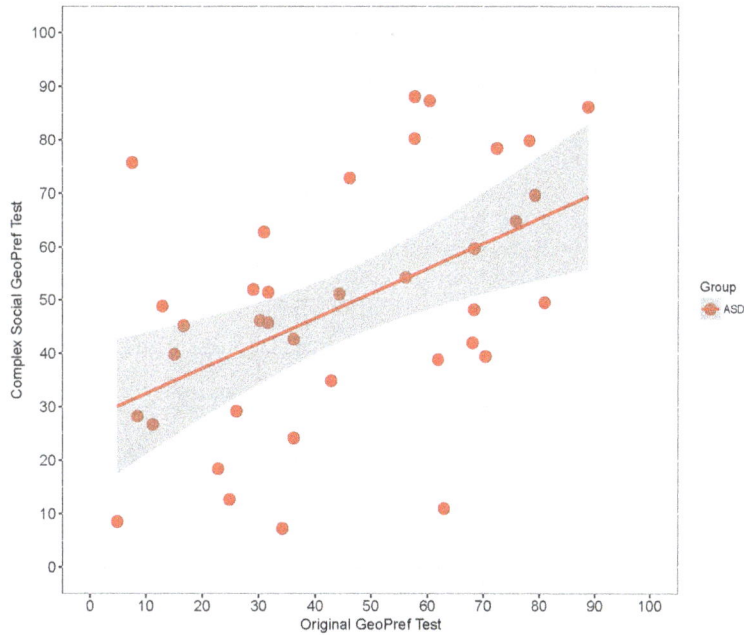

Fig. 3 Correlation between original and Complex Social GeoPref Tests. Scatterplot illustrating % Geo scores (summed fixation duration while viewing the dynamic geometric stimulus, divided by total fixation duration to the geometric and social stimuli combined) for each test for each subject in the ASD group who completed both eye tracking tests on separate visits across the span of the study

Clinical classification performance: combination of new and original GeoPref tests

AUC, sensitivity, specificity, and PPV and NPV values were then examined when using a two-test screening model on data from the 126 subjects who participated in both the Complex Social and original GeoPref tests in order to determine if use of two tests enhanced classification performance. Results are shown in Table 4 (see data

Table 3 Clinical classification performance, comparison of original and Complex Social Geopref tests

69% Geo threshold	All available subjects N = 444	All available subjects N = 227	Screening referred subjects only N = 122
True positive = ASD only	Original GeoPref test (2016)	Complex Social GeoPref test	Complex Social GeoPref test
True positive	35	14	10
False negative	117	62	36
False positive	4	4	3
True negative	288	147	73
Sensitivity (%)	23	18	22
Specificity (%)	99	97	96
Positive predictive value (%)	90	78	77
Negative predictive value (%)	71	70	67
Area under ROC curve	.71	.74	.73

in the left two columns). Sensitivity increased substantially from 18% for the Complex Social test alone (Table 3) to 35% with two tests, while specificity remained high. AUC calculated for this two-test model was 0.75. Pilot results in the Additional file 1 suggest this enhancement does not occur if the two tests are given immediately back-to-back but only if separated in time.

Classification performance of the combination of the two tests for screening referred toddlers only was also examined. Results are shown in Table 4 (data in the right two columns). Again, sensitivity increased substantially from 18% (Table 3) to 33%, while specificity remained high. AUC calculated for this two-test model applied to screening referred toddlers only was 0.73.

Discussion

Debate and controversy regarding the replication of findings from the biological sciences and psychology have been common in recent years [51, 52]. In contrast, the Geometric Preference effect in toddlers with autism has now been replicated multiple times in both direct, identical replication [39] and in this conceptual replication with varied social stimuli. Following our original report in 2011 [38], independent laboratories have also reported similar findings, e.g., [53, 54]. The Complex Social GeoPref test has 97% specificity for ASD in our sample, which is especially high given that our sample contains toddlers with a large variety of presentations beyond typical development and ASD, including

Table 4 Clinical classification, two tests: combined original and Complex Social Geopref Tests

69% Geo threshold	All available subjects N = 126	All available subjects N = 126	Screening referred subjects only N = 82	Screening referred subjects only N = 82
Positive = positive on either test	ASD only = true positive	ASD + ASD features = true positive	ASD only = true positive	ASD + ASD features = true positive
True positive	13	15	9	11
False negative	24	32	18	23
False positive	5	3	5	3
True negative	84	76	50	45
Sensitivity (%)	35	32	33	32
Specificity (%)	94	96	91	94
Positive predictive value (%)	72	83	64	79
Negative predictive value (%)	78	70	74	66
Area under ROC curve	.75	.78	.73	.76

language delay and global developmental delay. In comparison, genetic biomarkers of ASD are often pleiotropic and therefore also associated with a number of other neurodevelopmental disorders, so they can have poor specificity [1], as well as low sensitivity due to the large number of different genetic inputs that converge on the ASD phenotype [55]. Effective usage of GeoPref tests would involve prescreening such as we have done here using the CSBS at pediatrician offices; therefore, positive predictive value need not be measured against the 1/68 base rate of ASD in the general population [9]. Without high specificity tests, applied correctly, with results communicated appropriately, false positives do result in inadvertent harms in the process of early identification for infants at risk for ASD [56]. These harms include the family's exposure to stress and stigma and the unnecessary usage of somewhat scarce and costly intervention services [57]. It has been shown that pediatricians do not refer a significant portion of children who fail screenings for developmental delays, probably due in part to concern regarding the potential for false positive results [58]. Therefore, the availability of screening tools with few false positives could significantly impact the efficacy of screening procedures used for early identification of ASD.

Because the GeoPref tests, both the original and the Complex Social version, detect a subtype of ASD, sensitivity is considerably lower than specificity: at optimal specificity, the Complex Social GeoPref test will catch about 1 in 5 children with autism, while the rate for the original GeoPref test is about 1 in 4.However, here we show that when the two tests are used in combination across separate testing sessions, the correct detection rate is 1 in 3 and specificity remains high at about 94% (Table 4). Further, as can be seen in Fig. 2, the range of %Geo scores for ASD children does not extend as low as that of other groups, which is not a property of the

original GeoPref test. If borne out by further data, this could be of value clinically as a means of ruling out ASD in certain children who are exhibiting some ambiguous warning signs but have very low %Geo scores, in order to shift them away from unnecessary ASD services. This result is described in more detail in the Additional file 1. Future research will work toward creating a battery of multiple eye tracking tests in order to further increase sensitivity to ASD in general and to zero in on optimal procedures for detection of this GeoPref subtype of ASD and to elucidate its biological bases.

The ASD GeoPref subtype toddlers detected with GeoPref tests tend to be the most affected cases, as ADOS symptom severity is correlated with %Geo score. It has been observed that more severe presentations of ASD tend to be less studied [59], despite being arguably more in need of treatment. It is possible that the defects impacting the "social brain," particularly in the frontal regions that control attention and social interest [60], are more pronounced in this ASD subgroup. Since functional brain imaging began to be utilized to understand the operations of the brains of those on the autism spectrum about 20 years ago, abnormalities in virtually every social brain region examined have been reported [61]. However, in addition to the fact that such studies almost exclusively included only older and/or high functioning individuals, data was almost always presented at the group level. As such, previous studies made it hard to understand if reported "social brain" abnormalities were ubiquitous across all ASD individuals, or were being driven by certain subgroups or individuals with the most severe functional abnormalities. In an effort to parse the heterogeneity of social brain neural functional responding in ASD, our new resting state functional imaging study, which examined ASD GeoPref toddlers as a separate subgroup, found substantially weakened functional connectivity between the default mode network

(DMN) which includes key "social brain" regions such as the medial prefrontal cortex [62] and a visual network within the occipito-temporal cortex (OTC) in GeoPref ASD toddlers, but not in other toddlers (Lombardo et al., In Review). This finding is consistent with the previous theory that argues that ASD is a disorder wherein higher order social frontal systems are disconnected from more basic systems [63] and further underscores that the severity of this disconnection may be a driving factor in the social abilities of ASD individuals. Notably, ASD toddlers that did not show the GeoPref profile, i.e., SocPref ASD toddlers, did not show distinctly abnormal functional connectivity between the DMN and OTC (Lombardo et al., In Review). The implication of this work is that ASD SocPref toddlers may have stronger and more typical functional circuitry and, again, promise for a better long-term outcome.

Given the intrinsic heterogeneity in the loose category circumscribed by an ASD diagnosis, focusing on subgroups with phenotypic commonalities may be a key research strategy [64]. Another topic for future research is characterization of the GeoPref and SocPref subtypes in terms of traits that are prevalent but not defining characteristics of ASD, such as gastrointestinal issues, altered sensorimotor processing, or comorbid seizure disorder. If found, differences in rates of comorbid epilepsy, motor impairment, and sleep disturbance, because specific mutations have been associated with each [65], could point to genotypic differences between the phenotypic subgroups identified by GeoPref tests.

Consistent with previously reported findings [43], we hypothesized that our revised social stimuli that presented more than one person or social interactions between multiple people tend to magnify the differences between ASD and TD gaze behavior when compared to simpler social stimuli presenting a single person. We did not find this to be the case, as the Original GeoPref test that paired individual children dancing and dynamic geometric images elicited similar or even slightly larger differences between diagnostic groups than the current Complex Social GeoPref test. Alternately, other variables that differ between the Original and Complex Social stimuli, such as salience of biological motion, temporal dynamics of vignettes unfolding, or the overall length, or perhaps differences in low-level visual properties influencing salience (e.g., color or contrast), may account for this finding [66, 67].

One limitation of the current study is that because of differences between the stimuli that are unrelated to their content as social and geometric (e.g., basic feature salience), "geometric preference" is not the only reasonable explanation for the observed differences in behavior across groups. Although we have referred to ASD children who show the least interest in the social stimuli and the most interest in dynamic geometric images as

"Geometric Responders" or the "GeoPref" subtype, we have not yet manipulated the geometric images in a large study. It is conceivable that pronounced lack of interest in, or aversion to, the social stimuli alone is driving the geometric preferences, and one could replace the competing stimuli with another type of nonsocial stimuli with similar results. At least one new study suggests that aversion to gaze is not a driving factor in abnormal visual fixation patterns in ASD [68]. However, atypical amygdala responses when viewing eye gaze and faces and disrupted amygdala functional connectivity have been previously observed in ASD and related to gaze aversion and social anxiety [69–71]. It is also possible that the slow rate of saccades shown by the GeoPref subgroups (see Additional file 1) to geometric stimuli may indicate difficulty with attentional disengagement, which then causes longer percent total fixation duration to geometric images. This explanation may have little to do with social motivation, social reward, or "preference" for one stimulus type over the other. Interestingly, however, research studies examining attentional disengagement in ASD are inconclusive, with reports of both deficits [21] and typical responding [72], likely reflecting the wide range of stimuli and procedures used across studies.

The importance of finding the GeoPref profile in toddlers may go beyond its potential value as a screening or even diagnostic biomarker—it may be most importantly useful as a prognostic biomarker. Although it is currently unknown if the abnormal visual fixation patterns displayed during the Complex Social and original GeoPref tests generalize to the everyday life of ASD toddlers, it is at least theoretically plausible that ASD toddlers who display the GeoPref profile are experiencing socially impoverished visual input from their environment. As experience in the first few years of life crucially shapes the brain's organization, we hypothesize that a GeoPref profile in a toddler may predict distal functional and cognitive outcomes, and our future work intends to examine whether the GeoPref profile is associated with a worse long-term outcome than that of ASD toddlers who prefer social images. Importantly, experience-dependent mechanisms involved in early social learning may be amenable to intervention, and therefore, GeoPref tests may be useful for early identification of and differential intervention for toddlers who strongly attend to certain non-social stimuli, ignoring social information. Tailoring treatment according to ASD subtypes could potentially result in improved treatment responses and better long-term outcomes.

Conclusion

Across multiple types of social stimuli and temporal presentations, substantially increased viewing of geometric images during preferential looking tasks that pair dynamic social and geometric images robustly indicates ASD among toddlers. Furthermore, across multiple sorts of stimuli, the subset of ASD toddlers who strongly prefer geometric images have more severe scores on indicators of autism impairment compared to those who strongly prefer social images. In addition to replicating the original GeoPref phenomenon, the Complex Social GeoPref test finding shows potential as a valid behavioral biomarker, as it identifies ASD in toddlers at the individual subject level.

Acknowledgements
We thank Sunny Pence, Mee-Kyoung Kwon, and Linda Lopez for the assistance with the data collection, subject tracking, and research assistant supervision, Srinivasa Nalabolu for the data management, Elizabeth Bacon and Jessica Garcia for the assistance with the clinical testing, Josiah Faustino for the data quality confirmation, and Vahid Gazestani for the statistical consulting.

Funding
This work was supported by the National Institutes of Health grants R01-MH080134 and P50-MH081755.

Authors' contributions
AM collected the data, analyzed the data, and wrote and revised the manuscript. MW and AY collected the data and contributed to the data analysis. CCB and DC provided the diagnostic and standardized testing for the participants. EC interpreted the findings and revised the manuscript. KP designed the study, interpreted the findings, and revised the manuscript. All authors read and approved the final manuscript.

Competing interests
An invention disclosure form was filed by KP with the University of California, San Diego, on March 5, 2010, and the original GeoPref test is licensed by the University of California, San Diego, but free for research use. The other authors declare that they have no competing interests.

References
1. Walsh P, et al. In search of biomarkers for autism: scientific, social and ethical challenges. Nat Rev Neurosci. 2011;12(10):603–12.
2. Tager-Flusberg H, Kasari C. Minimally verbal school-aged children with autism spectrum disorder: the neglected end of the spectrum. Autism Res. 2013;6(6):468–78.
3. Bal VH, et al. Daily living skills in individuals with autism spectrum disorder from 2 to 21 years of age. Autism. 2015;19(7):774–84.
4. Newschaffer CJ, Curran LK. Autism: an emerging public health problem. Public Health Rep. 2003;118(5):393–9.
5. Dawson G, et al. Early behavioral intervention is associated with normalized brain activity in young children with autism. J Am Acad Child Adolesc Psychiatry. 2012;51(11):1150–9.
6. Dawson G, et al. Randomized, controlled trial of an intervention for toddlers with autism: the early start Denver model. Pediatrics. 2010;125(1):e17–23.
7. Anderson DK, Liang JW, Lord C. Predicting young adult outcome among more and less cognitively able individuals with autism spectrum disorders. J Child Psychol Psychiatry. 2014;55(5):485–94.
8. Bauman ML, Kemper TL. Neuroanatomic observations of the brain in autism: a review and future directions. Int J Dev Neurosci. 2005;23(2–3):183–7.
9. Anderson GM. Autism biomarkers: challenges, pitfalls and possibilities. J Autism Dev Disord. 2015;45(4):1103–13.
10. Stoner R, et al. Patches of disorganization in the neocortex of children with autism. N Engl J Med. 2014;370(13):1209–19.
11. Shic F, Macari S, Chawarska K. Speech disturbs face scanning in 6-month-old infants who develop autism spectrum disorder. Biol Psychiatry. 2014; 75(3):231–7.
12. Jones W, Klin A. Attention to eyes is present but in decline in 2-6-month-old infants later diagnosed with autism. Nature. 2013;504(7480):427–31.
13. Chawarska K, Macari S, Shic F. Decreased spontaneous attention to social scenes in 6-month-old infants later diagnosed with autism spectrum disorders. Biol Psychiatry. 2013;74(3):195–203.
14. Christensen DL, Baio J, Van Naarden Braun K, Bilder D, Charles J, Constantino JN, Daniels J, Durkin MS, Fitzgerald RT, Kurzius-Spencer M, Lee LC, Pettygrove S, Robinson C, Schulz E, Wells C, Wingate MS, Zahorodny W, Yeargin-Allsopp M. Prevalence and characteristics of autism spectrum disorder among children aged 8 years–autism and developmental disabilities monitoring network, 11 sites, United States, 2012. Centers for Disease Control and Prevention (CDC): MMWR. Surveillance Summaries; 2016.
15. Kapur S, Phillips AG, Insel TR. Why has it taken so long for biological psychiatry to develop clinical tests and what to do about it? Mol Psychiatry. 2012;17(12):1174–9.
16. Insel TR. The NIMH Research Domain Criteria (RDoC) project: precision medicine for psychiatry. Am J Psychiatry. 2014;171(4):395–7.
17. Bolte S, et al. How can clinicians detect and treat autism early? Methodological trends of technology use in research. Acta Paediatr. 2016; 105(2):137–44.
18. Gredebäck G, Johnson S, von Hofsten C. Eye tracking in infancy research. Dev Neuropsychol. 2010;35(1):1–19.
19. Rommelse NN, Van der Stigchel S, Sergeant JA. A review on eye movement studies in childhood and adolescent psychiatry. Brain Cogn. 2008;68(3):391–414.
20. Wass SV, et al. Shorter spontaneous fixation durations in infants with later emerging autism. Sci Rep. 2015;5:8284.
21. Sacrey LA, et al. Impairments to visual disengagement in autism spectrum disorder: a review of experimental studies from infancy to adulthood. Neurosci Biobehav Rev. 2014;47:559–77.
22. Falck-Ytter T, Bolte S, Gredeback G. Eye tracking in early autism research. J Neurodev Disord. 2013;5(1):28.
23. Insel TR. Translating scientific opportunity into public health impact: a strategic plan for research on mental illness. Arch Gen Psychiatry. 2009; 66(2):128–33.
24. Klin A, et al. Two-year-olds with autism orient to non-social contingencies rather than biological motion. Nature. 2009;459(7244):257–61.
25. Shic F, et al. Limited activity monitoring in toddlers with autism spectrum disorder. Brain Res. 2011;1380:246–54.
26. Chawarska K, Shic F. Looking but not seeing: atypical visual scanning and recognition of faces in 2 and 4-year-old children with autism spectrum disorder. J Autism Dev Disord. 2009;39(12):1663–72.
27. Thorup E, et al. Altered gaze following during live interaction in infants at risk for autism: an eye tracking study. Mol Autism. 2016;7:12.
28. Bedford R, et al. Precursors to social and communication difficulties in infants at-risk for autism: gaze following and attentional engagement. J Autism Dev Disord. 2012;42(10):2208–18.
29. Carpenter M, Nagell K, Tomasello M. Social cognition, joint attention, and communicative competence from 9 to 15 months of age. Monogr Soc Res Child Dev. 1998;63(4):i–vi. 1-143
30. Charman T. Why is joint attention a pivotal skill in autism? Philos Trans R Soc Lond Ser B Biol Sci. 2003;358(1430):315–24.
31. Jones W, Carr K, Klin A. Absence of preferential looking to the eyes of approaching adults predicts level of social disability in 2-year-old toddlers with autism spectrum disorder. Arch Gen Psychiatry. 2008;65(8):946–54.
32. Keehn B, Muller RA, Townsend J. Atypical attentional networks and the emergence of autism. Neurosci Biobehav Rev. 2013;37(2):164–83.
33. Elsabbagh M, et al. Social and attention factors during infancy and the later emergence of autism characteristics. Prog Brain Res. 2011;189:195–207.
34. Bedford R, et al. Additive effects of social and non-social attention during infancy relate to later autism spectrum disorder. Dev Sci. 2014;17(4):612–20.
35. Murza KA, et al. Joint attention interventions for children with autism spectrum disorder: a systematic review and meta-analysis. Int J Lang Commun Disord. 2016;51(3):236–51.

36. Chawarska K, Macari S, Shic F. Context modulates attention to social scenes in toddlers with autism. J Child Psychol Psychiatry. 2012;53(8):903–13.

37. Guillon Q, et al. Visual social attention in autism spectrum disorder: insights from eye tracking studies. Neurosci Biobehav Rev. 2014;42:279–97.

38. Pierce K, et al. Preference for geometric patterns early in life as a risk factor for autism. Arch Gen Psychiatry. 2011;68(1):101–9.

39. Pierce K, et al. Eye tracking reveals abnormal visual preference for geometric images as an early biomarker of an autism spectrum disorder subtype associated with increased symptom severity. Biol Psychiatry. 2016;79(8):657–66.

40. Hadjikhani N, et al. Abnormal activation of the social brain during face perception in autism. Hum Brain Mapp. 2007;28(5):441–9.

41. Grossman ED, Blake R. Brain areas active during visual perception of biological motion. Neuron. 2002;35(6):1167–75.

42. Lloyd-Fox S, et al. Selective cortical mapping of biological motion processing in young infants. J Cogn Neurosci. 2011;23(9):2521–32.

43. Chita-Tegmark M. Social attention in ASD: a review and meta-analysis of eye-tracking studies. Res Dev Disabil. 2016;48:79–93.

44. Pierce K, et al. Detecting, studying, and treating autism early: the one-year well-baby check-up approach. J Pediatr. 2011;159(3):458–65. e1-6

45. Wetherby AM, et al. Validation of the Infant-Toddler Checklist as a broadband screener for autism spectrum disorders from 9 to 24 months of age. Autism. 2008;12(5):487–511.

46. Luyster R, et al. The Autism Diagnostic Observation Schedule-Toddler Module: a new module of a standardized diagnostic measure for autism spectrum disorders. J Autism Dev Disord. 2009;39(9):1305–20.

47. Mullen E. Mullen Scales of Early Learning. Circle Pines: American Guidance Service; 1995.

48. Sparrow S. *Vineland Adaptive Behavior Scales: Survey Form Manual*, D. Balla, Editor. Circle Pines, MN: American Guidance Service; 1984.

49. Accuracy and precision test method for remote eye trackers. 2011 [cited Accessed 18 Feb 2017.

50. Wass SV, Smith TJ, Johnson MH. Parsing eye-tracking data of variable quality to provide accurate fixation duration estimates in infants and adults. Behav Res Methods. 2013;45(1):229–50.

51. Pashler H, Wagenmakers EJ. Editors' introduction to the special section on replicability in psychological science: a crisis of confidence? Perspect Psychol Sci. 2012;7(6):528–30.

52. Begley CG, Ellis LM. Drug development: raise standards for preclinical cancer research. Nature. 2012;483(7391):531–3.

53. Franchini M, et al. Brief report: a preference for biological motion predicts a reduction in symptom severity 1 year later in preschoolers with autism spectrum disorders. Front Psychiatry. 2016;7:143.

54. Franchini M, et al. Social orienting and joint attention in preschoolers with autism spectrum disorders. PLoS One. 2017;12(6):e0178859.

55. Goldani AA, et al. Biomarkers in autism. Front Psychiatry. 2014;5:100.

56. Rossi J, Newschaffer C, Yudell M. Autism spectrum disorders, risk communication, and the problem of inadvertent harm. Kennedy Inst Ethics J. 2013;23(2):105–38.

57. Sheldrick RC, et al. Thresholds and accuracy in screening tools for early detection of psychopathology. J Child Psychol Psychiatry. 2015;56(9):936–48.

58. Wissow LS, et al. Universal mental health screening in pediatric primary care: a systematic review. J Am Acad Child Adolesc Psychiatry. 2013;52(11):1134–47. e23

59. Jack A, Pelphrey KA. Annual research review: understudied populations within the autism spectrum—current trends and future directions in neuroimaging research. J Child Psychol Psychiatry. 2017;58(4):411–35.

60. Bicks LK, et al. Prefrontal cortex and social cognition in mouse and man. Front Psychol. 2015;6:1805.

61. Adolphs R. Cognitive neuroscience of human social behaviour. Nat Rev Neurosci. 2003;4(3):165–78.

62. Amodio DM, Frith CD. Meeting of minds: the medial frontal cortex and social cognition. Nat Rev Neurosci. 2006;7(4):268–77.

63. Courchesne E, Pierce K. Why the frontal cortex in autism might be talking only to itself: local over-connectivity but long-distance disconnection. Curr Opin Neurobiol. 2005;15(2):225–30.

64. Voineagu I, Yoo HJ. Current progress and challenges in the search for autism biomarkers. Dis Markers. 2013;35(1):55–65.

65. Jeste SS, Geschwind DH. Disentangling the heterogeneity of autism spectrum disorder through genetic findings. Nat Rev Neurol. 2014;10(2):74–81.

66. Bertone A, et al. Enhanced and diminished visuo-spatial information processing in autism depends on stimulus complexity. Brain. 2005;128(Pt 10):2430–41.

67. Perreault A, et al. Behavioral evidence for a functional link between low- and mid-level visual perception in the autism spectrum. Neuropsychologia. 2015;77:380–6.

68. Moriuchi JM, Klin A, Jones W. Mechanisms of diminished attention to eyes in autism. Am J Psychiatry. 2017;174(1):26–35.

69. Shen MD, et al. Functional connectivity of the amygdala is disrupted in preschool-aged children with autism spectrum disorder. J Am Acad Child Adolesc Psychiatry. 2016;55(9):817–24.

70. Kleinhans NM, et al. Association between amygdala response to emotional faces and social anxiety in autism spectrum disorders. Neuropsychologia. 2010;48(12):3665–70.

71. Baron-Cohen S, et al. The amygdala theory of autism. Neurosci Biobehav Rev. 2000;24(3):355–64.

72. Fischer J, et al. Unimpaired attentional disengagement in toddlers with autism spectrum disorder. Dev Sci. 2016;19(6):1095–103.

7

A cross-cultural study of autistic traits across India, Japan and the UK

Sophie Carruthers[1], Emma Kinnaird[1], Alokananda Rudra[2], Paula Smith[3], Carrie Allison[3], Bonnie Auyeung[4], Bhismadev Chakrabarti[5], Akio Wakabayashi[6], Simon Baron-Cohen[3], Ioannis Bakolis[1] and Rosa A Hoekstra[1*]

Abstract

Background: There is a global need for brief screening instruments that can identify key indicators for autism to support frontline professionals in their referral decision-making. Although a universal set of conditions, there may be subtle differences in expression, identification and reporting of autistic traits across cultures. In order to assess the potential for any measure for cross-cultural screening use, it is important to understand the relative performance of such measures in different cultures. Our study aimed to identify the items on the Autism Spectrum Quotient (AQ)-Child that are most predictive of an autism diagnosis among children aged 4–9 years across samples from India, Japan and the UK.

Methods: We analysed parent-reported AQ-Child data from India (73 children with an autism diagnosis and 81 neurotypical children), Japan (116 children with autism and 190 neurotypical children) and the UK (488 children with autism and 532 neurotypical children). None of the children had a reported existing diagnosis of intellectual disability. Discrimination indices (DI) and positive predictive values (PPV) were used to identify the most predictive items in each country.

Results: Sixteen items in the Indian sample, 15 items in the Japanese sample and 28 items in the UK sample demonstrated excellent discriminatory power (DI ≥ 0.5 and PPV ≥ 0.7), suggesting these items represent the strongest indicators for predicting an autism diagnosis within these countries. Across cultures, good performing items were largely overlapping, with five key indicator items appearing across all three countries (can easily keep track of several different people's conversations, enjoys social chit-chat, knows how to tell if someone listening to him/her is getting bored, good at social chit-chat, finds it difficult to work out people's intentions). Four items indicated potential cultural differences. One item was highly discriminative in Japan but poorly discriminative (DI < 0.3) in the UK and India, and a further item had excellent discrimination properties in the UK but poorly discriminated in the Indian and Japanese samples. Two additional items were highly discriminative in two cultures but poor in the third.

Conclusions: Cross-cultural overlap in the items most predictive of an autism diagnosis supports the general notion of universality in autistic traits whilst also highlighting that there can be cultural differences associated with certain autistic traits. These findings have the potential to inform the development of a brief global screening tool for autism. Further development and evaluation work is needed.

Keywords: Autism, Culture, Cross-cultural comparison, Positive predictive values

* Correspondence: rosa.hoekstra@kcl.ac.uk
Sophie Carruthers and Emma Kinnaird are joint first authors.
Ioannis Bakolis and Rosa A. Hoekstra are joint last authors.
[1]Institute of Psychiatry, Psychology and Neuroscience, King's College London, London, UK
Full list of author information is available at the end of the article

Background

Autism spectrum disorders (ASD), henceforth 'autism', are neurodevelopmental conditions, characterised by difficulties with social interaction and communication, unusually repetitive and restricted behaviours and interests and sensory hyper-sensitivity [1]. Despite a considerable amount of research into autism [2], the majority of studies have been conducted in Western, higher income countries [3–6]. Consequently, assumptions surrounding the epidemiology, diagnosis and treatment of autism have not been adequately tested across different cultures and socio-economic settings.

A diagnosis of autism is based on the behavioural characteristics of an individual. Though core autism characteristics are believed to be universal, there is preliminary evidence to suggest that cultural differences may exert subtle influence over the expression, identification and/or reporting of symptomatology [5, 7–9]. Culturally specific stigmas, norms and priorities may mask or emphasise relative distinctions between autistic traits and typically developing behaviours [3, 7, 9]. For example, previous work validating screening measures in Japan reported that parent judgements of whether their child is interested in their peers do not correlate with autism in Japanese communities as it does in the US [10]. If this example reflects a true cultural difference, such disparities could reflect a relative higher peer interest for Japanese children with autism, a relative lower peer interest for the Japanese typically developing children or that the salience of these symptoms is weaker for Japanese parents. Consequently, the profile of autism symptoms as measured by parent report may not be globally consistent [5, 7].

Tools developed for screening autism are increasingly being used outside their original cultural context [11, 12], with the majority developed in Europe and North America [13, 14]. Due to the emphasis on behavioural symptoms of such tools, if the presentation, salience and reporting of autistic characteristics are not globally consistent, this could impact the ability to use tools developed in one culture (typically the West) in other countries [15]. Developing new screening tools requires extensive resources and effort that may not be feasible for lower income countries. Existing Western screening tools have been translated into other languages [10, 16–20] but not always without difficulties [6, 21, 22], and validation studies of these screening tools in other cultures have typically examined overall mean group differences, rather than item-level analyses [16, 18–20, 23]. Moreover, the previous literature has often focused on toddlers [21, 24, 25]. However, children with autism without intellectual disability are less likely to exhibit salient symptoms at the preschool age and often only receive a diagnosis in mid-late childhood [26–28]. This is particularly problematic since behavioural expectations of children in different countries may differ according to age [29], suggesting that findings on toddler screening measures may neither be translatable to school-aged children, nor necessarily be equivalent across cultures.

There is thus a need for cross-cultural research exploring screening tools for this age group. An important consideration, particularly when aiming to develop a short screening tool, is whether the autistic traits that best predict an autism diagnosis are similar across different cultures. Initial research exploring such 'key indicators' has been conducted using the Autism Spectrum Quotient (AQ), a 50-item open-access and free to use questionnaire developed in the UK, adapted for different ages and validated in several languages [19, 24, 30–37]. Researchers developed shorter versions for different age groups (AQ-10) by examining which items best discriminate between cases and controls in UK samples, identifying ten highly predictive items [38]. The AQ-10 exhibited high test accuracy properties and internal consistency and is as effective as the original questionnaire in identifying high-risk autism cases across a range of different ages [38]. However, this analysis has so far only been conducted within a UK sample.

This study aimed to contribute towards a greater understanding of expression and recognition of childhood autism symptoms across cultures by identifying key indicator items across three distinct cultural settings: the UK, Japan and India.

Methods

Study sample

The sample from India has been described previously [23]. In brief, participants were recruited from Delhi and Kolkata, using Hindi and Bengali translations of the AQ-Child respectively. Children with a formal autism diagnosis were recruited from not-for-profit organisations in both cities that provide support for people with autism and their families. Typically developing children were recruited from mainstream schools and the general population through word of mouth. Overall, 75 children with autism and 81 typically developing children between the ages of four and eight were recruited from both locations. No children had a reported existing diagnosis of comorbid intellectual disability. Information on the AQ-Child was provided by either parent.

The sample of Japanese participants has not previously been reported; the data collection was coordinated through Chiba University in Japan. Children with a formal autism diagnosis were recruited through special education schools for children with developmental disorders in Tokyo and the surrounding area, typically developing children via mainstream schools. Overall, 116 children with autism and 190 typically developing children between the ages of four and nine were recruited.

No children had a comorbid diagnosis other than autism, including no diagnoses of intellectual disability. The AQ-Child was completed by the child's mother in all instances.

The UK sample was collected by the Autism Research Centre (ARC) at the University of Cambridge. Children with autism were recruited from the ARC's volunteer database and typically developing children through an epidemiological study of social and communication skills recruited via mainstream primary schools. Overall, the sample consisted of 488 children with autism and 532 typically developing children. The participants included in the current study partly overlaps with the sample reported in previous studies [32, 38]. In contrast to these previous studies, the current project only used data from children aged 4–9 years who resided in the UK. Since the publication of the previous studies, additional data from UK children with ASD has been collected through the volunteer database; these new data are also included in the current study. Further details on the methodology employed in the data collection in the three countries are presented in Table 1.

Autism Spectrum Quotient (AQ-Child)

The Autism Spectrum Quotient (AQ-Child) [32] consists of 50 statements relating to autistic traits, where parents indicate on a 4-point Likert scale whether they definitely disagree, slightly disagree, slightly agree or definitely agree with each statement. The AQ includes items assessing a range of autism-characteristic domains, including attention switching, attention to detail, communication, social skills and imagination. The AQ-Child has previously been translated into Japanese [19], Hindi and Bengali [23], with all three versions exhibiting similar psychometric properties to the original [32]. Translation involved blind back translation and multiple cycles of translations until all parties reached consensus. Further details can be found in the respective validation papers [19, 23].

Statistical analyses

Statistical analyses were conducted with the use of Stata 14.2. AQ item scores were converted from the Likert format into binary scoring for the purpose of these analyses in line with previous work [38]. Relevant items were inverse scored so that a score of 1 indicated the presence of an autistic trait and a score of 0 a negative response.

We randomly split the samples from each country into a derivation and validation sample (Table 2; [38]). Discrimination indices (DI) for each item were calculated using the derivation samples by subtracting the

Table 1 Inclusion criteria, recruitment and collection methods of the samples from UK, Japan and India

	UK	Japan	India
Inclusion criteria	*All* Aged 4–9 years Lives in UK No diagnosed ID No siblings in the study	*All* Aged 4–9 years Lives in Tokyo No diagnosed ID No siblings in the study	*All* Aged 4–9 years Lives in Kolkata or Delhi No diagnosed ID Primary language Hindi (if in Delhi) or Bengali (if in Kolkata) No visual, hearing, motor, neurological or mental health disorder No siblings in the study
	Cases Diagnosed by recognised clinical service, according to DSM-IV[a] or DSM-5[b] criteria.	*Cases* Diagnosis confirmed by school and/or clinic Diagnosis by DSM-IV[a]/ICD-10[c] No additional diagnosis other than ASD	*Cases* Diagnosis by DSM-IV[a]/ICD-10[c]
	Controls No neurodevelopmental disorder	*Controls* No diagnosable condition	*Controls* No formal diagnosis of any mental health condition
Autism recruitment	Via ARC's volunteer database	Special education schools for children with developmental disorders	Not-for-profit organisations providing support for people with ASD
Control recruitment	Mainstream schools in Cambridgeshire, UK	Mainstream schools in Tokyo	Mainstream schools in Kolkata and Delhi, general population
AQ-Child method of completion	Cases online; controls pen and paper	Pen and paper	Pen and paper
Informant	Either parent	Mothers	Either parent

ARC Autism Research Centre, University of Cambridge, *DSM* Diagnostic and Statistical Manual of Mental Disorders, *ICD* International Statistical Classification of Diseases and Related Health Problems, *UK* United Kingdom
[a]DSM-IV [48]
[b]DSM-5 [1]
[c]ICD-10 [49]

Table 2 Descriptive statistics of the study sample for each country

	Control derivation sample	Autism derivation sample	Control validation sample	Autism validation sample	Total
Japan					
n	88	65	102	51	306
Sex					
Female	37	8	60	11	116
Male	51	57	42	40	190
Mean age in years (SD)	7.74 (0.10) (*n* = 88)	7.55 (0.16) (*n* = 65)	7.88 (0.09) (*n* = 102)	7.82 (0.19) (*n* = 51)	
India					
n	36	42	45	33	156
Sex					
Female	9	3	12	0	24
Male	9	19	11	16	55
Missing	18	20	22	17	77
Mean age in years (SD)	6.24 (0.87) (*n* = 34)	5.11 (1.09) (*n* = 40)	6.14 (0.24) (*n* = 45)	6.69 (0.27) (*n* = 33)	
UK					
n	269	241	263	247	1020
Sex					
Female	152	44	143	42	381
Male	117	197	120	205	639
Mean age in years (SD)	8.84 (0.81)	6.26 (1.65)	8.76 (0.88)	6.49 (1.66)	

n Number of participants, *SD* standard deviation

percentage of controls who scored 1 (false positives) from the percentage of cases who scored 1 (true positives). Positive predictive values (PPV) were calculated for each item using the validation samples by dividing the number of true positives by the total number of positives (cases and controls scoring 1).

In order to identify a list of key indicator items most predictive of an autism diagnosis within each country, all items per country with a DI ≥ 0.5 (in line with Allison et al.'s previous paper with a UK-based sample [38]) and PPV ≥ 0.7 were selected. Receiver Operating Characteristic (ROC) curves were calculated and compared for these key indicator items and the original 50 items for each country. Optimal cut-offs were determined using the highest percentage correctly classified as guidelines. The area under the curve (AUC) indicates overall predictive validity, with AUC > 0.90 indicating excellent validity. Recommended sensitivity and specificity for developmental screening measures is 70–80% [39]. Cronbach's Alpha was calculated for each measure with a value of > 0.80 indicating excellent internal consistency. Independent *t* tests were used to assess whether the key indicator items exhibited the expected difference between cases and controls, and Pearson correlations were calculated between key indicator items and AQ-50 total scores for each country.

The relative discrimination properties of all AQ-50 items were compared cross-culturally using the following criteria: DI ≥ 0.5 and PPV ≥ 0.7 = 'excellent'

discrimination, DI ≥ 0.3 = 'acceptable' discrimination and DI < 0.3 = 'poor' discrimination [38, 40]. Any item that had 'excellent' discrimination in at least one country but 'poor' in the other(s) was considered to represent a potential cultural difference. In the UK dataset, there was a significant age difference between controls and cases (see Table 2 and the 'Results' section). Therefore, an additional sensitivity analysis was run on the UK dataset to examine whether this age difference could account for the findings.

Results

Children's demographic characteristics are summarised in Table 2. There were no age differences between cases and controls in the Japanese and Indian samples; in the UK, the autism group was younger than the control group ($p < .001$) (Table 2).

DI and PPV analyses for each item are summarised in Table 3, with a summary of case/control responses per country for each item included in Additional file 1. Inspection of the DI and PPV values revealed 16 items for the Indian sample with DI ≥ 0.5 and PPV ≥ 0.7 (cells labelled with 'a' in Table 3), indicating that these items provided excellent differentiation between autism cases and controls. Similarly, 15 AQ-Child items for the Japanese sample and 28 items for the UK sample surpassed the excellent item performance thresholds (in the middle and right-hand columns of Table 3).

Table 3 Item discrimination indices and PPV for each of the 50 items in the AQ across India, Japan and UK

	India		Japan		UK	
AQ item summary	DI	PPV	DI	PPV	DI	PPV
1. Prefers to do things with others rather than alone	.06[c]	.66[c]	.38[b]	.56[b]	.43[b]	.75[b]
2. Prefers to do things the same way over and over again	.52[b]	.60[b]	.54[b]	.59[b]	.62[a]	.70[a]
3. Finds it very easy to create a picture in her/his mind	.67[a]	.94[a]	.45[b]	.89[b]	.55[a]	.81[a]
4. Gets absorbed in one thing and loses sight of other things	.29[c]	.59[c]	.40[b]	.49[b]	.32[b]	.60[b]
5. Notices small sounds when others do not	.20[c]	.46[c]	.35[b]	.61[b]	.52[b]	.68[b]
6. Notices house numbers or similar strings of information	-.25[c]	.33[c]	.37[b]	.80[b]	.30[b]	.61[b]
7. Has difficulty understanding rules for polite behaviour	.58[a]	.78[a]	.44[b]	.96[b]	.80[a]	.89[a]
8. Can easily imagine what characters in a story look like	.86[a]	1[a]	.44[b]	.64[b]	.67[a]	.93[a]
9. Fascinated by dates	-.22[c]	.22[c]	.19[c]	.66[c]	.16[c]	.62[c]
10. Can easily keep track of different conversations	**.57[a]**	**.89[a]**	**.51[a]**	**.76[a]**	**.69[a]**	**.79[a]**
11. Finds social situations easy	.68[a]	.90[a]	.60[b]	.66[b]	.75[a]	.86[a]
12. Tends to notice details that others do not	.08[c]	.36[c]	.32[b]	.49[b]	.24[c]	.56[c]
13. Would rather go to a library than a birthday party	.17[c]	.50[c]	.26[c]	.60[c]	.40[b]	.91[b]
14. Finds making up stories easy	.87[a]	.81[a]	.38[b]	.45[b]	.59[a]	.79[a]
15. Drawn more strongly to people than to things	.39[b]	.50[b]	.36[b]	.49[b]	.55[a]	.74[a]
16. Has strong interests, gets upset if cannot pursue	.30[b]	.56[b]	.53[a]	.81[a]	.36[b]	.63[b]
17. Enjoys social chit-chat	**.75[a]**	**.75[a]**	**.52[a]**	**.97[a]**	**.71[a]**	**.90[a]**
18. When talking, it is not easy to get a word in edgeways	*.02[c]*	*.31[c]*	*.60[a]*	*.83[a]*	*.17[c]*	*.57[c]*
19. Fascinated	-.03[c]	.44[c]	.39[b]	.81[b]	.20[c]	.66[c]
20. Finds it difficult to work out characters' feelings in a story	.39[b]	.58[b]	.37[b]	.68[b]	.72[a]	.88[a]
21. Does not particularly enjoy fictional stories	.42[b]	.83[b]	.31[b]	.63[b]	.34[b]	.80[b]
22. Finds it hard to make new friends	.64[a]	.74[a]	.39[b]	.67[b]	.67[a]	.85[a]
23. Notices patterns in things all the time	.10[c]	.57[c]	.24[c]	.63[c]	.37[b]	.66[b]
24. Would rather go to the cinema than a museum	-.24[c]	.36[c]	.44[b]	.63[b]	.28[c]	.68[c]
25. Is not upset if daily routine is disturbed	.13[c]	.45[c]	.34[b]	.67[b]	.63[a]	.78[a]
26. Does not know how to keep a conversation going	.64[b]	.68[b]	.78[a]	1[a]	.86[a]	.92[a]
27. Finds it easy to "read between the lines" in conversation	.47[b]	.81[b]	.85[a]	.84[a]	.61[a]	.76[a]
28. Concentrates more on a whole picture, rather than details	.23[c]	.86[c]	.58[b]	.59[b]	.49[b]	.69[b]
29. Not very good at remembering phone numbers	.03[c]	.32[c]	-.08[c]	.26[c]	-.17[c]	.45[c]
30. Does not usually notice small changes	-.12[c]	.36[c]	-.13[c]	.35[c]	-.09[c]	.42[c]
31. Knows if someone listening is getting bored	**.65[a]**	**.72[a]**	**.80[a]**	**.87[a]**	**.66[a]**	**.74[a]**
32. Finds it easy to alternate between different activities	.58[a]	.92[a]	.52[b]	.54[b]	.72[a]	.81[a]
33. Not sure when it is her/his turn to speak on the phone	.48[b]	.62[b]	.52[a]	.93[a]	.69[a]	.84[a]
34. Enjoys doing things spontaneously	*.23[c]*	*.50[c]*	*.26[c]*	*.82[c]*	*.57[a]*	*.89[a]*
35. Often the last to understand the point of a joke	*.14[c]*	*.54[c]*	*.71[a]*	*1[a]*	*.62[a]*	*.81[a]*
36. Finds it easy to tell how someone feels from their face	.68[a]	.80[a]	.59[b]	.60[b]	.69[a]	.87[a]
37. Can switch back to what they were doing if interrupted	.30[b]	.80[b]	.51[a]	.87[a]	.63[a]	.84[a]
38. Good at social chit-chat	**.75[a]**	**.86[a]**	**.73[a]**	**.98[a]**	**.80[a]**	**.90[a]**
39. People say they go on and on about the same thing	.44[b]	.68[b]	.59[a]	.94[a]	.41[b]	.70[b]
40. Enjoyed playing pretend games with others in preschool	.78[a]	.87[a]	.38[b]	.69[b]	.71[a]	.86[a]
41. Likes to collect information about categories of things	-.40[c]	.34[c]	.26[c]	.52[c]	.22[c]	.61[c]
42. Finds it difficult to imagine being someone else	.38[b]	.55[b]	.79[a]	.85[a]	.62[a]	.79[a]
43. Likes to plan any activities s/he participates in carefully	-.51[c]	.25[c]	.08[c]	.30[c]	.18[c]	.56[c]

Table 3 Item discrimination indices and PPV for each of the 50 items in the AQ across India, Japan and UK *(Continued)*

	India		Japan		UK	
44. Enjoys social occasions	.23^c	.66^c	.51^a	.87^a	.56^a	.92^a
45. Finds it difficult to work out people's intentions	**.50^a**	**.72^a**	**.80^a**	**.83^a**	**.63^a**	**.76^a**
46. New situations make him/her anxious	.61^b	.59^b	.50^b	.59^b	.45^b	.65^b
47. Enjoys meeting new people	.40^b	.82^b	.25^c	.51^c	.49^b	.84^b
48. Is good at taking care not to hurt other people's feelings	.60^a	.79^a	.41^b	.61^b	.73^a	.88^a
49. Not very good at remembering people's date of birth	-.26^c	.27^c	.19^c	.42^c	-.18^c	.46^c
50. Finds it easy to play pretend games with children	.73^a	.93^a	.36^b	.63^b	.69^a	.89^a

^{a}Key indicator item: excellent item performance (DI ≥ 0.5 and PPV ≥ 0.7); ^{b}item performed acceptably (DI ≥ 0.3); ^{c}item performed poorly (DI < 0.3) Bold text: 'Universal' key indicator item with excellent performance across all three countries. Italics: 'Cultural Difference' item with variable item performance across countries

Psychometric properties

Internal consistency was very high for both the India AQ-16 (α = 0.94) and AQ-50 (α = 0.92). The AUC for both versions indicated excellent validity (AUC > 0.90). The AQ-16 and AQ-50 correlated strongly (r = 0.89, p < .001). At a cut-off point of 5 on the AQ-16, sensitivity was 0.96, specificity was 0.97 and the proportion of correctly classified cases was 0.97. Internal consistency was very high for both the Japanese AQ-15 (α = 0.95) and AQ-50 (α = 0.95). The AUC for both versions indicated excellent validity (AUC > 0.90), and both versions correlated strongly with each other(r = 0.95, p < .001). At a cut-off point of 12 on the AQ-15, sensitivity was 0.96, specificity was 0.96 and proportion correctly classified was 0.92. Internal consistency was very high for both the UK AQ-28 (α = 0.97) and UK AQ-50 (α = 0.96). The AUC for both versions indicated excellent validity (AUC > 0.90). There was a significant correlation between the AQ-28 and AQ-50 (r = 0.97, p < .001). At a cut-off point of 14 on the AQ-28, sensitivity was 0.98, specificity was 0.97 and proportion correctly classified was 0.97.

Cross-cultural comparisons

Five items were identified to be universal key indicators, as they were consistently excellent at discriminating between children with autism and controls in all three countries (see bold items in Table 3). In a social group, s/he can easily keep track of several different people's conversations; s/he enjoys social chit-chat; s/he knows how to tell if someone listening to him/her is getting bored; s/he is good at social chit-chat and s/he finds it difficult to work out people's intentions. There were an additional 23 items that performed excellently or acceptably across all three countries.

Four items were identified as indicating potential cultural differences (see items in italics in Table 3). Item 34 ('S/he enjoys doing things spontaneously') had excellent discrimination properties in the UK, but discriminated poorly in the Indian and Japanese samples. In contrast, item 18 ('When s/he talks, it isn't always easy for others to get a word in edgeways') performed well

in Japan, but poorly in the UK and India. A further two items (35, 'S/he is often the last to understand the point of a joke', and 44, 'S/he enjoys social occasions') were found to perform poorly in India whilst exhibiting excellent predictive value in the UK and Japan. Further information on how cases and controls in each country responded to the AQ items is available in Additional file 1: Tables S1–S3.

A subgroup analysis restricting the age group to 7–9 years for cases and controls in the UK sample, indicated that age differences between cases and controls in the full UK sample did not explain the pattern of results (Additional file 1: Table S4).

Discussion

This study aimed to identify which items on the AQ-Child were most predictive of an autism diagnosis among children from India, Japan and the UK. Sixteen items in the Indian sample, 15 in the Japanese sample and 28 items in the UK sample demonstrated high discriminant and predictive ability of ASD cases, excellent psychometric properties and similar sensitivity and specificity values to the original AQ-50. This suggests that at least within cultures, it is possible to adapt existing measures into psychometrically sound brief tools that successfully differentiate children with and without autism.

When comparing the 'key indicator' items across cultures, our findings suggest that there is substantial overlap in the items most predictive of an autism diagnosis cross-culturally. Overall, 28 items were found to have acceptable or excellent discrimination properties in all three countries. This suggests that a number of autistic traits are consistently expressed, salient for parents and thus reliably identified and reported across different countries. This provides support for the position that screening measures developed in one country can indeed be used in different cultures. Five items were identified to be consistently excellent at discriminating between children with autism and controls in all three countries and identified as universal key indicators. However, it should be noted that two of these universal items (item 17; s/he enjoys social chit-chat and item 38; s/he is good at social chit-chat) are similarly worded and therefore may be overlapping measurements of the same aspect of behaviour.

The present study also identified four autistic traits that may represent cultural differences. Item 34 (s/he enjoys doing things spontaneously) was a highly predictive item in the UK sample, but not in Japan or India. In the UK, two-thirds of the autism children in the derivation sample were reported to not enjoy spontaneity (in line with autism symptomatology). This ratio was much reduced in the Indian and Japanese samples, where only around 30% of the children with autism were reported to not enjoy spontaneity. By contrast, control children across all three countries were reported to enjoy spontaneity at similar levels (91–97%), suggesting that this difference is specific to the autism group. Cross-cultural studies show that societies differ in their tolerance for uncertainty. For instance, Japan is characterised as a highly uncertainty avoidant society, whereas India and the UK score much lower on uncertainty avoidance [41]. It is possible that as a result of Japanese society's tendency towards reducing uncertainty, any spontaneous activity is more structured in Japan than in the other cultures, resulting in relatively few children objecting to spontaneous activities. Indian children with autism also appear more accepting of spontaneity that could reflect the prevalence of an authoritarian parenting style in India, resulting in a general reduction in spontaneity across diagnostic groups and so accounting for the reduced predictive power of this item [42]. Alternatively, these differences may be due to linguistic variation rather than a cultural difference: in the Japanese translation of the AQ-Child, the meaning of item 34 was perceived ambiguously by parents and so had to be clarified with a supplemental explanation in addition to the original question [19]. In the supplemental explanation, more emphasis was placed on the meaning of spontaneous as 'doing something on your own initiative, without suggestions from others', rather than on 'doing something without much prior planning'. Similarly, the terms used in the Bengali and Hindi translations of the AQ-Child for 'spontaneous' are more common in written than in spoken language. Therefore, these differences in response patterns may reflect a lack of familiarity or ambiguity for parents interpreting the question.

Item 18 (when s/he talks, it is not always easy for others to get a word in edgeways) has strong predictive properties in the Japan sample but not in India or the UK. As expected from a highly predictive item, this item is endorsed (suggesting the presence of the autistic trait) in a larger proportion of the cases (64%) and very few controls (3%) in Japan. In contrast, although endorsed for a large proportion of UK cases (70%), it is also reported in a large proportion of UK controls (53%). For India, the proportion of children

for whom it is reported are very similar for both cases (61%) and controls (63%). While lack of qualitative research or cognitive interviewing data prevents us from drawing strong inferences on the causes of these differences, we speculate that parents in the UK and India may have interpreted the item to mean their child was very chatty. While excessive chatting by children is culturally acceptable in the UK and India, the stronger emphasis in Japanese society on social conformity [9, 43–45], politeness and respect for elders may make this characteristic much less acceptable and/or more salient to the reporting parents in Japan.

Items 35 (s/he is often the last to understand the point of a joke) and 44 (s/he enjoys social occasions) were both highly discriminative in the UK and Japan samples but not in India. Although these may be indicative of cultural differences, the smaller size of the Indian sample leads us to interpret these with caution. Moreover, these questions may represent a translation issue: in the versions for India, both 'joke' and 'social occasion' were translated using more formal language.

Strengths and limitations

The comparatively smaller number of key indicator items in the India and Japan samples ($n = 15$ and $n = 16$, respectively) in comparison to that of the UK sample ($n = 28$) may reflect the smaller size of the samples for Japan and India compared to the UK. Alternatively, it may indicate that cross-cultural differences generally limit the discriminating power of certain items when the instrument is used outside of the UK culture in which it was originally developed. Moreover, our three samples have come from different research studies, and therefore, subtle differences exist in their sampling characteristics and recruitment procedures. While in all three countries ASD diagnoses were made by a qualified professional using DSM-IV criteria, the exact diagnostic procedures may have varied both within and across country. No data were available on ethnicity, specific IQ information and socio-economic status; all of which may have influenced the results. Additionally, given the vast regional and cultural differences that exist in India, our findings based on relatively small urban population samples may not generalise across all Indian cultures and contexts, particularly rural areas which were not sampled in this study [46]. In all three countries, the autism samples were purposely selected, rather than derived from a population based survey and may therefore not be fully representative of the population of children with autism in each country. In India and Japan, children with autism were recruited from special schools; this sample may represent a subset of autistic trait profiles within the countries and the most predictive items reported in this study may not be as sensitive to more subtle presentations in the community [47]. This highlights the importance of future studies using population-based samples; although this is challenging in low resource contexts.

Across all three countries, data in clinical samples were collected in children in whom autism had previously been diagnosed. This may have resulted in enhanced awareness of parents of their child's autistic traits and thus increased likelihood of endorsement on corresponding autistic traits. It will be imperative for the development of effective screening tools that future studies explore cross-cultural differences in parent-reports prior to clinical autism diagnoses. It will also be important for comparisons to be conducted in the discrimination of children with ASD and other neurodevelopmental disorders, as this is the more informative contrast for clinicians.

A strength of this study is the exclusion of children with reported diagnoses of intellectual disability, resulting in a more homogenous group of children who are more likely to be left undiagnosed until this primary school age. However, it would also be important to confirm that any measure was equally effective across autism severity, intelligence level and age in each cultural setting. Any global screening initiative would also need to explore any cultural differences in the expression or latent structure of autistic symptomatology in this age group.

Evaluating the utility of the five universal items as a brief screener was beyond the scope of this paper as this would require a different type of psychometric evaluation on a multi-country population-based sample of participants, and we do not recommend use of these items in the place of current screening tools on the basis of these results. However, our findings are informative for the future development of a global screening tool for autism for early-mid childhood, the age when children with autism without intellectual disability are likely to still remain undetected and without formal diagnosis. We identified five items that show consistently excellent performance across all three cultures, suggesting these items hold promise as universal key indicators of autism. This study also identified four items suggesting subtle cultural differences, indicating that researchers should not assume that all autistic traits are equally salient across all cultures. An alternative explanation for the subtle cultural differences identified in this study is the semantic differences in the items concerned. In addition, some of the differences may be of socio-economic rather than cultural origin. To further explore whether the semantics or interpretation of items may be constraining their discriminating abilities and to identify any unique socio-economic or cultural nuances not currently captured by the AQ items, qualitative research (e.g. using cognitive interviews and focus groups) is needed.

Conclusions

Our analyses have demonstrated that taking the most discriminating items from the AQ-Child from three countries results in psychometrically sound brief measures that correctly classify children with autism and typically developing controls. Items with good discriminating power were, to a large extent, universal across the UK, Japan and India samples, but there were also some potential cultural differences. These findings suggest that five items included in the AQ-50 have consistent excellent power to discriminate autism from control children across three distinct cultures and thus hold promise as cross-cultural key indicators for autism. Additional research is needed to further advance our understanding of the cross-cultural nature of autism symptomatology before a 'universal' screening instrument for autism can be derived.

Abbreviations
AQ-Child: Autism Spectrum Quotient-Child Version; ARC: Autism Research Centre, University of Cambridge; ASD: Autism spectrum disorder; AUC: Area under the curve; DI: Discrimination indices; DSM-5: Diagnostic and Statistical Manual of Mental Disorders—5th edition; DSM-IV: Diagnostic and Statistical Manual of Mental Disorders—4th edition; ICD-10: International Statistical Classification of Diseases and Related Health Problems, tenth edition; ID: Intellectual disability; N: Number of participants; PPV: Positive predictive value; ROC: Receiver Operating Characteristic curve; SD: Standard deviation; UK: United Kingdom; US: United States

Acknowledgements
The authors would like to thank all of the participants for being involved in the study.

Funding
Sophie Carruthers and Emma Kinnaird are supported by the UK Medical Research Council (MRC) (MR/N013700/1) and King's College London member of the MRC Doctoral Training Partnership in Biomedical Sciences. The Indian data collection was funded by Autism Speaks, the Japanese data collection by The Grant-in-Aid for Scientific Research from the Japan Society for the Promotion of Science and the UK data collection by the Nancy Lurie-Marks Family Foundation and the MRC, UK. SBC, CA and PS were supported by the Autism Research Trust during the period of this work. IB is supported by the NIHR Biomedical Research Centre at South London and Maudsley NHS Foundation Trust and by the NIHR Collaboration for Leadership in Applied Health Research and Care South London at King's College Hospital NHS Foundation Trust, King's College London.

Authors' contributions
SC, EK, RH and IB designed the study and conducted the analyses. AR, BC, AW, BA, CA and SBC were involved in the original data collection. PS contributed to data analysis. SC and EK wrote the first and final draft of the manuscript. All authors read, contributed to and approved the final manuscript.

Competing interests

The authors declare that they have no competing interests.

Author details

[1]Institute of Psychiatry, Psychology and Neuroscience, King's College London, London, UK. [2]Psychology, Ben-Gurion University of the Negev, Beer Sheva, Israel. [3]Autism Research Centre, Department of Psychiatry, University of Cambridge, Cambridge, UK. [4]Department of Psychology, School of Philosophy, Psychology and Language Sciences, University of Edinburgh, Edinburgh, UK. [5]Centre for Autism, School of Psychology and Clinical Language Sciences, University of Reading, Reading, UK. [6]Chiba University, Chiba, Japan.

References

1. American Psychiatric Association. Diagnostic and statistical manual of mental disorders (DSM-5). Washington, DC: American Psychiatric Association; 2013.
2. Bishop DV. Which neurodevelopmental disorders get researched and why? PLoS One. 2010;5:e15112.
3. Daley TC. The need for cross-cultural research on the pervasive developmental disorders. Transcult Psychiatry. 2002;39:531–50.
4. Dyches TT, Wilder LK, Sudweeks RR, Obiakor FE, Algozzine B. Multicultural issues in autism. J Autism Dev Disord. 2004;34:211–22.
5. Freeth M, Sheppard E, Ramachandran R, Milne E. A cross-cultural comparison of autistic traits in the UK, India and Malaysia. J Autism Dev Disord. 2013;43:2569–83.
6. Durkin MS, Elsabbagh M, Barbaro J, Gladstone M, Happe F, Hoekstra RA, Lee LC, Rattazzi A, Stapel-Wax J, Stone WL, et al. Autism screening and diagnosis in low resource settings: challenges and opportunities to enhance research and services worldwide. Autism Res. 2015;8:473–6.
7. Norbury CF, Sparks A. Difference or disorder? Cultural issues in understanding neurodevelopmental disorders. Dev Psychol. 2013;49:45–58.
8. Caron KG, Schaaf RC, Benevides TW, Gal E. Cross-cultural comparison of sensory behaviors in children with autism. Am J Occup Ther. 2012;66:e77–80.
9. Freeth M, Milne E, Sheppard E, Ramachandran R. Autism across cultures: perspectives from non-Western cultures and implications for research. In: Handbook of Autism and Pervasive Developmental Disorders. 4th ed; 2014.
10. Inada N, Koyama T, Inokuchi E, Kuroda M, Kamio Y. Reliability and validity of the Japanese version of the modified checklist for autism in toddlers (M-CHAT). Res Autism Spectr Disord. 2011;5:330–6.
11. Soto S, Linas K, Jacobstein D, Biel M, Migdal T, Anthony BJ. A review of cultural adaptations of screening tools for autism spectrum disorders. Autism. 2015;19:646–61.
12. Stewart LA, Lee LC. Screening for autism spectrum disorder in low- and middle-income countries: a systematic review. Autism. 2017;21:527–39. https://doi.org/10.1177/1362361316677025.
13. Charman T, Gotham K. Measurement issues: screening and diagnostic instruments for autism spectrum disorders - lessons from research and practice. Child Adolesc Ment Health. 2013;18:52–63.
14. Charman T, Baird G, Simonoff E, Chandler S, Davison-Jenkins A, Sharma A, O'Sullivan T, Pickles A. Testing two screening instruments for autism spectrum disorder in UK community child health services. Dev Med Child Neurol. 2016;58:369–75.
15. Henrich J, Heine SJ, Norenzayan A. Most people are not WEIRD. Nature. 2010;466:29.
16. Perera H, Wijewardena K, Aluthwelage R. Screening of 18-24-month-old children for autism in a semi-urban community in Sri Lanka. J Trop Pediatr. 2009;55:402–5.
17. Seif Eldin A, Habib D, Noufal A, Farrag S, Bazaid K, Al-Sharbati M, Badr H, Moussa S, Essali A, Gaddour N. Use of M-CHAT for a multinational screening of young children with autism in the Arab countries. Int Rev Psychiatry. 2008;20:281–9.
18. Srisinghasongkram P, Pruksananonda C, Chonchaiya W. Two-step screening of the modified checklist for autism in toddlers in Thai children with language delay and typically developing children. J Autism Dev Disord. 2016;46:3317–29.
19. Wakabayashi A, Baron-Cohen S, Uchiyama T, Yoshida Y, Tojo Y, Kuroda M, Wheelwright S. The Autism-Spectrum Quotient (AQ) Children's Version in Japan: a cross-cultural comparison. J Autism Dev Disord. 2007;37:491–500.
20. Albores-Gallo L, Roldán-Ceballos O, Villarreal-Valdes G, Betanzos-Cruz BX, Santos-Sánchez C, Martínez-Jaime MM, Lemus-Espinosa I, Hilton CL. M-CHAT Mexican version validity and reliability and some cultural considerations. ISRN Neurol. 2012;2012:408694.
21. Samadi SA, McConkey R. Screening for autism in Iranian preschoolers: contrasting M-CHAT and a scale developed in Iran. J Autism Dev Disord. 2015;45:2908–16.
22. Brennan L, Fein D, Como A, Rathwell IC, Chen C-M. Use of the modified checklist for autism, revised with follow up-Albanian to screen for ASD in Albania. J Autism Dev Dis. 2016;46:3392–407 Advance online publication.
23. Rudra A, Banerjee S, Singhal N, Barua M, Mukerji S, Chakrabarti B. Translation and usability of autism screening and diagnostic tools for autism spectrum conditions in India. Autism Res. 2014;7:598–607.
24. Robins DL, Fein D, Barton ML, Green JA. The modified checklist for autism in toddlers: an initial study investigating the early detection of autism and pervasive developmental disorders. J Autism Dev Disord. 2001;31:131–44.
25. Siu A. Screening for autism spectrum disorder in young children: US Preventive Services Task Force recommendation statement. JAMA. 2016;315:691–6.
26. Kamio Y, Inada N, Koyama T. A nationwide survey on quality of life and associated factors of adults with high-functioning autism spectrum disorders. Autism. 2013;17:15–26.
27. Mandell DS, Novak MM, Zubritsky CD. Factors associated with age of diagnosis among children with autism spectrum disorders. Pediatrics. 2005;116:1480–6.
28. Shattuck PT, Durkin M, Maenner M, Newschaffer C, Mandell DS, Wiggins L, Lee LC, Rice C, Giarelli E, Kirby R, et al. Timing of identification among children with an autism spectrum disorder: findings from a population-based surveillance study. J Am Acad Child Adolesc Psychiatry. 2009;48:474–83.
29. Joshi MS, Maclean M. Maternal expectations of child development in India, Japan, and England. J Cross-Cult Psychol. 1997;28:219–34.
30. Hoekstra RA, Bartels M, Cath DC, Boomsma DI. Factor structure, reliability and criterion validity of the Autism-Spectrum Quotient (AQ): a study in Dutch population and patient groups. J Autism Dev Disord. 2008;38:1555–66.
31. Ruta L, Mazzone D, Mazzone L, Wheelwright S, Baron-Cohen S. The Autism-Spectrum Quotient--Italian version: a cross-cultural confirmation of the broader autism phenotype. J Autism Dev Disord. 2012;42:625–33.
32. Auyeung B, Baron-Cohen S, Wheelwright S, Allison C. The Autism Spectrum Quotient: Children's Version (AQ-Child). J Autism Dev Disord. 2008;38:1230–40.
33. Baron-Cohen S, Wheelwright S, Skinner R, Martin J, Clubley E. The Autism-Spectrum Quotient (AQ): evidence from Asperger syndrome/high-functioning autism, males and females, scientists and mathematicians. J Autism Dev Disord. 2001;31:5–17.
34. Baron-Cohen S, Hoekstra RA, Knickmeyer R, Wheelwright S. The Autism-Spectrum Quotient (AQ)–adolescent version. J Autism Dev Disord. 2006;36:343–50.
35. Murray AL, Allison C, Smith PL, Baron-Cohen S, Booth T, Auyeung B. Investigating diagnostic bias in autism spectrum conditions: an item response theory analysis of sex bias in the AQ-10. Autism Res. 2017;10(5)790-800.
36. James RJ, Dubey I, Smith D, Ropar D, Tunney RJ. The latent structure of autistic traits: a taxometric, latent class and latent profile analysis of the adult Autism Spectrum Quotient. J Autism Dev Disord. 2016;46:3712–28.
37. Ashwood KL, Gillan N, Horder J, Hayward H, Woodhouse E, McEwen FS, Findon J, Eklund H, Spain D, Wilson CE, et al. Predicting the diagnosis of autism in adults using the Autism-Spectrum Quotient (AQ) questionnaire. Psychol Med. 2016;46:2595–604.
38. Allison C, Auyeung B, Baron-Cohen S. Toward brief "Red Flags" for autism screening: the short Autism Spectrum Quotient and the short Quantitative Checklist for Autism in toddlers in 1,000 cases and 3,000 controls [corrected]. J Am Acad Child Adolesc Psychiatry. 2012;51:202–12 e207.
39. Glascoe FP. Parents' concerns about children's development: prescreening technique or screening test? Pediatrics. 1996;99:522–8.
40. Gillis JM, Callahan EH, Romanczyk RG. Assessment of social behavior in children with autism: the development of the behavioral assessment of social interactions in young children. Res Autism Spectr Disord. 2011;5:351–60.

41. Hofstede G. Culture's Consequences: Comparing Values, Behaviors, Institutions and Organizations Across Nations. 2nd ed. Thousand Oaks: Sage Publications; 2001.

42. Rose GM, Dalakas V, Kropp F. Consumer socialization and parental style across cultures: findings from Australia, Greece, and India. J Consum Psychol. 2003;13:366–76.

43. Aron A, Aron EN, Tudor M, Nelson G. Close relationships as including other in the self. J Pers Soc Psychol. 1991;60:241.

44. Fiske A, Kitayama S, Markus HR, Nisbett RE. The cultural matrix of social psychology. In: Gilbert SF D, Lindzey G, editors. The handbook of social psychology. 4th ed. San Francisco: McGraw-Hill; 1998. p. 915–81.

45. Rosenberger NR. Japanese sense of self. New York: Cambridge University Press; 1992.

46. Girimaji SC, Srinath S. Perspectives of intellectual disability in India: epidemiology, policy, services for children and adults. Curr Opin Psychiatry. 2010;23:441–6.

47. Whiting PF, Rutjes AW, Westwood ME, Mallett S, Deeks JJ, Reitsma JB, Leeflang MM, Sterne JA, Bossuyt PM. QUADAS-2: a revised tool for the quality assessment of diagnostic accuracy studies. Ann Intern Med. 2011; 155:529–36.

48. American Psychiatric Association. Diagnostic and statistical manual of mental disorders. 4th, text revision edn. Washington, DC: American Psychiatric Association; 2000.

49. World Health Organisation. The ICD-10 classification of mental and behavioural disorders: Clinical descriptions and diagnostic guidelines. Geneva: World Health Organisation; 1992.

8

Modeling the neuropsychiatric manifestations of Lowe syndrome using induced pluripotent stem cells: defective F-actin polymerization and WAVE-1 expression in neuronal cells

Jesse Barnes[1], Franklin Salas[2], Ryan Mokhtari[3], Hedwig Dolstra[4], Erika Pedrosa[2] and Herbert M. Lachman[1,2,5,6*]

Abstract

Background: Lowe syndrome (LS) is a rare genetic disorder caused by loss of function mutations in the X-linked gene, *OCRL*, which codes for inositol polyphosphate 5-phosphatase. LS is characterized by the triad of congenital cataracts, neurodevelopmental impairment (primarily intellectual and developmental disabilities [IDD]), and renal proximal tubular dysfunction. Studies carried out over the years have shown that hypomorphic mutations in *OCRL* adversely affect endosome recycling and actin polymerization in kidney cells and patient-derived fibroblasts. The renal problem has been traced to an impaired recycling of megalin, a multi-ligand receptor that plays a key role in the reuptake of lipoproteins, amino acids, vitamin-binding proteins, and hormones. However, the neurodevelopmental aspects of the disorder have been difficult to study because the mouse knockout (KO) model does not display LS-related phenotypes. Fortunately, the discovery of induced pluripotent stem (iPS) cells has provided an opportunity to grow patient-specific neurons, which can be used to model neurodevelopmental disorders in vitro, as demonstrated in the many studies that have been published in the past few years in autism spectrum disorders (ASD), schizophrenia (SZ), bipolar disorder (BD), and IDD.

Methods: We now report the first findings in neurons and neural progenitor cells (NPCs) generated from iPS cells derived from patients with LS and their typically developing male siblings, as well as an isogenic line in which the *OCRL* gene has been incapacitated by a null mutation generated using CRISPR-Cas9 gene editing.

Results: We show that neuronal cells derived from patient-specific iPS cells containing hypomorphic variants are deficient in their capacity to produce F-filamentous actin (F-actin) fibers. Abnormalities were also found in the expression of WAVE-1, a component of the WAVE regulatory complex (WRC) that regulates actin polymerization. Curiously, neuronal cells carrying the engineered OCRL null mutation, in which OCRL protein is not expressed, did not show similar defects in F-actin and WAVE-1 expression. This is similar to the apparent lack of a phenotype in the mouse *Ocrl* KO model, and suggests that in the complete absence of OCRL protein, as opposed to producing a dysfunctional protein, as seen with the hypomorphic variants, there is partial compensation for the F-actin/WAVE-1 regulating function of OCRL.

(Continued on next page)

* Correspondence: Herb.Lachman@einstein.yu.edu
[1]Department of Genetics, Albert Einstein College of Medicine, Bronx, New York, USA
[2]Department of Psychiatry and Behavioral Sciences, Albert Einstein College of Medicine, Bronx, New York, USA

(Continued from previous page)

Conclusions: Alterations in F-actin polymerization and WRC have been found in a number of genetic subgroups of IDD and ASD. Thus, LS, a very rare genetic condition, is linked to a more expansive family of genes responsible for neurodevelopmental disorders that have shared pathogenic features.

Keywords: Lowe syndrome, Dent disease, OCRL, INPP5B, Induced pluripotent stem cells, Autism, Developmental, Intellectual, Renal, Cataract

Background

Lowe syndrome (LS) (OMIM #300535) is a rare genetic disorder (~ 1/500,000 males) caused by loss of function mutations in the X-linked gene, *OCRL* (*OCRL-1; INPP5F*) [1–4]. It is characterized by the triad of congenital cataracts, neurodevelopmental impairment, and renal proximal tubular dysfunction [5]. Hypotonia, short stature, epilepsy, and behavioral problems (tantrums and stereotypy [complex repetitive behaviors]) are commonly found as well.

OCRL codes for a 901 amino acid protein, inositol polyphosphate 5-phosphatase, which is a key factor in endosome recycling and actin polymerization [6, 7]. A more moderate form of OCRL deficiency known as Dent-2 disease is dominated by the renal manifestations [8]. OCRL catalyzes the removal of the 5′ phosphate from phosphatidylinositol 4,5-bisphosphate (PI(4,5)P2), phosphatidylinositol 1,4,5-trisphosphate, and inositol 1,3,4,5-tetrakisphosphate [9–11].

There is extensive *OCRL* allelic heterogeneity in LS, which is primarily caused by hypomorphic missense mutations that lead to markedly reduced 5-phosphatase activity [12–14]. More than 90% of mutations occur in exons 9–14, and 18–24, which code for the phosphatase and ASH-RhoGAP domains, respectively [14, 15]. Hypomorphic variants in the ASH-RhoGAP domain affect the recruitment of OCRL to early endosomes by impaired binding to APPL1 and RAB5 [7]. Approximately 6% of LS cases are caused by deletions affecting the phosphatase domain [16, 17]. Complete *OCRL* deletions of the gene are rare. Paradoxically, one such deletion resulted in intellectual disability, but no renal disease [16]. On the other hand, a complete deletion in two other cases resulted in LS [18, 19]. In addition, Hichri et al. found a Dent disease patient with a frameshift deletion in exons 3 and 4 who did not have intellectual disability or congenital cataracts [14]. These findings suggest that genetic background and/ or compensation by OCRL paralogs, such as *INPP5B*, could affect the clinical presentation of individuals with *OCRL* deficiency. Compensation by *Inpp5b* has been suggested as a possible mechanism for the absence of LS-related clinical phenotypes in the mouse *Ocrl* knockout (KO) model [20].

The molecular basis of LS has been primarily investigated in fibroblasts and immortalized cell lines (e.g., HeLa;

Cos-7 cells). OCRL deficiency impairs the recycling of various receptors by reducing the trafficking of early endosomes to late endosomes [6, 7]. OCRL interacts with clathrin, and null and hypomorphic mutations lead to impaired clathrin-mediated endocytosis [2, 21, 22]. This can impair the recycling of various receptors, including megalin, which is responsible for the low molecular weight proteinuria and aminoaciduria seen in LS patients [6, 22].

So far, the effects of *OCRL* loss of function mutations on neuronal function and the brain have not been adequately investigated, but a few interesting clinical and preclinical findings are emerging. In LS children, delayed myelination, dilated perivascular spaces, and the development of multiple small cystic lesions in deep, periventricular white matter have been observed [23]. In zebrafish, *ocrl1* deficiency increases the susceptibility to heat-induced seizures, and causes cystic brain lesions and reduced Akt signaling. In addition, there is an increase in apoptosis and reduced proliferation in neural tissue. These effects appear to be due to deficits in clathrin-mediated membrane trafficking [24]. Mouse models have been developed, but, as noted above, *Ocrl* null mice are asymptomatic [20, 25].

Although these studies have been instrumental in helping to elucidate the molecular effects of OCRL deficiency and its pathological and clinical consequences in non-neuronal cells, there is a gap in understanding the effects of OCRL deficiency at a cellular level in neurons and, perhaps, other cell types found in the brain. In addition, because of the unique structure of neurons, loss of function *OCRL* mutations could lead to abnormalities and features not seen in non-neuronal cell types, such as neurite outgrowth, axonal transport, and dendritic spine morphology. This can now be addressed using induced pluripotent stem (iPS) cell technology, which is transforming the study of neurodevelopmental and neuropsychiatric disorders through the capacity to produce patient-specific neurons, astrocytes, oligodendrocytes, and microglia [26–40]. In addition, disease modeling using iPS cells can also be accomplished by altering the expression of relevant genes through KO or RNA interference (RNAi), as we and others have done for the autism spectrum disorders (ASD) and schizophrenia (SZ) candidate gene *CHD8* [32, 41, 42].

We now report preliminary findings on NPCs and neurons derived from iPS cells made from boys with LS and their typically developing siblings, as well as an *OCRL* KO iPS cell line generated from a control line using CRISPR-Cas9 gene editing. A defect in filamentous actin (F-actin) and WAVE-1 formation was found in neuronal cells derived from the patient samples.

Interestingly, in a finding similar to the absence of an observable phenotype in the mouse *Ocrl* KO model, a defect in WAVE-1 expression was not observed in the *OCRL* engineered KO line. This could be due to differences in the expression of OCRL-deficient phenotypes between hypomorphic variants, in which a mutated protein is produced, compared with the complete absence of OCRL protein, the latter of which allows for rescue by a compensatory pathway.

Methods
Subjects
The study and consent forms were approved by the Albert Einstein College of Medicine (AECOM). A diagnosis of LS was made during infancy in each patient based on clinical findings, fibroblast OCRL enzyme activity, and ultimately by genotyping.

Development of iPS cells from peripheral blood CD34+ cells
iPS cell lines were generated from human peripheral blood CD34+ cells with a CytoTune-iPS 2.0 Sendai Reprogramming Kit (Invitrogen) following the manufacturer's protocol. Briefly, frozen PBMCs were thawed 2 days before reprogramming (day – 2) and cultured in STIF medium [43]. On day 0, CD34+ cells were flow-sorted by FACSAria II (bipolar disorder; BD) and transduced with Sendai virus vectors containing Klf4–Oct3/4–Sox2, cMyc, and Klf4 in the presence of 4 µg/mL of polybrene. Three days after transduction, the transduced cells were plated on a Matrigel-coated 24-well plate in StemSpan SFEM medium (STEMCELL Technologies). On day 7, half of the StemSpan SFEM medium was replaced, and on day 8, the culture medium was completely replaced. Thereafter, culture medium was changed every 2 days from days 2–7, then changed daily from day 8. The iPS cell-like clones were picked and passaged by mechanical dissection from day 21 to day 28. FACS analysis of pluripotent markers (SSEA3, SSEA4, TRA-1-60, TRA-1-81), in vitro differentiation and immunohistochemical detection of three germ-layer markers (α-fetoprotein, α-smooth muscle actin and β-III tubulin), RT-PCR assay for virus gene integration, and karyotyping were performed on each iPS cell clone to ensure that integration-free iPS cells with the capacity to differentiate into all three germ layers were generated.

Generating neural progenitor cells (NPCs) and neurons from iPS cells
The NPC protocol was adapted from the STEMCELL Technologies, STEMdiff™ Neural Induction Protocol with slight modifications. Briefly, iPS cells were maintained in mTeSR1 with daily feeding until near confluence. At the start of the experiment, differentiated cells were manually removed and the remaining un-differentiated cells were washed with PBS. The cells were incubated with gentle dissociation reagent (Stemcell Tech) for 8–10 min at 37 °C. Cells were dislodged by pipetting with a sterile 1-ml pipet tip (using a P1000 pipet) and collected in a 15-ml tube. The cell culture plate was rinsed with DMEM/F12 and added to the tube containing the cell suspension. Viable cells were treated with Trypan Blue and counted manually using a hemocytometer. Cells were then centrifuged at 300×g for 5 min. Supernatant was carefully aspirated, and cell pellet was re-suspended in STEMdiff™ Neural Induction Medium + 10 uM Y-27632 (ROCK inhibitor) Medium + 10 uM Y-27632 (ROCK inhibitor) to obtain a final concentration of 10^6 cells/ml. Two milliliters of cell suspension were aliquoted into one well of a six-well plate, pre-coated with matrigel. Cells were fed daily for 6–7 days in STEMdiff™ Neural Induction medium without Y-27632. NPCs are ready for passage when cultures are approximately 90% confluent. NPCs are washed with DMEM/F12 and 1 ml of accutase was added to each well for 7 min at 37 °C. Cells were dislodged with a sterile 1-ml pipet tip and collected in a 15 ml tube. The cell culture plate was rinsed with DMEM/F12, and remaining NPCs were transferred to the bulk cell suspension. Viable cells were stained with Trypan Blue and counted using a hemocytometer. Cells were then centrifuged at 300×g for 5 min. Supernatant was carefully aspirated, and cell pellet was re-suspended in STEMdiff™ Neural Induction Medium + 10 uM Y-27632. Cells were plated at a density of 1.5×10^6 cells/well in a six-well plate, pre-coated with PORN/Laminin. They were subsequently fed daily with STEMdiff™ Neural Induction Medium without Y-27632. NPCs were induced to differentiate into neurons at passage four.

Once NPCs reached ~ 50% confluence, neural differentiation was initiated by withdrawing FGF2 and adding NBF media supplemented with fresh growth factors as follows: WNT3A (100 ng/ml) (R&D Systems), BDNF (10 ng/ml), GDNF (10 ng/ml), IGF-1 (10 ng/ml) (PeproTech), and cAMP 1 µM (Sigma), as previously described [32], which produces a heterogeneous mix of glutamatergic neurons and GABAergic neurons.

CRISPR-Cas9 gene editing
The *OCRL* KO line (690KO) was generated from a previously generated control (690C) unrelated to the LS

subjects using CRISPR-Cas9 gene editing, as described by Ran et al. [44]. Guide sequences coding for a region on exon 6 were cloned into the Bbs1 site of pSpCas9n(BB)-2A-Puro (Addgene catalog #48139) using the guide RNA encoding sequences CACCGTACC AGAAATTAGACACTA (top strand) and AAAC TAGTGTCTAATTTCTGGTAC (bottom strand), which were annealed prior to ligation into the linearized plasmid. Human iPS cells from a typically developing control were cultured and fed daily in mTeSR1 (Stem Cell technologies) on Matrigel (BD) coated plates at 37 °C/5% CO_2/85% in a humidified incubator. Cells were maintained in log phase growth, and differentiated cells were manually removed before starting the experiment. iPS cells were exposed to 10 uM ROCK Inhibitor for ~ 4 h to improve cell survival during nucleofection. After 4 h, growth medium was aspirated and the cells were rinsed with DMEM/F12. iPS cells were dissociated into single cells with accutase and harvested by centrifugation. Nucleofection was performed using the Amaxa-4D Nucleofector Basic Protocol for Human Stem Cells (Lonza) according to the manufacturer's instructions. Briefly, 8×10^5 cells and 5 µg of plasmid were nucleofected using the P3 Primary Cell 4D-Nucleofector X Kit L with program CA-137. Cells were re-suspended in mTeSR1 + 10 uM ROCK Inhibitor and placed in one well of a six-well Matrigel-coated plate. The following day, cells were fed with fresh mTeSR1 and were subsequently fed with fresh medium daily. On days 4–14, cells were exposed to 0.5 µg/ml puromycin for 6 h. Puromycin-resistant colonies were picked and expanded in mTeSR1 without further puromycin treatment. DNA was analyzed to identify clones with frame shift mutations (see below).

DNA and cDNA sequencing

Total cellular DNA was isolated using Gentra Puregene Blood Kit (Qiagen catalog# 158445). Total RNA was extracted using miRNeasy Mini Kit (Qiagen, catalog# 217004) according to the manufacturer's instructions (Qiagen). An additional treatment with DNase1 (Qiagen, Valencia, CA) was included to remove genomic DNA. cDNA for sequencing was generated from RNA by RT-PCR (OneStep RT-PCR Kit, Qiagen, catalog# 210210 Valencia, CA) (see primers below). Genomic DNA was amplified using Taq DNA Polymerase (Invitrogen, catalog# 18038–042) using primers that flank the patient-specific and KO alleles (OCRL_LS100/300 for LS100 and LS300; OCRL_LS500 for LS500; OCRL_KO for the CRISPR-engineered line; see below for primer sequences). For the splice junction analysis, cDNA was amplified using exon 22 and exon 24 primers (LS300cDNA), and exon 23 and exon 24 primers (LS100cDNA). Amplicons were purified using a QIAquick PCR Purification Kit (Qiagen, catalog# 28104) according

to the manufacturer's instructions. DNA and cDNA were sequenced by the standard Sanger dideoxy chain termination method using nested primers (LS100seq, LS300seq), or one of the PCR primers.

Western blotting

Proteins were prepared with ProteoExtract Complete Mammalian Proteome Extraction Kit (Millipore cat# 539779) according to the manufacturer's protocol. Protein concentrations were verified using the Qubit™ Protein Assay kit (Invitrogen cat#Q33211). Briefly, 20–100 µg of protein were denatured with the addition of Laemmli buffer and 2-mercaptoethanol and boiled for 5 min. Samples were loaded onto a 12% precast polyacrylamide gel (BIO-RAD cat#456-1044). Gel electrophoresis was set at constant voltage (80 V) for the first 30 min and 200 V for the remainder of the run. The running buffer was in 1X TrisGlycine/SDS buffer. After separation by electrophoresis, proteins were bound to a nitrocellulose membrane (BIO-RAD cat# 162-0146). Electrophoretic transfer was set at constant voltage (70 V) for 2 h at 4 °C in 1X TrisGlycine buffer containing 20% methanol. After transfer, membranes were blocked in 5% milk with gentle agitation for 1 h at room temperature. Membranes were then incubated overnight with gentle agitation at 4 °C with primary antibody of interest. Following primary antibody incubation, membranes were washed three times with gentle agitation in 1X TBS/T buffer (20 mM Tris Base, 0.136 M NaCl, 0.1% Tween-20). Membranes were then incubated with secondary antibody plus anti-biotin for 1 h at room temperature with gentle agitation. Membranes were washed again, as above, and subsequently incubated with SuperSignal™ West Dura Extended Duration Substrate (Thermo Scientific cat# 34075) for 5 min at room temperature with gentle agitation. Immediately thereafter, membranes were exposed to blue autoradiograph film for analysis.

Immunocytochemistry (ICC)

Cells were fixed in 10% buffered formalin phosphate for 10 min at 4 °C, then permeabilized at room temperature for 15 min in 1% Triton X-100 in PBS. Samples were blocked in 1% BSA (10 mg/ml), 5% donkey serum, and 0.1% Triton X-100 for 45 min at room temperature. Samples were then incubated for 1 h at room temperature with primary antibodies. Samples were washed seven times with Rinse Solution (5% donkey serum, 1% BSA; 5 min per wash). Secondary antibodies (Alexa Fluor 488 anti-rabbit, Alexa Fluor 568 anti-mouse, 1:300, Thermo Scientific) were applied for 45 min at room temperature in the dark (excluding F-actin, since conjugated phalloidin:FITC requires no secondary). Each sample was then washed five times with Rinse Solution for 5 min each. Coverslips were applied with ProLong Gold™ antifade reagent with DAPI (cat# P36931, Invitrogen) and visualized after 24 h.

Neurons were grown on 12-mm coverslips, and NPCs were grown on four-well chamber slides pre-coated with PORN/Laminin. All images were taken with AxioVert 200 M inverted fluorescence microscope equipped with a Plan-Apochromat × 63/1.40 Oil DIC Objective and HBO 100 microscope illumination system. Alexa-Fluor 488 fluorescence was measured with a GFP-470-nm excitation filter/509-nm emission filter. Alexa-Fluor 568 fluorescence was measured with a Rhodamine-540-nm excitation filter/ 580-nm emission filter. DAPI nuclear stain was observed with a 359-nm excitation filter/461-nm emission filter. Images were acquired with Zeiss AxioCam MR3 camera operating with Zeiss AxioVision FRET software. Brightness and contrast were adjusted with ImageJ software with identical changes for comparing image sets.

Quantification of OCRL and APPL-1 expression at axon/ soma junctions was carried out using ImageJ. Single channels from each image were converted into 8-bit greyscale images and equally adjusted to subtract background. Junctions were manually segmented, and total segment fluorescence was recorded. Segment fluorescence was adjusted based on corrected total cellular fluorescence.

Analysis of PI(4,5)P2 and WAVE-1 by quantitative immunocytochemistry (ICC)

PI(4,5)P2 was visualized in both NPCs and neurons using ICC. Images were captured using the same parameters for each channel. Random images (5–10) containing ~ 10 cells were captured from each section. The staining intensity was measured using ImageJ software. The background signals were removed using the thresholding tool. Then, the pixel intensities were measured, and the mean pixel intensity from each image was recorded. The signal was normalized to DAPI (LS samples and siblings) or cyclophilin (690C and 690KO). Statistical analysis of the normalized PI(4,5)P2 levels was determined using the Student's t test. A similar analysis was carried out for WAVE-1 in NPCs. All p values were two-tailed.

Antibodies

Antibody	Company	Catalogue #	Dilution
Anti-OCRL	Proteintech Group	17695-1-AP	WB, 1:200, ICC, 1:50
Anti-APPL1	OriGene	TA807768	1:500
Phalloidin:FITC	ECM Biosciences	PF7501	1:200
Anti-Actin	ECM Biosciences	AM2021	1:100
Anti-Wave1	Abcam	AB50356	WB, 1:2000; ICC, 1:200
Anti-TGN46	Sigma-Aldrich	SAB4200355	1:100
α-Fetoprotein	R&D Systems	MAB1369	1:50
α-Smooth Actin	R&D Systems	MAB1420	1:50

(Continued)			
β-III Tubulin	R&D Systems	MAB1195	1:50

PCR primers used in this study

Gene	Forward	Reverse
β2M	gctcgcgctactctctcttt	caatgtcggatggatgaaac
OCRL_LS500	cctgcatgaccagaatttga	ttaaaagcgctatgctgacg
OCRLexp-F	acaggtcctgcttcccacta	tggaggtggatgtctaggca
OCRLexp2-F	atccacctccagagcaacac	gctgtgggaaggagcaatag
OCRL_KO	agagctgccctcatttcctt	tgggcctggacttgataaaa
LS100cDNA	ttttcttggaagccctgcca	tgccataaggttgggtggag
LS300cDNA	agcgtcaatgccaacatgatc	aaggagggattaggaaacgctc
OCRL_LS100/300	attgtgttggccatgaggag	ggaggcctcaggagaagact

Sequencing primers

LS100seq		aatactcttagtgcattgtatc
LS300seq		tagaagttagacagatgaaatg

Results

Patient-specific iPS cell lines were developed from three boys with LS and their typically developing male siblings. LS100 is a 17-year-old boy who was delivered vaginally after a 36-week gestation. His mother was 34 years old at the time. Routine maternal alpha-fetoprotein (AFP) testing during pregnancy revealed a marked elevation, which resulted in an amniotic fluid analysis that also showed an increase. Ultrasound in the third trimester showed an excessive accumulation of amniotic fluid (polyhydramnios). At birth, mild hypotonia was noted. At the first postnatal visit, bilateral cataracts were detected, which were removed at 5 and 7 weeks. LS was suspected and confirmed at 10 months of age with an inositol polyphosphate 5-phosphatase OCRL-1 activity assay on fibroblasts (0.54 nmol/min/mg protein [normal controls were 8.18 and 10.10]). The child had delayed developmental milestones; he walked at 2 years, used single words at 2, and put together a string of a couple of words at age 3. Early educational intervention was begun in preschool, and the boy was educated in a regular school in a self-contained classroom. He was able to read individual words at age 5. From the ages of 3–7, he suffered from periodic grand mal seizures, which were controlled with medication. He was treated with human growth hormone because of short stature and hypotonia. He is currently being treated for renal tubular acidosis. The patient was diagnosed with OCD, which is well-controlled with escitalopram. LS200 is his typically developing older brother who was 22 years old when blood was provided to generate iPS cells.

LS300 is a 19-year-old boy diagnosed in infancy. He was a full-term breach delivered by C-section to his 29-year-old mother. Routine AFP screening of maternal blood during pregnancy showed elevated levels, which was confirmed by amniocentesis. He was born with severe hypotonia and bilateral cataracts, which were removed at 4 months. He contracted whooping cough only 2 weeks after birth. LS was diagnosed by analyzing skin fibroblasts for OCRL enzyme activity (results not available). There was a delay in major milestones. He walked at 2.5 years and spoke words at age 3. There was an episode of seizures at age 18, perhaps precipitated by a febrile illness, but subsequently, he has been free of seizure activity without medication. The patient has renal tubular acidosis, scoliosis and hypotonia, and is being treated with escitalopram for OCD and anxiety. LS400 is his typically developing older brother who was 21 years old when he provided blood for iPS cell development.

LS500 is a 9-year-old boy who was delivered vaginally at full term. His mother was 36-years-old. Cataracts were observed at birth, along with hypotonia. Cataracts were removed at 4 weeks, and a diagnosis of LS was made at ~ 8 weeks based on clinical features, which was confirmed by DNA analysis. The child walked at 3.5 years and began to talk at around the same time. There is no history of epilepsy. Renal tubular acidosis, hypotonia, and glaucoma are the primary persistent features. He is being educated in a regular public school with additional support and is able to read two grade levels below his chronological age. Cognitive function was assessed at age 8 using the Wechsler Intelligence Scale for Children—Fifth Edition (WISCV), which provides composite scores that represent intellectual functioning in specified cognitive domains (i.e., verbal comprehension, visual spatial, fluid reasoning, working memory, and processing speed). Each domain was below the fifth percentile, and the full-scale IQ (FSIQ) composite score was 65 (first percentile). LS600 is his typically developing older brother (age 13. iPS cells were also generated from another typically developing male siblihg (age 16), which has not yet been analyzed).

Analysis of patient-specific mutations

To identify the LS-causing mutations, DNA was sequenced at each OCRL exon and intron-exon junction by GeneDx (Gaithersburg, MD); disease-causing mutations were found in all three patient samples, which were confirmed and characterized in our lab. LS100 was found to have a G>T transversion at the canonical "AG" splice acceptor site in intron 23, one base pair upstream from cDNA position 2582 (c.2582-1 G>T). LS300 was found to have a canonical splice acceptor mutation in intron 22, an A>G transition two bases upstream from cDNA position 2470 (c.2470-2 A>G) (Fig. 1a). Finally, LS500 was found to have a "C" deletion in exon 20 at codon 727 (ChrX:128721069 [hg19]), which is cDNA position 2179 (2179delC). This leads to a predicted frame shift and a premature termination signal after 80 codons.

In order to understand how the LS100 and LS300 canonical splice acceptor mutations influence splicing, we sequenced cDNA using primers in the exons flanking the mutations. As seen in Fig. 1c, the control sample shows the expected connection between exons 22 and 23. By contrast, cDNA sequencing of LS300 shows that exon 22 is joined to exon 24; exon 23 is completely bypassed. The loss of exon 23 disrupts the reading frame in exon 24 and leads to the predicted loss of 78 amino acids in the C-terminal end, which contains the RhoGAP domain. Since the cDNA sequence strip shows no evidence of a mixture of mutant and normal splice variants, which would manifest as superimposed, out of frame bases and a chaotic sequencing strip following the frameshift, the c.2470-2 A>G splice site mutation results in the complete absence of normal splicing at exon 23.

The LS100 splice acceptor mutation is interesting. The mutation predicts that the intron 23/exon 24 splice acceptor site will not be recognized (AG/CT>AT/CT). In addition, the first 16 bases of exon 24 resembles a splice acceptor site (CTACTCTCTTCACTAG/TC), with an "AG" preceded by a putative polypyrimidine tract, which suggests that a cryptic slice site might be generated if the natural intron 23/exon24 slice site is bypassed (Fig. 1b). Indeed, as seen in Fig. 1c, the normal joining of exons 23 and 24 seen in the cDNA sequence of the control sample does not occur, and the predicted cryptic splice site in exon 24 is observed. This leads to the loss of 16 bases from the mRNA and a frame shift resulting in the addition of three novel amino acids followed by a premature termination codon, and the loss of 41 amino acids from the OCRL C-terminal end.

Finally, we engineered an *OCRL* null allele using CRISPR-Cas9 gene editing, targeting exon 6 (see "Methods"). This resulted in several lines, which contained in-frame deletions that have not been further characterized. One line with a null variant was recovered, 690KO, which contains an "A" nucleotide insert at codon 137 in exon 6 (position chrX:128691900 [hg19]; cDNA position 413) (Fig. 1a) that results in a predicted frame shift leading to premature termination after one codon.

Western blotting was carried out to examine OCRL protein and to establish that the 690KO frameshift mutation resulted in the loss of OCRL protein expression. As seen in Fig. 2, no protein was detected in NPCs derived from the KO line, whereas it is expressed in the isogenic control parent line. OCRL protein is detected in the patient-derived LS samples. Although

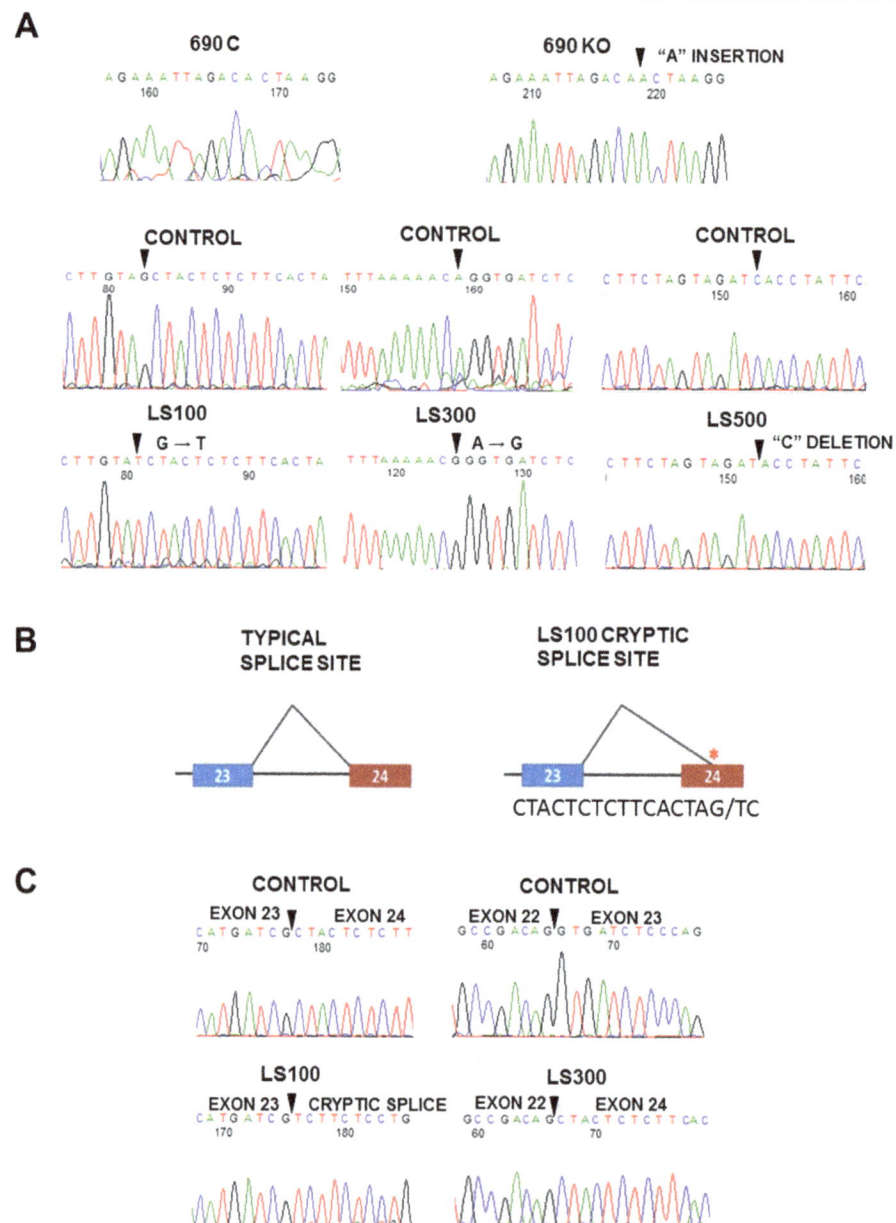

Fig. 1 DNA and cDNA sequencing. **a** Genomic DNA sequences showing mutations in the CRISPR-engineered knockout line (690KO) and the LS samples (LS100, LS300, and LS500) along with controls. The arrows point to the mutations. **b** The LS100 splice acceptor mutation predicts the loss of the natural splice site at the intron 23/exon 24 border, as well as a cryptic splice site 16 bases into exon 24. **c** cDNA sequencing showing normal exon 22/23 and exon 23/24 combinations in controls, and aberrant splicing in LS300, which leads to the exclusion of exon 23, thereby connecting exon 22 to 24; and the cryptic splice in LS100, as predicted in panel **b**

the mutant OCRL proteins are predicted to be somewhat smaller than the normal protein, the difference is not sufficient to be resolved on a 12% polyacrylamide for a protein as large as OCRL (104 kDa).

OCRL expression in NPCs and early differentiating neurons
Immunocytochemistry (ICC) was used to assess the intracellular OCRL expression pattern in early

differentiating neurons derived from iPS cells. As seen in Fig. 3, there is an asymmetric pattern of OCRL immunoreactivity in control samples (LS200 and LS400) in early differentiating neurons (day 14 after differentiation). A diffuse, low-level expression pattern is seen throughout the soma, along with a hyper-dense staining pattern occurring primarily at the junction between the soma and projections. The asymmetric pattern of expression suggests that OCRL may be involved

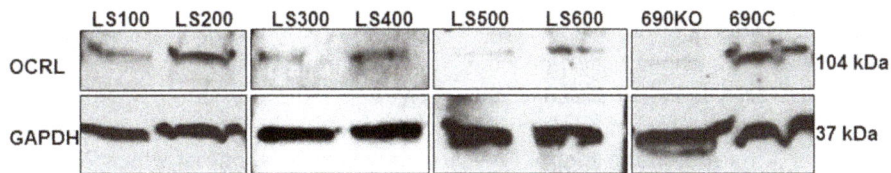

Fig. 2 Western blot showing OCRL and GAPDH proteins in NPCs. GAPDH was used as a loading control

in neuronal polarization and/or neurite outgrowth. It is interesting to note in this regard that depletion of OCRL in epithelial cells results in a failure to polarize apical markers [45].

In addition, a punctate pattern is detected in neuronal projections suggesting that OCRL could be involved in the axonal transport system that shuttles endosomes and other cargo to and from the soma and presynaptic terminal, a hypothesis that is currently under investigation.

By contrast, in patient samples (LS100 and LS300), OCRL immunoreactivity is more sparse compared with

controls at the hyper-dense regions. We quantified the OCRL signal at multiple soma/axon junctions in two LS samples and their sibling controls. As seen in Fig. 3a, some soma/axon junctions in the control samples show intense OCRL immunoreactivity; most are more modest. Overall, there was a statistically significant 41% decrease in OCRL immunoreactivity at soma/axon junctions in LS100 compared with LS200 (Student's t test, p value = 1.35E–05) and a 23% decrease in LS300 vs LS400 (p value = 8.03E–04) (Fig. 3b). The immunofluorescent signals were quantified for the same area at

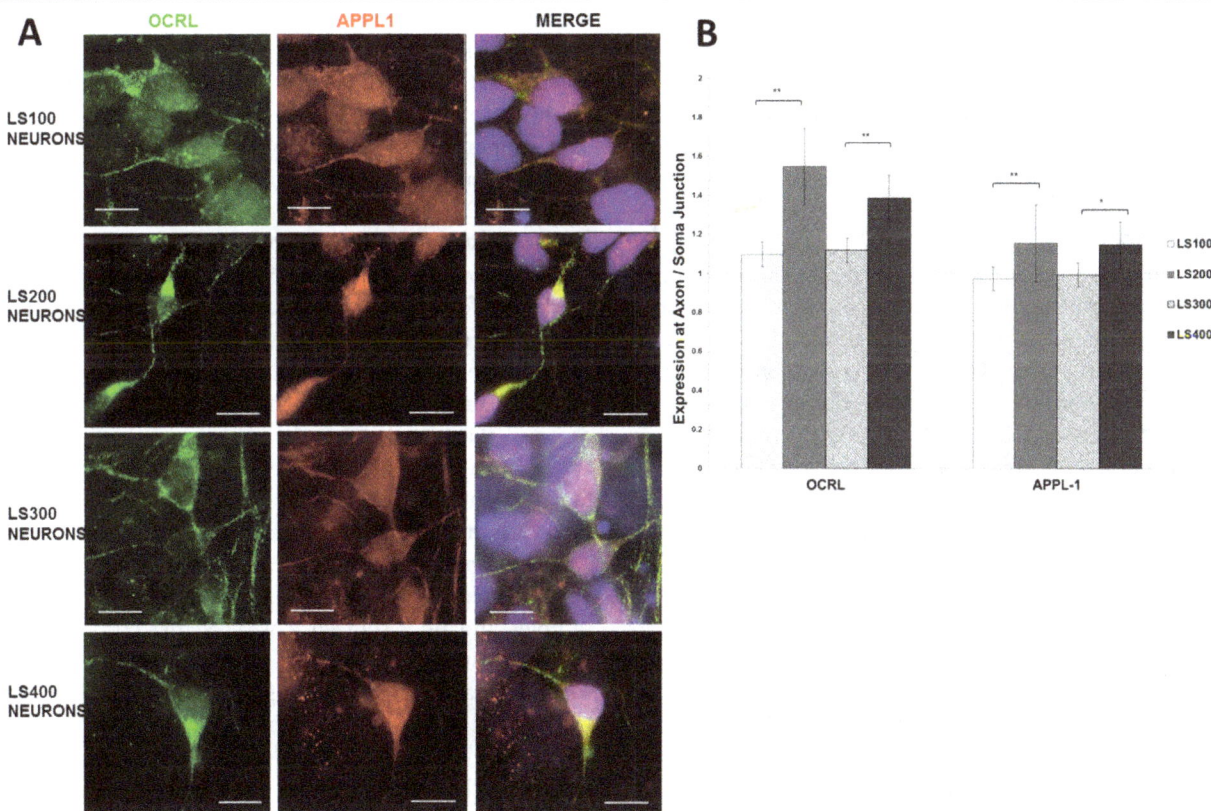

Fig. 3 a. OCRL and APPL-1 immunocytochemistry showing hyper-dense localization in control neuronal samples (LS200 and LS400) (arrows) compared with patient samples (LS100 and LS300). Neuronal differentiation was carried out once for each sample. All images were captured with the ×63 objective. A 10-μm bar is shown as a reference size marker. **b**. The immunofluorescent signals were quantified for the same area at a total of 66 soma/axon junctions for OCRL and 90 for APPL1. Differences in signal intensity were assessed between the LS samples vs their corresponding sibling controls and analyzed using a Student's t test. One asterisk denotes a two-tailed p value of < 0.05; two asterisks indicate a p value of < 0.01 (actual values are OCRL: LS100 vs LS200 [1.35E–05]; LS300 vs LS400 [8.03E–04]. APPL1: LS100 vs LS200 [3.91E–05]; LS300 vs LS400 [1.84E–02]). The error bars show the standard error of the mean a total of 66 soma/axon junctions for OCRL and 90 for APPL1 in a single neuronal induction for each set.

As noted above, *OCRL* mutations affecting the ASH-RhoGAP domain have been found to attenuate the interaction between OCRL and the endosome adaptor protein APPL1 in Cos-7 cells [7]. As seen in the control samples, APPL1 has a diffuse staining pattern similar to OCRL and accumulates in the hyper-dense regions of OCRL immunoreactivity. Furthermore, similar to OCRL, the expression level is lower in those regions in the LS samples. Overall, a statistically significant ~ 19% decrease was seen in LS100 and a ~ 15% decrease in LS300 compared to their controls (*p* value = 3.91E–05; *p* value = 1.84E–02, respectively. The pattern appears to be somewhat different from the findings described by McCrea et al. [7] in Cos-7 cells. In that study, APPL1-positive/OCRL-negative puncta were seen in some regions, consistent with the idea that APPL1 recruits OCRL to those areas. If the same mechanism was occurring in the hyper-dense regions, one would expect APPL1 accumulation in those regions to be the same in control and LS neurons. Our observation is more consistent with the idea that OCRL is drawn to these regions in an APPL1-independent manner, after which APPL1 is being recruited.

F-actin and WAVE-1 expression is altered in LS neuronal cells

OCRL is an important regulator of actin remodeling and cytoskeletal dynamics. In kidney cell lines, OCRL deficiency leads to the accumulation of PI(4,5)P2 in early endosomes, which induces N-WASP (Wiskott-Aldrich syndrome protein)-dependent increases in endosomal F-actin [6] and an increase in actin comets in endosomes [46], perhaps due to the presence of PI(4,5)P2 on intercellular bridges, which would lead to an increase in actin polymerization. However, in fibroblasts from patients with LS and Dent-2 disease, a decrease in actin stress fibers in fibroblasts has been observed [47, 48].

As seen in Fig. 4a, the NPCs from controls show a dense F-actin staining pattern with prominent fibers outlining the cytoskeleton. By contrast, the LS NPCs have a more diffuse pattern and an apparent decrease in signal intensity. This staining pattern was observed in duplicate NPC samples.

Quantitative ICC showed a significant, several-fold decrease in F-actin immunoreactivity (Fig. 4b). We also analyzed the F-actin expression pattern in the CRISPR/Cas9 engineered line (690KO) line, along with its isogenic control (690C). Interestingly, the F-actin staining pattern in control and KO NPCs is quite similar to each other; both show dense fibers, and no differences were detected between the two following quantitative ICC (Fig. 4b).

The findings suggest that the abnormal expression pattern seen in the LS samples, which express hypomorphic *OCRL* variants, is not recapitulated in *OCRL* null NPCs.

A key regulator of actin polymerization is the WAVE regulatory complex (WRC), which initiates F-actin nucleation through an interaction with the Arp2/3 complex [49–52]. One of the components of WRC is the Wiskott-Aldrich syndrome protein that includes several family members, one of which, WAVE-1, is expressed at high levels in the brain compared to other cells/tissue [53]. Consequently, we analyzed WAVE-1 by ICC. As seen in Fig. 5a, there is a marked difference in the pattern of WAVE-1 immunoreactivity in LS and control NPCs. In the control samples, the WAVE-1 expression pattern is similar to the F-actin pattern, with a robust, dense expression pattern. However, in the LS samples, this is not seen. Instead, there is a more disorganized expression pattern with large, patchy accumulations of WAVE-1. This was observed in duplicate NPC samples.

Quantitative ICC was used to quantify the WAVE-1 signal. No differences in the sibling sets were detected (Fig. 5b). Thus, the observed differences in WAVE-1 expression are qualitative rather than quantitative.

We also analyzed the WAVE-1 expression pattern in 690KO and 690C NPCs. Interestingly, similar to the F-actin findings, 690 and 690C NPCs show the same, robust WAVE-1 staining pattern similar to the control NPCs (LS200, LS400, LS600); the patchy inclusions seen in the LS samples are not observed in 690KO NPCs. This supports the idea that hypomorphic *OCRL* variants have a phenotype in NPCs that is not recapitulated in *OCRL* null NPCs. The F-actin and WAVE-1 findings were observed in replicate NPC samples.

WAVE-1 was also analyzed by Western blotting (WB); a marked difference was seen in the LS samples compared to controls (Fig. 6). In the control samples, a single band was observed at ~ 75 kDa in both. However, in the two LS neuronal samples, two lower molecular weight bands were detected. The nature of these bands is not known at this time, but we speculate that they represent WAVE-1 breakdown products. Similar to the findings shown in Fig. 5, there was no quantitative difference in WAVE-1 expression between the control and patient samples.

By contrast, the 690 KO line resembled the control samples and only showed a weak signal corresponding to the presumed degradation product. Thus, similar to the ICC analysis, WAVE-1 expression in the 690KO line resembles controls rather than the LS samples.

Overall, the F-actin and WAVE-1 findings suggest that similar to the mouse *Ocrl* KO, the complete absence of OCRL protein may be less detrimental than expressing a hypomorphic protein (see "Discussion").

PI(4,5)P2 expression is increased in OCRL-deficient NPCs

Since PI(4,5)P2 activates WRC and is a major OCRL substrate, we measured its relative level of expression by quantitative ICC by normalizing its expression in NPCs

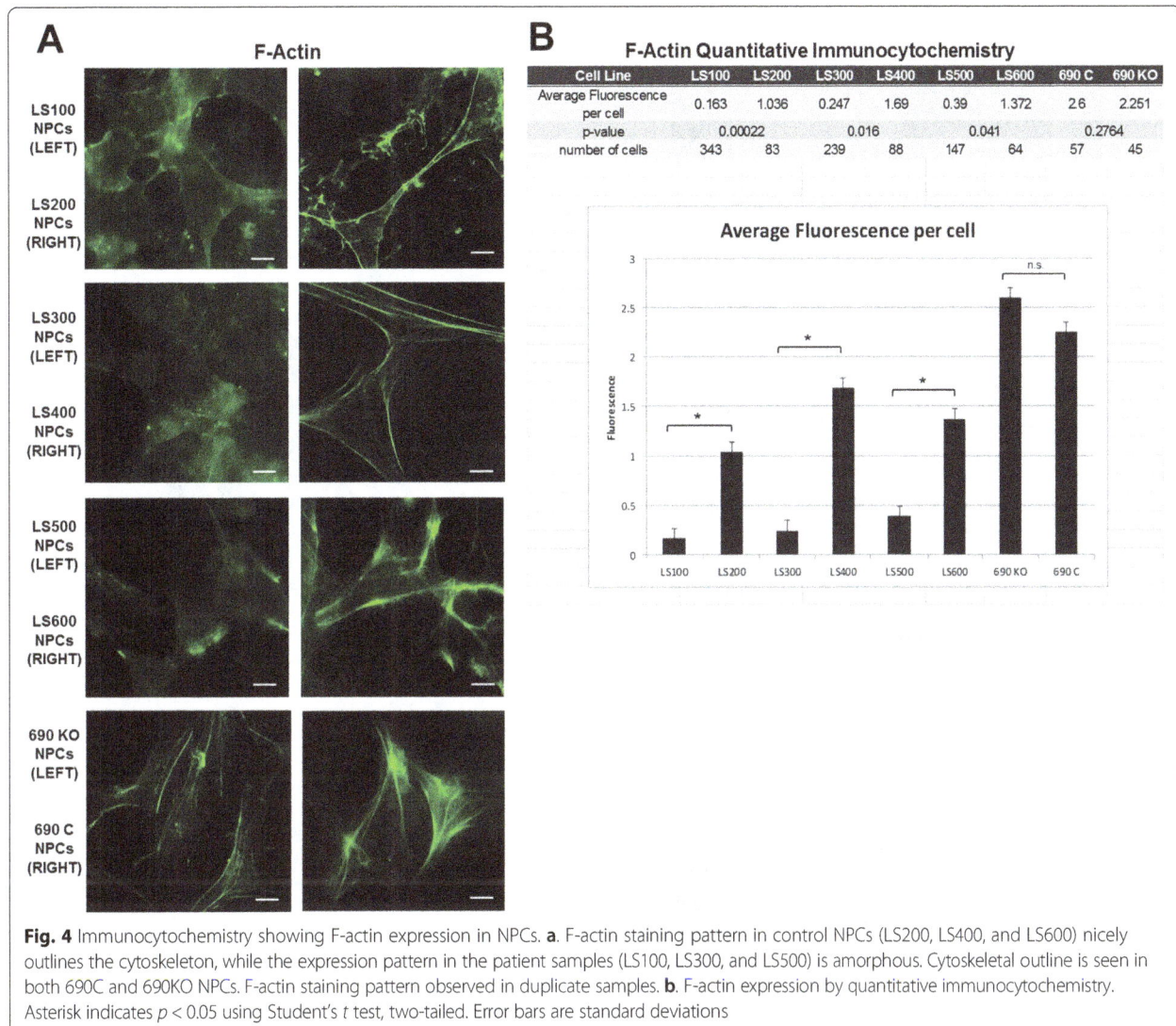

A

F-Actin

LS100 NPCs (LEFT)

LS200 NPCs (RIGHT)

LS300 NPCs (LEFT)

LS400 NPCs (RIGHT)

LS500 NPCs (LEFT)

LS600 NPCs (RIGHT)

690 KO NPCs (LEFT)

690 C NPCs (RIGHT)

B

F-Actin Quantitative Immunocytochemistry

Cell Line	LS100	LS200	LS300	LS400	LS500	LS600	690 C	690 KO
Average Fluorescence per cell	0.163	1.036	0.247	1.69	0.39	1.372	2.6	2.251
p-value	0.00022		0.016		0.041		0.2764	
number of cells	343	83	239	88	147	64	57	45

Average Fluorescence per cell

Fig. 4 Immunocytochemistry showing F-actin expression in NPCs. **a**. F-actin staining pattern in control NPCs (LS200, LS400, and LS600) nicely outlines the cytoskeleton, while the expression pattern in the patient samples (LS100, LS300, and LS500) is amorphous. Cytoskeletal outline is seen in both 690C and 690KO NPCs. F-actin staining pattern observed in duplicate samples. **b**. F-actin expression by quantitative immunocytochemistry. Asterisk indicates $p < 0.05$ using Student's t test, two-tailed. Error bars are standard deviations

against a nuclear marker. As seen in Fig. 7, there was a statistically significant, ~ 25% increase in PI(4,5)P2 levels in the patient samples compared with their unaffected siblings, as one would predict in OCRL-deficient cells. A significant increase was also seen in the KO line compared to its control. Thus, unlike the WAVE-1 findings, which are seen in the LS samples but not in 690KO, the increase in PI(4,5)P2 is similar in all OCRL-deficient NPCs and neurons. Between 88 and 128 cells were quantified for each sample in a single neuronal/NPC induction.

The finding supports the hypothesis that in the complete absence of OCRL, some cellular and molecular phenotypes can be rescued, but others are not. This is consistent with the clinical manifestations of some Dent-2 patients who have null mutations in the 5′ end of the gene who do have renal disease, but not neurodevelopmental problems. The findings in the patient samples also suggest that in neuronal cells, there is an inverse relationship between PI(4,5)P2 and F-actin/WAVE-1 dynamics, which is opposite the findings in kidney cell lines [6, 7], but similar to findings in fibroblasts from LS patients [47, 48].

Discussion

We have developed an iPS cell model for Lowe syndrome, which provides an opportunity to grow patient-specific neurons in vitro. Based on studies carried out on non-neuronal cells over the years, OCRL deficiency causes deficits in endosome recycling and transport, and endosomal actin dynamics. In this initial report, we were particularly interested in determining whether LS mutations affect F-actin polymerization in neuronal cells since this is a key regulator of neuronal migration, neurite outgrowth, dendritic spine formation and NMDA and AMPA receptor recycling, and defects in these phenomena have been found in many different

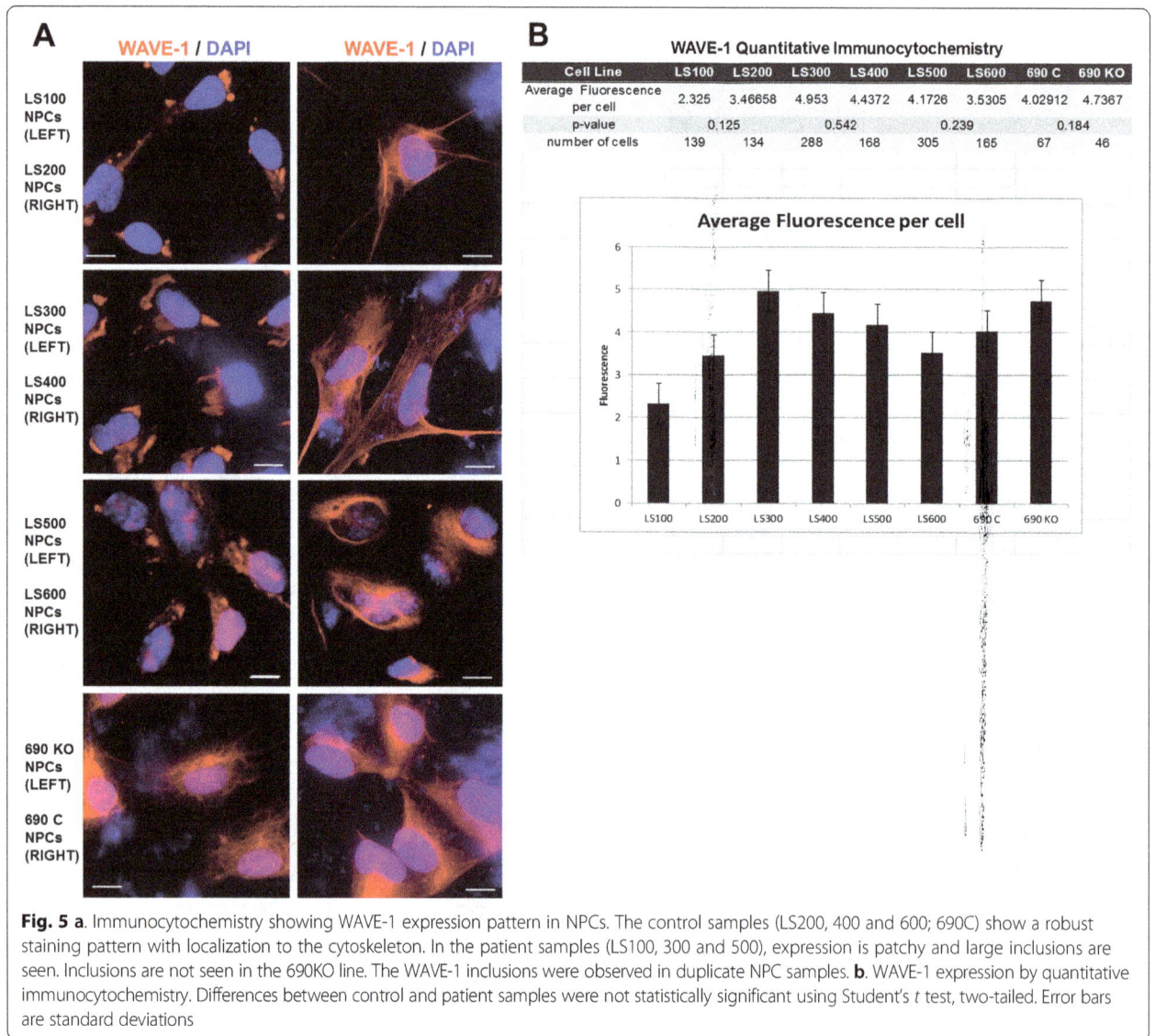

Fig. 5 a. Immunocytochemistry showing WAVE-1 expression pattern in NPCs. The control samples (LS200, 400 and 600; 690C) show a robust staining pattern with localization to the cytoskeleton. In the patient samples (LS100, 300 and 500), expression is patchy and large inclusions are seen. Inclusions are not seen in the 690KO line. The WAVE-1 inclusions were observed in duplicate NPC samples. **b**. WAVE-1 expression by quantitative immunocytochemistry. Differences between control and patient samples were not statistically significant using Student's *t* test, two-tailed. Error bars are standard deviations

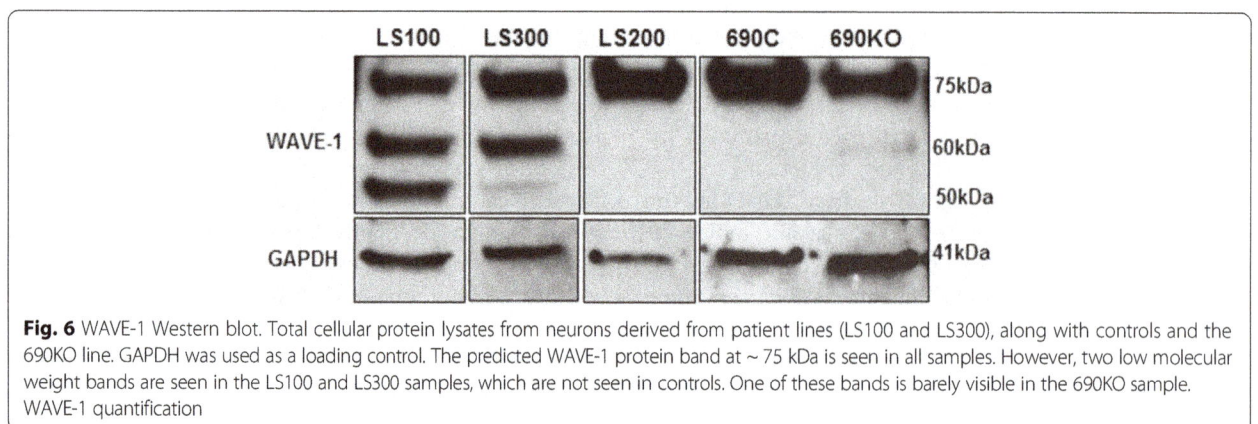

Fig. 6 WAVE-1 Western blot. Total cellular protein lysates from neurons derived from patient lines (LS100 and LS300), along with controls and the 690KO line. GAPDH was used as a loading control. The predicted WAVE-1 protein band at ~ 75 kDa is seen in all samples. However, two low molecular weight bands are seen in the LS100 and LS300 samples, which are not seen in controls. One of these bands is barely visible in the 690KO sample. WAVE-1 quantification

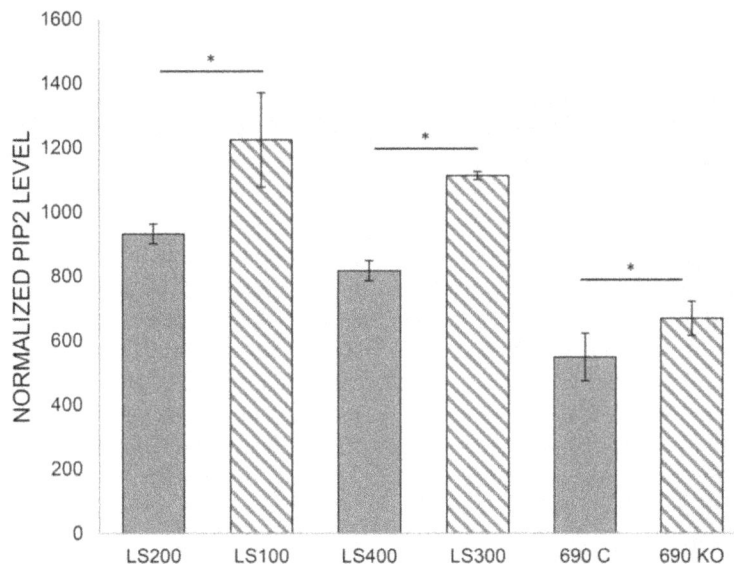

Fig. 7 PIP2 levels in neuronal cells by quantitative ICC. The relative level of PIP2 was normalized against a nuclear marker. The LS100/LS200 set was carried out on NPCs, while the analysis of the LS300/LS400 and 690KO/690C sets were carried out on day 14 neurons. The asterisk denotes statistical significance using the Student's *t* test, two-tailed: LS100 and LS200; $p = 0.025$, LS300 and LS400; $p = 0.003$, 690C and 690KO; $p = 0.0001$. Error bars are standard deviations. A single NPC or neuronal induction was carried out for each set, with between 88 and 128 cells quantified for each

genetic subgroups of SZ, ASD, and intellectual and developmental disabilities (IDD) [54–64]. Most studies show a decrease or disruption of F-actin expression, similar to our findings in LS neuronal cells. However, an increase in F-actin polymerization has been found in Fragile X [65]. Thus, altered F-actin dynamics—either increases or decreases in expression and structure—can lead to neurodevelopmental problems.

In the lines derived from LS patients, we found abnormalities in the expression of F-actin and WAVE-1 in neuronal cells. A decrease in the cytoskeletal organization of both was found. This is different from the effects of OCRL deficiency in other cell types where an increase in endosomal F-actin has been observed [6, 7]. This effect is likely due to an increase in endosomal PI(4,5)P2, which induces F-actin recruitment through the activation of N-WASP [6, 66]. However, in fibroblasts from patients with OCRL and Dent-2 disease, a decrease in actin stress fibers has been observed [47, 48]. This effect was not correlated with PI(4,5)P2 levels, similar to our findings, which show an inverse relationship between F-actin and PI(4,5)P2 in LS neuronal cells.

The disorganized expression of WAVE-1 was characterized by the formation of large inclusions, the cause of which is currently under investigation. One possibility being explored is the involvement of the autophagy-lysosome pathway. Recently, De Leo et al. showed that OCRL regulates autophagosome-lysosome fusion in HK-2 cells [67].

WAVE-1 is one of five proteins that constitute the WRC in neuronal cells, which include CYFIP1, ABI2, Nap1, and HSPC300 (BRK1) or their orthologs [68–70].

Consistent with the association between defective F-actin polymerization and neurodevelopmental disorders, several genes coding for WRC components have also been implicated in these disorders. For example, CYFIP1, which is an FMR1 interacting protein 1, plays a role in synaptic function and appears to be the gene responsible for 15q11.2-related neurodevelopmental disorders [56, 60, 69, 71, 72]. Further, shRNA-mediated knockdown (KD) of CYFIP1 leads to a significant decrease in WAVE-1 and F-actin expression in NPCs derived from iPS cells [56].

In addition, rare variants in *ABI2* have been found in an exome sequencing study in consanguineous families with intellectual disabilities [73]. Also, *NCKAP1*, which codes for a WAVE-1 regulatory protein, has been identified as a strong candidate gene for ASD and IDD [74, 75].

The disconnect we observe between PI(4,5)P2 expression with F-actin and WAVE-1 organization suggests that another aspect of OCRL deficiency, aside from its effect as a PI(4,5)P2 phosphatase, is responsible for the abnormalities we observed. An effect on Rac1, a Rho GTPase, is a possibility. Rac1 activates the WRC in the Arp2/3-mediated polymerization of actin [76, 77] (Additional file 1: Figure S1). Rac1 is an OCRL target; downregulation of OCRL has been found to cause aberrant activation of Rac1 in human chondrocytes [78]. This is likely due to the loss of the GTPase activating domain, which is found in the C-terminal end of OCRL. A reduction in Rac1 GTPase activity could conceivably cause constitutive Rac1 activation because of a reduction in the conversion of GTP (which is bound to the active form of Rac1), to GDP (which leads to Rac1 inactivation). The mutations in LS100, LS300, and LS500 all disrupt the RhoGAP domain. On the other hand, in LS fibroblasts, OCRL deficiency causes a reduction in active Rac1 [79], which would be consistent with the effect we observed on F-actin/WAVE-1 dynamics in LS neuronal cells. Clarifying the role of Rac1 in OCRL-deficient NPCs and neurons is currently under investigation.

It is important to note that Rac1 is dysregulated in certain neurodevelopmental disorders through an effect on synaptic plasticity and dendritic spines [80]. In addition, Rac1 has been found to be upregulated in fragile X syndrome [81, 82], and rare genetic variants in Rac1 regulators have been found in ASD, BD and SZ [57, 83, 84].

It is also interesting to note in the context of F-actin/WAVE-1 regulation that the expression of Arp2/3 complex subunits is significantly downregulated in the prefrontal cortex in SZ postmortem samples [85], and that DISC1 regulates Rac1 activation in response to NMDA receptor stimulation [62].

In summary, our findings suggest that LS, an extremely rare condition, is part of a larger functional subgroup of neurodevelopmental disorders that are caused by mutations that disrupt F-actin/WAVE-1 dynamics. How this disruption affects LS NPC and neuronal function is currently under investigation.

Considering the widespread effects of F-actin polymerization, altered neuronal migration, neurite branching and outgrowth, and dendritic spine formation and function are possible; this too is currently under investigation. However, it is also important to note that non-neuronal cells in the brain—specifically microglia and astrocytes—also require intact F-actin dynamics in their maintenance of synaptic function, which are accomplished by F-actin-dependent processes (e.g., migration and phagocytosis). The effect of abnormal F-actin formation on these cell types in LS and other genetic subgroups of neurodevelopmental disorders can now be studied in vitro using newly defined methods for converting iPS cells into functional astrocytes and microglia [86–88].

Finally, our preliminary findings show some differences between LS neuronal cells and those derived from an *OCRL* KO line we generated using CRISPR-Cas9. This is similar to the absence of an observable phenotype in the mouse *Ocrl* KO model, which has been attributed to rescue by the *OCRL* paralog, *INPP5B* [20]. It is also similar to the absence of a severe neurodevelopmental phenotype in a few patients with Dent-2 disease who have apparent null variants in the 5′ end of *OCRL* [14]. Although additional *OCRL* KO iPS cell lines are currently being generated to confirm our findings, our preliminary observations suggest that hypomorphic variants that produce dysfunctional OCRL proteins may cause more dramatic molecular and cellular alterations than those occurring in the complete absence of OCRL protein, perhaps by competitive inhibition at critical binding sites between dysfunctional OCRL proteins and INPP5B or another compensatory pathway. Whether our findings in KO neuronal cells extend to other cell types relevant to LS pathogenesis, such as renal tubules, remains to be seen. However, the finding that neurodevelopmental problems occur in some patients with OCRL deletions and null variants suggests that compensatory rescue in humans is not universal, owing perhaps to genetic background or polymorphic variation in *INPP5B*. Nevertheless, if our findings are replicated, it would suggest that in some individuals, completely blocking mutant OCRL protein might, paradoxically, have a positive therapeutic effect. The findings also suggest that a more effective approach for generating a mouse LS model would be to "knock in" a hypomorphic variant.

Conclusion

We have established an iPS cell model for Lowe syndrome, a rare X-linked disorders caused by loss of function mutations in *OCRL*, which codes for inositol polyphosphate 5-phosphatase, a regulator of endosome recycling and actin dynamics. In neuronal cells derived from patient-specific iPS cells, abnormalities were found in the formation of F-actin and WAVE-1, a component of the wave regulatory complex. This property is shared with other ASD and IDD candidate genes. Thus, Lowe syndrome, a rare cause of IDD, is part of a larger subgroup of patients who have a common underlying pathogenic process.

Abbreviations

AFP: Alpha-feto protein; ASD: Autism spectrum disorders; BD: Bipolar disorder; F-actin: Filamentous actin; FSIQ: Full-scale IQ; ICC: Immunocytochemistry; IDD: Intellectual and developmental disabilities; iPS: Induced pluripotent stem cell; IRB: Institutional Review Board; KD: Knockdown; KO: knockout; LS: Lowe syndrome; NPC: neural progenitor cell; N-WASP: Wiskott-Aldrich syndrome protein; PI(4,5)P2: Phosphatidylinositol 4,5-bisphosphate; SZ: Schizophrenia; WB: Western blotting; WRC: WAVE regulatory complex

Acknowledgements

The authors would like to thank the participating LS families.

Funding

This project was supported by pilot grants from the Lowe Syndrome Association and the Lowe Syndrome Foundation. HML is supported by a grant from NIMH National Institute of Mental Health (NIMH) (MH099427). We are grateful to the New York State Department of Health (NYSTEM Program) for supporting the Einstein Comprehensive Human Pluripotent Stem Cell Center (NYSTEM C029154). This work was also supported in part by a grant to The Rose F. Kennedy Intellectual and Developmental Disabilities Research Center (RFK-IDDRC) from the Eunice Kennedy Shriver National Institute of Child Health & Human Development (NICHD) at the NIH (1P30HD071593).

Authors' contributions

JB contributed the Western blots and ICC and prepared the manuscript. FS and RM took part in the ICC. HD contributed Western blots. EP is responsible for the iPS cell cultures, NPC, and neuron development HL took part in the data analysis, manuscript preparation, and conceived experiment. All authors read and approved the final manuscript.

Competing interests

The authors declare that they have no competing interests.

Author details

[1]Department of Genetics, Albert Einstein College of Medicine, Bronx, New York, USA. [2]Department of Psychiatry and Behavioral Sciences, Albert Einstein College of Medicine, Bronx, New York, USA. [3]Department of Neuroscience and Physiology, SUNY Upstate Medical University, Syracuse, New York, USA. [4]Swammerdam Institute of Life Sciences, University of Amsterdam, Amsterdam, Netherlands. [5]Department of Neuroscience, Albert Einstein College of Medicine, Bronx, New York, USA. [6]Department of Medicine, Albert Einstein College of Medicine, Bronx, New York, USA.

References

1. Silver DN, Lewis RA, Nussbaum RL. Mapping the Lowe oculocerebrorenal syndrome to Xq24-q26 by use of restriction fragment length polymorphisms. J Clin Invest. 1987;79(1):282–5.
2. Schurman SJ, Scheinman SJ. Inherited cerebrorenal syndromes. Nat Rev Nephrol. 2009;5(9):529–38.
3. Waugh MG. PIPs in neurological diseases. Biochim Biophys Acta. 2015; 1851(8):1066–82.
4. Staiano L, De Leo MG, Persico M, De Matteis MA. Mendelian disorders of PI metabolizing enzymes. Biochim Biophys Acta. 2015;1851(6):867–81.
5. Lewis RA, Nussbaum RL, Brewer ED. Lowe Syndrome. In: Adam MP, Ardinger HH, Pagon RA, Wallace SE, Bean LJH, Stephens K, Amemiya A, editors. Seattle: University of Washington; 1993.
6. Vicinanza M, Di Campli A, Polishchuk E, Santoro M, Di Tullio G, Godi A, Levtchenko E, De Leo MG, Polishchuk R, Sandoval L, Marzolo MP, De Matteis MA. OCRL controls trafficking through early endosomes via PtdIns4,5P(2)-dependent regulation of endosomal actin. EMBO J. 2011;30(24):4970–85.
7. McCrea HJ, Paradise S, Tomasini L, Addis M, Melis MA, De Matteis MA, De Camilli P. All known patient mutations in the ASH-RhoGAP domains of OCRL affect targeting and APPL1 binding. Biochem Biophys Res Commun. 2008;369(2):493–9.
8. Hoopes RR Jr, Shrimpton AE, Knohl SJ, Hueber P, Hoppe B, Matyus J, Simckes A, Tasic V, Toenshoff B, Suchy SF, Nussbaum RL, Scheinman SJ. Dent disease with mutations in OCRL1. Am J Hum Genet. 2005;76(2):260–7.
9. Nakatsu F, Messa M, Nandez R, Czapla H, Zou Y, Strittmatter SM, De Camilli P. Sac2/INPP5F is an inositol 4-phosphatase that functions in the endocytic pathway. J Cell Biol. 2015;209(1):85–95.
10. Zhang X, Jefferson AB, Auethavekiat V, Majerus PW. The protein deficient in Lowe syndrome is a phosphatidylinositol-4,5-bisphosphate 5-phosphatase. Proc Natl Acad Sci U S A. 1995;92(11):4853–6.
11. Zhang X, Hartz PA, Philip E, Racusen LC, Majerus PW. Cell lines from kidney proximal tubules of a patient with Lowe syndrome lack OCRL inositol polyphosphate 5-phosphatase and accumulate phosphatidylinositol 4,5-bisphosphate. J Biol Chem. 1998;273(3):1574–82.
12. Pasternack SM, Bockenhauer D, Refke M, Tasic V, Draaken M, Conrad C, Born M, Betz RC, Reutter H, Ludwig M. A premature termination mutation in a patient with Lowe syndrome without congenital cataracts: dropping the "O" in OCRL. Klin Padiatr. 2013;225(1):29–33.
13. Recker F, Zaniew M, Bockenhauer D, Miglietti N, Bokenkamp A, Moczulska A, Rogowska-Kalisz A, Laube G, Said-Conti V, Kasap-Demir B, Niemirska A, Litwin M, Siten G, Chrzanowska KH, Krajewska-Walasek M, Sethi SK, Tasic V, Anglani F, Addis M, Wasilewska A, Szczepanska M, Pawlaczyk K, Sikora P, Ludwig M. Characterization of 28 novel patients expands the mutational and phenotypic spectrum of Lowe syndrome. Pediatr Nephrol. 2015;30(6):931–43.
14. Hichri H, Rendu J, Monnier N, Coutton C, Dorseuil O, Poussou RV, Baujat G, Blanchard A, Nobili F, Ranchin B, Remesy M, Salomon R, Satre V, Lunardi J. From Lowe syndrome to Dent disease: correlations between mutations of the OCRL1 gene and clinical and biochemical phenotypes. Hum Mutat. 2011;32(4):379–88.
15. Utsch B, Bokenkamp A, Benz MR, Besbas N, Dotsch J, Franke I, Frund S, Gok F, Hoppe B, Karle S, Kuwertz-Broking E, Laube G, Neb M, Nuutinen M, Ozaltin F, Rascher W, Ring T, Tasic V, van Wijk JA, Ludwig M. Novel OCRL1 mutations in patients with the phenotype of Dent disease. Am J Kidney Dis. 2006;48(6):942. e1–942.14
16. Watanabe M, Nakagawa R, Kohmoto T, Naruto T, Suga KI, Goji A, Horikawa H, Masuda K, Kagami S, Imoto I. Exome-first approach identified a novel gloss deletion associated with Lowe syndrome. Human Genome Var. 2016;3:16037.
17. Peces R, Peces C, de Sousa E, Vega C, Selgas R, Nevado J. A novel and de novo deletion in the OCRL1 gene associated with a severe form of Lowe syndrome. Int Urol Nephrol. 2013;45(6):1767–71.
18. Peverall J, Edkins E, Goldblatt J, Murch A. Identification of a novel deletion of the entire OCRL1 gene detected by FISH analysis in a family with Lowe syndrome. Clin Genet. 2000;58(6):479–82.
19. Addis M, Meloni C, Congiu R, Santaniello S, Emma F, Zuffardi O, Ciccone R, Cao A, Melis MA, Cau M. A novel interstitial deletion in Xq25, identified by array-CGH in a patient with Lowe syndrome. Eur J Med Genetics. 2007;50(1):79–84.
20. Janne PA, Suchy SF, Bernard D, MacDonald M, Crawley J, Grinberg A, Wynshaw-Boris A, Westphal H, Nussbaum RL. Functional overlap between murine Inpp5b and Ocrl1 may explain why deficiency of the murine ortholog for OCRL1 does not cause Lowe syndrome in mice. J Clin Invest. 1998;101(10):2042–53.
21. Nandez R, Balkin DM, Messa M, Liang L, Paradise S, Czapla H, Hein MY, Duncan JS, Mann M, De Camilli P. A role of OCRL in clathrin-coated pit dynamics and uncoating revealed by studies of Lowe syndrome cells. eLife. 2014;3:e02975.
22. Sharma S, Skowronek A, Erdmann KS. The role of the Lowe syndrome protein OCRL in the endocytic pathway. Biol Chem. 2015;396(12):1293–300.
23. Allmendinger AM, Desai NS, Burke AT, Viswanadhan N, Prabhu S. Neuroimaging and renal ultrasound manifestations of Oculocerebrorenal syndrome of Lowe. J Radiol Case Rep. 2014;8(10):1–7.
24. Ramirez IB, Pietka G, Jones DR, Divecha N, Alia A, Baraban SC, Hurlstone AF, Lowe M. Impaired neural development in a zebrafish model for Lowe syndrome. Hum Mol Genet. 2012;21(8):1744–59.
25. Bothwell SP, Chan E, Bernardini IM, Kuo YM, Gahl WA, Nussbaum RL. Mouse model for Lowe syndrome/Dent disease 2 renal tubulopathy. J Am Soc Nephrol. 2011;22(3):443–8.
26. Boland MJ, Nazor KL, Tran HT, Szucs A, Lynch CL, Paredes R, Tassone F, Sanna PP, Hagerman RJ, Loring JF. Molecular analyses of neurogenic defects in a human pluripotent stem cell model of fragile X syndrome. Brain. 2017; 140(3):582–98.
27. Dezonne RS, Sartore RC, Nascimento JM, Saia-Cereda VM, Romao LF, Alves-Leon SV, de Souza JM, Martins-de-Souza D, Rehen SK, Gomes FC. Derivation of functional human astrocytes from cerebral organoids. Sci Rep. 2017;7:45091.
28. Sellgren CM, Sheridan SD, Gracias J, Xuan D, Fu T, Perlis RH. Patient-specific models of microglia-mediated engulfment of synapses and neural progenitors. Mol Psychiatry. 2017;22(2):170–7.
29. Chandrasekaran A, Avci HX, Leist M, Kobolak J, Dinnyes A. Astrocyte differentiation of human pluripotent stem cells: new tools for neurological disorder research. Front Cell Neurosci. 2016;10:215.
30. O'Shea KS, McInnis MG. Neurodevelopmental origins of bipolar disorder: iPSC models. Mol Cell Neurosci. 2016;73:63–83.
31. Mariani J, Coppola G, Zhang P, Abyzov A, Provini L, Tomasini L, Amenduni M, Szekely A, Palejev D, Wilson M, Gerstein M, Grigorenko EL, Chawarska K, Pelphrey KA, Howe JR, Vaccarino FM. FOXG1-dependent dysregulation of GABA/glutamate neuron differentiation in autism spectrum disorders. Cell. 2015;162(2):375–90.

32. Wang P, Lin M, Pedrosa E, Hrabovsky A, Zhang Z, Guo W, Lachman HM, Zheng D. CRISPR/Cas9-mediated heterozygous knockout of the autism gene CHD8 and characterization of its transcriptional networks in neurodevelopment. Mol Autism. 2015;6:55. 015–0048-6. eCollection 2015

33. Lancaster MA, Knoblich JA. Generation of cerebral organoids from human pluripotent stem cells. Nat Protoc. 2014;9(10):2329–40.

34. Yazawa M, Dolmetsch RE. Modeling Timothy syndrome with iPS cells. J Cardiovasc Transl Res. 2013;6(1):1–9.

35. Lin M, Zhao D, Hrabovsky A, Pedrosa E, Zheng D, Lachman HM. Heat shock alters the expression of schizophrenia and autism candidate genes in an induced pluripotent stem cell model of the human telencephalon. PloS one. 2014;9(4):e94968.

36. Brennand KJ, Simone A, Jou J, Gelboin-Burkhart C, Tran N, Sangar S, Li Y, Mu Y, Chen G, Yu D, McCarthy S, Sebat J, Gage FH. Modelling schizophrenia using human induced pluripotent stem cells. Nature. 2011;473(7346):221–5.

37. Tcw J, Wang M, Pimenova AA, Bowles KR, Hartley BJ, Lacin E, Machlovi SI, Abdelaal R, Karch CM, Phatnani H, Slesinger PA, Zhang B, Goate AM, Brennand KJ. An efficient platform for astrocyte differentiation from human induced pluripotent stem cells. Stem Cell Rep. 2017;9(2):600–14.

38. Zhang Y, Pak C, Han Y, Ahlenius H, Zhang Z, Chanda S, Marro S, Patzke C, Acuna C, Covy J, Xu W, Yang N, Danko T, Chen L, Wernig M, Sudhof TC. Rapid single-step induction of functional neurons from human pluripotent stem cells. Neuron. 2013;78(5):785–98.

39. Yang N, Chanda S, Marro S, Ng YH, Janas JA, Haag D, Ang CE, Tang Y, Flores Q, Mall M, Wapinski O, Li M, Ahlenius H, Rubenstein JL, Chang HY, Buylla AA, Sudhof TC, Wernig M. Generation of pure GABAergic neurons by transcription factor programming. Nat Methods. 2017;14(6):621–8.

40. Wilkinson B, Grepo N, Thompson BL, Kim J, Wang K, Evgrafov OV, Lu W, Knowles JA, Campbell DB. The autism-associated gene chromodomain helicase DNA-binding protein 8 (CHD8) regulates noncoding RNAs and autism-related genes. Transl Psychiatry. 2015;5:e568.

41. Knowles H, Li Y, Perraud AL. The TRPM2 ion channel, an oxidative stress and metabolic sensor regulating innate immunity and inflammation. Immunol Res. 2013;55(1–3):241–8.

42. Wang P, Mokhtari R, Pedrosa E, Kirschenbaum M, Bayrak C, Zheng D, Lachman HM. CRISPR/Cas9-mediated heterozygous knockout of the autism gene CHD8 and characterization of its transcriptional networks in cerebral organoids derived from iPS cells. Mol Autism. 2017;8:11. 017–0124-1. eCollection 2017

43. Olivier E, Qiu C, Bouhassira EE. Novel, high-yield red blood cell production methods from CD34-positive cells derived from human embryonic stem, yolk sac, fetal liver, cord blood, and peripheral blood. Stem Cells Transl Med. 2012;1(8):604–14.

44. Ran FA, Hsu PD, Lin CY, Gootenberg JS, Konermann S, Trevino AE, Scott DA, Inoue A, Matoba S, Zhang Y, Zhang F. Double nicking by RNA-guided CRISPR Cas9 for enhanced genome editing specificity. Cell. 2013;154(6):1380–9.

45. Grieve AG, Daniels RD, Sanchez-Heras E, Hayes MJ, Moss SE, Matter K, Lowe M, Levine TP. Lowe syndrome protein OCRL1 supports maturation of polarized epithelial cells. PloS one. 2011;6(8):e24044.

46. Ueno T, Falkenburger BH, Pohlmeyer C, Inoue T. Triggering actin comets versus membrane ruffles: distinctive effects of phosphoinositides on actin reorganization. Sci Sig. 2011;4(203):ra87.

47. Montjean R, Aoidi R, Desbois P, Rucci J, Trichet M, Salomon R, Rendu J, Faure J, Lunardi J, Gacon G, Billuart P, Dorseuil O. OCRL-mutated fibroblasts from patients with Dent-2 disease exhibit INPP5B-independent phenotypic variability relatively to Lowe syndrome cells. Hum Mol Genet. 2015;24(4):994–1006.

48. Suchy SF, Nussbaum RL. The deficiency of PIP2 5-phosphatase in Lowe syndrome affects actin polymerization. Am J Hum Genet. 2002;71(6):1420–7.

49. Murk K, Blanco Suarez EM, Cockbill LM, Banks P, Hanley JG. The antagonistic modulation of Arp2/3 activity by N-WASP, WAVE2 and PICK1 defines dynamic changes in astrocyte morphology. J Cell Sci. 2013;126(Pt 17):3873–83.

50. Daste F, Walrant A, Holst MR, Gadsby JR, Mason J, Lee JE, Brook D, Mettlen M, Larsson E, Lee SF, Lundmark R, Gallop JL. Control of actin polymerization via the coincidence of phosphoinositides and high membrane curvature. J Cell Biol. 2017;216(11):3745–65.

51. Chia PH, Chen B, Li P, Rosen MK, Shen K. Local F-actin network links synapse formation and axon branching. Cell. 2014;156(1–2):208–20.

52. Alekhina O, Burstein E, Billadeau DD. Cellular functions of WASP family proteins at a glance. J Cell Sci. 2017;130(14):2235–41.

53. Shah K, Rossie S. Tale of the good and the bad Cdk5: remodeling of the actin cytoskeleton in the brain. Mol Neurobiol. 2018;55(4):3426–38.

54. Bralten J, van Hulzen KJ, Martens MB, Galesloot TE, Arias Vasquez A, Kiemeney LA, Buitelaar JK, Muntjewerff JW, Franke B, Poelmans G. Autism spectrum disorders and autistic traits share genetics and biology. Mol Psychiatry. 2018;23(5):1205–12.

55. Deans PJM, Raval P, Sellers KJ, Gatford NJF, Halai S, Duarte RRR, Shum C, Warre-Cornish K, Kaplun VE, Cocks G, Hill M, Bray NJ, Price J, Srivastava DP. Psychosis risk candidate ZNF804A localizes to synapses and regulates neurite formation and dendritic spine structure. Biol Psychiatry. 2017;82(1):49–61.

56. Nebel RA, Zhao D, Pedrosa E, Kirschen J, Lachman HM, Zheng D, Abrahams BS. Reduced CYFIP1 in human neural progenitors results in dysregulation of schizophrenia and epilepsy gene networks. PloS one. 2016;11(1):e0148039.

57. Sadybekov A, Tian C, Arnesano C, Katritch V, Herring BE. An autism spectrum disorder-related de novo mutation hotspot discovered in the GEF1 domain of Trio. Nat Commun. 2017;8(1):601. 017–00472-0

58. Lilja J, Zacharchenko T, Georgiadou M, Jacquemet G, De Franceschi N, Peuhu E, Hamidi H, Pouwels J, Martens V, Nia FH, Beifuss M, Boeckers T, Kreienkamp HJ, Barsukov IL, Ivaska J. SHANK proteins limit integrin activation by directly interacting with Rap1 and R-Ras. Nat Cell Biol. 2017;19(4):292–305.

59. Yan Z, Kim E, Datta D, Lewis DA, Soderling SH. Synaptic actin dysregulation, a convergent mechanism of mental disorders? J Neurosci. 2016;36(45):11411–7.

60. Hsiao K, Harony-Nicolas H, Buxbaum JD, Bozdagi-Gunal O, Benson DL. Cyfip1 regulates presynaptic activity during development. J Neurosci. 2016; 36(5):1564–76.

61. Han K, Chen H, Gennarino VA, Richman R, Lu HC, Zoghbi HY. Fragile X-like behaviors and abnormal cortical dendritic spines in cytoplasmic FMR1-interacting protein 2-mutant mice. Hum Mol Genet. 2015;24(7):1813–23.

62. Hayashi-Takagi A, Takaki M, Graziane N, Seshadri S, Murdoch H, Dunlop AJ, Makino Y, Seshadri AJ, Ishizuka K, Srivastava DP, Xie Z, Baraban JM, Houslay MD, Tomoda T, Brandon NJ, Kamiya A, Yan Z, Penzes P, Sawa A. Disrupted-in-schizophrenia 1 (DISC1) regulates spines of the glutamate synapse via Rac1. Nat Neurosci. 2010;13(3):327–32.

63. Miyoshi K, Honda A, Baba K, Taniguchi M, Oono K, Fujita T, Kuroda S, Katayama T, Tohyama M. Disrupted-in-schizophrenia 1, a candidate gene for schizophrenia, participates in neurite outgrowth. Mol Psychiatry. 2003;8(7):685–94.

64. Lin YC, Frei JA, Kilander MB, Shen W, Blatt GJ. A subset of autism-associated genes regulate the structural stability of neurons. Front Cell Neurosci. 2016;10:263.

65. Pyronneau A, He Q, Hwang JY, Porch M, Contractor A, Zukin RS. Aberrant Rac1-cofilin signaling mediates defects in dendritic spines, synaptic function, and sensory perception in fragile X syndrome. Sci Signal. 2017;10(504) https://doi.org/10.1126/scisignal.aan0852.

66. Saarikangas J, Zhao H, Lappalainen P. Regulation of the actin cytoskeleton-plasma membrane interplay by phosphoinositides. Physiol Rev. 2010;90(1): 259–89.

67. De Leo MG, Staiano L, Vicinanza M, Luciani A, Carissimo A, Mutarelli M, Di Campli A, Polishchuk E, Di Tullio G, Morra V, Levtchenko E, Oltrabella F, Starborg T, Santoro M, Di Bernardo D, Devuyst O, Lowe M, Medina DL, Ballabio A, De Matteis MA. Autophagosome-lysosome fusion triggers a lysosomal response mediated by TLR9 and controlled by OCRL. Nat Cell Biol. 2016;18(8):839–50.

68. Chen Z, Borek D, Padrick SB, Gomez TS, Metlagel Z, Ismail AM, Umetani J, Billadeau DD, Otwinowski Z, Rosen MK. Structure and control of the actin regulatory WAVE complex. Nature. 2010;468(7323):533–8.

69. Abekhoukh S, Sahin HB, Grossi M, Zongaro S, Maurin T, Madrigal I, Kazue-Sugioka D, Raas-Rothschild A, Doulazmi M, Carrera P, Stachon A, Scherer S, Drula Do Nascimento MR, Trembleau A, Arroyo I, Szatmari P, Smith IM, Mila M, Smith AC, Giangrande A, Caille I, Bardoni B. New insights into the regulatory function of CYFIP1 in the context of WAVE- and FMRP-containing complexes. Dis Model Mech. 2017;10(4):463–74.

70. Mendoza MC. Phosphoregulation of the WAVE regulatory complex and signal integration. Semin Cell Dev Biol. 2013;24(4):272–9.

71. Oguro-Ando A, Rosensweig C, Herman E, Nishimura Y, Werling D, Bill BR, Berg JM, Gao F, Coppola G, Abrahams BS, Geschwind DH. Increased CYFIP1 dosage alters cellular and dendritic morphology and dysregulates mTOR. Mol Psychiatry. 2015;20(9):1069–78.

72. Napoli I, Mercaldo V, Boyl PP, Eleuteri B, Zalfa F, De Rubeis S, Di Marino D, Mohr E, Massimi M, Falconi M, Witke W, Costa-Mattioli M, Sonenberg N, Achsel T, Bagni C. The fragile X syndrome protein represses activity-dependent translation through CYFIP1, a new 4E-BP. Cell. 2008;134(6):1042–54.

73. Harripaul R, Vasli N, Mikhailov A, Rafiq MA, Mittal K, Windpassinger C, Sheikh TI, Noor A, Mahmood H, Downey S, Johnson M, Vleuten K, Bell L, Ilyas M, Khan FS, Khan V, Moradi M, Ayaz M, Naeem F, Heidari A, Ahmed I, Ghadami

S, Agha Z, Zeinali S, Qamar R, Mozhdehipanah H, John P, Mir A, Ansar M, French L, Ayub M, Vincent JB. Mapping autosomal recessive intellectual disability: combined microarray and exome sequencing identifies 26 novel candidate genes in 192 consanguineous families. Mol Psychiatry. 2018;23(4): 973–84.

74. Freed D, Pevsner J. The contribution of mosaic variants to autism spectrum disorder. PLoS Genetics. 2016;12(9):e1006245.

75. Anazi S, Maddirevula S, Salpietro V, Asi YT, Alsahli S, Alhashem A, Shamseldin HE, AlZahrani F, Patel N, Ibrahim N, Abdulwahab FM, Hashem M, Alhashmi N, Al Murshedi F, Al Kindy A, Alshaer A, Rumayyan A, Al Tala S, Kurdi W, Alsaman A, Alasmari A, Banu S, Sultan T, Saleh MM, Alkuraya H, Salih MA, Aldhalaan H, Ben-Omran T, Al Musafri F, Ali R, Suleiman J, Tabarki B, El-Hattab AW, Bupp C, Alfadhel M, Al Tassan N, Monies D, Arold ST, Abouelhoda M, Lashley T, Houlden H, Faqeih E, Alkuraya FS. Expanding the genetic heterogeneity of intellectual disability. Hum genetics. 2017; 136(11-12):1419–29.

76. Chen B, Chou HT, Brautigam CA, Xing W, Yang S, Henry L, Doolittle LK, Walz T, Rosen MK. Rac1 GTPase activates the WAVE regulatory complex through two distinct binding sites. eLife. 2017;6 https://doi.org/10.7554/eLife.29795.

77. Litschko C, Linkner J, Bruhmann S, Stradal TEB, Reinl T, Jansch L, Rottner K, Faix J. Differential functions of WAVE regulatory complex subunits in the regulation of actin-driven processes. Eur J Cell Biol. 2017;96(8):715–27.

78. Zhu S, Dai J, Liu H, Cong X, Chen Y, Wu Y, Hu H, Heng BC, Ouyang HW, Zhou Y. Down-regulation of Rac GTPase-activating protein OCRL1 causes aberrant activation of Rac1 in osteoarthritis development. Arthritis Rheumatol. 2015;67(8):2154–63.

79. van Rahden VA, Brand K, Najm J, Heeren J, Pfeffer SR, Braulke T, Kutsche K. The 5-phosphatase OCRL mediates retrograde transport of the mannose 6-phosphate receptor by regulating a Rac1-cofilin signalling module. Hum Mol Genet. 2012;21(23):5019–38.

80. Tejada-Simon MV. Modulation of actin dynamics by Rac1 to target cognitive function. J Neurochem. 2015;133(6):767–79.

81. Huang GH, Sun ZL, Li HJ, Feng DF. Rho GTPase-activating proteins: regulators of rho GTPase activity in neuronal development and CNS diseases. Mol Cell Neurosci. 2017;80:18–31.

82. Bongmba OY, Martinez LA, Elhardt ME, Butler K, Tejada-Simon MV. Modulation of dendritic spines and synaptic function by Rac1: a possible link to fragile X syndrome pathology. Brain Res. 2011;1399:79–95.

83. Katrancha SM, Wu Y, Zhu M, Eipper BA, Koleske AJ, Mains RE. Neurodevelopmental disease-associated de novo mutations and rare sequence variants affect TRIO GDP/GTP exchange factor activity. Hum Mol Genet. 2017;26(23):4728–40.

84. Lelieveld SH, Reijnders MR, Pfundt R, Yntema HG, Kamsteeg EJ, de Vries P, de Vries BB, Willemsen MH, Kleefstra T, Lohner K, Vreeburg M, Stevens SJ, van der Burgt I, Bongers EM, Stegmann AP, Rump P, Rinne T, Nelen MR, Veltman JA, Vissers LE, Brunner HG, Gilissen C. Meta-analysis of 2,104 trios provides support for 10 new genes for intellectual disability. Nat Neurosci. 2016;19(9):1194–6.

85. Datta D, Arion D, Roman KM, Volk DW, Lewis DA. Altered expression of ARP2/3 complex signaling pathway genes in prefrontal layer 3 pyramidal cells in schizophrenia. Am J Psychiatry. 2017;174(2):163–71.

86. Redlich S, Ribes S, Schutze S, Eiffert H, Nau R. Toll-like receptor stimulation increases phagocytosis of Cryptococcus neoformans by microglial cells. J Neuroinflammation. 2013;10:71. 2094–10-71

87. Guerra CR, Seabra SH, de Souza W, Rozental S. Cryptococcus neoformans is internalized by receptor-mediated or 'triggered' phagocytosis, dependent on actin recruitment. PloS one. 2014;9(2):e89250.

88. Johnston SA, May RC. Cryptococcus interactions with macrophages: evasion and manipulation of the phagosome by a fungal pathogen. Cell Microbiol. 2013;15(3):403–11.

9

Alterations in electrophysiological indices of perceptual processing and discrimination are associated with co-occurring emotional and behavioural problems in adolescents with autism spectrum disorder

Virginia Carter Leno[1]* (iD), Susie Chandler[1], Pippa White[1], Isabel Yorke[1], Tony Charman[1,2], Andrew Pickles[1] and Emily Simonoff[1,2]

Abstract

Background: Many young people with autism spectrum disorder (ASD) experience emotional and behavioural problems. However, the causes of these co-occurring difficulties are not well understood. Perceptual processing atypicalities are also often reported in individuals with ASD, but how these relate to co-occurring emotional and behavioural problems remains unclear, and few studies have used objective measurement of perceptual processing.

Methods: Event-related potentials (ERPs) were recorded in response to both standard and deviant stimuli (which varied in pitch) in an auditory oddball paradigm in adolescents (mean age of 13.56 years, SD = 1.12, range = 11.40–15.70) with ASD (n = 43) with a wide range of IQ (mean IQ of 84.14, SD = 24.24, range 27–129). Response to deviant as compared to standard stimuli (as indexed by the mismatch negativity (MMN)) and response to repeated presentations of standard stimuli (habituation) were measured. Multivariate regression tested the association between neural indices of perceptual processing and co-occurring emotional and behavioural problems.

Results: Greater sensitivity to changes in pitch in incoming auditory information (discrimination), as indexed by increased MMN amplitude, was associated with higher levels of parent-rated behaviour problems. MMN amplitude also showed a trend positive correlation with parent-rated sensory hyper-sensitivity. Conversely, greater habituation at the later N2 component was associated with higher levels of emotional problems. Upon more detailed analyses, this appeared to be driven by a selectively greater ERP response to the first (but not the second or third) standard stimuli that followed deviant stimuli. A similar pattern of association was found with other measures of anxiety. All results remained in covariation analyses controlling for age, sex and IQ, although the association between MMN amplitude and behaviour problems became non-significant when controlling for ASD severity.

Conclusions: Findings suggest that alterations in mechanisms of perceptual processing and discrimination may be important for understanding co-occurring emotional and behavioural problems in young people with ASD.

Keywords: IAMHealth, EEG, ERP, ASD, Perceptual processing, Sensory, Comorbidity, Psychopathology

* Correspondence: virginia.m.carter_leno@kcl.ac.uk
[1]Institute of Psychiatry, Psychology & Neuroscience, King's College London, 16 De Crespigny Park, London SE5 8AF, UK
Full list of author information is available at the end of the article

Background

Co-occurring psychopathology is highly prevalent in children and adolescents with ASD [1–6]; however, the aetiology of these additional emotional and behavioural problems in ASD is not well known. Rates of psychopathology are higher in ASD populations as compared to populations of individuals with intellectual disability (ID) [7, 8], suggesting that ASD is a risk factor, over and above having ID. One approach is to test whether performance in certain cognitive domains, thought to be impaired in individuals with ASD, is also associated with the presence of psychopathology. This will inform future longitudinal studies, where the predictive role of domains can be fully tested. Understanding ASD-specific risk factors will allow novel, targeted interventions to be developed, promoting improved quality of life and better long-term outcomes.

At a group level, ASD is characterised by specific neurocognitive impairments, thought to contribute to the core symptoms of social communication difficulties and restricted, repetitive behaviours [9, 10]. However, few studies have considered how variability in these domains of cognitive functioning may also be important in understanding the preponderance of additional psychopathology in individuals with ASD. The current manuscript focuses upon the domain of sensory or perceptual processing, where individuals with ASD often show atypical functioning. Previous research has highlighted that individuals with ASD experience both hypo- and hyper-sensitivity to perceptual inputs from auditory, tactile and visual sources [11–15] and that alterations in underlying neural processes may underpin these atypical perceptual experiences [16–18]. One of the most well-studied neural indices of perceptual processing in electroencephalography (EEG) paradigms is the mismatch negativity (MMN) component [19]. This is a fronto-central negative component found around 100–200 ms after stimulus presentation, which, in typically developing individuals, is of greater amplitude in response to deviant, as compared to standard stimuli. As MMN amplitude is found to be associated with individual discrimination skill [19–21], some have suggested it is an index of individual sensitivity to changes in incoming information (i.e., discrimination).

In terms of MMN alterations in individuals with ASD, findings are mixed (for a review see [22]). Some have found increased MMN amplitude in individuals with ASD [23–25], and decreased latency [26, 27], which have been interpreted as indexing hyper-sensitivity to unpredictable changes [17]. However, others have found decreased MMN amplitude [28–31] and increased MMN latency [32]. Furthermore, some have reported an association between MMN attenuation and higher sensory sensitivity scores [28, 31]. Differences in findings may be due to variation in the samples (e.g., with/without concurrent ID,

older vs. younger children) and experimental paradigms used, as one study found attenuated MMN in children with ASD during non-attended conditions, but when participants were instructed to listen to the sounds, there was no difference between the ASD and typically developing group [33].

Another, albeit less researched area of perceptual processing in ASD is that of habituation. In the types of oddball paradigms used to study discrimination between deviant and standard stimuli reviewed above, one can also study habituation to the standard stimuli, where the neural response exponentially decreases over repeated presentations of the same stimuli. This is thought to allow the brain to filter out irrelevant repetitive stimuli and conserve attentional resources [34]. Research has found reduced neural habituation to repeated presentations of the same stimuli in individuals with ASD [35, 36], and in 9-month old infants at higher genetic risk of developing ASD [37], and some suggest that this reduced habituation may underlie both the hypo- and hyper-sensitivity to sensory input found in individuals with ASD [37].

Although no study has directly looked at how neural indices of perceptual processing are related to emotional and behavioural problems in ASD, there are a small number of studies that used questionnaire measures of sensory/perceptual processing. A small sample pilot study ($n = 22$) found that caregiver-rated sensory processing atypicalities were significantly correlated ($r = 0.49$) with behavioural problems in children with ASD [38]. Another study of young children with ASD found parent-rated sensory avoidance was significantly associated with internalising problems, whereas sensory sensitivity was significantly associated with externalising problems [39]. Similar associations were found in a study that used teacher-rated questionnaires, where a significant correlation was found between tactile and movement sensitivity, and oppositional behaviour in children with ASD [40]. However, the specificity of this association was unclear, as tactile sensitivity was also correlated with ADHD-type symptoms. In the same study, the authors also found an association between difficulties with auditory filtering and internalising problems. A number of studies have reported an association between parent-rated sensory hyper-sensitivity and anxiety symptoms in individuals with ASD [41–44], including one that used physiological reactivity to a sensory challenge as an index of sensitivity [41]. One longitudinal study of toddlers with ASD found sensory over-sensitivity predicted increases in anxiety over and above child age, ASD symptom severity, cognitive ability, and maternal anxiety, but anxiety did not predict changes in sensory over-sensitivity [45], suggesting a potential causal pathway between sensory processing atypicalities and anxiety in ASD.

No study has specifically explored the association between habituation and co-occurring emotional and behavioural problems in individuals with ASD. However, in typically developing adolescents, decreased neural habituation was found to be associated with higher levels of trait anxiety [46]. In terms of how habituation could theoretically relate to anxiety, impaired habituation may lead to repeated and predictable perceptual inputs being experienced as novel and unpredictable, and neuroimaging research has found temporally unpredictable stimuli provoke anxiety behaviours in mice and humans [47].

Aims

In summary, it appears that individuals with ASD are characterised not only by alterations in neural response to deviant stimuli, but also by decreased habituation to repeated presentation of the same stimuli. Questionnaire studies from individuals with ASD and neuroimaging studies from typically developing individuals suggest that both of these domains may be linked to emotional and behavioural problems. However, no study has specifically tested how neural indices of perceptual processing relate to emotional and behavioural problems in individuals with ASD. The aim of this study was to investigate whether neural responses to (a) deviant vs. standard stimuli and (b) repeated presentation of the standard stimuli were associated with co-occurring emotional and behavioural problems in adolescents with ASD. Based on prior literature, it was hypothesised that greater sensitivity to changes in perceptual information, as indexed by increased MMN amplitude, would be associated with higher levels of emotional and behaviour problems. In terms of habituation, it was hypothesised that decreased habituation would be associated with increased emotional difficulties. Finally, correlations between neural measures of perceptual processing and parent-rated sensory sensitivities were calculated to understand how the selected neural measures related to real-life sensory behaviours.

Methods

Participants

Forty-three adolescents with ASD, consisting of 29 males and 14 females, with a mean age of 13.56 years (SD = 1.12, range = 11.40–15.70) and mean IQ of 84.14 (SD = 24.24, range 27–129; $n = 3$ with IQ < 50) completed an auditory oddball paradigm. Participants were part of the QUEST follow-up study, a longitudinal community sample recruited at age 4–8 years [3], which in turn was part of the wider IAMHealth project (https://iamhealthkcl.net//). The target population for the study was all children born between September 01, 2000, and August 31, 2004, living in two London boroughs (one inner and one outer London), who had a clinical diagnosis of ASD. More information about the sampling structure is given

in Additional file 1. Although participants had a clinical diagnosis of ASD, the 'intensively studied' (hereafter intensive) group ($n = 83$) included at present had their diagnosis confirmed at age 10–16 years with the Autism Diagnostic Observation Schedule-2 (ADOS-2) ([48]) and a subset also with the Autism Diagnostic Interview-Revised (ADI-R) [49]. Both the recommended autism cutoff [49] and the recommended ASD cutoff [50] were applied to the ADI-R data. All participants were above threshold on either or both instruments. Participants in the intensive group were selected to over-represent females, as one of the main aims of the study included sex comparisons. This sample completed a selection of neurocognitive assessments and parent-rated questionnaires. The larger 'extensively studied' (extensive) sample ($n = 128$) only completed a selection of parent-rated questionnaires online. The extensive sample did not complete any neurocognitive assessments, but for the purpose of this paper were included to allow for examination of the psychometric properties of the Sensory Experiences Questionnaire—brief version (see below for further details). From the original intensive QUEST sample ($n = 83$, which had an IQ range of 19–120), only those who were able to complete the auditory oddball paradigm ($n = 43$) were included in present analyses. All participating families gave their written informed consent, and the study was approved by Camden and King's Cross Ethics Sub-Committee (14/LO/2098). Table 1 gives demographic information for the sample, and comparison of key outcome measures between the total sample (intensive + extensive combined), the intensive sample and those who completed the auditory oddball paradigm is given in Additional file 1. All participating families gave their written informed consent.

Parent-rated questionnaires

As ASD is a broad spectrum, we intentionally used a variety of questionnaires to best capture the different

Table 1 Sample characteristics

Mean (SD, range) ($N = 43$ unless otherwise indicated)	
Age	13.56 (1.12, 11.4–15.7)
% male	67%
IQ	84.14 (24.24, 27–129)
ADOS-2 severity	6.05 (2.65, 1–10)
ARI ($n = 41$)	4.51 (3.21, 0–12)
DBC total behaviour problem score ($n = 41$)	53.56 (24.59, 16–127)
SCAS ($n = 41$)	27.90 (17.91, 4–77)
SDQ emotional problems ($n = 41$)	4.29 (2.69, 0–10)
SDQ ADHD symptoms ($n = 41$)	5.15 (2.58, 0–10)
SDQ conduct problems ($n = 41$)	2.12 (1.65, 0–6)

ADOS-2 Autism Diagnostic Observation Schedule, *ARI* Affective Reactivity Index, *DBC* Developmental Behaviour Checklist, *SCAS* Spence's Child Anxiety Scale, *SDQ* Strengths and Difficulties Questionnaire types of emotional and behavioural problems exhibited by this population. The details of these are given below.

Affective Reactivity Index (ARI)

The ARI [51] was used to assess participants' level of irritability and includes six items relating to feelings/behaviours specific for irritability and one question assessing impairment due to irritability. Internal consistency is reported to be good in samples of young people with ASD ($\alpha = 0.82$) [52].

Developmental Behaviour Checklist (DBC)

The DBC [53, 54] is a 96-item questionnaire designed to assess emotional and behavioural problems in young people with developmental disabilities and ID. Excellent internal consistency ($\alpha = 0.94$) is reported from large epidemiological samples, along with high correlations ($r = 0.70$–0.86) with other measures of emotional and behavioural disturbance [53, 54].

Spence's Child Anxiety Scale (SCAS)

The SCAS [55] is a 38-item questionnaire used to assess current symptoms of anxiety in 6–18-year-olds. Excellent internal consistency ($\alpha = .92$–$.93$) [56, 57] and convergent validity with DSM-IV-defined anxiety disorders [58] have been reported from samples of young people with ASD.

Strengths and Difficulties Questionnaire (SDQ)

The SDQ [59] is a 25-item questionnaire used to measure psychiatric symptoms. The SDQ comprises three psychiatric subscales of hyperactivity/inattention (ADHD symptoms), conduct problems and emotional problems (including both anxiety and depression symptoms), along with further subscales of peer-relationship problems and prosocial behaviour. The SDQ maintains good psychometric properties when used with individuals with ID [60] and has been shown to successfully detect change in additional mental health problems following intervention in populations of young people with ASD [61]. Current analyses focused upon the three psychiatric subscales of ADHD symptoms, conduct problems and emotional problems.

Sensory Experiences Questionnaire 3.0 (SEQ)—brief version for 10–14-year-olds

The SEQ 3.0—brief version for 10–14 year olds (Grace T. Baranek, copyright 2014) is an 18-item questionnaire designed to measure sensory features in young people with ASD. This shortened version, using a subset of items from the original SEQ 3.0, was created specifically for use with the QUEST sample and was based on a factor analysis of the original measure [62]. The SEQ is designed to capture four constructs and enhanced perception, hyper-responsiveness, hypo-responsiveness, and sensory interests, repetitions and seeking behaviour. Comparison of the brief version and the full SEQ found strong correlations between the two for all four constructs (enhanced perception $r = 0.84$, hyper-responsiveness $r = 0.85$, hypo-responsiveness $r = 0.86$, and sensory interests, repetitions and seeking behaviour $r = 0.81$) (Baranek, 2014. unpublished data). However, given the limited number of items measuring each construct in the brief version of the SEQ, the authors recommend grouping responses into two subscales: hyper-responsiveness + enhanced perception and hypo-responsiveness + sensory seeking (Grace T. Baranek, personal correspondence). In previous work with a larger sample ($n = 311$) of 10–14-year-olds with ASD, internal consistency was found to be acceptable for the total score ($\alpha = 0.75$) and for the hyper-responsiveness + enhanced perception subscale ($\alpha = 0.73$), however lower for the hypo-responsiveness + sensory seeking subscale ($\alpha = 0.64$) (Baranek, 2014. unpublished data). In the current total pooled QUEST sample (which included both the extensive sample, and all participants from the intensive sample, including those who completed questionnaire measures but not neurocognitive tasks) ($n = 198$), internal consistency was good for the total score ($\alpha = 0.85$) and the hypo-responsiveness + sensory seeking subscale ($\alpha = 0.80$) and acceptable for the hyper-responsiveness + enhanced perception subscale ($\alpha = 0.76$).

Direct assessments

ASD symptoms

The ADOS-2 [48] is considered a gold-standard instrument for assessing current ASD symptoms and consists of a semi-structured assessment designed to elicit certain ASD behaviours, which are then coded and scored. Based on the total score, a calibrated severity score is calculated, scored 0–10, which takes into account age and language level [63]. A higher score is indicative of a more severe level of ASD symptoms. Participants were assessed with either the ADOS-2 Module 1 ($n = 2$), 2 ($n = 2$), or 3 ($n = 39$), dependent upon their verbal abilities. All ADOS-2 assessments were administered by a trained researcher and co-scored by a second trained researcher, and final scores reflected consensus scores between the two coders.

Cognitive ability

IQ was estimated using either the Wechsler Abbreviated Scale of Intelligence (WASI) ([64]) ($n = 38$) or the Wechsler Preschool and Primary Scale of Intelligence (WPPSI) ([65]) ($n = 5$), depending on the child's age and developmental level. As the WPPSI was used out of age range, age-equivalents were calculated and a ratio IQ derived [ratio IQ = (age equivalent/chronological age) × 100] [66].

EEG paradigm
Stimuli
Auditory stimuli were presented in an oddball paradigm (adapted from [37]). Stimuli were two tones, each of 100 ms in duration with a rise and fall time of 5 ms, and an inter-stimulus interval of 700 ms. The infrequently presented deviant tone (8% probability) consisted of a 1200 Hz tone. The frequently presented standard tone (92% probability) consisted of a 1000 Hz tone. All tones were presented at 70 dB SPL. Stimuli were presented randomly, with the restriction that at least three standard tones (S1, S2 and S3) followed each deviant tone. To avoid substantial differences in trial numbers, analyses focused only on S1, S2 and S3 rather than all standard tones.

Procedure
Participants were seated within a sound-attenuated EEG suite, where sounds were presented through two speakers, located approximately 1 m in front of the participant. Participants watched two soundless movies whilst the auditory stimuli were presented. High-density scalp EEG was recorded continuously using a 128-channel HydroCel Geodesic Sensor Net system (Electrical Geodesics, Eugene, OR) at a 500-Hz sampling rate, with the NetAmps 400 amplifier which employs a 4 KHz antialiasing filter. Voltages were referenced online to the vertex electrode (Cz). Impedances checked to be below 40 kΩ before recording began. All electrophysiological data were recorded with NetStation 5.1 software (Electrical Geodesics, Eugene, OR), and all tasks were delivered through E-Prime 2.0 experimental design software (Psychology Software Tools, Pittsburgh, PA). Data were stored and analysed offline.

EEG recording and pre-processing
EEG data were processed offline using BrainVision Analyser 2.0 software (Brain Products, Munich, Germany). Data were down-sampled to 256 Hz, re-referenced to the average reference and filtered using 0.1 Hz high-pass and 30 Hz low-pass infinite impulse response (IIR) phase-shift free Butterworth 24 dB/Oct filters. The data were manually inspected to identify bad channels, which when possible were interpolated using spherical splines. Noisy segments of data were removed by visual inspection prior to running independent component analysis (ICA) ([67]). Visual inspection of the component map was used to identify and remove components representing ocular movement. Semi-automatic artefact detection was subsequently performed to remove any segments with any additional artefacts greater than maximum-minimum values of 200 μV. Epochs of 600 ms, including a – 100 ms prestimulus period, were extracted and averaged for each stimulus category (deviant, S1, S2 and S3). Data were baseline corrected using the 100 ms prior to stimuli presentation.

ERP analysis
The average amount of trials per condition was 68 (SD = 12.85) for all standard stimuli (S1 = 68, S2 = 69 and S3 = 68) and 69 (SD = 12.64) for deviant stimuli. Electrodes of interest were selected based on prior literature [33, 68, 69] and confirmed with visual inspection of the grand average waveform (see Fig. 1). Semi-automatic peak detection was used to mark specific components, and the amplitude and latency of components were extracted for statistical analysis. Each participant's individual waveform data were inspected to confirm that components of interest fell within the allotted temporal window. The MMN was extracted from a cluster of five electrodes (7, 31, 80, 106, Cz) corresponding to the Cz area. Peak amplitude of the most prominent negative deflection was measured in each participant in the 80–200 ms latency range, consistent with previous literature [19]. Amplitudes for all electrodes in a cluster were averaged.

For MMN analysis, responses to S1, S2 and S3 were averaged, and analyses compared response to deviant vs. standard stimuli. For analysis of habituation, responses to the first (S1), second (S2) and third (S3) standard tone after a deviant tone were averaged separately. From inspection of the grand averages (Fig. 1), it was clear that the ERP response to stimuli was characterised by two negative deflections, one early and one late. Thus, habituation analyses were conducted not only at the early N1 component (using the same latency window as was used in the MMN analysis, 80–200 ms), but also a later negative component (N2, 210–300 ms). Peak amplitude of the most prominent negative deflection in these latency ranges for S1, S2 and S3 was measured in each participant.

Analytic strategy
All analyses were completed in Stata 14 [70]. To ensure that the paradigm had reliably elicited the MMN component, amplitudes to deviant and standard tones at the early component were compared using planned pairwise comparisons. MMN amplitude was measured as the difference waveform obtained by subtracting response to the standard tones from response to the deviant tones. A habituation index was measured as the difference waveform obtained by subtracting response to S1 from response to S3. A higher value indicates a greater decrease in ERP response between S1 and S3 (i.e., greater habituation). Where significant associations were found with the habituation index, planned follow-up analyses looked at responses to each standard tone (S1, S2, S3) separately to clarify whether response to a specific standard tone was driving effects. Before beginning analyses,

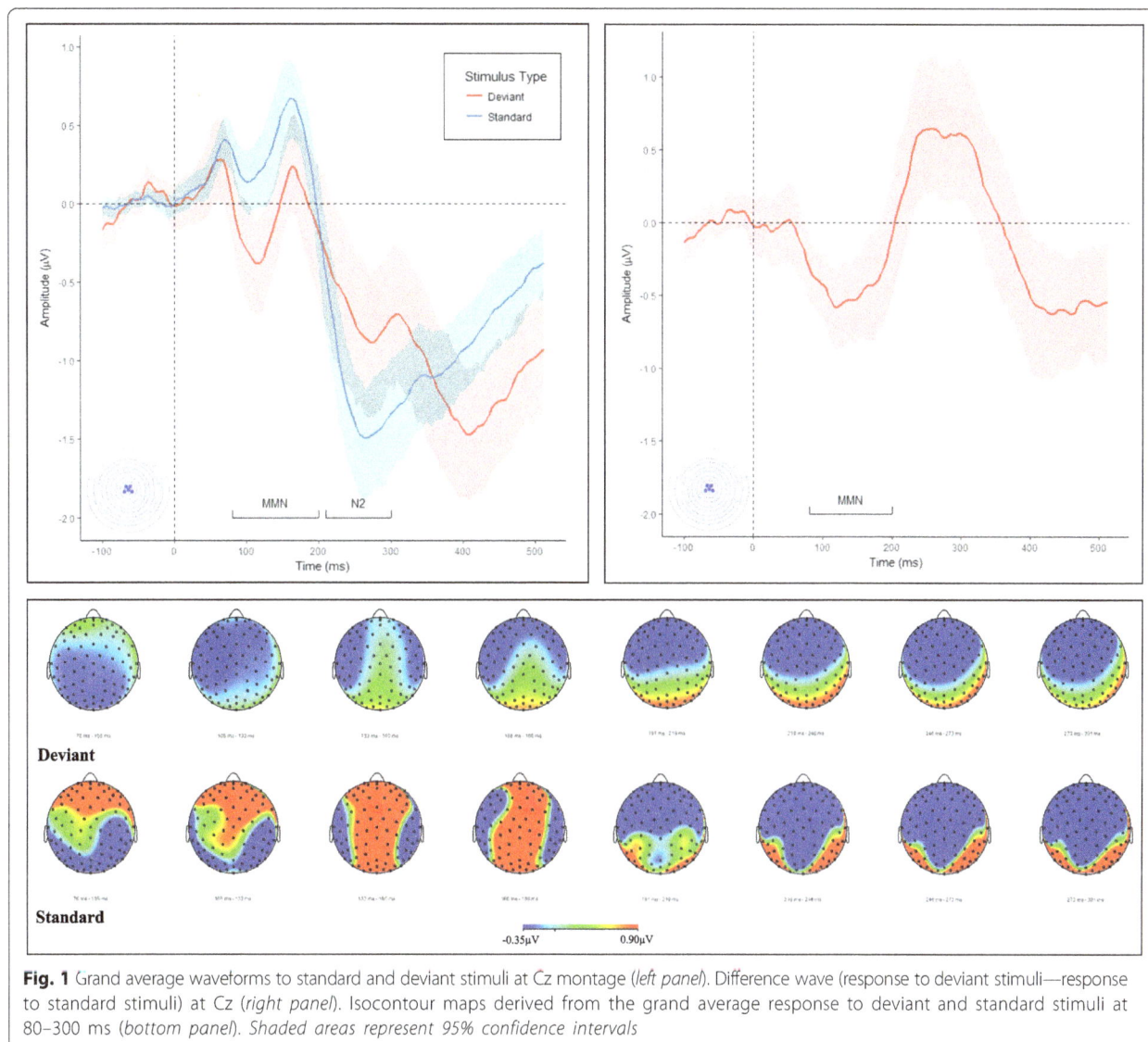

Fig. 1 Grand average waveforms to standard and deviant stimuli at Cz montage (*left panel*). Difference wave (response to deviant stimuli—response to standard stimuli) at Cz (*right panel*). Isocontour maps derived from the grand average response to deviant and standard stimuli at 80–300 ms (*bottom panel*). *Shaded areas represent 95% confidence intervals*

data were checked for skewness and outliers. As the S1 and S3 variables were negatively skewed, they were square root transformed. Outliers in EEG data were identified using box and whisker plots (Stata command graph box). This identifies outliers as values outside 1.5 × the interquartile range ± the value of the upper/lower quartile [71]. One outlier was identified in the MMN difference wave data and two outliers in the habituation index data. These were removed before conducting each analysis. For completeness, analyses were also conducted on the full dataset (including outliers). These are reported in Additional file 1, along with additional post hoc analyses adjusting for the overall number of available trials per participant, and using the mean, rather than peak, ERP amplitude.

Bi-variate correlations were calculated between all parent-rated predictor variables and EEG outcome variables to gain an initial understanding of the data. These are listed in Additional file 1. Following this, analyses used multivariate regression to test for an association between ERP response and SDQ subscales of emotional problems and ADHD symptoms and conduct problems, along with the ARI irritability scale. A separate regression was run to test for an association between ERP response and DBC total behaviour problem score. Questionnaires were grouped in this manner in the analyses as the SDQ and ARI were developed in non-ASD populations and demarcate well-defined domains of psychopathology (e.g., emotional problems, ADHD, conduct problems, irritability). Conversely, the DBC was designed for people with developmental disorders, including ASD and ID. Here, the total score indexes a range of emotional and behavioural problems which are often found in individuals with developmental disorders. The multivariate approach was selected as it is statistically parsimonious and takes account of multiple testing amongst correlated outcomes. Where trend or significant associations were found, results were first adjusted for age, sex and IQ, and then for age, sex, IQ and ASD severity, as measured by the ADOS calibrated severity score. Two separate sensitivity analyses were conducted, first excluding those using medication known to affect brain functioning ($n = 5$) and second excluding those with epilepsy ($n = 2$). Finally, to assess how brain indices related to real-life sensory sensitivities, bi-variate correlations were computed between key ERP components and the two SEQ subscales.

Results
Perceptual sensitivity as measured by the MMN
The ERP response to deviant tones was significantly greater than the response to the standard tones (mean standard amplitude = $- 0.39$, SD = 0.78, range $- 3.40$–1.27; mean deviant amplitude = $- 0.93$, SD = $- 1.07$, range $- 3.71$–1.11; $t(42) = 3.90$, $p < 0.01$), confirming the presence of the MMN.

No significant associations were found between the SDQ subscales or ARI total and MMN amplitude ($ps = 0.22$–0.99). A significant association was found between MMN amplitude and DBC total behaviour problem score ($\beta = 9.51$, $p < 0.05$), and this association remained at a trend level when controlling for age, sex and IQ ($\beta = 9.40$, $p = 0.07$), but became non-significant when controlling for age, sex, IQ and ASD severity ($\beta = 8.77$, $p = 0.11$). The association remained significant in sensitivity analyses, first excluding those using medication ($\beta = 10.10$, $p < 0.05$), and then excluding participants with epilepsy ($\beta = 10.39$, $p < 0.05$). Figure 2 depicts the association between MMN

amplitude and DBC total behaviour problem scores, in that those with greater MMN amplitude had higher DBC total behaviour problem scores. This association was not specifically driven by response to either standard or deviant ones as neither was significantly associated with DBC total behaviour problem score ($p = 0.18$ and $p = 0.78$ respectively).

Habituation
No significant association was found between behaviour and the habituation index at the early N1 component ($ps = 0.09$–0.99).

At the later N2 component, the SDQ emotional problem subscale was positively associated with the habituation index ($\beta = 1.47$, $p < 0.01$), in that those with higher habituation had a greater SDQ emotional problems score, and this association remained when controlling for age, sex and IQ ($\beta = 1.77$, $p < 0.01$) and controlling for age, sex, IQ and ASD severity ($\beta = 1.80$, $p < 0.01$), and in sensitivity analyses excluding participants using medication ($\beta = 1.53$, $p < 0.01$), and excluding participants with epilepsy ($\beta = 1.49$, $p < 0.01$). No association was found between the habituation index and the other SDQ subscales, ARI total, DBC total behaviour problem score ($ps = 0.16$–0.55).

Given that the directionality of association between habituation and anxiety was not what was expected (hypotheses predicted *decreased* habituation would be associated with greater anxiety, but in instead, the opposite was found), validation analyses were conducted with other measures of anxiety that were available. A comparable significant association was found with the SCAS total ($\beta = 9.01$, $p < 0.01$), and this remained when

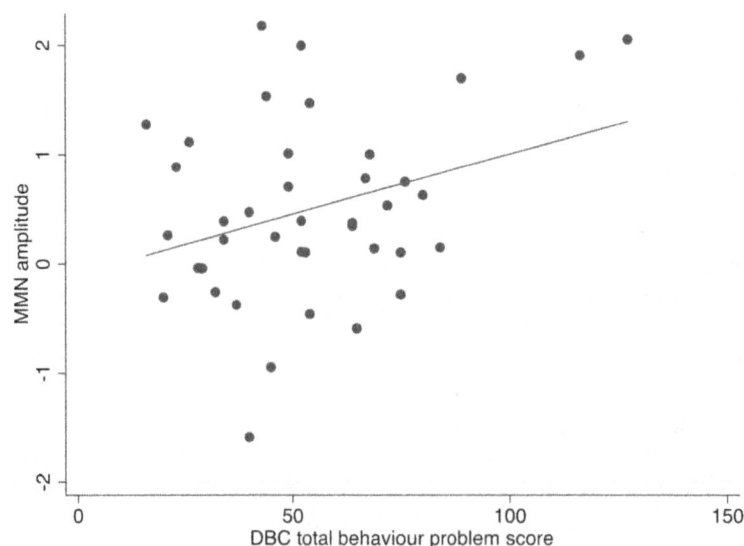

Fig. 2 Association between behaviour problems, rated by the Developmental Behavior Checklist, and MMN difference wave (response to deviant stimuli—response to standard stimuli)

adjusting for age, sex and IQ ($\beta = 10.64$, $p < 0.01$), and age, sex, IQ and ASD severity ($\beta = 10.71$, $p < 0.01$), and when excluding participants using medication ($\beta = 9.36$, $p < 0.01$), and excluding participants with epilepsy ($\beta = 9.12$, $p < 0.01$).

Response to S1, S2 and S3

To aid in the interpretation of the association between emotional problems and habituation, analyses next tested how SDQ emotional problems predicted response to S1, S2 and S3. There was a selective association with S1, in that higher levels of SDQ emotional problems were associated with greater S1 amplitude ($\beta = 2.09$, $p < 0.05$), but were not associated with the S2 ($p = 0.78$) or S3 ($p = 0.32$) (see Fig. 3). This association with S1 remained significant when controlling for age, sex and IQ ($\beta = 2.60$, $p < 0.05$), controlling for age, sex, IQ and ASD severity ($\beta = 2.65$, $p < 0.05$), and when excluding those using medication ($\beta = 2.06$, $p < 0.05$), and participants with epilepsy ($\beta = 1.87$, $p < 0.05$). The same selective association with S1 was found using the SCAS ($\beta = 17.53$, $p < 0.01$) and remained in all covariation and sensitivity analyses. Post estimation tests (controlling for age, sex, IQ and ASD severity) found the SDQ emotional problems—S1 association was not significantly different as compared against the SDQ emotional problems—S2 association ($p = 0.65$), but was at a trend level when compared against the SDQ emotional problems—S3 association ($p = 0.07$). The SCAS—S1 association was at a trend level when compared against the SCAS—S2 association ($p = 0.07$), and significantly different when compared against the SCAS—S3 association ($p = 0.03$).

Thus, although analyses began with a focus on habituation, results suggest that the habituation-anxiety association was likely driven by a selective association between anxiety symptoms and the first standard stimulus presented after the deviant stimulus.

Correlations between key ERP components and parent-rated sensory sensitivities

A trend positive correlation was found between MMN amplitude and the SEQ hyper-responsiveness + enhanced perception subscale ($r = 0.29$, $p = 0.07$). The correlation between MMN amplitude and the SEQ hypo-responsiveness + sensory seeking subscale was non-significant ($r = 0.25$, $p = 0.12$). No significant correlations were found between N2 response to S1 and either SEQ subscale.

Discussion

This study investigated whether alterations in neural indices of perceptual processing and discimination were associated with emotional and behavioural problems in young people with ASD. Results showed that increased sensitivity to deviant stimuli was associated with increased behaviour problems, whereas heightened response to standard stimuli following a deviant stimulus was associated with increased emotional problems, and this appeared to be mainly driven by anxiety symptoms.

The current finding of increased sensitivity to deviant stimuli, as measured by MMN amplitude, being associated with higher levels of challenging behaviours, as rated by the DBC total behaviour problem score, builds on prior work that has found comparable relationships in ASD populations using care-giver ratings of perceptual sensitivity [38–40]. In the current study, the association remained at a trend when adjusting for age, sex and IQ, and in sensitivity analyses excluding those taking psychotropic medication and those with a diagnosis of epilepsy. However, the association became non-significant when ASD severity was also accounted for, in addition to age, sex and IQ. Nevertheless, when ASD severity was added as a covariate, the standardised coefficients were not drastically changed, dropping from 9.51 to 8.77, and this change may be due to an increase in standard error with the inclusion of an additional covariate. Theoretically, the overlap between MMN amplitude and ASD severity is unsurprising given that sensory atypicalities are part of the diagnostic criteria for ASD, and MMN amplitude appeared to be tapping some form of sensory sensitivity, as shown by the trend correlation with the SEQ hyper-responsiveness + enhanced perception subscale. It is not possible to know from cross-sectional data, as was used as the current study, whether higher ASD severity leads to more atypical perceptual processing, or vice versa. It should also be noted that the few individuals with particularly high levels of reported behaviour problems (an established clinical characteristic of individuals with ASD; [7]) could have substantially contributed to the reported association between MMN amplitude and DBC behaviour problems (see Fig. 2). The present study is unable to disentangle whether the association between MMN amplitude and behaviour problems only applies to individuals with particularly high levels of behaviour problems (in a categorical manner) or is relevant to individuals with ASD with a range of behaviour problems (in a continuous manner). This requires further examination in a larger sample.

Additionally, results showed that the association with MMN amplitude was not driven by response to either the standard or the deviant in isolation, but the relative difference in neural response between the two (i.e., discrimination). Given that the MMN is correlated with individual discrimination ability [19–21], and is a relatively early component in the processing pathway, these results suggest that early, pre-attentive sensitivity to changes in perceptual input may be an important factor to consider in the aetiology of co-occurring psychopathology in individuals with ASD. Additionally, the MMN response appeared to be tapping perceptual processes that related to

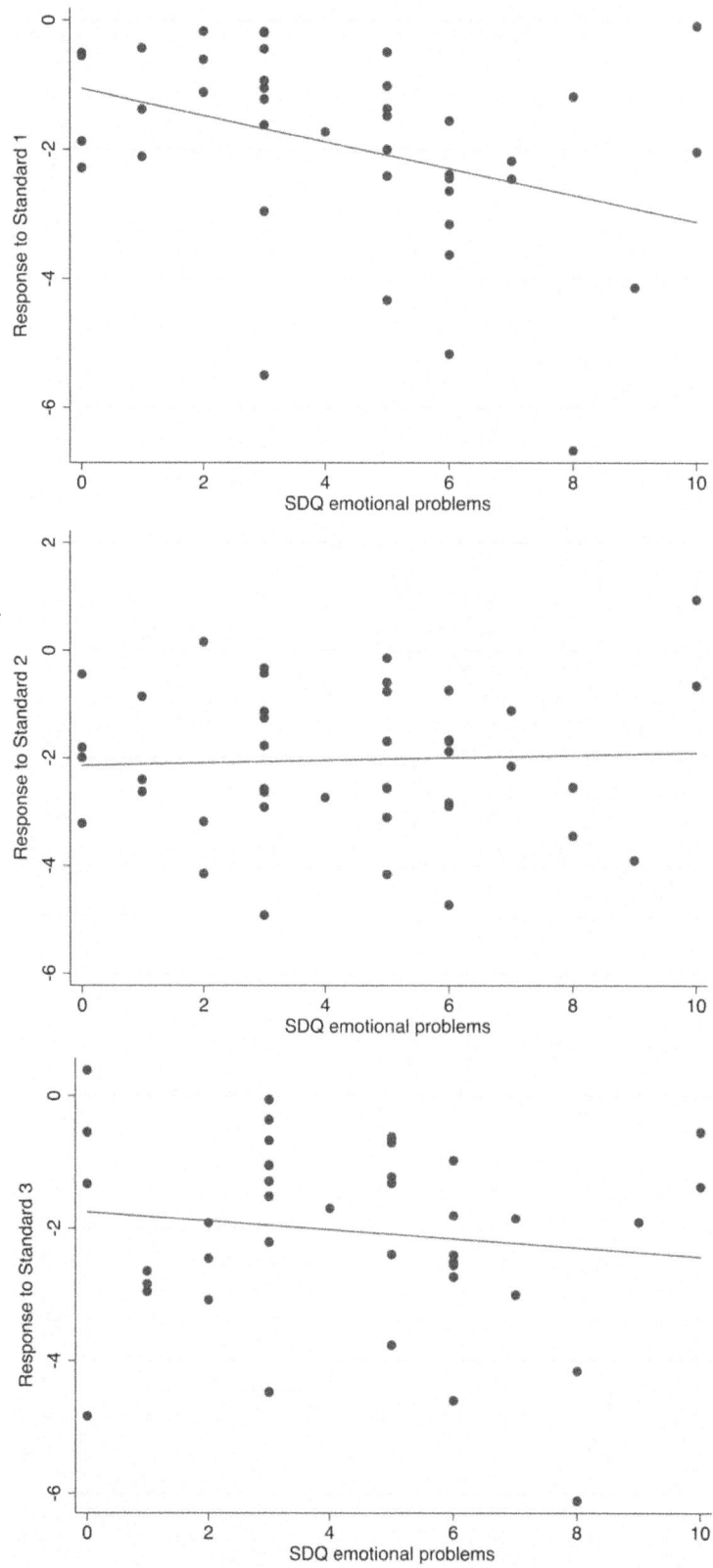

Fig. 3 Association between emotional problems, as rated by the Strengths and Difficulties Questionnaire, and N2 amplitude to the first (S1), second (S2) and third (S3) standard presented directly after a deviant stimulus

real-life sensory sensitivities, as shown by the association with the parent-rated SEQ subscale that indexed hyper-responsiveness and enhanced perception. Results are thus in line with clinical guidelines that recommend taking into account individual sensory sensitivities when designing interventions for use with young people with ASD [72]. However, it should be held in mind that the DBC is a broad-brushstroke measure and indexes a variety of types of challenging behaviours. From the association with the DBC total behaviour problem score, it cannot be determined exactly what type of behavioural problems hyper-sensitivity to perceptual input relates to, as prior literature has found associations to a variety of difficulties [39–41, 43, 44].

Although analyses began with showing that increased habituation was associated with increased emotional problems, this appeared to be driven by a selectively greater neural response to the first standard stimulus (S1) following a deviant stimulus. It should be stressed that these analyses were exploratory and require replication, as the results were not hypothesised a priori. However, a comparable association was found using multiple measures of anxiety, suggesting first that this was unlikely to be due to a type 1 error and second that the association with the SDQ emotional problems subscale was likely to be driven by items indexing anxiety. Current findings build on prior work, which has used questionnaire ratings to find associations between sensory over-responsivity and anxiety in individuals with ASD [15, 41–44]. Thus, although speculative, results are interpretable using the 'intolerance of uncertainty' framework [73], which has been conceptualised as a tendency to react negatively to uncertain situations and events [74]. Higher levels of parent and self-rated intolerance of uncertainty have been found in children and adolescents with ASD as compared to typically developing youth [73, 75, 76], and in both ASD and typically developing youth, greater intolerance of uncertainty are associated with higher levels of parent-rated anxiety, as measured by the SCAS [73]. In addition to the link between intolerance to uncertainty and anxiety, research has found that sensory sensitivity is related to both of these concepts [75, 77, 78]. Thus, in the current study when uncertainty was introduced (by the deviant stimuli), this may have led to a heightened state of arousal in participants who were rated as being more anxious. Conversely, biases in local perceptual processing may have led the incoming stimuli being perceived as more unpredictable, thus provoking heightened anxiety in participants with these perceptual biases. These interpretations are supported by existing literature, for example where temporally unpredictable auditory stimuli have been found to induce anxiety in mice and humans [47], and biases in perceptual processing (specifically in

hyper-sensitivity to local details) are associated with greater levels of compulsive-like behaviours (for example insistence on sameness) in children [79]. We propose the hyper-arousal induced by uncertainty was captured by the increased neural response to stimuli presented directly after the deviant (S1), but once it was recognised as one of the standard repeated stimuli, arousal decreased, thus explaining the lack of effect for S2 or S3. However, currently, the field remains unclear about directionality of pathways between sensory processing/sensitivities, intolerance of uncertainty and anxiety [75, 77]. The present data cannot make claims about the directionality of effects or indeed if a different, unacknowledged factor is driving the association between these concepts. It should be noted that the current study did not have a measure intolerance of uncertainty, and so, the link to this concept is speculative at present. Future work should use comprehensive measures of intolerance of uncertainty and follow a priori hypotheses, to better disentangle pathways between sensory sensitivity, intolerance of uncertainty and anxiety, in individuals with ASD.

Strengths and limitations

The first strength is the novelty of the approach taken. There is a limited body of research focused on understanding how variation in neurocognitive functioning may underpin variation in the behavioural phenotype of ASD, and despite the high prevalence of emotional and behavioural problems in individuals with ASD [1, 2, 4, 5], there is a paucity of ASD-specific models of psychopathology. Given the persistence of this psychopathology in youth with ASD [80], research is required to understand how to best predict and treat these co-occurring problems. Although previous work has looked at characteristics such as IQ, age, sex and ASD severity, few studies have looked specifically at domains of cognitive functioning. Focusing on carefully selected cognitive domains such as perceptual processing gives a deeper understanding of potential drivers of psychopathology beyond that of broad characteristics such as IQ and age and may offer clues as to the specific neurocognitive mechanisms at play. Additionally, the current study builds on prior work that has used parent-report of both cognitive functioning and behaviour, where shared method variance may have contributed to significant associations.

Another strength is the use of a community sample, where the target population was all individuals with a diagnosis with ASD in a specified geographical area (as opposed to using an opportunity sample of individuals with ASD who present to clinic with emotional and behavioural difficulties), thus making the sample more representative of ASD as a whole. Although the sample who completed EEG assessments had a higher IQ (as was expected) and lower scores on the SEQ hypo-responsiveness + sensory seeking subscale than the full sample, in all other key descriptive variables (ASD severity, age, co-occurring mental health problems), there were no significant differences (see Additional file 1). The sample also deliberately over-sampled females, meaning we had increased power to detect sex differences (unlike many other studies). Finally, the use of EEG meant that completing the paradigm did not require an overt response and thus allowed collection of data from a broader sample of participants (IQ range of 27–129). This approach is in line with recent commentaries calling for the inclusion of historically understudied populations within ASD [81].

In terms of limitations, the current study only measured one type of perceptual processing, and future research is needed to investigate if hyper-sensitivities in other modalities (e.g., proprioceptive, vestibular) are also associated with emotional and behaviour problems in individuals with ASD. Additionally, although the primary research aim was to test which neurocognitive domains are associated with psychopathology within individuals with ASD, the lack of control groups limits interpretation of results. Whether similar associations between cognition and behaviour are found in non-ASD samples, or if the current associations are specific to ASD, remains a question for future research. A further limitation of the current work is the use of a moderately sized sample, which could have led to limited power to detect associations of smaller effect. Current analyses also included multiple statistical tests, which should be held in mind when interpreting results, especially those that were not hypothesised a priori. Further work is required using larger sample sizes, to allow for more rigorous statistical testing and potential replication of the unpredicted results.

Implications

Current results suggest that alterations in sensory processing and discrimination could be considered as potential drivers of co-occurring emotional and behaviour problems in individuals with ASD (although this requires empirical testing using longitudinal studies, including studies starting at a younger age). Clinically, a comprehensive sensory assessment could be helpful when planning interventions with individuals with ASD and challenging behaviours and anxiety symptoms. Although surveys have found sensory-based interventions are commonly used in individuals with ASD [82], the specific targets of sensory interventions often differ, along with the methodologies used. Better characterisation of perceptual processing atypicalities in individuals with ASD would guide the development of more targeted interventions. The present results also suggest that a focus on intolerance of uncertainty may be helpful, especially as there is some preliminary evidence to suggest interventions targeting this concept may be efficacious in typically developing adolescents with anxiety disorders [83, 84].

Conclusions

The current study highlights how specific aspects of perceptual processing and discrimination are associated with the presence of additional emotional and behavioural problems in young people with ASD. Although the directionality of the pathway between cognition and behaviour cannot be assessed without longitudinal designs, the current work suggests alterations in perceptual processing and discrimination are important to consider when formulating a mechanistic understanding of additional psychopathology in people with ASD. This in turn will inform the design of novel, targeted interventions, and improve long-term outcomes for people with ASD.

Abbreviations

ADI: Autism Diagnostic Interview; ADOS: Autism Diagnostic Observation Schedule; ARI: Affective Reactivity Index; ASD: Autism spectrum disorder; DBC: Developmental Behavior Checklist; EEG: Electroencephalography; ERP: Event-related potential; ID: Intellectual disability; IQ: Intelligence quotient; MMN: Mismatch negativity; S1: First standard after the deviant tone; S2: Second standard after the deviant tone; S3: Third standard after the deviant tone; SCAS: Spence's Child Anxiety Scale; SDQ: Strengths and Difficulties Questionnaire; SEQ: Sensory Experiences Questionnaire (brief version); WASI: Wechsler Abbreviated Scale of Intelligence; WPPSI: Wechsler Preschool and Primary Scale of Intelligence

Acknowledgements

We thank Drs. Jacqueline Bold and Mark O'Leary for assistance with the QUEST follow-up study and all families who participated. We also thank Dr. Grace Baranek (USC) and the Sensory Experiences Laboratory team at UNC for the creation and use of the SEQ 3.0—brief version for 10–14-year-olds, and for on-going consultation regarding the measure, and Drs Elizabeth Shephard and Charlotte Tye for advice regarding EEG pre-processing and analysis.

Funding

The original QUEST sample was funded by Clothworkers' Foundation, brokered by Research Autism (R011217 Autism M10 2011/12). The IAMHealth research programme was funded by the National Institute for Health Research (NIHR) under its Programme Grants for Applied Research programme (RP-PG-1211-20016). This research was also in part funded by the NIHR Biomedical Research Centre at South London and Maudsley NHS Foundation Trust and King's College London. We also acknowledge support from the Guy's & St. Thomas' Charity (STR130505) and Maudsley Charity (grant reference 980). VCL was supported by a Medical Research Council (MRC) DTP Studentship. The views expressed in this presentation are those of the authors and not necessarily those of the NHS, the NIHR or the Department of Health.

Authors' contributions

VCL contributed to data collection, analysed and interpreted the data, and wrote the manuscript. PW, IY and SC contributed to study design, methods and data collection. ES, AP, TC and GB all oversaw the conception and design of the study, and ES and AP made substantial contributions to the analysis and interpretation of data. All authors were involved in drafting the manuscript, and read and approved the final manuscript.

Competing interests

AP receives royalties from the Social Communication Questionnaire. The other authors declare that they have no competing interests.

Author details

[1]Institute of Psychiatry, Psychology & Neuroscience, King's College London, 16 De Crespigny Park, London SE5 8AF, UK. [2]South London and Maudsley NHS Foundation Trust (SLaM), London, UK.

References

1. Lundström S, Reichenberg A, Melke J, Råstam M, Kerekes N, Lichtenstein P, Gillberg C, Anckarsäter H. Autism spectrum disorders and coexisting disorders in a nationwide Swedish twin study. J Child Psychol Psychiatry. 2014;56:702–10.
2. Gjevik E, Eldevik S, Fjæran-Granum T, Sponheim E. Kiddie-SADS reveals high rates of DSM-IV disorders in children and adolescents with autism spectrum disorders. J Autism Dev Disord. 2011;41:761–9.
3. Salazar F, Baird G, Chandler S, Tseng E, O'sullivan T, Howlin P, Pickles A, Simonoff E. Co-occurring emotional and behavioral disorders in preschool and elementary school-aged children with autism spectrum disorder. J Autism Dev Disord. 2015;45:2283–94.
4. Simonoff E, Pickles A, Charman T, Chandler S, Loucas T, Baird G. Psychiatric disorders in children with autism spectrum disorders: prevalence, comorbidity, and associated factors in a population-derived sample. J Am Acad Child Adolesc Psychiatry. 2008;47:921–9.
5. Leyfer OT, Folstein SE, Bacalman S, Davis NO, Dinh E, Morgan J, Tager-Flusberg H, Lainhart JE. Comorbid psychiatric disorders in children with autism: interview development and rates of disorders. J Autism Dev Disord. 2006;36:849–61.
6. Gadow KD, DeVincent CJ, Drabick DA. Oppositional defiant disorder as a clinical phenotype in children with autism spectrum disorder. J Autism Dev Disord. 2008;38:1302–10.
7. Brereton AV, Tonge BJ, Einfeld SL. Psychopathology in children and adolescents with autism compared to young people with intellectual disability. J Autism Dev Disord. 2006;36:863–70.
8. Farmer C, Aman M. Aggressive behavior in a sample of children with autism spectrum disorders. Res Autism Spectr Disord. 2011;5:317–23.
9. Frith U. Why we need cognitive explanations of autism. Q J Exp Psychol. 2012;65:2073–92.
10. Brunsdon VEA, Colvert E, Ames C, Garnett T, Gillan N, Hallett V, Lietz S, Woodhouse E, Bolton P, Happé F. Exploring the cognitive features in children with autism spectrum disorder, their co-twins, and typically developing children within a population-based sample. J Child Psychol Psychiatry. 2015;56:893–902.
11. Leekam SR, Nieto C, Libby SJ, Wing L, Gould J. Describing the sensory abnormalities of children and adults with autism. J Autism Dev Disord. 2007; 37:894–910.
12. Liss M, Saulnier C, Fein D, Kinsbourne M. Sensory and attention abnormalities in autistic spectrum disorders. Autism. 2006;10:155–72.
13. Crane L, Goddard L, Pring L. Sensory processing in adults with autism spectrum disorders. Autism. 2009;13:215–28.
14. Baranek GT, David FJ, Poe MD, Stone WL, Watson LR. Sensory Experiences Questionnaire: discriminating sensory features in young children with autism, developmental delays, and typical development. J Child Psychol Psychiatry. 2006;47:591–601.
15. Green D, Chandler S, Charman T, Simonoff E, Baird G. Brief report: DSM-5 sensory behaviours in children with and without an autism spectrum disorder. J Autism Dev Disord. 2016;46:3597–606.
16. Pellicano E, Burr D. When the world becomes 'too real': a Bayesian explanation of autistic perception. Trends Cog Sci. 2012;16:504–10.
17. Gomot M, Wicker B. A challenging, unpredictable world for people with autism spectrum disorder. Int J Psychophysiol. 2012;83:240–7.
18. Sinha P, Kjelgaard MM, Gandhi TK, Tsourides K, Cardinaux AL, Pantazis D, Diamond SP, Held RM. Autism as a disorder of prediction. Proc Natl Acad Sci U S A. 2014;111:15220–5.
19. Näätänen R, Alho K. Mismatch negativity - a unique measure of sensory processing in audition. Int J Neurosci. 1995;80:317–37.
20. Amenedo E, Escera C. The accuracy of sound duration representation in the human brain determines the accuracy of behavioural perception. Eur J Neurosci. 2000;12:2570–4.
21. Kujala T, Kallio J, Tervaniemi M, Näätänen R. The mismatch negativity as an index of temporal processing in audition. Clin Neurophysiol. 2001;112:1712–9.
22. O'Connor K. Auditory processing in autism spectrum disorder: a review. Neurosci Biobehav Rev. 2012;36:836–54.
23. Lepistö T, Kujala T, Vanhala R, Alku P, Huotilainen M, Näätänen R. The discrimination of and orienting to speech and non-speech sounds in children with autism. Brain Res. 2005;1066:147–57.
24. Lepistö T, Kajander M, Vanhala R, Alku P, Huotilainen M, Näätänen R, Kujala T. The perception of invariant speech features in children with autism. Biol Psychol. 2008;77:25–31.
25. Ferri R, Elia M, Agarwal N, Lanuzza B, Musumeci SA, Pennisi G. The mismatch negativity and the P3a components of the auditory event-related potentials in autistic low-functioning subjects. Clin Neurophysiol. 2003;114: 1671–80.
26. Gomot M, Belmonte MK, Bullmore ET, Bernard FA, Baron-Cohen S. Brain hyper-reactivity to auditory novel targets in children with high-functioning autism. Brain. 2008;131:2479–88.
27. Gomot M, Blanc R, Clery H, Roux S, Barthelemy C, Bruneau N. Candidate electrophysiological endophenotypes of hyper-reactivity to change in autism. J Autism Dev Disord. 2011;41:705–14.
28. Ludlow A, Mohr B, Whitmore A, Garagnani M, Pulvermüller F, Gutierrez R. Auditory processing and sensory behaviours in children with autism spectrum disorders as revealed by mismatch negativity. Brain Cogn. 2014; 86:55–63.
29. Vlaskamp C, Oranje B, Madsen GF, Møllegaard Jepsen JR, Durston S, Cantio C, Glenthøj B, Bilenberg N. Auditory processing in autism spectrum disorder: mismatch negativity deficits. Autism Res. 2017;10:1857–65.
30. Andersson S, Posserud M-B, Lundervold AJ. Early and late auditory event-related potentials in cognitively high functioning male adolescents with autism spectrum disorder. Res Autism Spectr Disord. 2013;7:815–23.
31. Donkers FCL, Schipul SE, Baranek GT, Cleary KM, Willoughby MT, Evans AM, Bulluck JC, Lovmo JE, Belger A. Attenuated auditory event-related potentials and associations with atypical sensory response patterns in children with autism. J Autism Dev Disord. 2015;45:506–23.
32. Jansson-Verkasalo E, Ceponiene R, Kielinen M, Suominen K, Jäntti V, Linna S-L, Moilanen I, Näätänen R. Deficient auditory processing in children with Asperger Syndrome, as indexed by event-related potentials. Neurosci Lett. 2003;338:197–200.
33. Dunn MA, Gomes H, Gravel J. Mismatch negativity in children with autism and typical development. J Autism Dev Disord. 2008;38:52–71.
34. Rankin CH, Abrams T, Barry RJ, Bhatnagar S, Clayton DF, Colombo J, Coppola G, Geyer MA, Glanzman DL, Marsland S, et al. Habituation revisited: an updated and revised description of the behavioral characteristics of habituation. Neurobiol Learn Mem. 2009;92:135–8.
35. Kleinhans NM, Johnson LC, Richards T, Mahurin R, Greenson J, Dawson G, Aylward E. Reduced neural habituation in the amygdala and social impairments in autism spectrum disorders. Am J Psychiatry. 2009;166: 467–75.

36. Swartz JR, Wiggins JL, Carrasco M, Lord C, Monk CS. Amygdala habituation and prefrontal functional connectivity in youth with autism spectrum disorders. J Am Acad Child Adolesc Psychiatry. 2013;52:84–93.

37. Guiraud JA, Kushnerenko E, Tomalski P, Davies K, Ribeiro H, Johnson MH. British Autism Study of Infant Siblings team: differential habituation to repeated sounds in infants at high risk for autism. Neuroreport. 2011;22: 845–9.

38. Baker AEZ, Lane A, Angley MT, Young RL. The relationship between sensory processing patterns and behavioural responsiveness in autistic disorder: a pilot study. J Autism Dev Disord. 2008;38:867–75.

39. Tseng M-H, Fu C-P, Cermak SA, Lu L, Shieh J-Y. Emotional and behavioral problems in preschool children with autism: relationship with sensory processing dysfunction. Res Autism Spectr Disord. 2011;5:1441–50.

40. Ashburner J, Ziviani J, Rodger S. Sensory processing and classroom emotional, behavioral, and educational outcomes in children with autism spectrum disorder. Am J Occup Ther. 2008;62:564–73.

41. Lane SJ, Reynolds S, Dumenci L. Sensory over-responsivity and anxiety in typically developing children and children with autism and attention deficit hyperactivity disorder: cause or coexistence? Am J Occup Ther. 2012;66: 595–603.

42. Lidstone J, Uljarević M, Sullivan J, Rodgers J, McConachie H, Freeston M, Le Couteur A, Prior M, Leekam S. Relations among restricted and repetitive behaviors, anxiety and sensory features in children with autism spectrum disorders. Res Autism Spectr Disord. 2014;8:82–92.

43. Mazurek MO, Vasa RA, Kalb LG, Kanne SM, Rosenberg D, Keefer A, Murray DS, Freedman B, Lowery LA. Anxiety, sensory over-responsivity, and gastrointestinal problems in children with autism spectrum disorders. J Abnorm Child Psychol. 2013;41:165–76.

44. Pfeiffer B, Kinnealey M, Reed C, Herzberg G. Sensory modulation and affective disorders in children and adolescents with Asperger's disorder. Am J Occup Ther. 2005;59:335–45.

45. Green SA, Ben-Sasson A, Soto TW, Carter AS. Anxiety and sensory over-responsivity in toddlers with autism spectrum disorders: bidirectional effects across time. J Autism Dev Disord. 2012;42:1112–9.

46. Hare TA, Tottenham N, Galvan A, Voss HU, Glover GH, Casey BJ. Biological substrates of emotional reactivity and regulation in adolescence during an emotional go-nogo task. Biol Psychiatry. 2008;63:927–34.

47. Herry C, Bach DR, Esposito F, Di Salle F, Perrig WJ, Scheffler K, Lüthi A, Seifritz E. Processing of temporal unpredictability in human and animal amygdala. J Neurosci. 2007;27:5958–66.

48. Lord C, Rutter M, PC DL, Risi S, Gotham K, Bishop SL, Luyster RJ, Guthrie W. The Autism Diagnostic Observation Schedule, second edition (ADOS-2). San Antonio: Pearson Assessments; 2012.

49. Rutter M, Couteur A, Lord C. Autism diagnostic interview-revised (ADI-R). Los Angeles: Western Psychological Services; 2003.

50. Risi S, Lord C, Gotham K, Corsello C, Chrysler C, Szatmari P, Cook EH, Leventhal BL, Pickles A. Combining information from multiple sources in the diagnosis of autism spectrum disorders. J Am Acad Child Adolesc Psychiatry. 2006;45:1094–103.

51. Stringaris A, Goodman R, Ferdinando S, Razdan V, Muhrer E, Leibenluft E, Brotman MA. The Affective Reactivity Index: a concise irritability scale for clinical and research settings. J Child Psychol Psychiatry. 2012;53:1109–17.

52. Mikita N, Hollocks MJ, Papadopoulos AS, Aslani A, Harrison S, Leibenluft E, Simonoff E, Stringaris A. Irritability in boys with autism spectrum disorders: an investigation of physiological reactivity. J Child Psychol Psychiatry. 2015; 56:1118–26.

53. Einfield SL, Tonge BJ. Manual for the Developmental Behaviour Checklist. Clayton, Melbourne: Monash University Centre for Developmental Psychiatry and Psychology; 1992.

54. Einfield SL, Tonge BJ. Manual for the Developmental Behaviour Checklist: primary carer version (DBC-P) & teacher version (DBC-T) (2nd. ed.). Clayton: Monash University Centre for Developmental Psychiatry and Psychology; 2002.

55. Nauta MH, Scholing A, Rapee RM, Abbott M, Spence SH, Waters A. A parent-report measure of children's anxiety: psychometric properties and comparison with child-report in a clinic and normal sample. Behav Res Ther. 2004;42:813–39.

56. Sofronoff K, Attwood T, Hinton S. A randomised controlled trial of a CBT intervention for anxiety in children with Asperger syndrome. J Child Psychol Psychiatry. 2005;46:1152–60.

57. Russell E, Sofronoff K. Anxiety and social worries in children with Asperger syndrome. Aust N Z J Psychiatry. 2005;39:633–8.

58. Zainal H, Magiati I, Tan JW-L, Sung M, Fung DSS, Howlin P. A preliminary investigation of the Spence Children's Anxiety Parent Scale as a screening tool for anxiety in young people with autism spectrum disorders. J Autism Dev Disord. 2014;44:1982–94.

59. Goodman R, Ford T, Simmons H, Gatward R, Meltzer H. Using the Strengths and Difficulties Questionnaire (SDQ) to screen for child psychiatric disorders in a community sample. Br J Psychiatry. 2000;177:534–9.

60. Emerson E. Use of the Strengths and Difficulties Questionnaire to assess the mental health needs of children and adolescents with intellectual disabilities. J Intellect Develop Disabil. 2005;30:14–23.

61. Chalfant AM, Rapee R, Carroll L. Treating anxiety disorders in children with high functioning autism spectrum disorders: a controlled trial. J Autism Dev Disord. 2007;37:1842–57.

62. Ausderau K, Sideris J, Furlong M, Little LM, Bulluck J, Baranek GT. National survey of sensory features in children with ASD: factor structure of the sensory experience questionnaire (3.0). J Autism Dev Disord. 2014;44:915–25.

63. Shumway S, Farmer C, Thurm A, Joseph L, Black D, Golden C. The ADOS calibrated severity score: relationship to phenotypic variables and stability over time. Autism Res. 2012;5:267–76.

64. Wechsler D. The Wechsler abbreviated scale of intelligence. San Antonio: The Psychological Corporation; 1999.

65. Wechsler D. Wechsler preschool and primary scale of intelligence—fourth edition. San Antonio: The Psychological Corporation; 2012.

66. Terman L, Maude M. Stanford–Binet intelligence scale: manual for the third revision form. Boston: Houghton Mifflin; 1960.

67. Jung TP, Makeig S, Humphries C, Lee TW, Mckeown MJ, Iragui V, Sejnowski TJ. Removing electroencephalographic artifacts by blind source separation. Psychophysiology. 2000;37:163–78.

68. Gomot M, Giard M-H, Roux S, Barthélémy C, Bruneau N. Maturation of frontal and temporal components of mismatch negativity (MMN) in children. Neuroreport. 2000;11:3109–12.

69. Banaschewski T, Brandeis D. Annotation: what electrical brain activity tells us about brain function that other techniques cannot tell us–a child psychiatric perspective. J Child Psychol Psychiatry. 2007;48:415–35.

70. StataCorp. Stata Statistical Software Release 14. College Station: Stata Press; 2015.

71. Tukey JW. Exploratory data analysis. Reading: Addison–Wesley; 1977.

72. National Institute for Health and Clinical Excellence. Autism spectrum disorder in under 19s: support and management [CG170]. London: NICE; 2013.

73. Boulter C, Freeston M, South M, Rodgers J. Intolerance of uncertainty as a framework for understanding anxiety in children and adolescents with autism spectrum disorders. J Autism Dev Disord. 2014;44:1391–402.

74. Buhr K, Dugas MJ. The intolerance of uncertainty scale: psychometric properties of the English version. Behav Res Ther. 2002;40:931–45.

75. Neil L, Olsson NC, Pellicano E. The relationship between intolerance of uncertainty, sensory sensitivities, and anxiety in autistic and typically developing children. J Autism Dev Disord. 2016;46:1962–73.

76. Chamberlain PD, Rodgers J, Crowley MJ, White SE, Freeston MH, South M. A potentiated startle study of uncertainty and contextual anxiety in adolescents diagnosed with autism spectrum disorder. Mol Autism. 2013;4:31.

77. Wigham S, Rodgers J, South M, McConachie H, Freeston M. The interplay between sensory processing abnormalities, intolerance of uncertainty, anxiety and restricted and repetitive behaviours in autism spectrum disorder. J Autism Dev Disord. 2015;45:943–52.

78. Black KR, Stevenson RA, Segers M, Ncube BL, Sun SZ, Philipp-Muller A, Bebko JM, Barense MD, Ferber S. Linking anxiety and insistence on sameness in autistic children: the role of sensory hypersensitivity. J Autism Dev Disord. 2017;47:2459–70.

79. Evans D, Elliott JM, Packard MG. Visual organization and perceptual closure are related to compulsive-like behaviour in typically developing children. Merrill Palmer Q. 2001;47:323–35.

80. Simonoff E, Jones CR, Baird G, Pickles A, Happé F, Charman T. The persistence and stability of psychiatric problems in adolescents with autism spectrum disorders. J Child Psychol Psychiatry. 2013;54:186–94.

81. Jack A, Pelphrey K. Annual research review: understudied populations within the autism spectrum – current trends and future directions in neuroimaging research. J Child Psychol Psychiatry. 2017;58:411–35.

82. Green VA, Pituch KA, Itchon J, Choi A, O'Reilly M, Sigafoos J. Internet survey of treatments used by parents of children with autism. Res Dev Disabil. 2006;27:70–84.

10

Role of *miR-146a* in neural stem cell differentiation and neural lineage determination: relevance for neurodevelopmental disorders

Lam Son Nguyen[1,2*], Julien Fregeac[1,2], Christine Bole-Feysot[1], Nicolas Cagnard[1], Anand Iyer[3], Jasper Anink[3], Eleonora Aronica[3], Olivier Alibeu[1], Patrick Nitschke[1] and Laurence Colleaux[1,2]

Abstract

Background: MicroRNAs (miRNAs) are small, non-coding RNAs that regulate gene expression at the post-transcriptional level. miRNAs have emerged as important modulators of brain development and neuronal function and are implicated in several neurological diseases. Previous studies found *miR-146a* upregulation is the most common miRNA deregulation event in neurodevelopmental disorders such as autism spectrum disorder (ASD), epilepsy, and intellectual disability (ID). Yet, how *miR-146a* upregulation affects the developing fetal brain remains unclear.

Methods: We analyzed the expression of *miR-146a* in the temporal lobe of ASD children using Taqman assay. To assess the role of *miR-146a* in early brain development, we generated and characterized stably induced H9 human neural stem cell (H9 hNSC) overexpressing *miR-146a* using various cell and molecular biology techniques.

Results: We first showed that *miR-146a* upregulation occurs early during childhood in the ASD brain. In H9 hNSC, *miR-146a* overexpression enhances neurite outgrowth and branching and favors differentiation into neuronal like cells. Expression analyses revealed that 10% of the transcriptome was deregulated and organized into two modules critical for cell cycle control and neuronal differentiation. Twenty known or predicted targets of *miR-146a* were significantly deregulated in the modules, acting as potential drivers. The two modules also display distinct transcription profiles during human brain development, affecting regions relevant for ASD including the neocortex, amygdala, and hippocampus. Cell type analyses indicate markers for pyramidal, and interneurons are highly enriched in the deregulated gene list. Up to 40% of known markers of newly defined neuronal lineages were deregulated, suggesting that *miR-146a* could participate also in the acquisition of neuronal identities.

Conclusion: Our results demonstrate the dynamic roles of *miR-146a* in early neuronal development and provide new insight into the molecular events that link *miR-146a* overexpression to impaired neurodevelopment. This, in turn, may yield new therapeutic targets and strategies.

Keywords: Autism spectrum disorders, microRNA, Human neural stem cell, Transcriptome

* Correspondence: lamson.nguyen@inserm.fr; lam-son.nguyen@inserm.fr
[1]INSERM UMR 1163, Laboratory of Molecular and pathophysiological bases of cognitive disorders, Imagine Institute, Necker-Enfants Malades Hospital, 24 Boulevard du Montparnasse, 75015 Paris, France
[2]Paris Descartes–Sorbonne Paris Cité University, 12 Rue de l'École de Médecine, 75006 Paris, France
Full list of author information is available at the end of the article

Background

Studies now indicate that epigenetic modifications play a role in neurodevelopmental disorders. The heritability rate of autism spectrum disorder (ASD) is over 50% with the remaining attributed to environmental/epigenetic factors [1]. MicroRNA (miRNA), one such factor, fine-tunes gene expression required for the development and function of cells and organs. Previously, our group and others implicated upregulation of *miR-146a* as the most common miRNA deregulation event in ASD [2, 3] and related neurodevelopmental disorders such as epilepsy [4] and intellectual disability (ID) [2]. In ASD, studies reported *miR-146a* upregulation in olfactory mucosal stem cells [2], skin fibroblasts [2], and a lymphoblastoid cell line [5] sampled from living patients and the frontal cortex of adult post-mortem brain samples [6]. In post mortem samples from ASD brains [7], *miR-146a* promoter correlates with an increased level of the active H3K27ac histone mark suggesting that the observed upregulation is due to transcriptional deregulation. In epilepsy, *miR-146a* is upregulated in astrocytes in region proximal to the lesions [4, 8]. Importantly, treatment with either an *anti-miR-146a* [9] or a *miR-146a* mimic [10] can ameliorate the latency, frequency, and duration of induced seizures in a rat model of temporal lobe epilepsy, emphasizing the causality and the reversibility of *miR-146a* effects. Understanding the functions of this miRNA in the brain may thus offer opportunities to develop treatments that are currently not available for neurodevelopmental disorders.

miR-146a is independently transcribed and processed and evolutionary conserved to lower vertebrates such as zebrafish and fruit fly. In the mouse brain, it is expressed ubiquitously during embryonic development [2]. In postnatal stages, its expression becomes restricted to neurons in regions important for higher cognitive and social functions including frontal cortex, amygdala, and hippocampus [2]. *miR-146a* is well known as a suppressor of inflammatory response by targeting *TRAF6* and *IRAK1* [11]. Its role in brain development is less well explored. In vitro data demonstrate that *miR-146a* regulates the homeostasis and function of brain cells in a developmental stage and cell type-specific manner. In primary mouse neural stem cell (NSC) cultured in EGF and FGF2, *miR-146a* overexpression promoted neuronal differentiation and cell cycle exit by targeting *Notch1* [12]. In mature primary mouse neurons, its overexpression altered dendritic arborization [2] and induced AMPA receptor endocytosis [13], while transfection with the *anti-miR-146a* reduced the frequency and amplitude of synaptic transmission [13]. In rat primary NSC cultured in N2 and bFGF, overexpression of *miR-146a* promoted astrocyte differentiation by inhibiting *Syt1* and *Nlgn1* expression [14]. In primary mouse astrocyte culture,

miR-146a overexpression hindered migration [12] and proliferation rate and increased glutamate uptake capacity [2].

Collectively, these studies suggest that *miR-146a* contributes to the maintenance and differentiation of NSC. Yet, how *miR-146a* controls the equilibrium among key genes that promote or inhibit entry into the neurogenic program in human NSC remains unclear. We also do not know how this extrapolates to human brain development. To address these issues, we combined expression analyses in human brain samples and in vitro studies on H9-derived human NSC (H9 hNSC) modified to overexpress *miR-146a*.

Methods

Patient information

Freshly frozen brain samples were acquired from the NIH Neurobiobank from donors with ASD diagnosis and normal controls. There was no difference in the distribution of sex, ethnicity, average age, nor post-mortem interval (PMI) between the ASD and the control groups (results not shown). The causes of death vary; more ASD donors died from accidents, and more control donors died from infection and heart failure (see Additional file 1: Table S1).

Whole exome sequencing technique and analysis

DNA was extracted from frozen brain samples using QIAamp DNA Mini Kit (51304, QIAGEN) with RNAse A treatment (19101, QIAGEN) following the manufacturer's instruction. WES libraries were prepared from 3 μg of genomic DNA sheared with a Covaris S2 Ultrasonicator. Exome capture was performed as recommended by the manufacturer with the 51 Mb SureSelect Human All Exon kit V5 (Agilent technologies). Sequencing of the WES libraries was carried on a pool of barcoded exome libraries on a HiSeq2500 (Illumina) using the HighOutput mode (48 WES libraries per FlowCell). 76+76 paired-end reads were generated. After demultiplexing, paired-end sequences were mapped on the human genome reference (NCBI build37/hg19 version) using BWA. The depth of coverage obtained for each sample was > 80× with > 90% of the exome covered at least by 15×. SNPs and indels calling were made using GATK tools. An in-house software (PolyWeb) was used to annotate and filter the variants. Variant filtering was performed as previously described. Following a published protocol [2], we performed whole exome sequencing (WES) to identify possible deleterious single nucleotide variants (SNVs) in known ASD genes (as collated in SFARI Database) and intellectual disability genes (Necker ID-Panel) in patients (see Additional file 1: Table S2). SNVs in two patients (5308 and 4721) are known single nucleotide polymorphism (SNPs) and unlikely to be pathogenic. We could not confidently establish a genetic cause for most patients, except one. Patient 1349 carried a heterozygous SNV leading to premature termination codon in *SEMA5A* (OMIM 209850), which could explain his phenotype.

Extraction and analysis of miRNAs

Approximately 50 mg of frozen brain samples were lysed in 600 µl of Lysis/Binding solution from the miRVana™ miRNA isolation kit (AM1560, ThermoFisher Scientific) using FastPrep Lysing Matrix D (116913500, MP Biomedicals) on a FastPrep®-24 Instrument (MP Biomedicals). The samples were spinned for 30 s at 13,000 RPM to reduce bubbles, after which extraction was performed according to the instruction of the manufacturer to obtain total RNA. The concentration was checked by NanoDrop 2000 (ThermoFisher Scientific). Expression profiles of *miR-146a* and 2 housekeeping miRNAs (*miR-106a* and *miR-17*) were assessed using Taqman assays on Fluidigm 98.98 array in technical quadruplicates. The qPCR analysis was carried out on the qPCR-HD-GPC core facility of the ENS and was supported by grants from Région Ile de France. The analysis was performed using mean of housekeeping miRNAs and average of all controls as references.

Human neural stem cell culture and differentiation

GIBCO® hNSC (H9 hESC-Derived) was purchased commercially (N7800100, ThermoFisher Scientific). Cells were cultured in flasks or plates previously coated for at least 1H with GelTrex™ LDEV-Free, hESC-qualified, reduced growth factor basement membrane matrix (A1413302, ThermoFisher Scientific). Cells were maintained in Complete StemPro® NSC SFM medium (growth media) consisting of KnockOut™ D-MEM/F-12 (12660012, ThermoFisher Scientific) supplemented with 2% StemPro® Neural Supplement (A1050901, ThermoFisher Scientific), 20 ng/mL EGF (PHG0315, ThermoFisher Scientific), 20 ng/mL bFGF (GF003, ThermoFisher Scientific), 2 mM GlutaMax™-I (35050038, ThermoFisher Scientific), and 10 µg/mL Penicillin-Streptomycin (15,140,122, ThermoFisher Scientific). For passaging, cells were washed once with DPBS (14190169, ThermoFisher Scientific) and detached from the surface by StemPro™ Accutase (A1110501, ThermoFisher Scientific), centrifuged at 1500 RPM for 5 min and replated in fresh growth media. To initiate spontaneous differentiation, H9 cells were plated at a density of 20,000 cells/cm^2 in growth media for 24 h, after which media was replaced with differentiating media (growth media without growth factors). Differentiating media was changed every 2–3 days during the course of the differentiation process.

Infection and selection of stably integrated H9 cells

The seed of the *miR-146a-5p* in the pLenti-III-miR-146a-GFP construct (mm10082, ABM) 5′-T(GAGAACTG)AATTCCATGGGTT-3′ was destroyed using the QuikChange site-directed mutagenesis kit (200515, Agilent) to produce to *miR-146a-Mut* construct 5′-T(_ATAGGAG)AATTCCATGGGTT-3′. Lentivirus were then produced from the construct by the Plateforme Vecterus Viraux et Transfert de Gènes from Hospital Necker as a paid service. Viral titer was determined by FACS of GFP signal. Virus infection was performed at the multiplicity of infection (MOI) of 5 in growth media, which was replaced after 24 h. Cells were grown in growth media for 72 h; Puromycin (11113802, ThermoFisher Scientific) at 1 µg/ml was then added to the media for 72 h to eliminate all cells without stable integration of the viral DNA containing the transgene and the Puromycin resistance gene. Cells were recovered in normal growth media until reaching confluence. All experiments were performed at the earliest passages possible.

Proliferation and apoptosis rate analysis

Cells were plated on coated 96-well plate (92096, TPP) in normal growth media. Twenty-four hours after, media was replaced with growth media containing 1/200 Annexin V Incucyte reagent (4641, Essen Bioscience). Cells were cultured inside the Incucyte® Live Cell Analysis System (Essen Bioscience), and images were taken at determined interval consecutively during several days using × 20 objective and at multiple spots per well. In post-analysis, a mask was designed using an inbuilt apoptosis analysis module to count the red apoptotic cells and the cell confluence percentage, which was used to normalize for cell numbers (see Additional file 2: Figure S2a). The same mask was applied to all time points and all repeats.

Differentiation analysis

Cells were plated on coated 24-well plate (92024, TPP) in normal growth media. Twenty-four hours after, growth media was replaced with differentiating media, which was refreshed every 2–3 days. Cells were cultured inside the IncuCyte® Live Cell Analysis System (Essen Bioscience), and images were taken every 3 h for 14 days using × 20 objective and at 25 different spots per well. In post analysis, a mask was designed using the inbuilt neurite analysis module to detect neurites and cell body. The same mask was applied to all time points and all repeats to record neurite extension over time.

FACS analysis

Cells were plated on coated T25 tissue flask (90025, TPP) in normal growth media. Twenty-four hours after, growth media was replaced with differentiating media, which was refreshed every 2–3 days. Cells were collected at 1 and 2 weeks into the differentiation process by scraping the surface of the vessels. Cells were then washed once with DPBS and incubated on ice for 30 min with the blue fluorescent reactive dye from the Live/dead fixable dead cell stain kit (L23105, Thermo-Fisher Scientific). Cells were washed once with DPBS and fixed in 1 ml of IC Fixation Buffer (FB001, Thermo-Fisher Scientific) for 5 min followed by 2 washes in IC Permeabilization Buffer (PB001, ThermoFisher Scientific) + 1% BSA. Cells were resuspended into 100 μl of IC Permeabilization Buffer + 1% BSA and primary antibodies at the desired concentrations for 1 h on ice. Cells were washed twice in IC Permeabilization Buffer + 1% BSA and incubated in the same media with the secondary antibodies at desired concentrations for 1 h on ice. Cells were washed twice with DPBS + 1% BSA and analyzed immediately on the BD FACS Aria II machine (BD Biosciences). Primary antibody list: polyclonal rabbit anti-NESTIN (N5413, Sigma), monoclonal mouse anti-TUB-III eFluor® 570 conjugated (41-4510, eBioscience), monoclonal mouse anti-GFAP eFluor® 660 (50-9892, eBioscience); secondary antibody list: donkey anti-rabbit Alexa Fluor 555 (A31572, ThermoFisher Scientific).

RNA sequencing technique and analysis

We tested cells from three independent experiments using three consecutive passages. Total RNA was extracted using TRizol reagent (15596026, ThermoFisher Scientific) and RNeasy Mini Kit (74104, QIAGEN) with DNase I treatment step (79254, QIAGEN) following the manufacturer's protocol. The integrity of RNA was determined by RNA ScreenTape (5067-5576, Agilent Technologies) on the Agilent 4200 TapeStation (Agilent Technologies). RNA-seq libraries were prepared starting from 600 ng of total RNA using the TruSeq Stranded mRNA LT Sample Prep Kit (Illumina) as recommended by the manufacturer. Half of the oriented cDNA produced from the poly-A+ fraction were PCR amplified (11 cycles). RNA-seq libraries were sequenced on an Illumina HiSeq2500 (Paired-End sequencing 130×130 bases, High Throughput Mode). A minimum of 10 million of paired-end reads was produced per library sample. Sequence reads were aligned to the human HG19 reference genome using the Burrows-Wheeler Alignment version 0.6.2.13. Raw and processed data for all samples are available for download from Gene Expression Omnibus (https://www.ncbi.nlm.nih.gov/geo/) under accession number GSE100670. RNA-Seq data were analyzed using a combination of three different tools namely limma [15], DESeq2 [16], and edgeR [17].

Quantitative reverse transcription PCR analysis (RT-qPCR)

To validate the RNA-Seq results, we selected 27 genes with relevant neuronal function or corresponding to known *miR-146a* targets and tested their expression by quantitative RT-PCR (RT-qPCR) on the Fluidigm 48.48 chip. As six of these genes were identified as DEGs in both conditions, this analysis included 33 comparisons. The qPCR analysis was performed at the qPCR-HD-GPC core facility of the ENS and was supported by grants from Région Ile de France. The analysis was performed using geometric mean of four housekeeping genes (*CYC1*, *GPBP1*, *RPL13A*, and *SDHA*) and average of the *miR-146a-Mut* repeats as references. No significant difference was detected for the 4 housekeeping genes. Lists of primers can be found in Additional file 1: Table S5.

In silico analyses

Known targets of *miR-146a* were extracted from miR-TarBase [18]. Predicted targets were extracted from miR-DIP [19]; only genes predicted by at least three different programs were considered. Target prediction of miR-146a-mut was performed using miRDB [20]. Pathway and function enrichment was analyzed using Ingenuity Pathway Analysis (QIAGEN). Protein-protein interaction map was extracted from STRING database [21] and further analyzed using Cytoscape V3.4.0 (http://www.cytoscape.org). Protein interaction enrichment was identified by ClusterOne Plugin downloaded from Cytoscape database. Analyses of expression in different brain regions throughout lifespan and brain cell type enrichment were performed using published code [22] in R program; please refer to the original publication for detailed description. Graphs and statistical analyses were generated by Partek Genomics Suite V6.0.

Dual luciferase assay

The 3′ untranslated region (UTR) of *DCX*, *GAD1*, and *PAK3* were subcloned into the psiCheck2 plasmid (Promega). Due to their size, the 3′UTR of *DCX* and *PAK3* were cloned into 2 (924 and 810 bp) and 3 parts (1106, 673, and 524 bp), respectively; each of these parts contains at least 3 predicted *miR-146a* binding sites. For luciferase assay, 2×10^5 HEK293T cells were plated in each well of a 6-well plate the day before transfection. Cells were transfected with the psiCheck2 3′UTR clones and the synthetic *miR-146a* (4464067, ThermoFisher Scientific) or *miR-mimic* for control (4464058, ThermoFisher Scientific) using JetPRIME® Polyplus Transfection Reagent (Ozyme) following the manufacturer's instruction. Assay were performed using the Dual-Luciferase® Reporter Assay System (Promega) 48 h after transfection. Ratio of Renilla to Firefly luciferase was taken as mean

Role of miR-146a in neural stem cell differentiation and neural lineage...

127

of technical triplicates. Three independent transfections were performed to confirm the results.

Results

miR-146a overexpression occurs early during human brain development

ASD, which is diagnosed before the age of 3, is associated with brain defects arising during early development, including enlarged brain volume (2–5%) that ameliorates in later stages [23] and disorganized cortical layers [24]. As a first step to understand how *miR-146a* overexpression may contribute to ASD, we asked whether it could be detected early during brain development. Using a Taqman assay, we analyzed the expression of *miR-146a* and two housekeeping miRNAs (*miR-106a* and *miR-17*) in the temporal lobe (Brodmann's Area 21) of ASD children (4–9 years old) (see the "Methods" section and Additional file 1: Tables S1, S2 for detailed sample description). We observed a 1.3-fold increase in *miR-146a* expression in the patient samples compared to controls (see Fig. 1a), demonstrating that *miR-146a* upregulation is observed during the early stages of ASD progression/emergence.

Generation and validation H9 hNSC lines overexpressing miR-146a

To elucidate the role of *miR-146a* in neural development, we used integrating viral approach to establish two H9 hNSC lines stably overexpressing a wild-type *miR-146a* gene or its mutant form, *miR-146a-Mut* (see Fig. 1b). Transgene expression was validated by either Taqman assay for *miR-146a* (see Fig. 1c) or measurement of the GFP transcript level by RT-qPCR for the *miR-146a-Mut cell* (see Fig. 1d). These lines were also validated using RNA-Seq, which showed a significant downregulation of known *miR-146a* target transcripts [18], including *ICAM1, FAS, IRAK2, CFH, CDKN1A, TLR4, L1CAM,* and *CARD10* (see Fig. 1e). Predicted targets of *miR-146a* were more frequently downregulated compared to those of *miR-146a-Mut* (20 vs. 5 targets with fold change > 1.5 and $P < 0.05$ in undifferentiated cells; $P < 0.01$ by Fisher's Exact Test), suggesting that off-target effect due to *miR-146a-Mut* overexpression was minimal. In addition, array comparative genomic hybridization analysis did not identify any copy number variation, indicating that the genomes of the newly established lines were stable (results not shown).

miR-146a promotes hNSC differentiation

We then assessed the effects of *miR-146a* overexpression using live cell imaging (see Additional file 2: Figure S1a). In normal growth conditions, overexpression of *miR-146a* had no effect on the proliferation rate or the apoptotic rate of the cells (see Additional file 2: Figures

S1b ,c). In contrast, upon induction of differentiation by withdrawal of EGF and bFGF growth factors, we observed a significant decrease in the proliferation rate (see Fig. 2a). The apoptotic rates of the *miR-146a* and *miR-146a-Mut* lines increased during cell differentiation, but there was no difference between them (see Fig. 2b). Importantly, over the 2-week course of differentiation, we observed increased dendritic branching (see Fig. 2c) and extension (see Fig. 2d) in the *miR-146a* line compared to control. Undifferentiated H9 hNSC co-express NESTIN, β-III-TUBULIN (TUB-III), and GFAP [25], which are markers for progenitor, differentiated neuron and astrocyte, respectively. As differentiation proceeded, some cells lost their NESTIN expression and increased TUB-III expression, while GFAP level remained unchanged (see Additional file 2: Figure S2a,b). We calculated the ratio of cells expressing high level/low level of TUB-III and the number of NESTIN positive/negative cells after differentiation. We found that *miR-146a* overexpression induces enhanced level of TUB-III and reduced levels of NESTIN (see Fig. 2e). Collectively, these results suggest that *miR-146a* overexpression favors differentiation of H9 hNSC into neurons in response to neurogenic cue.

miR-146a overexpression alters the balance between neural progenitor cell renewal and neuronal differentiation

miRNAs regulate multiple signaling pathways through their interaction with hundreds of different transcripts. To identify the mechanisms that could contribute to neural differentiation in *miR-146a* overexpressing hNSC, we performed expression analyses. Proteomic analysis is a valuable approach to identify changes in protein levels regulated by *miR-146a*, yet, it presents important limitations including limited access to low abundant proteins which expression is triggered during differentiation. Thus, we decided to perform RNA-Seq analyses in both undifferentiated and differentiated cells to identify differentially expressed genes (DEGs) and corresponding affected pathways that may mediate the effect of *miR-146a* overexpression on neural differentiation. Compared to *miR-146a-Mut* using a threshold of $P < 0.05$ and fold change > 1.5, we detected 1185 DEGs (10% of total detected transcripts, 54% downregulated, and 46% upregulated) in undifferentiated cells (see Fig. 3a and Additional file 1: Table S3) and 1039 DEGs (9% of total detected transcripts, 59% down, and 41% upregulated) in differentiated cells (see Fig. 3a and Additional file 1: Table S4). We obtained a 97% validation rate by RT-qPCR (32/33 genes validated, $R^2 = 0.978$; see the "Methods" section; see Fig. 3b and Additional file 1: Table S5). We further validated the downregulation of PAK3 in undifferentiated and differentiated H9 NSC,

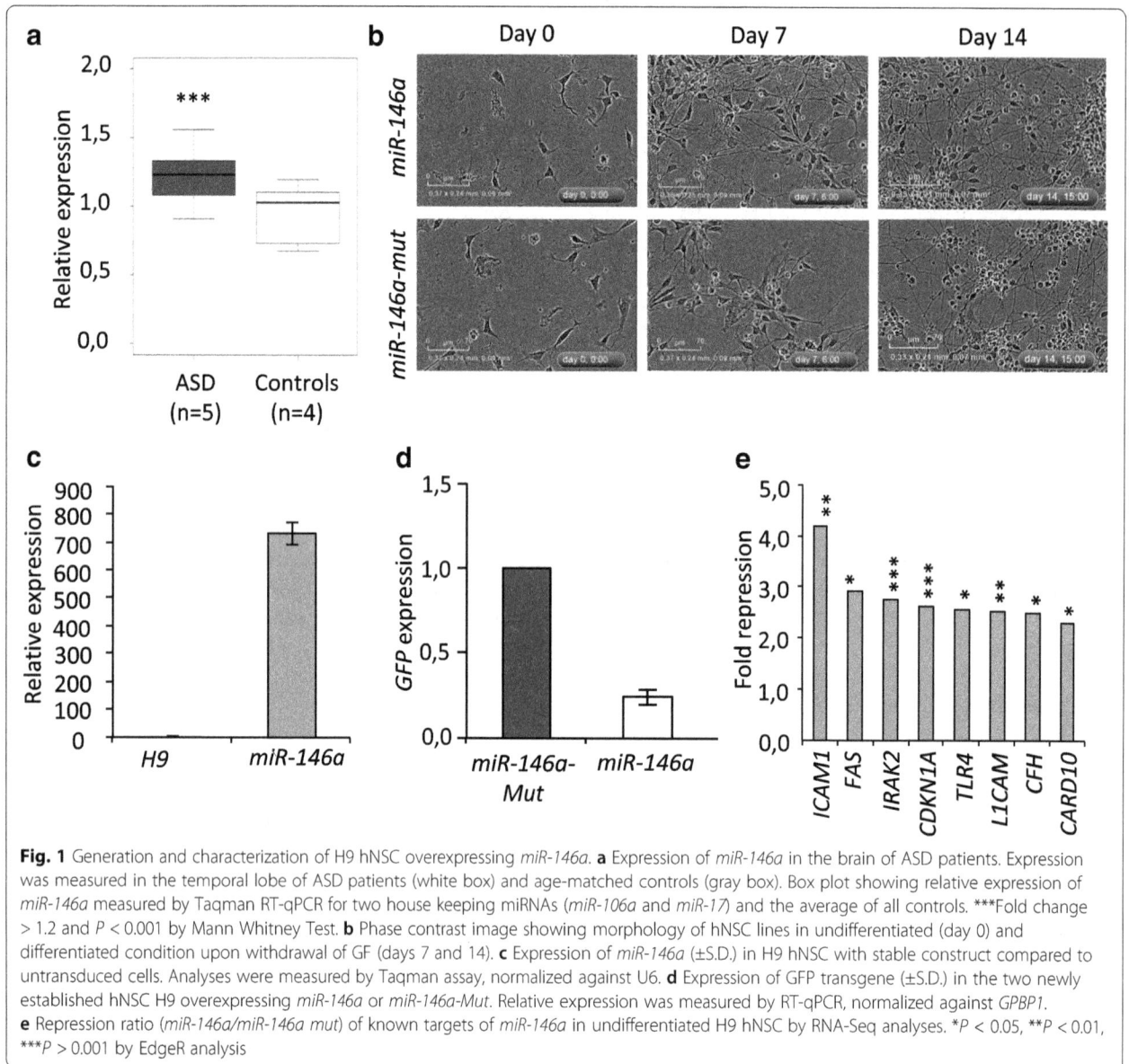

Fig. 1 Generation and characterization of H9 hNSC overexpressing *miR-146a*. **a** Expression of *miR-146a* in the brain of ASD patients. Expression was measured in the temporal lobe of ASD patients (white box) and age-matched controls (gray box). Box plot showing relative expression of *miR-146a* measured by Taqman RT-qPCR for two house keeping miRNAs (*miR-106a* and *miR-17*) and the average of all controls. ***Fold change > 1.2 and $P < 0.001$ by Mann Whitney Test. **b** Phase contrast image showing morphology of hNSC lines in undifferentiated (day 0) and differentiated condition upon withdrawal of GF (days 7 and 14). **c** Expression of *miR-146a* (±S.D.) in H9 hNSC with stable construct compared to untransduced cells. Analyses were measured by Taqman assay, normalized against U6. **d** Expression of GFP transgene (±S.D.) in the two newly established hNSC H9 overexpressing *miR-146a* or *miR-146a-Mut*. Relative expression was measured by RT-qPCR, normalized against *GPBP1*. **e** Repression ratio (*miR-146a/miR-146a mut*) of known targets of *miR-146a* in undifferentiated H9 hNSC by RNA-Seq analyses. *$P < 0.05$, **$P < 0.01$, ***$P > 0.001$ by EdgeR analysis

and the upregulation of NOTCH1 in differentiated cells by western blot (Additional file 2: Figure S3).

Next, we sought to identify the deregulated pathways. We first extracted high confident known and predicted interactions from STRING database [21]. In undifferentiated cells, pathway analyses suggested that DEGs affect very different classes of biological processes including axonal guidance, colorectal cancer, germ Cell-Sertoli Cell Junction Signaling (see Additional file 1: Table S6). Moreover, gene/protein interacting network was random and did not organize into functional modules (see Additional file 2: Figure S4). In contrast, analysis on data obtained from differentiated cells revealed enrichment for two networks (see Fig. 3c). Using Cytoscape with ClusterOne plugin, we found that the first network consisted of 155 genes comprising of four modules (see

Additional file 2: Figure S5 and Additional file 1: Table S7). Remarkably, all genes from this network except one are downregulated (154/155 DEGs, $P = 0$ by Fisher's Exact Test) and were enriched for cell cycle control pathways (Cell Cycle Module; see Fig. 3d and Additional file 1: Table S8). We further analyzed the remaining 884 genes by filtering out those encoding proteins with no or only one interaction (those in the outer edge). This created a second list of 350 genes with an equal distribution of up or downregulated DEGs (195 down, 153 upregulated, $P > 0.05$ by Fisher's Exact Test). Importantly, a significant enrichment for pathways related to neuronal differentiation was observed in this dataset (Neuronal Module; see Fig. 3c and Additional file 1: Table S9). To identify the drivers that could mobilize the observed interactions, we search for known and predicted *miR-146a*

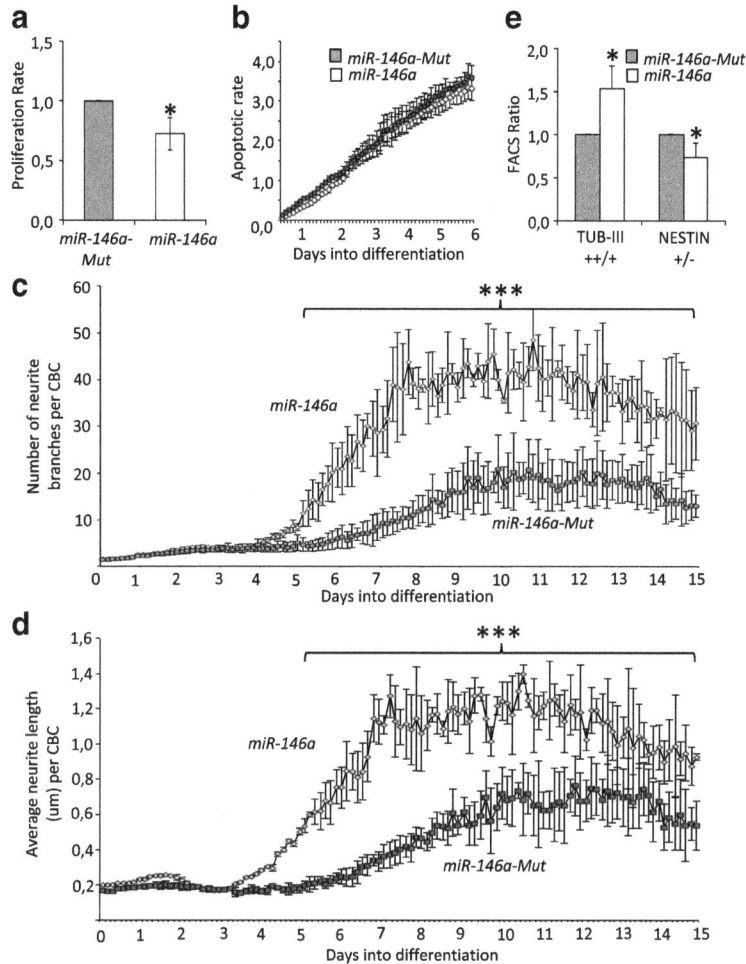

Fig. 2 *miR-146a* controls responses of H9 hNSC to neurogenic cues. **a** Cell proliferation rates measured using the Incucyte machine over 48 h after induction of differentiation. Graph shows the average ratio (±S.D.) of proliferation slopes from 3 independent experiments. *$P < 0.05$ by Student's 2-tail unpaired T test. **b** Apoptotic cell rates measured by the number of Annexin V labeled cells over the confluence percentage using the Incucyte machine. Graph shows average ratio (±S.D.) of four technical replicates and are representative of two independent repeats showing the same results. **c** Average number of neurite branching (±S.D.) and average neurite length **d** (±S.D.) in cells undergoing differentiation over 2 weeks. Analyses were performed using an analysis mask (see Additional file 2: Fig. S1a) on images taken at 25 different spots every 3 h over 15 days by the Incucyte machine. Results are representative of three independent repeats showing similar results. ***$P < 0.001$ by Student's 2-tailed unpaired T test. **e** FACS analysis was performed on differentiated cells labeled by TUB-III or NESTIN antibodies (see Additional file 2: Figure S2 for details). Graph shows average ratio (±S.D.) of three independent repeats. *$P < 0.05$ by Student's 2-tail unpaired T test

targets (as collated in miRTarBase [18] and using at least 3 different programs as collated by miRDiP [19]) that co-localized to this network (see Additional file 2: Figure S6). We chose to test the interaction between *miR-146a* and *PAK3*, *DCX* and *GAD1* by luciferase assays for their crucial roles in NSC differentiation and neuronal migration. This analysis revealed that *miR-146a* directly targets the 3′UTR of all three genes (see Fig. 3e). Taken together, our results suggested that *miR-146a* promotes cell cycle exit and neuronal differentiation by targeting 11 key cell cycle genes (*CHEK1*, *BRCA1*, *BRCA2*, *CCNA2*, *CDKN1A*, *CDKN3*, *TIMELESS*, *CDK1*, *CDCA5*, *E2F2* & *KIF18A*) and 9 neuronal genes (*DCX*, *PAK3*,

IRS1, *GAD1*, *SLC17A8*, *EPB41*, *MYBL1*, *IQGAP3* & *LIN28B*), 9 of which are validated targets while 11 are predicted targets of *miR-146a* (see Fig. 3f).

miR-146a overexpression affects specific regions in early human brain development

To identify the developmental stages and regions of the human brain potentially affected by the overexpression of *miR-146a*, we investigated the expression of the DEGs in a comprehensive dataset on the human brain transcriptome previously described [22, 26]. We found that expression of genes in the Cell Cycle Module is specifically restricted to early stages of fetal development in the

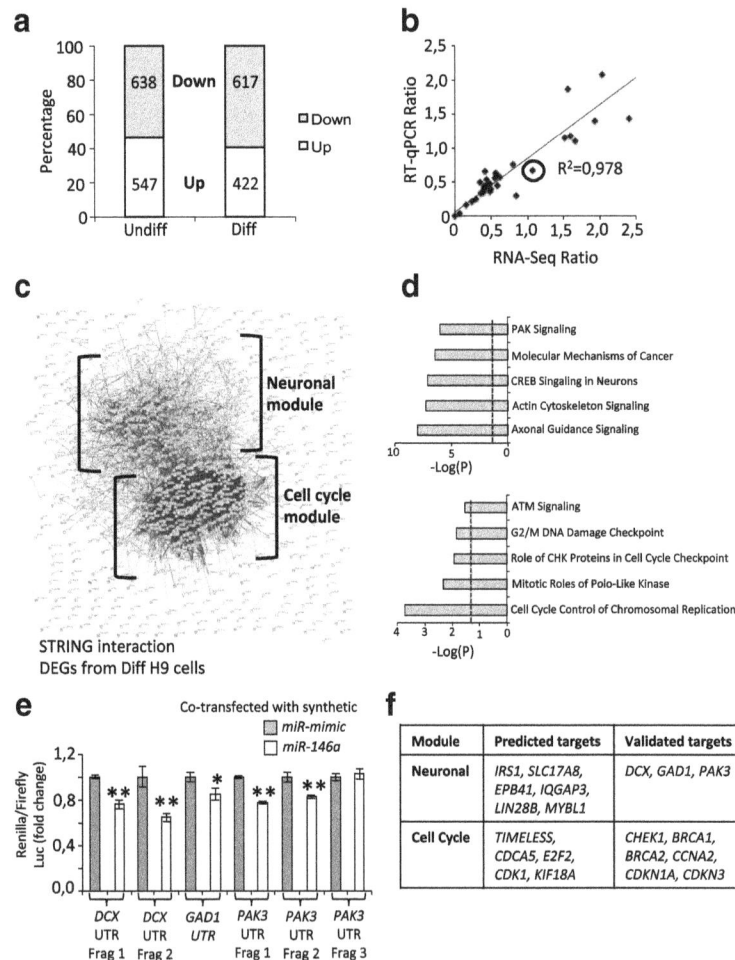

Fig. 3 *miR-146a* targets key genes to promote hNSC differentiation. **a** Distribution of DEGs identified by RNA-Seq in undifferentiated (Undiff) and differentiated (Diff) conditions. **b** Graph shows expression ratios of DEGs measured by RNA-Seq and RT-qPCR. Circle indicates only incompatible/non-validated DEGs. **c** Protein interaction network of all DEGs identified in differentiated cells mapped by STRING. Two modules are identified: Neuronal Module (top) contains 350 genes and Cell Cycle Module (bottom) contains 155 genes. **d** Top 5 pathways identified by Ingenuity Pathway Analysis of the 2 modules (see Additional file 1: Tables S8, S9 for extended lists). **e** *miR-146a* directly targets *DCX*, *GAD1*, and *PAK3* 3'UTR. Due to their size, the 3'UTR of *DCX* and *PAK3* were cloned into 2 and 3 fragments (frag), respectively. Each 3'UTR construct contains at least 3 predicted *miR-146a* binding sites. Ratio of Renilla/Firefly luciferase (±SD of 3 technical triplicates) was measured in cell lines co-transfected with either the synthetic *miR-mimic* (control) or the *miR-146a*. Graphs are representative of 3 independent assays showing the same results. *$P < 0.05$, **$P < 0.01$ by Student's 2 tailed paired t test. **f** List of known and predicted *miR-146a* targets that are downregulated in each respective module

hippocampus, amygdala, visual cortex, medial prefrontal cortex, and cerebellum (see Fig. 4a). By contrast, we observed a developmental gradient of expression of genes from the Neuronal Module that increases during fetal development in the hippocampus and amygdala, peaks at an early infancy stage in all regions of the brain and persists throughout the life. Cerebellar expression seems restricted to prenatal stages (see Fig. 4b). Notably, this Neuronal Module, but not Cell Cycle Module, is significantly enriched for ASD-associated genes ($P < 0.001$ by Fisher's Exact Test, see Additional file 1: Table S4).

To further explore the contribution of *miR-146a* upregulation on the transcriptome of ASD brain, we compared the DEGs identified in differentiated H9 hNSC to the published DEGs identified in ASD adult post-mortem brains (cortex, temporal lobe, and frontal cortex) [27]. We identified 42 overlapping genes that share the same trend of deregulation between the two studies (6.3% of published DEGs detectable in H9 hNSC) (see Additional file 1: Table S4). Half of these genes (20/42) belong to the Neuronal Module, whereas only two belong to the Cell Cycle Module. This analysis suggested that upregulation of *miR-146a* could be responsible for a portion of transcriptomic changes seen in ASD brains and that the use of H9 hNSC could provide relevant insights into both early processes of neural differentiation and later stages of neuronal development.

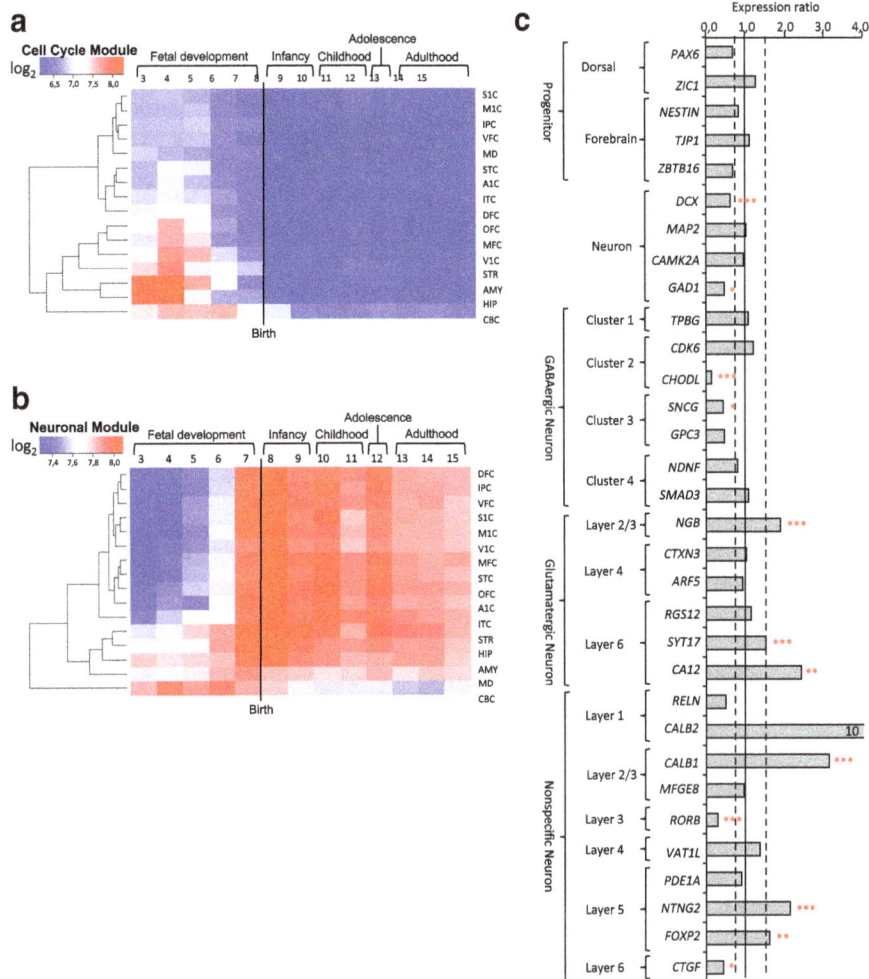

Fig. 4 *miR-146a* determines neuronal lineage identities. Heatmap of gradient of expression from the Cell Cycle (**a**) and Neuronal (**b**) Modules spanning human fetal development to late adulthood in distinct brain regions. A1C, auditory cortex; AMY, amygdala; CBC, cerebellar cortex; DFC, dorsolateral prefrontal cortex; HIP, hippocampus; IPC, posterior inferior parietal cortex; ITC, inferior temporal cortex; M1C, primary motor cortex; MD, mediodorsal nucleus of thalamus; MFC, medial prefrontal cortex; OFC, orbital prefrontal cortex; S1C, primary somatosensory cortex; STC, superior temporal cortex; STR, striatum; V1C, primary visual cortex; VFC, ventrolateral prefrontal cortex. Period labels: 3—Early fetal (10 ≤ Age ≤ 13 Post conception week, PCW); 4—Early midfetal (13 ≤ Age ≤ 16 PCW); 5—Early midfetal (16 ≤ Age ≤ 19 PCW); 6—Late midfetal (19 ≤ Age ≤ 24 PCW); 7—Late fetal (24 ≤ Age ≤ 38 PCW); 8—Neonatal and early infancy (Birth ≤ Age ≤ 6 Postnatal months, M); 9—Late infancy (6 ≤ Age ≤ 12 M); 10—Early childhood (1 ≤ Age ≤ 6 Postnatal years, Y); 11—Middle and late childhood (6 ≤ Age ≤ 12 Y); 12—Adolescence (12 ≤ Age ≤ 20 Y); 13—Young adulthood (20 ≤ Age ≤ 40 Y); 14—Middle adulthood (40 ≤ Age ≤ 60 Y); 15—Late adulthood (60 Y ≤ Age). **c** Expression difference of detectable neuronal specific markers in differentiated H9 hNSC. Dotted lines indicate expression difference threshold (fold change ≥ 1.5). *$P < 0.05$, **$P < 0.01$ and ***$P < 0.001$ by EdgeR analysis (as representative of 3 different RNA-Seq analyses)

miR-146a overexpression correlates with abnormal lineage-specific gene expression

The central nervous system contains many diverse neuronal subtypes that have been classified into 50 different groups based on single-cell gene expression profiles [28]. Since *miR-146a* overexpression alters hNSC differentiation, we asked whether it also affects neural cell fate programming and impacts neuronal specialization. Our RNA-seq data indicated that the Neuronal Module is enriched for genes expressed in pyramidal neurons and interneurons ($P < 0.05$; see Additional file 1: Table S10) [22], even though the Cell Cycle Module is broadly expressed

in all cell types (see Additional file 1: Table S10). When examining the expression of all 87 established cortical layer-specific, neuronal-specific, and progenitor-specific markers from published sources [24, 28, 29], we observed that 40% (13/32) of detectable markers for differentiated H9 cells were significantly deregulated in hNSC overexpressing *miR-146a* (see Fig. 4c). These markers were for GABAergic neurons (*CHODL*, *GAD1*, *SNCG*), glutamatergic neurons (*NGB*, *SYT17*, *CA12*), layers 2/3 (*CALB1*, *CALB2*), layer 4 (*RORB*), layers 5/6 (*NTNG2*, *FOXP2*, *CTGF*), and migrating neurons (*DCX*) (see Fig. 4c). These results strongly suggest that regulation of *miR-146a* expression level is important to correctly acquire neuronal lineage identities.

Discussion

In this study, we provided insight into the role of *miR-146a* in brain development and its relevance for neurodevelopmental disorders by combining the analyses of post-mortem human brain samples and in vitro models. We demonstrated that *miR-146a* overexpression in the brain of ASD patient is an early event detectable from childhood at an age when ASD are typically diagnosed (see Fig. 1a). Albeit the limited number of samples tested, this is the fifth time that this miRNA has been found upregulated in an independent cohort [2, 3, 5, 6]. In neural-relevant cell types, upregulation of *miR-146a* has been reported in adult cortex BA10 [6] and in adult olfactory mucosal stem cells (OMSC) [2]. These results collectively suggest that *miR-146a* upregulation is an event that occurs during embryogenesis and continues throughout development.

Our in vitro analyses on hNSC suggest that *miR-146a* contributes to the regulation of balancing cell-cycle exit/ cell-cycle re-entry of neural progenitors and committing to neural differentiation pathways. These results are in agreement with previously published studies. Indeed, overexpression of *miR-146a* has been shown to induce cell cycle arrest in normal [2] or malignant mouse astrocytes [12], in human non-small cell lung cancer cells [30] and in mouse NSC [12]. Increased *miR-146a* level also enhanced neuronal differentiation in mouse NSC through suppression of *Notch1* [12]. However, in our study, we found that NOTCH1 was upregulated in differentiated H9 NSC. This can be explained by two major differences: (i) unlike the mouse *Notch1*, the human *NOTCH1* gene is not predicted to be a target of *miR-146a*, and (ii) activation and not suppression of NOTCH1 is required for human NSC differentiation [31]. This emphasizes the relevance of using human H9 NSC to model early neuronal development of patients with ASD. In addition, we propose that *miR-146a* modulates the homeostasis of NSC by targeting directly and concurrently at least 20 different key neuronal and cell cycle genes, 9 of which are validated targets while 11 are predicted targets (see Fig. 3f). Thus, while inhibition of vesicular glutamate transporters (VGLUTs) promotes neuronal differentiation and migration of NPCs [32], we observed that *miR-146a* overexpression caused downregulation of the vesicular glutamate transporter gene *SLC17A8*. Similarly, RNA-Seq data revealed downregulation of the *LIN28B* gene; the RNA binding protein LIN28B plays essential functions in neuroblast proliferation by maintaining neural progenitors in an early state [33]. Lastly, *miR-146a* overexpression downregulates several CDK genes including *CDKN1A*, *CDKN3*, and *CDK1*, which encode for key proteins controlling the length of G_1 phase during cell-cycle and the balance between progenitor maintenance and generation of differentiated neurons [34].

Cortical cytoarchitecture relies on the spatiotemporal coordination of neuronal production rate, precursors cell-cycle control, and neuronal radial migration toward the cortical plate. Radial glial cells (RGC), the key progenitor cells in the developing CNS, divide asymmetrically to generate a new RGC as well as a post-mitotic neuron or an intermediate progenitor daughter cell. Neurons migrate toward the cortical plate along the fibers of RGC to reach their final position within the nascent neocortex and acquire their specific identity. Migration and final laminar positioning of neurons relies the fine-tuning of cell type- and layer-specific transcription factors [35]. Our results suggest that upregulation of *miR-146a* could disturb these transcriptional programs and may contribute to the disorganization of cortical layers [24] and the increase in number of neurons [36] and dendritic spine density [37] observed in ASD brains.

Data from RNA-Seq indicate that DEGs in H9 hNSC are significantly enriched for markers for pyramidal and interneurons, as well as markers for GABAergic (up regulated) and glutamatergic neurons (down regulated) (see Fig. 4c and Additional file 1: Table S10), suggesting that *miR-146a* may also contribute to the adequate distribution of these neurons. In mouse, artificially enhanced number of pyramidal neurons in the upper neocortical layers impaired neurite extension and laminar distribution of interneurons, ultimately leading to autism-like phenotype [38]. In human, Wegiel et al. examined post-mortem brains of 14 subjects with ASD and reported localized deficit of pyramidal neurons in the CA1 sector in 3 subjects and thickening of pyramidal layer in the CA1 sector in another [39]. The number of PVALB positive interneurons, a GABAergic subtype, was also found significantly reduced in prefrontal cortex BA46, BA47, and BA9 in 11 ASD cases [40]. As such, our results will direct future investigations into the role of *miR-146a* in the signaling cascade mediating the determination and acquisition of neuronal lineage identities.

Conclusion

The accurate generation of an appropriate number of different neuronal and glial subtypes is fundamental for normal brain functions. It requires tightly orchestrated, spatial, and temporal developmental programs to maintain the balance between neural progenitor cell proliferation and differentiation. While ASD is often considered as caused by synaptic dysfunction [41], several evidence from human neuropathology, systems biology, and developmental biology implicated dysregulation of the cell cycle and cortical lamination in the developing brain as a potential common pathophysiological mechanism underlying ASD [42–45]. Based on our results, we speculate that *miR-146a* plays a dynamic role to shape brain development from early neurogenesis to synaptic maturation and propose that *miR-146a* overexpression could provide a potential unifying explanation for brain dysfunctions observed in neurodevelopmental disorders.

Additional file

Additional file 1: Table S1. Detailed information of all patients and controls whose brain samples were used in this study. **Table S2.** Possibly deleterious variants in known ASD and ID genes. **Table S3.** DEGs identified in undifferentiated cells. **Table S4.** DEGs identified in differentiated cells. **Table S5.** Validation of RNA-Seq using RT-qPCR on Fluidigm array. **Table S6.** Top 20 cannonical pathways deregulated in undifferentiated cells. **Table S7.** Top 4 nodes enriched for protein-protein interaction as calculated by ClusterOne Plugin. **Table S8.** Top 20 cannonical pathways deregulated in the cell cycle modules of differentiated cells. **Table S9.** Top 20 cannonical pathways deregulated in the cell neuronal modules of differentiated cells. **Table S10.** Cell type enrichment analysis of DEGs from the Cell Cycle and Neuronal Modules. (XLSX 888 kb)

Additional file 2: Figure S1. Characteristics of undifferentiated H9 hNSC. **Figure S2.** FACS analyses of cell type specific markers NESTIN, GFAP and TUB-III in undifferentiated and differentiated conditions. **Figure S3.** Western blot validation of PAK3 and NOTCH1 expression in undifferentiated and differentiated H9 NSC. **Figure S4.** Protein interaction network of all DEGs in undifferentiated cells predicted by STRING. **Figure S5.** Top four interacting networks corresponding to the cell cycle module in differentiated cells. **Figure S6.** Co-localization of known and predicted targets of miR-146a in the protein interaction network of DEGs in differentiated cells. (PPTX 7099 kb)

Abbreviations
ASD: Autism spectrum disorder; CNS: Central nervous system; DEG: Differentially expressed gene; hNSC: Human neural stem cell; ID: Intellectual disability; miRNA: MicroRNA; MOI: Multiplicity of infection; OMSC: Adult olfactory mucosal stem cell; PMI: Post-mortem interval; RGC: Radial glial cell; RT-qPCR: Quantitative reverse transcription polymerase chain reaction; SNP: Single nucleotide polymorphism; SNV: Single nucleotide variant; TUB-III: β-III-TUBULIN; WES: Whole exome sequencing

Acknowledgements
Human tissues were obtained from University of Maryland Brain and Tissue Bank, which is a Brain and Tissue Repository of the NIH Neurobiobank. We would like to thank Bertrand Ducos, Juliette Pouch, and Elise Diaz for their help with the Fluidigm analysis. We would like to thank the core platforms of the Imagine Institute, notably the Cell Imagining Platform, the Gene Transfer Vector Platform for the virus production, the Cell Sorting Facility for their help with performing the FACS analyses and the Histology and Morphology Facility for their help with paraffin inclusion of brain samples and advice on analyses.

Funding
This work received a state subsidy managed by the National Research Agency under the "Investments for the Future" program bearing the reference ANR-10-IHU-01 and the "ANR-SAMENTA 2012" program. This work was also supported by the Fondation pour la Recherche Médicale (DEQ20160334938), the Fondation de France and the MSDAvenir Fund (Devo-Decode Project). LC is supported by the Centre National de la Recherche Scientifique. JF is supported by Crédit Agricole d'Ile-de-France Mécénat. We thank Life Science Editors for editing assistance.

Authors' contributions
LSN and LC designed and supervised the research. LSN performed all the experiments unless specified otherwise. JF cloned the miRNA expression constructs. CBF and OA performed the next generation sequencing experiments. NC and PN analyzed the next generation sequencing data. AI, JA, and EA helped analyze the human tissue biopsies. LSN and LC wrote the manuscript. All the authors reviewed the manuscript and approved the final manuscript.

Competing interests
The authors declare no competing interests.

Author details
[1]INSERM UMR 1163, Laboratory of Molecular and pathophysiological bases of cognitive disorders, Imagine Institute, Necker-Enfants Malades Hospital, 24 Boulevard du Montparnasse, 75015 Paris, France. [2]Paris Descartes–Sorbonne Paris Cité University, 12 Rue de l'École de Médecine, 75006 Paris, France. [3]Department of (Neuro) Pathology, Academic Medical Center, University of Amsterdam, 1105 AZ Amsterdam, The Netherlands.

References
1. Sandin S, Lichtenstein P, Kuja-Halkola R, Larsson H, Hultman CM, Reichenberg A. The familial risk of autism. JAMA. 2014;311:1770–7.
2. Nguyen LS, Lepleux M, Makhlouf M, Martin C, Fregeac J, Siquier-Pernet K, Philippe A, Feron F, Gepner B, Rougeulle C, et al. Profiling olfactory stem cells from living patients identifies miRNAs relevant for autism pathophysiology. Mol Autism. 2016; https://doi.org/10.1186/s13229-015-0064-6.
3. Fregeac J, Colleaux L, Nguyen LS. The emerging roles of MicroRNAs in autism spectrum disorders. Neurosci Biobehav Rev. 2016;71:729–38.
4. Iyer A, Zurolo E, Prabowo A, Fluiter K, Spliet WG, van Rijen PC, Gorter JA, Aronica E. MicroRNA-146a: a key regulator of astrocyte-mediated inflammatory response. PLoS One. 2012;7:e44789.
5. Talebizadeh Z, Butler MG, Theodoro MF. Feasibility and relevance of examining lymphoblastoid cell lines to study role of microRNAs in autism. Autism Res. 2008;1:240–50.
6. Mor M, Nardone S, Sams DS, Elliott E. Hypomethylation of miR-142 promoter and upregulation of microRNAs that target the oxytocin receptor gene in the autism prefrontal cortex. Mol Autism. 2015;6:46.
7. Sun W, Poschmann J, Cruz-Herrera Del Rosario R, Parikshak NN, Hajan HS, Kumar V, Ramasamy R, Belgard TG, Elanggovan B, Wong CC, et al. Histone Acetylome-wide Association Study of Autism Spectrum Disorder. Cell. 2016; 167:1385–97. e1311
8. Aronica E, Fluiter K, Iyer A, Zurolo E, Vreijling J, van Vliet EA, Baayen JC, Gorter JA. Expression pattern of miR-146a, an inflammation-associated microRNA, in experimental and human temporal lobe epilepsy. Eur J Neurosci. 2010;31:1100–7.
9. He F, Liu B, Meng Q, Sun Y, Wang W, Wang C. Modulation of miR-146a/complement factor H mediated inflammatory responses in a rat model of temporal lobe epilepsy. Biosci Rep. 2016;36(6):e00433.
10. Tao H, Zhao J, Liu T, Cai Y, Zhou X, Xing H, Wang Y, Yin M, Zhong W, Liu Z, et al. Intranasal delivery of miR-146a mimics delayed seizure onset in the lithium-pilocarpine mouse model. Mediat Inflamm. 2017;2017:6512620.
11. Taganov KD, Boldin MP, Chang KJ, Baltimore D. NF-kappaB-dependent induction of microRNA miR-146, an inhibitor targeted to signaling proteins of innate immune responses. Proc Natl Acad Sci U S A. 2006;103:12481–6.
12. Mei J, Bachoo R, Zhang CL. MicroRNA-146a inhibits glioma development by targeting Notch1. Mol Cell Biol. 2011;31:3584–92.
13. Chen YL, Shen CK. Modulation of mGluR-dependent MAP1B translation and AMPA receptor endocytosis by microRNA miR-146a-5p. J Neurosci. 2013;33: 9013–20.
14. Jovicic A, Roshan R, Moisoi N, Pradervand S, Moser R, Pillai B, Luthi-Carter R. Comprehensive expression analyses of neural cell-type-specific miRNAs identify new determinants of the specification and maintenance of neuronal phenotypes. J Neurosci. 2013;33:5127–37.

15. Ritchie ME, Phipson B, Wu D, Hu Y, Law CW, Shi W, Smyth GK. Limma powers differential expression analyses for RNA-sequencing and microarray studies. Nucleic Acids Res. 2015;43:e47.

16. Love MI, Huber W, Anders S. Moderated estimation of fold change and dispersion for RNA-seq data with DESeq2. Genome Biol. 2014;15:550.

17. Robinson MD, McCarthy DJ, Smyth GK. edgeR: a Bioconductor package for differential expression analysis of digital gene expression data. Bioinformatics. 2010;26:139–40.

18. Chou CH, Chang NW, Shrestha S, Hsu SD, Lin YL, Lee WH, Yang CD, Hong HC, Wei TY, Tu SJ, et al. miRTarBase 2016: updates to the experimentally validated miRNA-target interactions database. Nucleic Acids Res. 2016;44:D239–47.

19. Shirdel EA, Xie W, Mak TW, Jurisica I. NAViGaTing the micronome–using multiple microRNA prediction databases to identify signalling pathway-associated microRNAs. PLoS One. 2011;6:e17429.

20. Wong N, Wang X. miRDB: an online resource for microRNA target prediction and functional annotations. Nucleic Acids Res. 2015;43:D146–52.

21. Szklarczyk D, Morris JH, Cook H, Kuhn M, Wyder S, Simonovic M, Santos A, Doncheva NT, Roth A, Bork P, et al. The STRING database in 2017: quality-controlled protein-protein association networks, made broadly accessible. Nucleic Acids Res. 2017;45:D362–8.

22. Johnson MR, Shkura K, Langley SR, Delahaye-Duriez A, Srivastava P, Hill WD, Rackham OJ, Davies G, Harris SE, Moreno-Moral A, et al. Systems genetics identifies a convergent gene network for cognition and neurodevelopmental disease. Nat Neurosci. 2016;19:223–32.

23. Amaral DG, Schumann CM, Nordahl CW. Neuroanatomy of autism. Trends Neurosci. 2008;31:137–45.

24. Stoner R, Chow ML, Boyle MP, Sunkin SM, Mouton PR, Roy S, Wynshaw-Boris A, Colamarino SA, Lein ES, Courchesne E. Patches of disorganization in the neocortex of children with autism. N Engl J Med. 2014;370:1209–19.

25. Koch P, Opitz T, Steinbeck JA, Ladewig J, Brustle O. A rosette-type, self-renewing human ES cell-derived neural stem cell with potential for in vitro instruction and synaptic integration. Proc Natl Acad Sci U S A. 2009;106:3225–30.

26. Kang HJ, Kawasawa YI, Cheng F, Zhu Y, Xu X, Li M, Sousa AM, Pletikos M, Meyer KA, Sedmak G, et al. Spatio-temporal transcriptome of the human brain. Nature. 2011;478:483–9.

27. Voineagu I, Wang X, Johnston P, Lowe JK, Tian Y, Horvath S, Mill J, Cantor RM, Blencowe BJ, Geschwind DH. Transcriptomic analysis of autistic brain reveals convergent molecular pathology. Nature. 2011;474:380–4.

28. Tasic B, Menon V, Nguyen TN, Kim TK, Jarsky T, Yao Z, Levi B, Gray LT, Sorensen SA, Dolbeare T, et al. Adult mouse cortical cell taxonomy revealed by single cell transcriptomics. Nat Neurosci. 2016;19:335–46.

29. Pasca SP, Portmann T, Voineagu I, Yazawa M, Shcheglovitov A, Pasca AM, Cord B, Palmer TD, Chikahisa S, Nishino S, et al. Using iPSC-derived neurons to uncover cellular phenotypes associated with Timothy syndrome. Nat Med. 2011;17:1657–62.

30. Li YL, Wang J, Zhang CY, Shen YQ, Wang HM, Ding L, Gu YC, Lou JT, Zhao XT, Ma ZL, Jin YX. MiR-146a-5p inhibits cell proliferation and cell cycle progression in NSCLC cell lines by targeting CCND1 and CCND2. Oncotarget. 2016;7:59287–98.

31. Lowell S, Benchoua A, Heavey B, Smith AG. Notch promotes neural lineage entry by pluripotent embryonic stem cells. PLoS Biol. 2006;4:e121.

32. Sanchez-Mendoza EH, Bellver-Landete V, Arce C, Doeppner TR, Hermann DM, Oset-Gasque MJ. Vesicular glutamate transporters play a role in neuronal differentiation of cultured SVZ-derived neural precursor cells. PLoS One. 2017;12:e0177069.

33. Hennchen M, Stubbusch J, Abarchan-El Makhfi I, Kramer M, Deller T, Pierre-Eugene C, Janoueix-Lerosey I, Delattre O, Ernsberger U, Schulte JB, Rohrer H.

Lin28B and Let-7 in the control of sympathetic neurogenesis and neuroblastoma development. J Neurosci. 2015;35:16531–44.

34. Hindley C, Philpott A. Co-ordination of cell cycle and differentiation in the developing nervous system. Biochem J. 2012;444:375–82.

35. Kwan KY, Sestan N, Anton ES. Transcriptional co-regulation of neuronal migration and laminar identity in the neocortex. Development. 2012;139:1535–46.

36. Courchesne E, Mouton PR, Calhoun ME, Semendeferi K, Ahrens-Barbeau C, Hallet MJ, Barnes CC, Pierce K. Neuron number and size in prefrontal cortex of children with autism. JAMA. 2011;306:2001–10.

37. Hutsler JJ, Zhang H. Increased dendritic spine densities on cortical projection neurons in autism spectrum disorders. Brain Res. 2010;1309:83–94.

38. Fang WQ, Chen WW, Jiang L, Liu K, Yung WH, Fu AK, Ip NY. Overproduction of upper-layer neurons in the neocortex leads to autism-like features in mice. Cell Rep. 2014;9:1635–43.

39. Wegiel J, Kuchna I, Nowicki K, Imaki H, Wegiel J, Marchi E, Ma SY, Chauhan A, Chauhan V, Bobrowicz TW, et al. The neuropathology of autism: defects of neurogenesis and neuronal migration, and dysplastic changes. Acta Neuropathol. 2010;119:755–70.

40. Hashemi E, Ariza J, Rogers H, Noctor SC, Martinez-Cerdeno V. The number of parvalbumin-expressing interneurons is decreased in the medial prefrontal cortex in autism. Cereb Cortex. 2017;27:1931–43.

41. Zoghbi HY, Bear MF. Synaptic dysfunction in neurodevelopmental disorders associated with autism and intellectual disabilities. Cold Spring Harb Perspect Biol. 2012;4. https://doi.org/10.1101/cshperspect.a009886.

42. Courchesne E, Pierce K, Schumann CM, Redcay E, Buckwalter JA, Kennedy DP, Morgan J. Mapping early brain development in autism. Neuron. 2007;56:399–413.

43. Vaccarino FM, Smith KM. Increased brain size in autism—what it will take to solve a mystery. Biol Psychiatry. 2009;66:313–5.

44. Casanova EL, Casanova MF. Genetics studies indicate that neural induction and early neuronal maturation are disturbed in autism. Front Cell Neurosci. 2014;8:397.

45. Casanova MF. Autism as a sequence: from heterochronic germinal cell divisions to abnormalities of cell migration and cortical dysplasias. Med Hypotheses. 2014;83:32–8.

11

Objective measurement of head movement differences in children with and without autism spectrum disorder

Katherine B. Martin[1][*], Zakia Hammal[2], Gang Ren[3], Jeffrey F. Cohn[4], Justine Cassell[5], Mitsunori Ogihara[6], Jennifer C. Britton[1], Anibal Gutierrez[1] and Daniel S. Messinger[1]

Abstract

Background: Deficits in motor movement in children with autism spectrum disorder (ASD) have typically been characterized qualitatively by human observers. Although clinicians have noted the importance of atypical head positioning (e.g. social peering and repetitive head banging) when diagnosing children with ASD, a quantitative understanding of head movement in ASD is lacking. Here, we conduct a quantitative comparison of head movement dynamics in children with and without ASD using automated, person-independent computer-vision based head tracking (Zface). Because children with ASD often exhibit preferential attention to nonsocial versus social stimuli, we investigated whether children with and without ASD differed in their head movement dynamics depending on stimulus sociality.

Methods: The current study examined differences in head movement dynamics in children with ($n = 21$) and without ASD ($n = 21$). Children were video-recorded while watching a 16-min video of social and nonsocial stimuli. Three dimensions of rigid head movement—pitch (head nods), yaw (head turns), and roll (lateral head inclinations)—were tracked using Zface. The root mean square of pitch, yaw, and roll was calculated to index the magnitude of head angular displacement (quantity of head movement) and angular velocity (speed).

Results: Compared with children without ASD, children with ASD exhibited greater yaw displacement, indicating greater head turning, and greater velocity of yaw and roll, indicating faster head turning and inclination. Follow-up analyses indicated that differences in head movement dynamics were specific to the social rather than the nonsocial stimulus condition.

Conclusions: Head movement dynamics (displacement and velocity) were greater in children with ASD than in children without ASD, providing a quantitative foundation for previous clinical reports. Head movement differences were evident in lateral (yaw and roll) but not vertical (pitch) movement and were specific to a social rather than nonsocial condition. When presented with social stimuli, children with ASD had higher levels of head movement and moved their heads more quickly than children without ASD. Children with ASD may use head movement to modulate their perception of social scenes.

Keywords: Head movement, Motor movement, Autism spectrum disorder, Social processing

* Correspondence: kmartin@psy.miami.edu
[1]Department of Psychology, University of Miami, 5665 Ponce de Leon Blvd, Coral Gables, FL 33146, USA
Full list of author information is available at the end of the article

Background

Autism spectrum disorder (ASD) is characterized by persistent impairments in social interaction and communication, as well as repetitive and stereotyped behaviors [1]. Previous research has identified deficits in motor development [2] and higher levels of motor stereotypies in children with ASD than children without ASD [3]. Atypical movement patterns, such as abnormalities in eye contact and body posture, and motor stereotypies are used in the evaluation of ASD, but little attention has focused on characterizing these motor differences through automated, objective measurement [1, 3, 4]. The current study examined whether head movement dynamics differentiated children with and without ASD, and contrasted head movement while watching video of nonsocial and social stimuli.

While movement stereotypies are common in typically developing infants, they decrease rapidly over the first 2 years of life [3]. Atypical head movements in young children have garnered little attention, even though this stereotypy is clinically viewed as highly suggestive of ASD [3, 5, 6]. Descriptively, clinicians have noted that children with ASD exhibit atypical head movements as they stare at their fingers or objects closely from a "strange angle" [3], repetitively peer at objects "from the side" [7], and examine objects from "odd angles or peripheral vision" [8]. Goldman et al. [3] found that this stereotypy is rare, but seemingly specific to children with ASD.

Head movement stereotypy may be an adaptive strategy that facilitates perception or social communication [9, 10]. Turning away from over-stimulating stimuli often marks a child's need to self-regulate [11]. By engaging in head movement stereotypies or similar movements, individuals with ASD may be regulating incoming visual and social information that is perceived as over-arousing [9].

On the other hand, atypical head movements in children with ASD may contribute to the social impairments that characterize children with ASD. Motor movement is crucial for verbal and nonverbal communication, formation of friendships, and the maintenance of social interactions. Head nods and turns, for example, serve to influence turn-taking between social partners [12]. In successful social interactions, motor movements must be initiated and coordinated [13] as typical motor control functions link the perception of other's actions and one's own actions [14]. Motor delays in ASD, such as the inability to coordinate functional head and arm movements, may prevent head turning in response to one's name and gaze following, and contribute to failures to engage in gestural nonverbal communication such as joint attention [11]. Better quantification of these motor movements will further our understanding of their role in the development of ASD.

Motor movement in ASD has typically been assessed descriptively via parent report and trained human observers.

While parents have opportunities to observe their children in multiple contexts, their reports are prone to bias [4, 15]. Coding schemes of motor movement and stereotypies conducted by trained observers are frequently study-specific and receive little or no independent validation [3, 16]. In response to the limitations of qualitative efforts, automated measurement has been used to objectively document atypical motor movement and stereotypies [3, 4, 16–18]. ASD is associated with atypical gait in toddlers and children [19–22], reduced postural stability in children [23–26], and increased repetitive and stereotypic behaviors in children [3, 27, 28]. A recent meta-analysis revealed that motor impairments in movement preparation, upper extremity motor function, and gait were significantly more pronounced in individuals with ASD than individuals without ASD [4].

Automated measurement and machine-learning algorithms have been used to examine motor movements to both enhance clinical assessment [29, 30] and to elucidate the mechanisms and heterogeneity of ASD [22, 31–33]. Machine learning algorithms have successfully distinguished children with severe ASD (age 2–4 years) from children without ASD during a reach-to-grasp task [29]. Machine learning analysis of motor patterns of children playing with smart tablet computers correctly identified children with ASD from children without ASD [30]. Children with ASD contacted the table with greater force, had different distributions of force within a gesture, and displayed faster and larger movements than children without ASD [30, 32].

An initial report on postural sway examined head movement differences between children with and without ASD. Children with ASD exhibited greater head movement and sway while standing than children without ASD, and both groups reduced their postural sway during performance of a nonsocial task [23]. However, with the exception of postural sway tasks [23], investigations of motor movement have not focused on head movements in children with and without ASD. Taken together, previous research supports the importance of head movement atypicalities in ASD and suggests they warrant further exploration.

Current study

We conducted a quantitative comparison of head movement dynamics in children with and without ASD, matched on mental age, between 2.5- and 6.5-years-old, using an automated head tracking system. In lieu of subjective, manual coding, automated tracking provided objective measurement to quantify differences in head movement dynamics. We hypothesized that children with ASD would exhibit greater and more rapid head movement than children without ASD. As children with ASD typically exhibit preferential attention to nonsocial versus social stimuli [34–36], we conducted an *a priori* analysis to ascertain whether differences in head movement dynamics between children with and without ASD varied by social and nonsocial stimulus presentation.

Methods

Participants

Participants were 2.5–6.5-year-old children (*mean* = 4.72 years, SD = 1.14 years, *range* = 4.25 years) with (*n* = 21) and without (*n* = 21) ASD. Children with ASD were the older siblings of infants recruited from a longitudinal study of high-risk development. Children without ASD were typically developing children, with no reported risks or diagnoses at the time of study, and were recruited from a longitudinal study of high-risk development and from the community, through recruitment flyers. Children were excluded from the study if they had a gestational age below 37 weeks or major birth complications. Parents were reimbursed $50 for their child's participation in the study. Recruitment and procedures were approved by the University's Internal Review Board and written, parental consent was obtained before participation.

Measures and procedure

Clinical diagnosis of ASD or the absence of ASD was determined at study entry. The Autism Diagnostic Observation Schedule [37] and Autism Diagnostic Interview-Revised [38] were used to inform the DSM-IV-based best estimate diagnosis from a licensed psychologist, who was unfamiliar with the child's previous diagnosis. To assess children's mental age, children were administered with either the Wechsler Preschool and Primary Scale of Intelligence (*n* = 33; WPPSI-III, [39]) or the Mullen Scales of Early Learning (*n* = 6; Mullen, [40]). The Mullen was typically administered when children were 37 months of age or younger. Except for two 36-month-olds (1 ASD, 1 No ASD), the WPPSI was administered when children were older than 37 months. Three children (2 ASD, 1 No ASD) did not receive a cognitive assessment. Groups were comparable on the assessments administered, $\chi^2(2) = 1.27, p = .53$.

Groups were matched a priori on mental age [41]. Groups did not differ on chronological age, $F(1,41) = 4.00, p > .05$; mental age, $F(1,38) = .007, p > .05$ (Table 1); or gender, Fisher's exact test $p = .58$ (Table 2).

Table 1 Chronological age and mental age by ASD group

		N	Mean	SD
Age at visit (months)	No ASD	21	51.23	15.35
	ASD	21	60.80	16.52
Mental age (months)	No ASD	20	54.58	14.59
	ASD	19	54.08	22.95

Children with ASD did not differ from children without ASD on chronological or mental age

Table 2 Gender by ASD group

	Males	Females
No ASD	14	7
ASD	17	4

Children with ASD did not differ from children without ASD on gender

Children were seated approximately 65 cm in front of a 19-in. video monitor. They were asked to watch a short video, while a camera positioned on top of the monitor recorded their face and upper body at 29.971 frames/s. The protocol consisted of a 16-min video, composed of both social and nonsocial stimuli. The monitor displayed six videos of stimuli designed to elicit joint-attention and emotion expression in children. Video 1 was a 3-min social stimulus presentation of an actual boy pointing in a virtual environment to a side television of an animated character (SpongeBob), which was designed to elicit looks from the boy to the television (joint attention). Video 2 was a 2-min presentation of a non-social, audio-visual screensaver. Video 3 was a 3-min social stimulus presentation of an animated boy pointing in a virtual environment to a side television of an animated character (SpongeBob), which was designed to elicit looks from the boy to the television (joint attention). Video 4 was a social, 6-min emotion-eliciting story of a birthday party told by a woman. Video 5 was a social, 1-min Wonder Pets cartoon clip, and video 6 was a social, 1-min Mickey Mouse cartoon clip (Fig. 1).

Based on an a priori hypothesis, video 2 served as the nonsocial stimulus and the first 2-min of video 4 served as the social stimulus (the same pattern of results was observed when analyzing the full 6-min of video 4). Other videos contained a mixture of actual and animated figures and were not appropriate for sociality contrasts.

Head tracking

To quantify head movement dynamics, a fully automatic, person-independent computer-vision algorithm was used to track pitch, yaw, and roll of head movement (http://zface.org/, Zface, [42]). For each video frame, the algorithm registered a dense 3D face shape in real-time. This was accomplished using a fast cascade regression framework trained on high-resolution 3D face-scans of posed and spontaneous face and head motion. Zface was computationally efficient but delivered high precision tracking. Experimental findings strongly support the validity of real-time, 3D registration and reconstruction from 2D video [42]. Compared to 10 other computer-vision based approaches for head tracking, Zface achieved the lowest absolute angular error for head pitch and the second lowest angular error for yaw (2.66 and 3.93 degrees, respectively) [43].

For each video frame, the algorithm outputted 3° of rigid head movement—pitch (vertical movement; head nods), yaw (horizontal movement; head turns), and roll (lateral

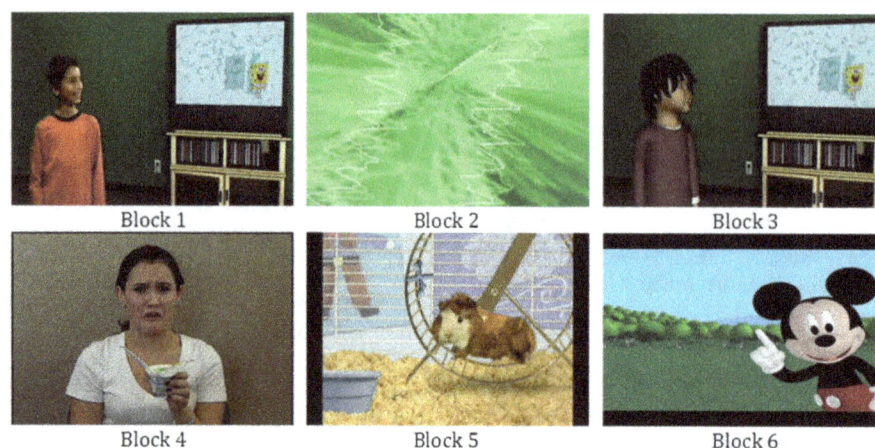

Fig. 1 Stimuli presentation by video. The 16-min video consisted of social and nonsocial stimuli, designed to elicit joint-attention and emotion expression in young children

head inclinations toward the shoulder) (Fig. 2) or a failure message when a frame could not be tracked (see Table 3 for the range of pitch, yaw, and roll).

17.4% of the frames could not be tracked, which is comparable with previous work in this area [44]. Several conditions contributed to tracking failure, including self-occlusion (hands on the face), extreme head movement, and location change (e.g., i.e., child moved out of the frame). Proportions of successfully tracked frames were examined for ASD group differences.

Data reduction

To ensure that missing data would not bias measurements, head movement dynamics were measured separately for each consecutively tracked segment (epoch). Epochs were defined as successfully tracked consecutive frames within a video (mean epoch length = 577.35 frames, at 29.971 frames per second). A 2 (group) by 6 (video) repeated-measures ANOVA indicated that the number of epochs per video did not differ significantly between groups, $F(40) = 2.70$, $p = .11$, Marginal Mean$_{ASD}$ = 18.1, Marginal Mean$_{NonASD}$ = 8.0. A 2 (group) by 6 (video) showed that the mean duration of an epoch also did not differ significantly between groups, $F(40) = 1.89$, $p = .18$, Marginal Mean$_{ASD}$ = 747.98 frames/epoch, Marginal Mean$_{NonASD}$ = 1049.04 frames/epoch (Table 4). Nevertheless, children with ASD tended to have more epochs of briefer duration than children without ASD.

Within each epoch, head movement dynamics were quantified with respect to the three principal axes of pitch, yaw, and roll. For each of these axes, angular displacement and angular velocity were calculated for each frame of video. Angular values in displacement and velocity of pitch, yaw, and roll were measured in radians and radians/frame, respectively. For pitch, yaw, and roll, angular displacement was calculated as the difference between each observed head angle value and the overall mean of head angle within each epoch. Similarly, for pitch, yaw, and roll, angular velocity was calculated as the temporal derivative of the angular displacement for

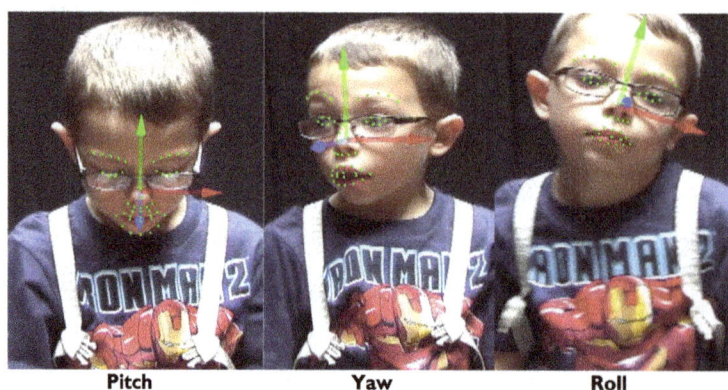

Fig. 2 Head orientation. The 3° of rigid head movement (pitch, yaw, and roll) are indexed above by the x, y, and z arrows. The green arrow indexes pitch, the blue arrow indexes yaw, and the red arrow indexes roll

Table 3 Range of pitch, yaw, and roll

	Minimum (radians)	Maximum (radians)	Minimum (degrees)	Maximum (degrees)
Pitch	−.75	1.16	42.97 down	66.46 up
Yaw	−.85	.84	48.70 left	48.13 right
Roll	−1.05	1.13	60.16 left shoulder	64.74 right shoulder

each movement direction using the finite difference method (the location difference between successive video frames).

The root mean square (RMS) then was used to measure the magnitude of angular displacement and angular velocity of pitch, yaw, and roll, respectively [44–47]. The RMS value was calculated as the square root of the arithmetic mean of the squares of the original values, in our case the angular displacements and the angular velocities. To account for the varying lengths of epochs caused by untracked frames, the RMS value for each epoch was weighted by its epoch duration. These weighted values were averaged across epochs to obtain a normalized RMS value (nRMS; Eq. 1). The obtained nRMS for angular displacement and angular velocity for pitch, yaw, and roll are used in subsequent analyses and are referred to as angular displacement and angular velocity for simplicity.

$$\mathrm{nRMS}_x = \sqrt{\frac{1}{n}\left(x_1^2 + x_2^2 + \dots + x_n^2\right)} \tag{1}$$

where $x_1^2 \dots x_n^2$ are the squared differences between the value of a frame and the mean value of frames within an epoch.

Analytic approach
Preliminary analyses
A preliminary 2 (group) × 6 (video) repeated-measures analysis of variance (ANOVA) compared the proportion of successfully tracked frames by ASD group to determine whether children with and without ASD differed in levels of automated tracking.

ASD group differences
A second 2 (group) × 6 (video) repeated-measures ANOVA was used to test for differences between

Table 4 Number of epochs and mean epoch duration by ASD Group

		Marginal Mean	F	p value
Number of Epochs	No ASD	8.00	2.70	.11
	ASD	18.00		
Mean Epoch Duration (frames)	No ASD	1049.04	1.89	.18
	ASD	747.98		

children with and without ASD in the angular displacement and angular velocity of pitch, yaw, and roll respectively. We hypothesized that children with ASD would exhibit greater angular displacement and angular velocity of pitch, yaw, and roll than children without ASD.

ASD group by stimulus type interaction
Planned contrasts were then used to test for the interaction between stimulus type (social versus nonsocial) and group (ASD versus no ASD). A 2 (group) × 2 (Nonsocial$_{Video2}$ vs. Social$_{Video4}$) repeated-measures ANOVAs examined whether children with and without ASD differed in pitch, yaw, and roll angular displacement and angular velocity separately between nonsocial (video 2) and social stimuli (video 4). All main analyses were then repeated covarying chronological age to determine the degree to which differences between the mental-age-matched groups might be due to chronological age. (Analyses of supplementary head movement variables, which yielded results similar to those outlined below, are found in Additional file 1.)

Results
Preliminary analyses
A one-way analysis of the proportion of successfully tracked frames over the entire course of the protocol revealed no group differences, $F(39) = .08$, $p = .77$, partial $\eta^2 = .003$ (Fig. 3). A repeated-measures ANOVA indicated a main effect of video, $F(3.58, 38) = 3.01$, $p = .03$ partial $\eta^2 = .07$, and no interaction of video by group, $F(3.58, 38) = .15$, $p = .95$, partial $\eta^2 = .004$. There were no

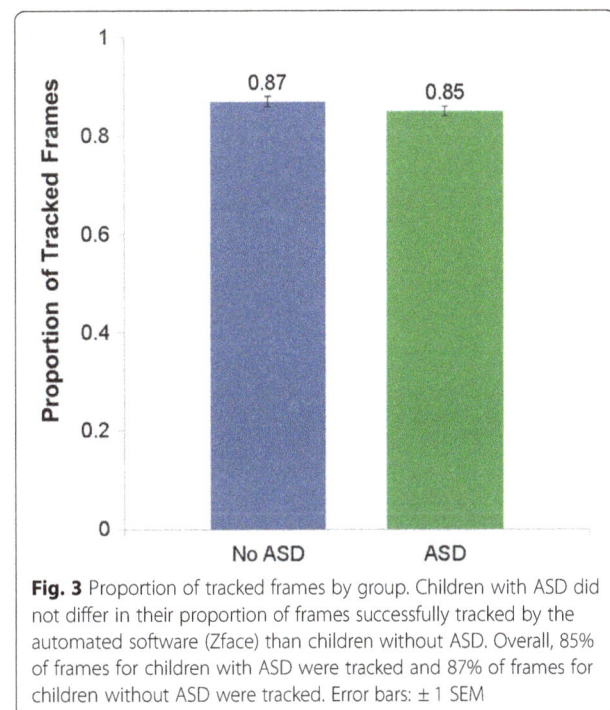

Fig. 3 Proportion of tracked frames by group. Children with ASD did not differ in their proportion of frames successfully tracked by the automated software (Zface) than children without ASD. Overall, 85% of frames for children with ASD were tracked and 87% of frames for children without ASD were tracked. Error bars: ± 1 SEM

group differences in proportion of successfully tracked frames by video, $ps > .69$.

ASD group differences

For angular displacement, a 2 (group) × 6 (video) repeated-measures analysis of variance (ANOVA) revealed main effects of video for pitch and yaw. No significant interactions of video and group were found for the angular displacement of pitch, yaw, and roll. Children with ASD exhibited greater angular displacement of yaw than children without ASD, indicating greater head turning, F (1, 37) = 4.36, $p = .04$, partial $\eta_p^2 = .11$ (Fig. 4, Table 5). Children with ASD did not differ from children without ASD on pitch and roll angular displacement, $ps > .05$.

For angular velocity, repeated-measures ANOVA revealed a main effect of video for pitch and roll. No significant interactions of video and group were found for angular velocity of yaw, pitch, and roll. Children with ASD exhibited greater angular velocity of yaw, F (1, 37) = 4.01, $p = .050$, partial $\eta_p^2 = .10$, and roll, F (1, 37) = 7.35, $p = .010$, partial $\eta_p^2 = .17$ than children without ASD, indicating greater head movement (Fig. 5, Table 5). Pitch angular velocity did not differ between children with and without ASD, $p > .05$.

ASD group by stimulus type (social versus nonsocial video) interaction

Planned contrasts revealed an interaction between video and group for yaw angular displacement, F (1,40) = 7.86, $p < .01$, $\eta_p^2 = 16$, and a significant between-subjects effect of group, F (1) = 5.99, $p = .019$, $\eta_p^2 = .13$ (Fig. 6). Children with ASD had greater angular displacement of yaw in the social video (video 4), than children without ASD, and did not differ in their angular displacement of yaw in the nonsocial video (video 2) than children without ASD. There were no interactions between video and group for angular displacement of pitch and roll, $ps > .05$.

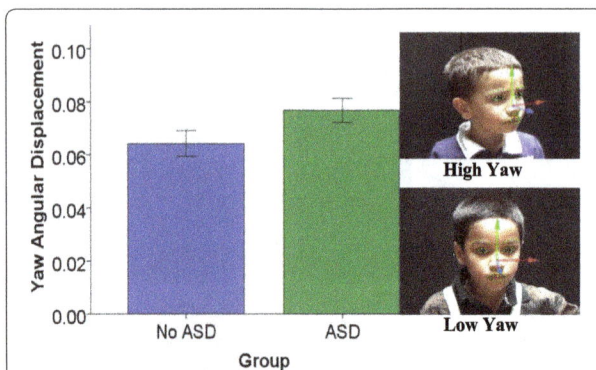

Fig. 4 Between-group differences in yaw angular displacement. Children with ASD have greater yaw angular displacement than children without ASD. Note. Error bars: ± 1 SEM

Table 5 Repeated-measures ANOVA of pitch, yaw, and roll

		df	F	p	η_p^2
ADis_Pitch	Video	3.74	3.21	.02*	.08
	Video*Group	3.74	0.40	.79	.01
	Group	1.00	1.81	.19	.05
ADis_Yaw	Video	4.85	3.97	<.01*	.10
	Video*Group	4.85	1.39	.23	.04
	Group	1.00	4.36	.04*	.11
ADis_ Roll	Video	2.71	0.42	.72	.01
	Video*Group	2.71	1.26	.29	.03
	Group	1.00	3.33	.08	.08
AVel_Pitch	Video	3.31	3.27	.02*	.08
	Video*Group	3.31	0.68	.58	.02
	Group	1.00	0.77	.39	.02
AVel_Yaw	Video	3.60	1.90	.12	.05
	Video*Group	3.60	0.57	.67	.02
	Group	1.00	4.01	.05*	.10
AVel_Roll	Video	3.46	2.58	.06	.07
	Video*Group	3.46	0.56	.67	.02
	Group	1.00	7.35	.01*	.17

*p < .05

ADis angular displacement, AVel angular velocity

For angular velocity of yaw, there was an interaction between video and group, F (1,40) = 8.35, $p < .01$, $\eta_p^2 = .17$, and a significant between-subjects effect of group, F (1,40) = 4.90, $p = .033$, $\eta_p^2 = .11$ (Fig. 6). There was also an interaction between video and group for angular velocity of roll F (1,40) = 4.27, $p = .045$, $\eta_p^2 = .10$, with a significant between-subjects effect of group, F (1,40) = 4.69, $p = .036$, $\eta_p^2 = .11$ (Fig. 6). Children with ASD had greater angular velocity of yaw and roll in video 4 (social video) than children without ASD and did not differ in their angular velocity of yaw and roll in video 2 (nonsocial video). There was no interaction between video and group for angular velocity of pitch, $p > .05$.

Controlling for age

A 2 (group) × 6 (video) repeated-measures analysis of variance (ANOVA) was conducted with chronological age as a covariate. As when not considering this covariate, children with ASD exhibited greater angular displacement of yaw than children without ASD, indicating greater head turning, F (1, 36) = 5.36, $p = .02$, $\eta_p^2 = .13$. As when not considering the age covariate, children with ASD exhibited greater angular velocity of roll, F (1, 36) = 5.45, $p = .02$, $\eta_p^2 = .13$, than children without ASD, indicating greater head rolling motion. Unlike previous findings without age, children with ASD did not exhibit greater angular velocity of yaw, F (1, 36) = .73, $p = .40$,

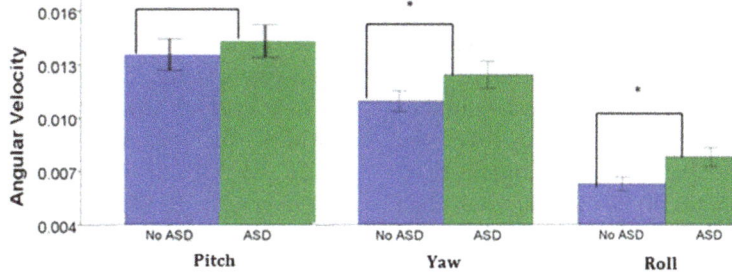

Fig. 5 Between-group differences in yaw and roll angular velocity. Children with ASD had greater yaw and roll angular velocity than children without ASD. Note. Error bars: ± 1 SEM

$\eta_p^2 = .02$ when controlling for chronological age. All other findings were unchanged.

The planned contrast models (social versus nonsocial video) were repeated with angular velocity including chronological age as a covariate. As in previous findings without age as a covariate, there was an interaction between video and group for angular velocity of yaw, F (1,39) = 4.83, $p < .03$, $\eta_p^2 = .11$, but there was no between subject's effect of group, F (1,39) = 1.72, $p = .20$, $\eta_p^2 = .04$. Children with ASD had greater angular velocity of yaw in the social video (video 4) than children without ASD, and the two groups did not differ in the angular velocity of yaw and roll in the nonsocial video (video 2). Unlike previous analyses without age as a covariate, no interaction between group and video was found for angular

velocity of roll when chronological age was included in the model, F (1,39) = 2.97, $p = .09$, $\eta_p^2 = .07$. All other findings were unchanged.

Discussion

Using automated, objective measurement, we quantified differences in head movement dynamics between children with and without ASD, shedding light on head movement atypicalities previously described by clinicians. Children with ASD showed greater angular displacement of yaw and greater angular velocity of yaw and roll than children without ASD. Angular displacement is interpreted as head movement *quantity*, and angular velocity is interpreted as the *speed* of head movement. Thus, children with ASD exhibited greater

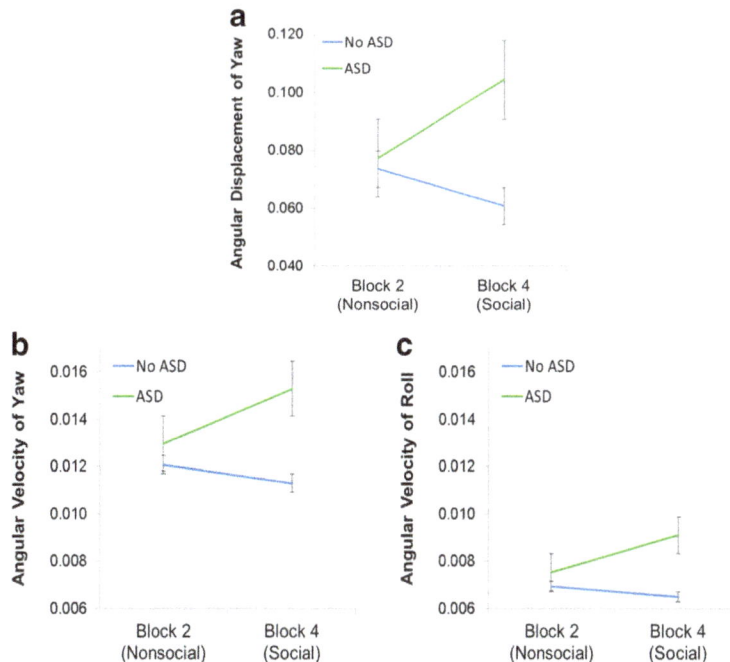

Fig. 6 Video (nonsocial vs. social) by group interaction. Compared to children without ASD, children with ASD differed in angular displacement of yaw (**a**) and angular velocity of yaw (**b**) and roll (**c**) only during the social stimulus (video 4), but not the nonsocial stimulus (video 2). Error bars: ± 1 SEM

head turning (yaw)—and turned their heads (yaw) and inclined their heads (roll) with greater speed—than children without ASD. Differences in head movement dynamics between children with and without ASD were specific to the presentation of a social stimulus. That is, children with ASD exhibited greater yaw angular displacement and yaw and roll angular velocity during presentation of the social stimulus than children without ASD.

Analyses were repeated including chronological age as a covariate—groups were matched a priori on mental age—to disentangle age and ASD differences [3, 48]. When controlling for chronological age, children with ASD continued to exhibit greater head turning (yaw) and inclined their heads (roll) with greater speed than children without ASD. When controlling for chronological age, differences in head movement dynamics between children with and without ASD remained specific to the presentation of a social stimulus for angular displacement of yaw and angular velocity of yaw, but not angular velocity of roll. Comparison of models, with and without statistical controls for chronological age, highlight angular displacement of yaw and angular velocity of yaw and roll as consistent signatures of ASD.

The current findings add to a small but growing body of literature utilizing automated measurement of body and head movement to objectively quantify the ASD phenotype [32, 49]. In a previous investigation, for example, 9-year-old children with ASD exhibited greater sway while standing in both the anterior-posterior (front-to-back) and medial-lateral (side-to-side) axes than did children without ASD, but sway was reduced during the search task, suggesting better movement control when pursuing a goal [23]. By contrast, we measured 3° of rigid head movement (pitch, yaw, and roll) from video-recordings of younger, seated children. Younger children with ASD exhibited greater head displacement and velocity in the horizontal (yaw) and lateral (roll) but not vertical (pitch) axes than children without ASD. These differences in displacement and velocity were specific to social stimuli presentation. Together, these findings suggest that nonsocial engagement constrains excess head movement dynamics in children with ASD, while spontaneous activity, particularly in reaction to social stimuli, is associated with increased head movement dynamics.

Children with ASD may use head movement as a way to modulate their sensory experience [50]. Previous primary research [4] and meta-analytic results of observational measures [51] indicate that infants and children with ASD displayed higher levels of motor impairments than infants and children without ASD. Motor impairments may constitute a core feature of ASD, a finding supported by the current studies comparisons of

children with and without ASD [4, 32]. However, when head movement was compared during the presentation of social and nonsocial stimuli, head movement differences were specific to the presentation of social stimuli. Previous research using eye-tracking indicates that children with ASD look less at social stimuli than nonsocial stimuli [36, 51, 52], suggesting that children with ASD shift their gaze to regulate overstimulating social information. Viewing faces and engaging with social partners requires complex timing and attunement, which may be effortful for children with ASD [53]. Together, these findings suggest that increased head movement in reaction to social stimuli may reflect increased sensitivity to social scenes among children with ASD.

Children with ASD may engage in more extreme and quicker head movement than children without ASD because they are unable to regulate incoming social information. Possible disruptions in motor planning and head movements early in development may have cascading effects in later social engagement [54, 55]. Given early associations between motor experience and the development of social behaviors [56], early disruptions in head movement may index atypical developmental trajectories [6, 57].

Limitations and future directions

Differences between children with and without ASD in head displacement and velocity were obtained in a small sample, highlighting the need for replication. The current study tested specific *a priori* hypotheses regarding head movement dynamic differences by nonsocial and social stimuli. Future research could build upon this research and explore whether head movement dynamics varies proportionally as a result of the degree of sociality of the stimulus. Future research with larger sample sizes and a fully counterbalanced protocol will allow researchers to examine more nuanced research questions.

While use of automated measurement marks progress in objectively quantifying head movement dynamics, there were limitations associated with this approach. The inability of the automated software to track extreme head movement and self-occlusion resulted in missing data (∼ 17%). Although missing data did not vary by group, the presence of missing data necessitated using epochs of continuous data collection as a unit of analysis. Moreover, although not significant, children with ASD tended to have more epochs of briefer duration than children without ASD. It is possible that an inability to quantify head movement between epochs yielded a conservative assessment of group differences.

Angular displacement and velocity of pitch, yaw, and roll were moderately correlated in our data, and we chose to examine these dynamics separately. An alternative approach could be to model these movements together to assess differences in children with and without ASD. The addition of postural adjustments and muscle tension measurements to the model would allow for examination of coupling between head, neck, and torso in human movement, and potential differences in coupling associated with ASD.

Conclusions

Using automated measurement, we quantified differences in the quantity and speed of head movement between children with and without ASD, finding differences in the lateral (yaw and roll) but not vertical (pitch) domain. Children with ASD had greater yaw angular displacement and greater yaw and roll angular velocity, and these differences were most pronounced during social stimulus presentation. The results are consistent with the hypothesis that children with ASD use head movement to regulate their direct exposure to potentially arousing social situations. The study reports on a promising advance in objectively characterizing head movement dynamics. Our findings highlight the possibility of using automated measurement of head motion to supplement current diagnostic approaches for ASD. Automated measurement of head motion in varied contexts could provide an objective method of differentiating children with and without ASD. In contrast to previous approaches to head movement quantification, the computer-vision based approach we used here is non-invasive, may be applied to already collected video of children, and may be well suited for use in monitoring change over the course of the disorder and in response to interventions.

Abbreviations
ANOVA: Analyses of variance; ASD: Autism spectrum disorder; nRMS : Normalized root mean square; RMS: Root mean square

Acknowledgements
Not applicable

Funding
Autism Speaks National Institute of General Medical Sciences (1R01GM105004).

Authors' contributions
KM analyzed and interpreted the head movement data and drafted the manuscript for submission. ZH tracked the videotaped participants using Zface, compiled a dataset of head movement, and revised the manuscript critically. JCohn oversaw the measurement of head movement and was a major contributor in writing the manuscript and revising it critically. JCassell made substantial contributions to the design of the study and contributed video stimuli. AG contributed to the acquisition of data. GR analyzed the head movement data and MO contributed to the analytic approach and

interpretation of the data. JB contributed to the analytic approach of the data and revised the manuscript critically. DM contributed to the conception and design of the study, oversaw the acquisition of data, reviewed the analytic approach, and was a major contributor in the writing of the manuscript. All authors read and approved the final manuscript.

Authors' information
JCohn leads efforts to develop methods for the automatic analysis of facial expression and automated tracking of rigid and non-rigid head motion and applied those tools to research in psychopathology. ZH is part of the JCohn's interdisciplinary group and has applied computer vision and machine learning to improve measurement of and theoretical advances in mother-infant interaction, depression, pain, and social interaction. JCassell is the director of the Human-Computer Interaction Institute, in the school of Computer Science at Carnegie Mellon University, and focuses on applying computer vision systems to the study of human interactions. GR is a postdoctoral fellow at the Center for Computational Science and is part of the Big Data Mining and Data Analytics team, and MO is a professor in the Department of Computer Science at the University of Miami. Together, GR and MO have expertise in computational approaches to big-data. JB is an assistant professor in the Department of Psychology at the University of Miami with expertise in interdisciplinary research that utilizes advancements in technology to study the intersection of human development and clinical outcomes. AG is the assistant director for the Center for Autism and Related Disabilities (CARD) at the University of Miami. DM's research uses objective measurement of body movement, facial expression, and vocalization to better understand communicative development in typically developing children and those affected by ASD.

Consent for publication
Parents consented to the following:
"VIDEOTAPES: When the researcher plays with your child and when your child watches the children's videos, we will be videotaping your child. The videotapes of your child will be coded by experts, undergraduate students, and other parents. Additionally, the videos will be measured using computer software at the University of Miami, University of Pittsburgh, and the University of Denver. They may also be used in publications and at scientific conferences. You agree to all of these uses by taking part in this study...."
"CONFIDENTIALITY: Your child's videotaped images will be rated by other people, analyzed by computer at the University of Pittsburgh, and presented in scientific reports. The images will not be linked to personal identifiers in any way. These videotaped images are scientifically valuable and will be stored permanently by the investigators as a record of this study. At your request, the images will be immediately destroyed. The US Department of Health and Human Services (DHHS) may request to review and obtain copies of your records. Your records may also be reviewed for audit purposes by authorized University employees or other agents who will be bound by the same provisions of confidentiality."

Competing interests
The authors declare that they have no competing interests.

Author details
[1]Department of Psychology, University of Miami, 5665 Ponce de Leon Blvd, Coral Gables, FL 33146, USA. [2]Robotics Institute, Carnegie Mellon University, 5000 Forbes Ave, Pittsburgh, PA 15213, USA. [3]Center for Computational Science, University of Miami, 1320 S Dixie Hwy, Miami, FL 33146, USA. [4]Department of Psychology, University of Pittsburgh, 210 S. Bouquet St., Pittsburgh, PA 15260, USA. [5]Human Computer Interaction, Carnegie Mellon University, 5000 Forbes Avenue, Pittsburgh, PA 15213, USA. [6]Department of Computer Science, University of Miami, 1365 Memorial Drive, Coral Gables, FL 33146, USA.

References

1. American Psychiatric Association. Diagnostic and statistical manual of mental disorders: *DSM-5*. 5th ed. Arlington: American Psychiatric Publishing; 2013.
2. Provost B, Lopez B, Heimerl S. A comparison of motor delays in young children: autism spectrum disorder, developmental delay, and developmental concerns. J Autism Dev Disord. 2007;37(2):321–8.
3. Goldman S, et al. Motor stereotypies in children with autism and other developmental disorders. Dev Med Child Neurol. 2009;51(1):30–8.
4. Fournier, et al. Motor coordination in autism spectrum disorders: a synthesis and meta-analysis. J Autism Dev Disord. 2010;40(10):1227–40.
5. Freeman BJ, et al. The behavior observation scale for autism: initial methodology, data analysis, and preliminary findings on 89 children. J Am Acad Child Psychiatry. 1978;17(4):576–88.
6. Zwaigenbaum L, et al. Behavioral manifestations of autism in the first year of life. Int J Dev Neurosci. 2005;23(2–3):143–52.
7. Kim SH, Lord C. Restricted and repetitive behaviors in toddlers and preschoolers with autism spectrum disorders based on the autism diagnostic observation schedule (ADOS). Autism Res. 2010;3(4):162–73.
8. Ozonoff S, et al. A prospective study of the emergence of early behavioral signs of autism. J Am Acad Child Adolesc Psychiatry. 2010;49(3):256–66. e2
9. Mottron, et al. Lateral glances toward moving stimuli among young children with autism: early regulation of locally oriented perception? Dev Psychopathol. 2007;19(1):23–36.
10. Hellendoorn A, et al. The relationship between atypical visual processing and social skills in young children with autism. Res Dev Disabil. 2014;35(2):423–8.
11. Mundy P, Newell L. Attention, joint attention, and social cognition. Curr Dir Psychol Sci. 2007;16(5):269–74.
12. Duncan S. Some signals and rules for taking speaking turns in conversations. J Pers Soc Psychol. 1972;23(2):283.
13. Piek JP, Dyck MJ. Sensory-motor deficits in children with developmental coordination disorder, attention deficit hyperactivity disorder and autistic disorder. Hum Mov Sci. 2004;23(3):475–88.
14. Wolpert DM, Doya K, Kawato M. *A unifying computational framework for motor control and social interaction*. Philosophical Transactions of the Royal Society of London. Series B: Biological Sciences. 2003;358(1431):593–602.
15. Mooney E, Gray K, Tonge B. Early features of autism. Eur Child Adolesc Psychiatry. 2006;15(1):12–8.
16. Ozonoff S, et al. Gross motor development, movement abnormalities, and early identification of autism. J Autism Dev Disord. 2008;38(4):644–56.
17. Bryson SE, et al. A prospective case series of high-risk infants who developed autism. J Autism Dev Disord. 2007;37(1):12–24.
18. Loh A, et al. Stereotyped motor behaviors associated with autism in high-risk infants: a pilot videotape analysis of a sibling sample. J Autism Dev Disord. 2007;37(1):25–36.
19. Calhoun M, Longworth M, Chester VL. Gait patterns in children with autism. Clin Biomech. 2011;26(2):200–6.
20. Esposito G, et al. Analysis of unsupported gait in toddlers with autism. Brain Dev. 2011;33(5):367–73.
21. Rinehart NJ, et al. Gait function in newly diagnosed children with autism: cerebellar and basal ganglia related motor disorder. Dev Med Child Neurol. 2006;48(10):819–24.
22. Rinehart NJ, et al. Gait function in high-functioning autism and Asperger's disorder. Eur Child Adolesc Psychiatry. 2006;15(5):256–64.
23. Chang C-H, et al. Visual tasks and postural sway in children with and without autism spectrum disorders. Res Dev Disabil. 2010;31(6):1536–42.
24. Chen FC, et al. Postural responses to a suprapostural visual task among children with and without developmental coordination disorder. Res Dev Disabil. 2011;32(5):1948–56.
25. Fournier, et al. Decreased static and dynamic postural control in children with autism spectrum disorders. Gait & Posture. 2010;32(1):6–9.
26. Memari AH, et al. Postural sway patterns in children with autism spectrum disorder compared with typically developing children. Res Autism Spectr Disord. 2013;7(2):325–32.
27. Rodgers J, et al. Anxiety and repetitive behaviours in autism spectrum disorders and Williams syndrome: a cross-syndrome comparison. J Autism Dev Disord. 2012;42:175–80.
28. Singer HS. Motor stereotypies. Semin Pediatr Neurol. 2009;16(2):77–81.
29. Crippa A, et al. Use of machine learning to identify children with autism and their motor abnormalities. J Autism Dev Disord. 2015;45(7):2146–56.
30. Anzulewicz A, Sobota K, Delafield-Butt JT. Toward the autism motor signature: gesture patterns during smart tablet gameplay identify children with autism. Sci Rep. 2016;6:31107
31. Rinehart NJ, et al. Movement preparation in high-functioning autism and Asperger disorder: a serial choice reaction time task involving motor reprogramming. J Autism Dev Disord. 2001;31(1):79–88.
32. Torres E, et al. Autism: the micro-movement perspective. Front Integr Neurosci. 2013;7:32.
33. Torres EB, et al. Toward precision psychiatry: statistical platform for the personalized characterization of natural behaviors. Front Neurol. 2016;7:8.
34. Pierce K, et al. Preference for geometric patterns early in life as a risk factor for autism. Arch Gen Psychiatry. 2011;68(1):101–9.
35. Klin A, et al. Visual fixation patterns during viewing of naturalistic social situations as predictors of social competence in individuals with autism. Arch Gen Psychiatry. 2002;59:809–16.
36. Chawarska K, Macari S, Shic F. Decreased spontaneous attention to social scenes in 6-month-old infants later diagnosed with autism Spectrum disorders. Biol Psychiatry. 2013;74(3):195–203.
37. Lord C, et al. The autism diagnostic observation schedule—generic: a standard measure of social and communication deficits associated with the spectrum of autism. J Autism Dev Disord. 2000;30(3):205–23.
38. Lord C, Rutter M, Le Couteur A. Autism diagnostic interview-revised: a revised version of a diagnostic interview for caregivers of individuals with possible pervasive developmental disorders. J Autism Dev Disord. 1994;24(5):659–85.
39. Wechsler D. The Wechsler Primary and Preschool Scale of Intelligence. San Antonio, TX: The Psychological Corporation; 2002.
40. Mullen EM. Mullen scales of early learning. MN: AGS Circle Pines; 1995.
41. Staples KL, Reid G. Fundamental movement skills and autism spectrum disorders. J Autism Dev Disord. 2010;40(2):209–17.
42. Jeni, L.A., J.F. Cohn, and T. Kanade, Dense 3D face alignment from 2D videos in real-time. 2015, FG.
43. Jeni LA, Cohn JF. Person-independent 3d gaze estimation using face frontalization. In: Proceedings of the IEEE Conference on Computer Vision and Pattern Recognition Workshops. Las Vegas: 2016. p. 87-95.
44. Hammal Z, et al. Head movement dynamics during normal and perturbed parent-infant interaction. In: Humaine Association Conference on Affective Computing and Intelligent Interaction (ACII), 2013. Geneva: 2013. p. 276-282.
45. Hammal Z, Cohn JF, George DT. Interpersonal coordination of headmotion in distressed couples. Affective Computing, IEEE Transactions on. 2014;5(2):155–67.
46. Barnes G, Asselman P. The mechanism of prediction in human smooth pursuit eye movements. J Physiol. 1991;439(1):439–61.
47. McLean L, et al. The effect of head position, electrode site, movement and smoothing window in the determination of a reliable maximum voluntary activation of the upper trapezius muscle. J Electromyogr Kinesiol. 2003;13(2):169–80.
48. Mahone EM, et al. Repetitive arm and hand movements (complex motor stereotypies) in children. J Pediatr. 2004;145(3):391–5.
49. Cohen I, et al. Rating scale measures are associated with Noldus EthoVision-XT video tracking of behaviors of children on the autism spectrum. Mol Autism. 2014;5(1):15.
50. Dunn W. The impact of sensory processing abilities on the daily lives of young children and their families: a conceptual model. Infants & Young Children. 1997;9(4):23–35.
51. Shic F, et al. Limited activity monitoring in toddlers with autism spectrum disorder. Brain Res. 2011;1380:246–54.
52. Klin A, et al. Two-year-olds with autism orient to non-social contingencies rather than biological motion. Nature. 2009;459(7244):257–61.
53. Happé F, Frith U. The weak coherence account: detail-focused cognitive style in autism Spectrum disorders. J Autism Dev Disord. 2006;36(1):5–25.
54. Trevarthen C, Delafield-Butt JT. Autism as a developmental disorder in intentional movement and affective engagement. Front Integr Neurosci. 2013;7:49.
55. Cook J. From movement kinematics to social cognition: the case of autism. Phil Trans R Soc B. 2016;371(1693):20150372.
56. Libertus K, Needham A. Reaching experience increases face preference in 3-month-old infants. Dev Sci. 2011;14(6):1355–64.
57. Landa R, Garrett-Mayer E. Development in infants with autism spectrum disorders: a prospective study. J Child Psychol Psychiatry. 2006;47(6):629–38.

12

Loss of the Chr16p11.2 ASD candidate gene *QPRT* leads to aberrant neuronal differentiation in the SH-SY5Y neuronal cell model

Denise Haslinger[1], Regina Waltes[1], Afsheen Yousaf[1], Silvia Lindlar[1], Ines Schneider[2], Chai K. Lim[3], Meng-Miao Tsai[4], Boyan K. Garvalov[4,5], Amparo Acker-Palmer[6], Nicolas Krezdorn[7], Björn Rotter[7], Till Acker[4], Gilles J. Guillemin[3], Simone Fulda[2], Christine M. Freitag[1] and Andreas G. Chiocchetti[1]* iD

Abstract

Background: Altered neuronal development is discussed as the underlying pathogenic mechanism of autism spectrum disorders (ASD). Copy number variations of 16p11.2 have recurrently been identified in individuals with ASD. Of the 29 genes within this region, *quinolinate phosphoribosyltransferase* (*QPRT*) showed the strongest regulation during neuronal differentiation of SH-SY5Y neuroblastoma cells. We hypothesized a causal relation between this tryptophan metabolism-related enzyme and neuronal differentiation. We thus analyzed the effect of *QPRT* on the differentiation of SH-SY5Y and specifically focused on neuronal morphology, metabolites of the tryptophan pathway, and the neurodevelopmental transcriptome.

Methods: The gene dosage-dependent change of *QPRT* expression following Chr16p11.2 deletion was investigated in a lymphoblastoid cell line (LCL) of a deletion carrier and compared to his non-carrier parents. Expression of *QPRT* was tested for correlation with neuromorphology in SH-SY5Y cells. QPRT function was inhibited in SH-SY5Y neuroblastoma cells using (i) siRNA knockdown (KD), (ii) chemical mimicking of loss of QPRT, and (iii) complete CRISPR/Cas9-mediated knock out (KO). *QPRT-KD* cells underwent morphological analysis. Chemically inhibited and *QPRT-KO* cells were characterized using viability assays. Additionally, *QPRT-KO* cells underwent metabolite and whole transcriptome analyses. Genes differentially expressed upon KO of *QPRT* were tested for enrichment in biological processes and co-regulated gene-networks of the human brain.

Results: *QPRT* expression was reduced in the LCL of the deletion carrier and significantly correlated with the neuritic complexity of SH-SY5Y. The reduction of *QPRT* altered neuronal morphology of differentiated SH-SY5Y cells. Chemical inhibition as well as complete KO of the gene were lethal upon induction of neuronal differentiation, but not proliferation. The QPRT-associated tryptophan pathway was not affected by KO. At the transcriptome level, genes linked to neurodevelopmental processes and synaptic structures were affected. Differentially regulated genes were enriched for ASD candidates, and co-regulated gene networks were implicated in the development of the dorsolateral prefrontal cortex, the hippocampus, and the amygdala.

(Continued on next page)

* Correspondence: andreas.chiocchetti@kgu.de
[1]Department of Child and Adolescent Psychiatry, Psychosomatics and Psychotherapy, University Hospital Frankfurt, JW Goethe University Frankfurt, Frankfurt am Main, Germany
Full list of author information is available at the end of the article

(Continued from previous page)

Conclusions: In this study, *QPRT* was causally related to in vitro neuronal differentiation of SH-SY5Y cells and affected the regulation of genes and gene networks previously implicated in ASD. Thus, our data suggest that *QPRT* may play an important role in the pathogenesis of ASD in Chr16p11.2 deletion carriers.

Keywords: Autism, 16p11.2, Quinolinate phosphoribosyltransferase, Quinolinic acid, Kynurenine, CRISPR/Cas9, Sholl analysis

Background

Altered neuronal development is suggested to be one of the major drivers in the etiology of autism spectrum disorders (ASD). Neuropathological studies based on postmortem brains of ASD patients reported aberrant neuronal development including reduced dendritic branching in the hippocampus [1], smaller pyramidal neurons in the language associated Broca's area [2], abnormal minicolumnar organization in the cerebral cortex leading to decreased inter-areal connectivity [3], and disorganized layers of the cortical areas [4]. The underlying etiology of ASD is mainly based on different genetic findings including de novo copy number variations (CNVs). These CNVs, in particular deletions, have been recurrently shown to alter genic regions in ASD individuals [5], specifically affecting neurodevelopmental genes [6].

One of the most recurrent CNVs in ASD resides within Chr16p11.2 spanning ~ 600 kb. Overall, duplications and deletions of 16p11.2 can be identified in 0.8% of ASD cases [7]. A deletion of this region is associated with a nine times higher likelihood of developing ASD, and the duplication is associated with a nine times higher risk of both ASD and schizophrenia [8]. While developmental delay or intellectual disability can occur in some cases of 16p11.2 duplication carriers, they are more common in deletions [9, 10].

The 16p11.2 CNV region spans 29 genes which showed gene dosage-dependent expression in lymphoblastoid cell lines (LCLs) of CNV carriers, leading to a differential expression of genes implicated in biological processes such as synaptic function or chromatin modification [11].

A study in zebrafish showed that the majority of the human Chr16p11.2 homologous genes are involved in nervous system development: loss of function of these genes led to an altered brain morphology for 21 of 22 tested genes [12]. Double heterozygous knockouts of the Chr16p11.2 homologs *double C2 domain alpha (DOC2A)* and *family with sequence similarity 57, member Ba (FAM57BA)* induced hyperactivity, increased seizure susceptibility and increased body length and head size in zebrafish [13]. In mice, CNVs of the homologous 16p11.2 region induced differing phenotypes. Two studies reported the deletion to result in a reduction of the skull [14] or brain size [15], accompanied by

gene dosage-sensitive changes of behavior and synaptic plasticity [14] as well as altered cortical cytoarchitecture, and reduction of downstream extracellular signaling-related kinase (ERK/MAPK) effectors [15]. Comparing individual brain regions in mice with deletions to wild-type animals, Horev and associates identified six regions with an increased volume, which were not altered in duplication carriers (see Dataset S04 in the original publication [16]). In another study, mice carrying a heterozygous microduplication of the region showed increased dendritic arborization of cortical pyramidal neurons [17]. Via network analysis of protein-protein-interaction, the authors identified the gene coding for mitogen-activated protein kinase 3 (MAPK3) as hub gene. MAPK3 plays a role in signaling cascades involved in proliferation and differentiation. A recent study focused on different effects of 16p11.2 deletions in male and female mice and reported impairments of reward-directed learning in male mice accompanied by male-specific overexpression of *dopamine receptor D2 (DRD2)* and *adenosine receptor 2a (ADORA2A)* in the striatum [18]. Both genes have been discussed in the context of ASD [19, 20].

While the functional validation of the entire CNV models the genomic status of the patients, investigating gene dosage effects of single genes located in Chr16p11.2 is useful to understand their individual contribution to the complex and diverse pathologies of ASD. In zebrafish, the suppression of *potassium channel tetramerization domain containing 13 (KCTD13)* was associated with macrocephaly whereas overexpression led to microcephaly [21]. In mice, the same study showed a reduction of *KCTD13* to result in increased proliferation of neuronal progenitors, which is also suggested to result in macrocephaly. Further, a heterozygous deletion of the gene coding for major vault protein (*MVP*) induced a reduction of functional synapses in mice [22]. *TAO kinase 2 (TAOK2)*, also located in 16p11.2, was found to be essential for the development of basal dendrites and axonal projections in cortical pyramidal neurons of mice [23]. Chr16p11.2 genes *DOC2A*, *KIF22*, and *T-box 6 (TBX6)* are required for the development of neuronal polarity in mouse hippocampal cultures [24].

In ASD patients, multiple brain measures such as the thalamic or total brain volume were reported to be increased in 16p11.2 deletion carriers and reduced in duplication carriers [25, 26]. Another study integrated physical interactions of 16p11.2 proteins with spatiotemporal gene expression of the human brain. The authors identified the KCTD13-Cul3-RhoA pathway as being crucial for controlling brain size and connectivity [27]. Still, only few genes of the Chr16p11.2 region have been investigated for their specific role in neuronal differentiation in human models.

Here, we investigated the SH-SY5Y neuroblastoma cell model as a well-studied and feasible model for neuronal differentiation in vitro. Previously, we reported that a continuous application of brain-derived neurotrophic factor (BDNF) and retinoic acid (RA) leads to neuronal cells of most likely cortical identity with a transcriptomic signature reminiscent of that of neocortical brain tissue developed for 16–19 weeks post-conception [28]. In addition, we showed expressed genes in the differentiated SH-SY5Y model to be co-regulated within modules, several of which were associated with neurodevelopmental disorders such as the orange module. We then implemented three complementary statistical methods to identify genes that were (i) differentially regulated upon differentiation, (ii) significantly involved in the independent processes active during differentiation and/or (iii) that were significantly changed over time. Finally, we described a list of 299 robustly regulated genes that appeared to be significant in all three analyses [28].

We here report that of the 29 genes located within Chr16p11.2, a total of 10 genes were identified by at least one of the three implemented statistical approaches. However, only the gene coding for *quinolinate phosphoribosyltransferase (QPRT)* was identified by all three analyses. In addition, *QPRT* was one of the most highly expressed genes of the Chr16p11.2 region and showed the highest regulatory fold change (FC) after induction of neuronal differentiation. Also, *QPRT* was co-regulated with an early upregulated gene module (MEorange) which showed significant enrichment for ASD candidate genes [28].

QPRT codes for an enzyme of the kynurenine pathway, the primary route for tryptophan catabolism, which results in the production of nicotinamide adenine dinucleotide (NAD^+). In addition, it is the only enzyme catabolizing quinolinic acid (QUIN), a potent excitotoxin acting as N-methyl-D-aspartate receptor (NMDA-R) agonist. QUIN is also linked to astroglial activation and cell death as originally identified in the context of Alzheimer's disease [29]. *QPRT-KO* mice showed increased QUIN levels in the brain [30] and increased excretion of QUIN in urine [31]. A significant increase of QUIN was observed in blood plasma of children with ASD when compared to their age-matched healthy control siblings [32]. Furthermore, QPRT was identified as an interaction partner of the ASD candidate neuroligin 3 (NLGN3; [33]), suggesting an involvement of QPRT in the formation of the postsynaptic density.

Here, we hypothesized that *QPRT* is implicated in neuronal differentiation and that reduced *QPRT* expression following its deletion results in alterations of neuromorphological development. We first tested the gene dosage-dependent expression of *QPRT* in a patient-specific LCL of one Chr16p11.2 deletion carrier. We then analyzed the expression of *QPRT* and its co-regulated gene set for correlation with the development of neuronal morphology in SH-SY5Y wild-type (WT) cells. To study the effects on neuronal morphology, we inhibited QPRT function in SH-SY5Y cells using (i) siRNA knockdown (KD), (ii) chemical mimicking of loss of QPRT, and (iii) complete CRISPR/Cas9-mediated knock out (KO). *QPRT-KD* cells underwent morphological analysis. Chemically inhibited and *QPRT-KO* cells were characterized using viability assays. To understand the effects of QPRT loss on the kynurenine pathway and QUIN levels, we additionally performed a metabolite analysis of the generated *QPRT-KO* cells. To explore the systems-wide interaction network of QPRT, we investigated the transcriptomic signature of *QPRT-KO* cells. Finally, to understand the role of *QPRT* in neural development, we tested the genes associated with *QPRT-KO* for enrichment among gene-networks implicated in human brain development [34].

Methods
Cellular models
Patient-specific lymphoblastoid cell lines (LCLs)
Lymphoblastoid cell lines (LCLs) were generated as previously published [35, 36]. We investigated LCLs generated from one Chr16p11.2 heterozygous deletion carrier and his non-carrier parents. The child was diagnosed with autism (ICD10: F84.0) based on both the Autism Diagnostic Interview-Revised (ADI-R; [37, 38]) and the Autism Observation Schedule (ADOS; [39]). The patient presented with a severe impairment of social interaction, hyperactive and aggressive behavior as well as language delay, and an average non-verbal IQ = 90. The deletion was identified in a screen of 710 children with ASD and their parents using the Illumina Human OmniExpress Microarray and validated via real-time PCR (unpublished data). To investigate *QPRT* gene expression at transcriptional level in exponentially growing cell cultures of the Chr16p11.2 deletion carrier compared to his non-carrier parents, 1×10^6 viable cells were inoculated into 5 ml RPMI medium supplied with 10% fetal bovine serum (FBS), 100 U/ml penicillin, 100 μg/ml streptomycin, 1X GlutaMAX (all from GIBCO®, Life Technologies, Paisley, UK). Volume was doubled when cultures reached a density of 1×10^6 cells/ml. Finally, cells were

harvested with a total volume of 20 ml at a density of again 1×10^6 cells/ml. Whole RNA was extracted, including DNase treatment, and reversely transcribed using the GeneJet RNA Purification Kit and the RevertAid H Minus first strand cDNA synthesis kit (both from Thermo Fisher Scientific) following the manufacturer's protocols. Real-time RT-PCR was performed using the Universal Probe Library (UPL; Roche) and a StepOne Plus device (Applied Biosystems) and normalized to *glucuronidase beta* (*GUSB*; see Additional file 1: Supplementary Methods and Table S1).

Neuroblastoma cell line SH-SY5Y

Out of possible cell types to investigate neuronal differentiation, SH-SY5Y is well studied, feasible, and with an optimized protocol shows reproducible differentiation of cells into cortical-like neurons [28]. For proliferation, cells were cultured in Dulbecco's modified Eagle's medium (DMEM) supplemented with 10% FBS, 1% sodium pyruvate (all from Life Technologies), and 1% penicillin/streptomycin (PAA). As described in our previous study [28], SH-SY5Y cells were differentiated using a continuous application of retinoic acid (RA) and brain-derived neurotrophic factor (BDNF). Differentiation media consisted of Neurobasal®-A medium supplemented with 1x GlutaMAX, 1x B-27 supplement (all from Life Technologies), 10 μM RA, 2 mM cAMP (both from Sigma-Aldrich), 50 ng/ml hBDNF (Immunotools), 1% penicillin/streptomycin (PAA), and 20 mM KCl. Cells were differentiated for 11 days changing the medium every other day. The time points for extraction of mRNA or protein and imaging were set 24 h after media changes (0/undifferentiated cells, 1, 3, 5, 7, 9, and 11 days of in vitro differentiation).

To study the morphological development of WT SH-SY5Y cells during neuronal differentiation, we transfected proliferating cells with pmaxGFP (Lonza) using Metafectene Pro (Biontex) according to the manufacturer's protocol. One day after transfection, cells were seeded 1:2 in co-cultures with untransfected cells with a density of 1×10^4 cells/cm^2 to allow imaging of individual transfected cells. Cultures were imaged using a Motic AE31 fluorescence microscope (Motic). Images were analyzed using custom macros in ImageJ [40] available on request. In short, all images were equalized, despeckled, and the background was subtracted using the rolling ball method prior to binarization (Auto threshold "Otsu-dark"). Sholl analysis [41], a concentric circle method, was performed using the respective ImageJ plugin with manual selection of the cells' center and with fitting polynomial regression of the fifth degree, as suggested by the manual [42]. The following morphological parameters were assessed: maximum intersections (maximum number of neuritic intersections for one radius), sum of intersections (sum of all intersections of one

cell), enclosing radius (the outer radius intersecting the cell, describing the longest distance between soma and neurites), intersecting radii (number of radii intersecting a cell, also describing the distance between soma and neurites), average number of intersections (the number of intersections analyzed divided by the number of intersecting radii; a measure describing neuritic complexity) and maximum intersections radius (the distance from the soma where most neurites are present, i.e., the site of the highest branching density; also reflecting neuritic complexity). Morphological parameters have been assessed in parallel during the previous transcriptomic analysis [28].

We made use of the previously published whole transcriptome data of differentiating SH-SY5Y cells (gene expression omnibus repository (GEO) under the accession number GSE69838 [28]) and analyzed *QPRT* expression as well as regulation of modules of co-expressed genes for correlation with the simultaneously assessed morphological parameters of SH-SY5Y neuronal differentiation (see also the "Statistical analysis" section below). Furthermore, *QPRT* expression during neuronal differentiation was validated in the same mRNA extracts using real-time RT-PCR. RNA extraction, cDNA generation, and real-time RT-PCR were performed as described above and in Additional file 1: Supplementary Methods. Expression values were normalized to *GUSB* and *glyceraldehyde-3-phosphate dehydrogenase* (*GAPDH*).

Reduction of QPRT in neuroblastoma cell line SH-SY5Y
siRNA-mediated knockdown (KD) of QPRT

QPRT expression in SH-SY5Y was reduced using three different siRNAs (siQ1–siQ3) and compared to a non-targeting control siRNA (siCtrl) using the Ambion Silencer Select siRNAs (Thermo Fisher; Additional file 1: Supplementary Methods). siRNA-generated KD of QPRT after 11 days of differentiation was proven in parallel to the morphological analysis on protein level via Western Blot as described in Additional file 1: Supplementary Methods. In short, QPRT (mouse anti-QPRT, Abcam) and control β-Actin (ACTB; mouse anti-β-Actin, Sigma) were detected using the secondary antibody anti-mouse IgG HRP-conjugated (Santa Cruz), the ECL Prime Western Blot Detection Reagent, and the Amersham Hyperfilm ECL (both from GE Healthcare). To allow imaging of fluorescent single cells in order to study morphological effects of *QPRT* knockdown, we co-transfected SH-SY5Y cells with mCherry (Plasmid #30125; Addgene). In a 96-well format, 5.2×10^4 cells/cm^2 were reversely transfected with 120 ng of mCherry and 5 nM siRNA using Lipofectamine RNAi Max and OptiMEM (Thermo Fisher).

CRISPR/Cas9 mediated knock out (KO) of QPRT
CRISPR/Cas9 gene editing was performed as described elsewhere [43]. In short, sgRNAs were designed [44] and

oligos were ordered from Sigma-Aldrich and cloned into pSpCas9(BB)-2A-Puro (PX459) V2.0 (Plasmid #62988; Addgene). Two sgRNAs targeting different sequences of *QPRT* were designed to generate homozygous knock out in addition to the non-targeting empty control vector (see Additional file 1: Supplementary Methods and Supplementary Results). Validated plasmids (Sanger sequencing) were transfected into SH-SY5Y cells using Metafectene Pro (Biontex) according to the manufacturer's protocol with subsequent puromycin (Sigma-Aldrich) selection using 750 ng/ml for 7 to 14 days. After low-density seeding, single clones were isolated using 5 μl of Trypsin-EDTA (Thermo Fisher Scientific) and expanded in 96-well plates. Overall, we sequenced at least ten clones per construct and confirmed homozygous single cell clones at least twice by Sanger sequencing including the empty control vector. Clones were named as follows: del268T (*QPRT* NM_014298 del268T; Ex2.1), ins395A (*QPRT* NM_014298 ins395A; Ex2.2), eCtrl (empty control vector). Both indels induced premature stop codons as validated in silico and by Sanger sequencing. KO of *QPRT* was further shown on RNA and protein level using real-time RT-PCR and Western Blot, respectively. RNA extraction, cDNA generation, and real-time RT-PCR as well as protein extraction and Western Blots were performed as described above and in Additional file 1: Supplementary Methods. RNA expression values were normalized to *GUSB* and *GAPDH*, and protein expression was descriptively compared to GAPDH expression.

Functional analyses in neuroblastoma cell line SH-SY5Y

siRNA-mediated KD of QPRT

The day after transfection (see above), media were changed from proliferation to differentiation media. After changing the media every other day for a time course of 11 days, cells were imaged using an ImageXPress Micro XLS (Molecular Devices). Images were pre-processed in MetaXPress and analyzed in ImageJ using Sholl analysis (as described above).

Chemical mimicking of QPRT loss

To measure the effect of chemical QPRT inhibition, we seeded WT SH-SY5Y cells with a density of 2.5×10^4 cells/cm^2. After cells have attached overnight, media were changed to either fresh proliferation or differentiation media containing 0 (reference), 5, or 10 mM of the QPRT inhibitor phthalic acid (PA; Sigma; directly diluted in the respective media; [45]) and incubated for 3 days followed by propidium iodide (PI) viability assays. PI and Hoechst33342 (both from Sigma) were pre-diluted in DPBS (Life Technologies) and used with final concentrations of 1 μg/ml and 10 μg/ml for the assay, respectively. Prior to analysis, supernatant including detached and dead cells was removed and attached cells were washed with DPBS. Next, attached cells were incubated with PI and Hoechst33342 for 5 min at 37 °C and imaged using the ImageXPress Micro XLS microscope (Molecular Devices). Images were acquired through DAPI and TRITC channels and analyzed using the MetaXPress macro "Cell Scoring". Percentage of dead cells after application of 5 and 10 mM PA was compared to the 0 mM reference for proliferating and differentiating cells, respectively.

To test if the observed cell death upon chemical inhibition of QPRT during differentiation is driven by an accumulation of the QPRT substrate quinolinic acid (QUIN; Sigma), we exposed WT cells to this neurotoxin. Cells were seeded with a density of 2.5×10^4 cells/cm^2 and media were changed after 24 h to either fresh proliferation or differentiation media containing 0 (reference; vehicle H$_2$O only), 5, or 250 μM of QUIN [46] and incubated for 3 days followed by PI viability-assays (as described above). Percentage of dead cells after application of 5 and 250 μM QUIN was compared to the 0 μM reference for proliferating and differentiating cells, respectively.

CRISPR/Cas9-mediated KO of QPRT

Viability assay To measure the effect of *QPRT-KO* on the viability of differentiating SH-SY5Y, KO and eCtrl cells were seeded at a density of 2.5×10^4 cells/cm^2. The following day, media were changed to differentiation media. After 3 days, PI viability-assays were performed (as described above).

Rescue experiments of *QPRT-KO* cells We further aimed to rescue the effects of a potential *QPRT-KO*-driven increase of QUIN by inhibiting downstream pathways. Cells were seeded with a density of 2.5×10^4 cells/cm^2. After 24 h, media were changed to differentiation media containing (i) 0 (reference; vehicle H$_2$O only), 6, and 12 μM of the NMDA-R antagonist MK801 [47], (ii) 0 (reference; vehicle H$_2$O only), 0.5, and 1 mM of nitric oxide synthase 1 (NOS1) inhibitor L-NAME [48], and (iii) 0 (reference; vehicle H$_2$O only), 5, and 10 mM of NAD$^+$ [49]. PI viability assays were performed after an incubation of 3 days (as described above). All rescue experiments were performed with differentiating *QPRT-KO* cell lines compared to the eCtrl.

Metabolite analysis To characterize *QPRT-KO* at the level of the kynurenine pathway, i.e., tryptophan catabolism, we analyzed its metabolites in cell culture supernatants using ultra-high-performance liquid chromatography (UHPLC; for tryptophan (TRP), kynurenine (KYN), 3-hydroxykynurenine (3HK), 3-hydroxyanthranilic acid (3HAA), anthranilic acid (AA) and kynurenic acid (KA)), and gas chromatography-mass spectrometry (GC/MS; for picolinic acid (PIC) and QUIN). Cell lines were seeded with a density of 2×10^4 cells/cm^2 and grown in proliferation or differentiation media for 3 days as described above. Supernatants of replicates were harvested and stored at -80 °C until further proceedings. UHPLC and GC/MS were performed as described previously [32, 50] (see also Additional file 1: Supplementary Methods).

Massive analysis of cDNA ends (MACE) To investigate the transcriptomic changes induced by *QPRT-KO*, we performed a whole transcriptome analysis using the RNA-Seq approach MACE. MACE sequencing in contrast to RNA sequencing reads cDNA ends only rather than whole transcripts, i.e., poly-A tails. The output values of MACE-Seq are absolute counts per cDNA end. This approach is more sensitive compared to classical RNA-Seq. This method allows the detection of low abundant transcripts and differentiation between alternative 3′UTRs with high accuracy [51, 52]. However, it does not allow to identify alternative exon usage.

Cell lines (three biological replicates of each WT, eCtrl, and KO cells) were seeded with a density of 2×10^4 cells/cm^2 in proliferation medium. After 3 days, media were changed to differentiation and cells were differentiated for 3 days without media changes. RNA was prepared as described above. RNA integrity number (RIN) was analyzed using the LabChip GX system and only samples with RINs above 9.7 underwent further analysis. MACE analysis including quality control was outsourced to GenXPro (Frankfurt) [53]. Reads were mapped to the human genome version hg38 using the Bowtie2 algorithm implementing the "--sensitive-local" parameter and standard settings as published [54].

A total of 12 genes found to be significantly differentially expressed in KO cells with an absolute log2 fold change (FC) above 2.5 were chosen for validation via real-time RT-PCR using the UPL system as described above with *GAPDH*, *GUSB*, and *proteasome 26S subunit, non-ATPase 7* (*PSMD7*) as housekeeping genes. Additionally, the GOIs *QPRT*, *nicotinamide nucleotide adenylyltransferase 2* (*NMNAT2*; only downstream enzyme of *QPRT* differentially regulated upon KO of *QPRT*), and *NLGN3* were included for validation (Additional file 1: Table S1).

Statistical analysis

If not stated otherwise, statistical analyses were performed using R version 3.2.3.

Group differences

Group differences between mRNA expression in LCLs of a deletion carrier compared to his non-carrier parents were tested using t test. Group differences of morphological parameters were tested using ANOVA and pairwise ANOVA (type III error) with Tukey's honest significant difference (HSD) correcting for multiple testing; Tukey's FDRs were considered significant below a threshold of FDR $\leq$ 0.05. Group differences between treated and untreated samples (e.g., PI assays) were tested using t test; uncorrected p values are reported. All samples were compared to their respective control (e.g., non-targeting siRNA) or reference (e.g., 0 mM of inhibitor).

Correlations

Correlation between morphological parameters and gene expression or eigengene expression was tested based on the Pearson's product moment correlation coefficient following a t-distribution. Reported p values are Bonferroni corrected for 126 tests (6 morphological parameters, 20 gene modules, 1 gene expression).

Targeted mRNA expression

Data of real-time RT-PCR experiments were analyzed using the $2^{\Delta\Delta Ct}$ method [55]. Group differences were tested using t test. For validation of RNA-Seq data, real-time RT-PCR data and RNA-Seq (MACE) normalized reads were tested for correlation as described above using Pearson's correlation tests.

Transcriptome analysis

Overall 32,739 transcripts were targeted by MACE analysis and defined as the gene universe (reference gene panel). Differentially expressed genes were identified using the "DESeq2" pipeline [56] with the gene expression as the dependent variable and the respective groups as the independent variable. No additional covariates have been included since the samples did not differ with respect to RIN, number of total counts, or batch. Hierarchical cluster analysis using the top 2000 genes based on variance was performed to exclude any technical outlier samples (for detailed quality checks see Additional file 1: Figure S6). Four different cell lines underwent MACE analysis: the untreated wild-type (WT), the empty control vector (eCtrl), the KO cell line *QPRT$^{-/-}$* del268T, and the KO cell line *QPRT$^{-/-}$* ins395A. Three technical replicates were sequenced for each cell line. Differential gene expression induced by *QPRT-KO* was assessed by comparing (i) WT vs eCtrl, (ii) eCtrl vs KO del268T as well as (iii) eCtrl vs KO ins395A independently. A gene was considered to be significantly associated with *QPRT-KO* if (i) no significant change was identified between the WT and the eCtrl cell line (FDR > 0.1), (ii) if a significant (FDR < 0.05) difference was observed between both the eCtrl and KO del268T and between eCtrl and KO ins395A, and (iii) the direction of the effect was the same in both of the comparisons eCtrl vs KO del268T and eCtrl vs KO ins395A, respectively. For the differential expression analysis between two groups, raw counts of the respective replicates were loaded into DESeq2 using the "DESeqDataSetFromMatrix" function. Differential expression was estimated using the function "DESeq" with the option "fitType = 'local'". Significantly up and downregulated genes underwent GO term analysis (Additional file 1: Supplementary Methods). Genes surviving quality check (more than 10 reads per gene in at least 6 of the 12 samples) were subjected to weighted gene co-expression network analysis (WGCNA; Additional file 1: Supplementary Methods).

Gene list enrichment test in gene networks of brain development

To gain a deeper insight into the brain-specific effects of up and downregulated genes from MACE analysis, we used part of a framework proposed by Yousaf et al. [57]. In short, this framework uses the Allen Brain Atlas dataset of Kang and colleagues, who have identified 29 co-regulated gene sets using the spatiotemporal transcriptome of the human brain from early embryonal development to late adulthood [34]. Each module corresponds to specific biological processes involved in brain development and aging. We tested these modules for enrichment with the sets of genes up or downregulated upon QPRT-KO in SH-SY5Y using Fisher's exact tests. Expression patterns of the enriched modules were then visualized using heatmaps of the eigenvalues of the respective modules for each human brain region over time.

Results

Patient-specific lymphoblastoid cell lines (LCLs)

To replicate previous reports [11] of altered QPRT expression in 16p11.2 CNV carriers, we compared QPRT expression in a patient-specific LCL of a deletion carrier and his unaffected parents. We confirmed a dosage dependent expression of QPRT at mRNA level (16p11.2 deletion carrier vs. non-carrier parents; logFC = − 0.68, $p = 0.014$; Additional file 1: Figure S1a).

Correlation of QPRT and neuritic complexity in SH-SY5Y wild-type cells

RNA expression of QPRT during SH-SY5Y differentiation significantly correlated between microarray [28] and real-time RT-PCR ($\rho = 0.88$; $p = 0.0098$; Additional file 1: Figure S1b). Further, we used the expression data of QPRT as well as of the modules of genes co-regulated during neuronal differentiation and tested them for their correlation with morphological parameters using Sholl analysis during 11 days of neuronal differentiation (Additional file 1: Figure S1c and d). Both QPRT expression and the eigenvalue of its associated module (MEorange) significantly

correlated with the average number of intersections (QPRT microarray: $\rho = 0.86$, FDR = 8.16E−05; QPRT RT-PCR: $\rho = 0.54$, FDR = 0.020; MEorange: $\rho = 0.93$, FDR = 1.71E−07; Additional file 1: Figure S1d).

In summary, we report a correlative association between QPRT expression and a measure for the development of neurite complexity during in vitro neuronal differentiation of wild-type SH-SY5Y cells. To investigate if the correlation of QPRT expression with neuritic complexity is causal or secondary, i.e., due to the progressive neurite growth over time, we performed functional inhibition analysis of QPRT.

Functional validation in neuroblastoma cell line SH-SY5Y
siRNA mediated knockdown (KD) of QPRT

All three siRNAs targeting three different sites of QPRT (named here siQ1–siQ3) induced a decrease in QPRT protein after 11 days of differentiation as confirmed by Western Blot (Fig. 1a). At neuromorphological level, KD cell lines compared to control cell lines (siCtrl) showed a significant decrease of the maximum intersections radius, altering neuritic complexity in that the site of highest branching density was shifted closer towards the soma (p siQ1 0.027, siQ2 0.001, siQ3 3.8E−04; means [SD] siCtrl 103.98[115.54]; siQ1 56.50[80.53]; siQ2 56.29[97.17]; siQ3 41.51[76.70]). The overall cell size or the enclosing radius, did not change upon KD of QPRT (all $p > 0.6$; means [SD] siCtrl 349.60[223.68]; siQ1 286.98[125.05]; siQ2 270.06 [135.62]; siQ3 293.81[176.86]; Fig. 1a; Additional file 1: Figure S2).

Mimicking of QPRT loss

Cells exposed to an inhibitor of QPRT, the chemical phthalic acid (PA), showed an increased cell death upon induction of differentiation, and thus no end-point morphological analysis was performed. Application of PA for 3 days led to a dosage-dependent increase of cell death during differentiation (5 mM PA: FC = 1.81, $p = 0.019$; 10 mM PA: FC = 4.21, $p = 0.039$) but not during proliferation (5 mM PA: FC = 0.73, $p = 0.432$; 10 mM PA: FC = 0.68, $p = 0.355$; Fig. 1b).

We further hypothesized that inhibition of QPRT might lead to increased levels of its neurotoxic substrate quinolinic acid (QUIN). Thus, we exposed wild-type cells to elevated QUIN levels. However, we did neither observe an increase in cell death during proliferation (all $p > 0.3$ for 5 μM and 250 μM QUIN) nor during differentiation (all $p > 0.3$ for 5 μM and 250 μM QUIN; Additional file 1: Figure S5a) compared to vehicle only (0 μM). Since the findings from chemical inhibition and mimicking of QPRT inhibition suggested that QPRT is causally linked to differentiation deficits independent of its substrate QUIN, we aimed at elucidating the

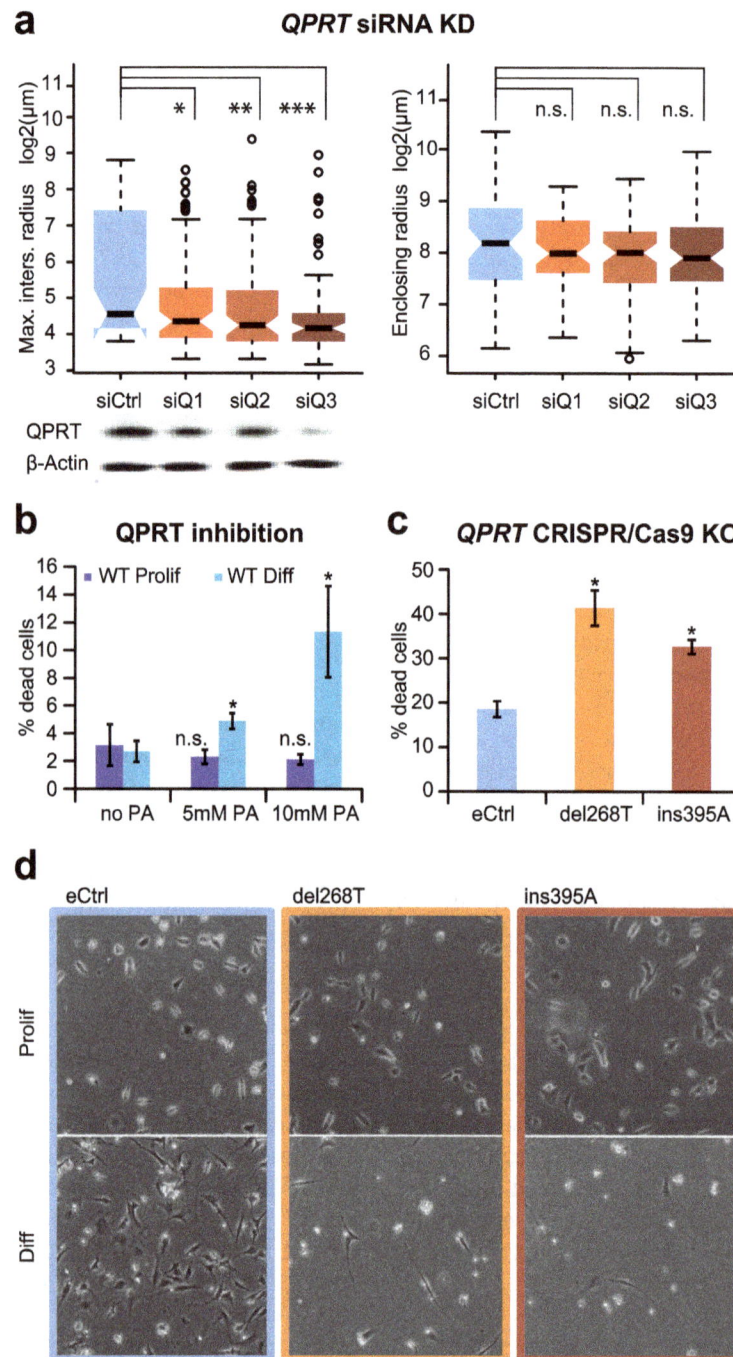

Fig. 1 Functional analysis of *QPRT* in SH-SY5Y cells. **a** siRNA-mediated knockdown (KD) of *QPRT*. Cells were transfected with a non-targeting siRNA (siCtrl) and three different siRNAs targeting *QPRT* (siQ1–siQ3). Transfected cells were differentiated for 11 days followed by morphological analysis. Knockdown of QPRT was confirmed at protein level. Upon *QPRT-KD*, cells showed a significant decrease of the maximum intersections radius when compared to the non-targeting control, i.e., the maximum complexity of neurites was significantly closer to the cell soma. None of the three KDs differed with respect to the enclosing radius when compared to the non-target control, i.e., the length of the neurites was not different (Additional file 1: Figure S2). Maximum intersections radius: radial distance of the maximum number of intersections from the cell body. Enclosing radius: outer radius intersecting the cell. All *p* values were corrected for multiple testing using Tukey's HSD correction. **b** Chemical inhibition of *QPRT*. Application of the QPRT inhibitor phthalic acid (PA) for 3 days led to a dose-dependent significant increase of cell death in differentiating wild-type SH-SY5Y cells. In proliferating cells, QPRT inhibition did not change the rate of cell death. **c** Viability assays of CRISPR/Cas9 mediated *QPRT-knock out* (KO) cells. Percentage of cell death was assessed performing viability assays after 3 days of differentiation showing a significant increase of cell death in both generated *QPRT-KO* cell lines. **d** Representative images of *QPRT-KO* cells after differentiation. KO of *QPRT* led to observable cell death during 9 days of differentiation but not during proliferation

underlying processes in SH-SY5Y cells with a stable loss of *QPRT*.

CRISPR/Cas9 mediated knock out (KO) of QPRT

Generation and viability Using two separate sgRNA sequences (see Additional file 1: Supplementary Methods and Supplementary Results), we generated two homozygous *QPRT-KO* cell lines, del268T and ins395A (NM_014298), both of which showed a nearly complete loss of expression of *QPRT* mRNA expression (proliferating cell lines: del268T: below detection limits, ins395A: FC = 0.17, p = 0.046; 2 days of differentiation: del268T: FC = 0.13, p = 0.003; ins395A: FC = 0.15, p = 0.003; all compared to the proliferating empty control vector (eCtrl); Additional file 1: Figures S3 and S4). For proliferating cells, QPRT-KO was furthermore descriptively confirmed at protein level (Additional file 1: Figure S4). While the eCtrl and both *QPRT-KO* cell lines were growing comparably during proliferation, both KO cell lines died upon differentiation. After 3 days of differentiation, we observed a significant increase of cell death in the KO cell lines when compared to eCtrl cells harboring the empty control vector (eCtrl to del268T: FC = 2.23, p = 8.2E−04; eCtrl to ins395A: FC = 1.76, p = 5.2E−04; Fig. 1c), and after 9 days of differentiation, merely no differentiating KO cells were detected under the microscope (Fig. 1d).

Rescue experiments using small compounds We tried to rescue the *QPRT-KO* effect by inhibiting the effector pathways downstream of QUIN, i.e., inhibit a potentially induced neurotoxicity by hyperactivation of NMDA-R as well as replenish NAD$^+$, which is the downstream metabolite of QPRT as well as the final outcome of the kynurenine pathway. Neither the NMDA-R antagonist MK801 (both *QPRT-KO* compared to eCtrl: FC > 1.7, p < 3.9E−03 for 0 μM; FC > 1.6, p < 0.04 for 6 μM; FC > 1.6, p < 1.5E−03 for 12 μM) nor the inhibition of the NMDA-R downstream enzyme NOS1 by L-NAME (both *QPRT-KO* compared to eCtrl: FC > 1.3, p < 0.05 for 0 mM; FC > 1.3, p < 0.02 for 0.5 mM; FC > 1.5, p < 0.01 for 1 mM) nor supplying NAD$^+$, the downstream product of tryptophan catabolism (both *QPRT-KO* compared to eCtrl: FC > 1.3, p < 9E−03 for 0 mM; FC > 1.3, p < 1.6E−03 for 5 mM; del268T compared to eCtrl: FC = 1.20, p = 0.1; ins395A compared to eCtrl: FC = 1.54, p = 0.009 for 10 mM), resulted in a significant reduction of cell death for both of the KO cell lines upon differentiation (Additional file 1: Figure S5b).

Metabolite analysis To test if the loss of *QPRT* results in an altered metabolite profile of the kynurenine pathway, we implemented UHPLC and GC/MS analysis. We

were able to detect tryptophan (TRP), kynurenine (KYN), kynurenic acid (KA), 3-hydroxykynurenine (3HK), anthranilic acid (AA), and picolinic acid (PA). QUIN could not be detected in any of the samples, while 3-hydroxyanthranilic acid (3HAA) could only be detected in the differentiated (eCtrl and both of the KO) cell lines only. However, no significant changes could be observed in any of the metabolites when comparing both of the *QPRT-KO* cell lines to the control cell lines (Additional file 1: Figure S5c).

MACE transcriptome analysis of QPRT-KO Since in our cell model the effect of *QPRT-KO* on neuronal differentiation was not related to changes in the kynurenine pathway or the neurotoxic effects of QUIN, we aimed to further elucidate the effect of the KO on differentiating cells implementing a transcriptome-wide analysis. Overall, we were able to measure the expression of 32,739 transcripts (Additional file 2: Table S2). Statistical analysis identified 269 differentially regulated genes (103 upregulated and 166 downregulated; Fig. 2a; Additional file 2: Table S2) expressed in all three replicates of both KO cell lines, all with an FDR ≤ 0.05. The 12 genes (Table 1) with an absolute log2FC > 2.5 were technically validated using real-time RT-PCR with an average correlation between RNA sequencing data and real-time RT-PCR of ρ = 0.91 (SD = 0.10). *QPRT-KO* was also confirmed (eCtrl vs del268T: log2FC = − 2.44, FDR = 1.07E−207; eCtrl vs ins395A: log2FC = − 3.17, FDR = 9.88E−291). Of the genes coding for components of the kynurenine pathway, only *NMNAT2* was significantly downregulated upon *QPRT-KO* (eCtrl vs del268T: log2FC = − 0.70, FDR = 2.10E−07; eCtrl vs ins395A: log2FC = − 1.51, FDR = 6.70E−28). The ASD-implicated protein NLGN3 was differentially downregulated in the del268T only (eCtrl vs del268T: log2FC = − 0.43, FDR = 6.58E−02; eCtrl vs ins395A log2FC = − 0.09, FDR = 9.15E−01) and was thus not considered to be regulated upon KO of *QPRT*.

The genes upregulated upon KO of *QPRT* were enriched (all p values < 0.05, Fig. 2b; Additional file 3: Table S3) for GO annotated biological processes involved in neurotransmitter secretion, regulation of synapse structure, or activation (Fig. 2b) but also negative regulation of cell growth and negative regulation of cytoskeleton organization among others (Additional file 3: Table S3). In addition, upregulated genes were enriched for the GO term apoptotic process involved in morphogenesis via the genes *BCL2 antagonist/killer 1* (*BAK1*) and *scribbled planar cell polarity protein* (*SCRIB*). Genes downregulated in KO cell lines showed enrichment for GO terms including synapse organization, modulation of excitatory postsynaptic potentials, or glutamate secretion (Fig. 2b) or positive regulation of neuron differentiation, positive regulation of dendritic spine development as

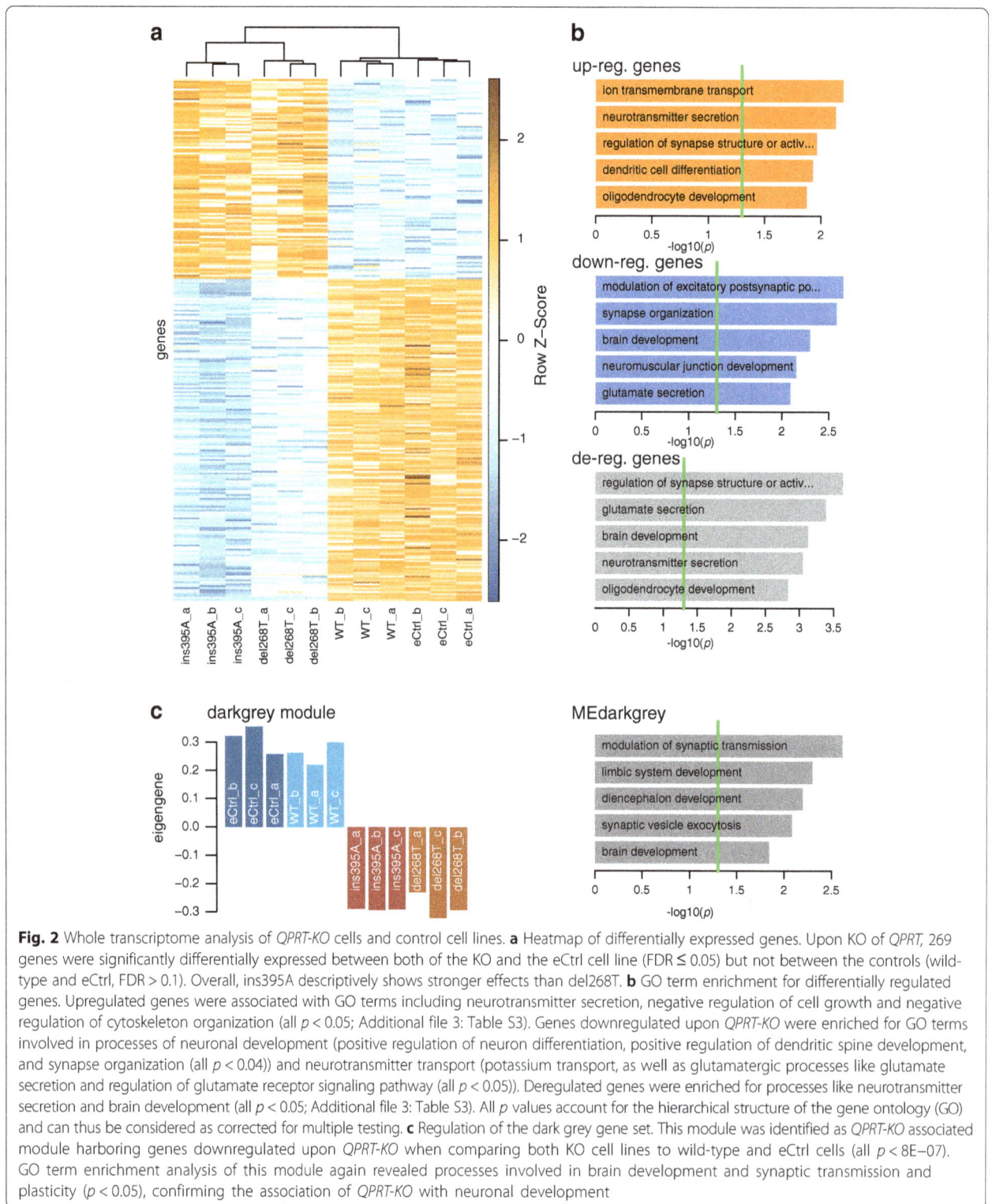

Fig. 2 Whole transcriptome analysis of *QPRT-KO* cells and control cell lines. **a** Heatmap of differentially expressed genes. Upon KO of *QPRT,* 269 genes were significantly differentially expressed between both of the KO and the eCtrl cell line (FDR ≤ 0.05) but not between the controls (wild-type and eCtrl, FDR > 0.1). Overall, ins395A descriptively shows stronger effects than del268T. **b** GO term enrichment for differentially regulated genes. Upregulated genes were associated with GO terms including neurotransmitter secretion, negative regulation of cell growth and negative regulation of cytoskeleton organization (all $p < 0.05$; Additional file 3: Table S3). Genes downregulated upon *QPRT-KO* were enriched for GO terms involved in processes of neuronal development (positive regulation of neuron differentiation, positive regulation of dendritic spine development, and synapse organization (all $p < 0.04$)) and neurotransmitter transport (potassium transport, as well as glutamatergic processes like glutamate secretion and regulation of glutamate receptor signaling pathway (all $p < 0.05$)). Deregulated genes were enriched for processes like neurotransmitter secretion and brain development (all $p < 0.05$; Additional file 3: Table S3). All p values account for the hierarchical structure of the gene ontology (GO) and can thus be considered as corrected for multiple testing. **c** Regulation of the dark grey gene set. This module was identified as *QPRT-KO* associated module harboring genes downregulated upon *QPRT-KO* when comparing both KO cell lines to wild-type and eCtrl cells (all $p < 8E-07$). GO term enrichment analysis of this module again revealed processes involved in brain development and synaptic transmission and plasticity ($p < 0.05$), confirming the association of *QPRT-KO* with neuronal development

well as ion transmembrane transport (Fig. 2b; Additional file 3: Table S3). We also observed significant enrichment for ASD genes among highly differentially regulated candidates. Of the 269 differentially regulated genes, 15 were listed in the SFARI gene [58] with an evidence score of 4 or better ($p = 9.2E-04$, odds ratio OR [95% confidence interval] = 2.68 [1.47–4.54]), for example *gamma-aminobutyric acid type A receptor beta 3 subunit (GABRB3), potassium voltage-gated channel subfamily Q member 3 (KCNQ3), syntrophin*

Table 1 Differentially expressed genes upon *QPRT-KO* with |log2FC| > 2.5

Gene	Chr	del268T vs eCtrl		ins395A vs eCtrl		WT vs eCtrl		SFARI score	ASD literature
		FDR	log2FC	FDR	log2FC	FDR	log2FC		
COX17	3q13.33	3.33E−138	− 5.94	1.78E−154	− 5.63	0.30	− 0.13	/	/
GUCA1A	6p21.1	4.56E−41	− 5.38	3.97E−46	− 5.88	0.20	0.26	/	/
COX17P1	13q14.13	1.09E−84	− 5.19	5.82E−93	− 5.28	0.59	− 0.11	/	/
VSTM2A	7p11.2	1.81E−10	− 5.00	6.36E−12	− 5.28	0.61	− 0.27	/	/
KCNQ3	8q24.22	5.77E−04	− 4.76	1.25E03	− 3.04	0.46	0.49	3	Role for KCNQ3 in epilepsy and autism [75]
CCK	3p22.1	2.56E−04	− 3.18	5.97E−05	− 3.13	0.17	0.68	/	Candidate gene for Asperger's in a microdeletion case study [76]
GABRB3	15q12	3.04E−43	− 3.00	9.43E−54	− 3.58	0.80	0.04	2	CNV Chr15q11-13 implicated in ASD; polymorphisms associated with ASD [62, 77]
BRINP1	9q33.1	8.93E−09	− 2.92	2.09E−09	− 2.85	0.20	− 0.53	/	−/− mice: autism-like behavior including reduced sociability and altered vocalization [78]
LINC01760	1p21.3	1.02E−02	2.74	4.93E−03	2.62	0.95	− 0.30	/	/
SNTG2	2p25.3	7.04E−04	− 2.71	5.06E−07	− 5.58	0.72	0.22	4	Region linked with ID [64], associated with ASD [65]; interaction partner of neuroligins, interaction altered by ASD associated mutations [66]
ARHGAP20	11q23.1	1.63E−09	− 2.65	4.08E−15	− 3.93	0.45	− 0.30	/	/
SRRM4	12q24.23	1.29E−18	− 2.61	2.25E−26	− 3.40	0.54	− 0.20	/	−/+ mice: multiple autistic-like features [79]

Chr chromosomal region, *del268T* CRISPR/Cas9 induced mutation (deletion of one nucleotide) in exon 2 of QPRT, *ins395A* CRISPR/Cas9-induced mutation (insertion of one nucleotide) in exon 2 of QPRT, *eCtrl* control cell line with empty CRISPR/Cas9 control vector, *WT* wild-type SH-SY5Y cell line untreated, *FDR* False discovery rate, *log2 FC* log2 fold change, *SFARI score* score in the SFARI database [58] (a smaller score means higher evidence), *ASD references* Pubmed was searched for "gene and autism" and "gene and ASD"

gamma 2 (*SNTG2*), or *contactin associated protein-like 2* (*CNTNAP2*).

A total of eleven out of 166 downregulated genes and one gene of 103 upregulated genes showed a |log2FC| > 2.5 (Table 1). Literature search for these twelve highly regulated genes revealed that six had been published in the context of ASD before (Table 1).

Gene network analysis At gene network level, we identified 20 co-regulated modules upon KO. Here, *QPRT* was co-regulated within a module associated with modulation of synaptic transmission, synaptic vesicle exocytosis, or limbic system and diencephalon development (Fig. 2c) as well as neurotransmitter secretion or negative regulation of neurogenesis ($p < 0.04$). Overall, the eigenvalue of this module was not different between controls and KOs. We identified one co-regulated gene set (dark grey, Fig. 2c) to be associated with *QPRT-KO* as it was significantly downregulated in both KO cell lines when compared to the control cell lines (KOs versus eCtrl or WT, all $p < 8E-07$). GO term enrichment analysis of this module again revealed processes involved in brain development and synaptic transmission and plasticity ($p < 0.05$; Fig. 2c; Additional file 3: Table S3), confirming the association of *QPRT-KO* with neuronal development.

Translation to developmental brain expression data Finally, we aimed to translate the effects of *QPRT-KO* onto the spatial and temporal gene expression network

of the brain using previously published data [34]. In this previous work, the authors report 29 gene modules (termed "Kang-Module" in the following) that are co-regulated during the development of human brain regions. We observe that the *QPRT-KO*-induced downregulated genes were strongly enriched in the Kang-Modules number 1 (odds ratio OR [95% confidence interval] = 8.86 [3.12–20.45], $p = 5.76E-04$), number 2 (OR = 5.96 [3.55–9.75], $p = 2.21E09$), number 10 (OR = 69.92 [20.70–188.44], $p = 2.64E-07$), number 15 (OR = 14.58 [6.00–30.72], $p = 1.57E-06$) and number 20 (OR = 7.13 [4.40–11.40], $p = 7.74E-13$) while the *QPRT-KO* up-regulated genes were enriched in Kang-Modules number 2 (OR = 23.20 [11.25–49.97], $p = 1.07E-16$) and number 20 (OR = 3.54 [1.46–7.76], $p = 4.18E-02$). Kang-Module 17 was enriched for *QPRT-KO*-induced deregulated genes in general, i.e., for the merged lists of up and downregulated genes (OR = 20.41 [2.33–82.57], $p = 2.45E-02$; Fig. 3a). By plotting the eigengene value of the Kang-Module over time for each region, we observed that number 1 shows strong early upregulation in the hippocampus (HIP) and the amygdala (AMY) during embryonal development while it is downregulated in all tested brain regions after birth (Fig. 3b). Kang-Module 1 is also slightly upregulated in embryonal development in parts of the frontal cortex (orbitofrontal cortex (OFC), dorsolateral prefrontal cortex (DFC) and medial prefrontal cortex (MFC)), the striatum (STR), and the cerebellar cortex (CBC). Kang-Module 2 is overall

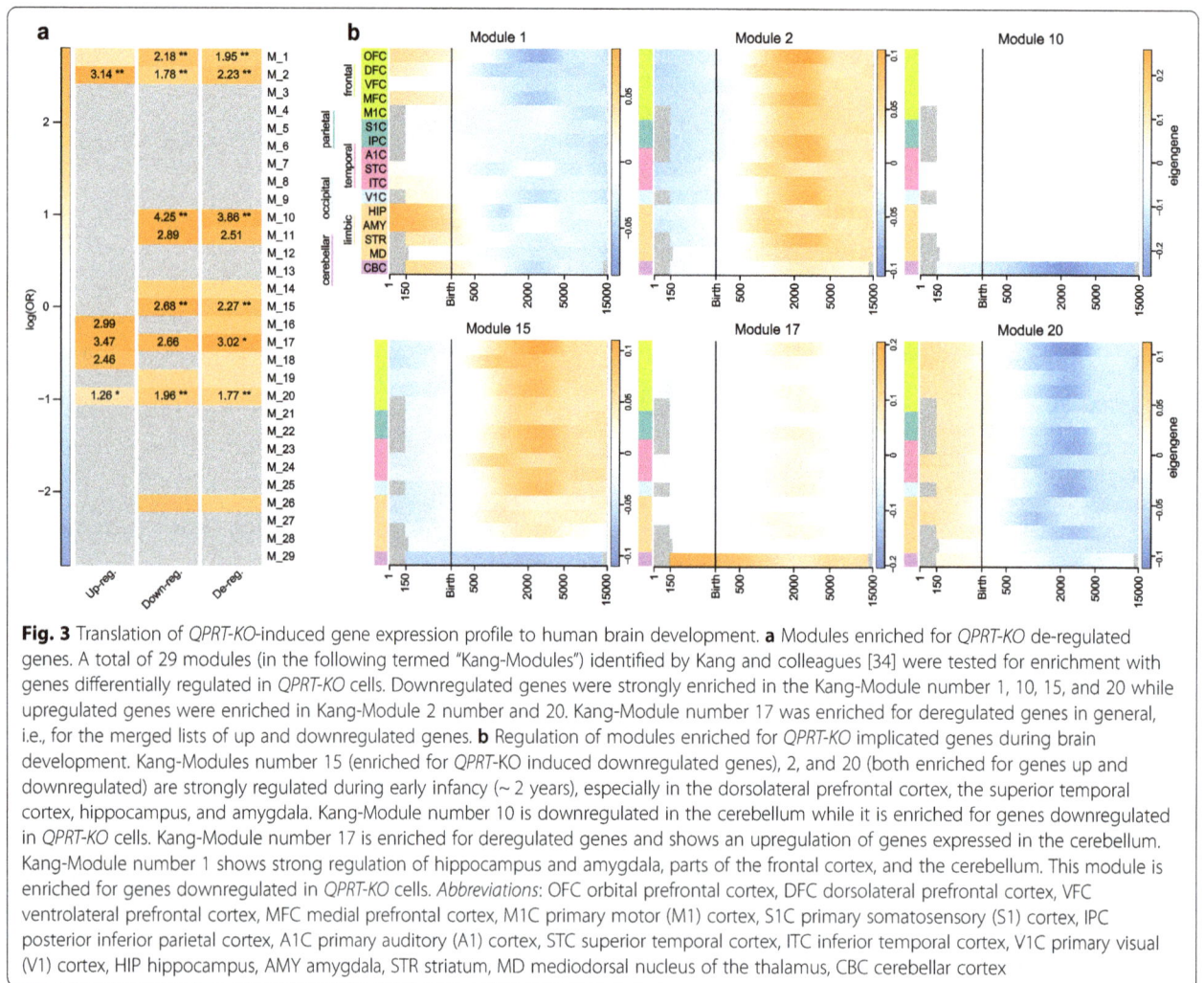

Fig. 3 Translation of *QPRT-KO*-induced gene expression profile to human brain development. **a** Modules enriched for *QPRT-KO* de-regulated genes. A total of 29 modules (in the following termed "Kang-Modules") identified by Kang and colleagues [34] were tested for enrichment with genes differentially regulated in *QPRT-KO* cells. Downregulated genes were strongly enriched in the Kang-Module number 1, 10, 15, and 20 while upregulated genes were enriched in Kang-Module 2 number and 20. Kang-Module number 17 was enriched for deregulated genes in general, i.e., for the merged lists of up and downregulated genes. **b** Regulation of modules enriched for *QPRT-KO* implicated genes during brain development. Kang-Modules number 15 (enriched for *QPRT*-KO induced downregulated genes), 2, and 20 (both enriched for genes up and downregulated) are strongly regulated during early infancy (~ 2 years), especially in the dorsolateral prefrontal cortex, the superior temporal cortex, hippocampus, and amygdala. Kang-Module number 10 is downregulated in the cerebellum while it is enriched for genes downregulated in *QPRT-KO* cells. Kang-Module number 17 is enriched for deregulated genes and shows an upregulation of genes expressed in the cerebellum. Kang-Module number 1 shows strong regulation of hippocampus and amygdala, parts of the frontal cortex, and the cerebellum. This module is enriched for genes downregulated in *QPRT-KO* cells. *Abbreviations*: OFC orbital prefrontal cortex, DFC dorsolateral prefrontal cortex, VFC ventrolateral prefrontal cortex, MFC medial prefrontal cortex, M1C primary motor (M1) cortex, S1C primary somatosensory (S1) cortex, IPC posterior inferior parietal cortex, A1C primary auditory (A1) cortex, STC superior temporal cortex, ITC inferior temporal cortex, V1C primary visual (V1) cortex, HIP hippocampus, AMY amygdala, STR striatum, MD mediodorsal nucleus of the thalamus, CBC cerebellar cortex

downregulated prenatally and shows upregulation after birth, with maximum expression between the ages of 6 and 14, i.e., during middle and late childhood in OFC, MFC, posterior inferior parietal cortex (IPC), primary auditory (A1) cortex (A1C), inferior temporal cortex (ITC), primary visual (V1) cortex (V1C), and STR. Kang-Module 10 is only expressed in the CBC with a peak around the age of 6 years, while Kang-Module 15 is strongly downregulated during embryonal development in the CBC. The low expression of Kang-Module 15 in the CBC is stable across the tested time course, and it is slightly upregulated in other brain regions, showing peaks between the years 6 and 14 in OFC, DFC, ventrolateral prefrontal cortex (VFC), MFC, IPC, A1C, ITC, and V1C. Kang-Module 17 shows a constant active expression in the CBC over time with a peak during early development in the CBC. Kang-Module 20 is an overall early upregulated gene network downregulated after the age of ~ 2 years, showing the

strongest downregulation between the years 6 and 14 in OFC, MFC, IPC, A1C, ITC, V1C, and STR.

Discussion

Based on our differential analysis, we report a causal relation between *QPRT*, located in the ASD-associated CNV region Chr16p11.2 and neuronal differentiation of SH-SY5Y cells. A gene dosage reduction or inhibition of QPRT affects morphological parameters during neuronal differentiation as well as the regulation of genes and gene networks that were previously implicated in ASD. This includes processes like synapse organization or brain development. In summary, our findings suggest a neurodevelopmental role for *QPRT* in the etiology of ASD in 16p11.2 deletion carriers.

As expected from previous findings [11], in one deletion carrier with ASD, we confirmed that *QPRT* was expressed in a gene dosage-dependent manner strengthening the role of *QPRT* as a potential risk gene in the pathology of Chr16p11.2 deletion syndrome. By comparing our previously published transcriptome data of SH-SY5Y wild-type cells [28] to the morphological changes during neuronal differentiation described in the present study, we found *QPRT* to be correlated with the development of the neuritic complexity. These results suggest a potential regulatory link between *QPRT* and neuronal maturation. Our findings of the KD and KO cell models further underline this interpretation: the KD of *QPRT* led to subtle changes of SH-SY5Y neuronal complexity in line with previous reports using mouse models of Chr16p11.2 [17] as well as iPS cells generated from 16p11.2 CNV carriers [59] and post-mortem studies of ASD individuals [1]. Inhibition of QPRT activity as well as genetic KO both led to cell death of differentiating but not proliferating cells. These findings suggest that enough protein is left for the survival of differentiating cells upon KD of QPRT while the loss of QPRT is lethal for differentiating SH-SY5Y cells. Interestingly, the administration of the QPRT substrate QUIN, which is a potent excitotoxin, did not show any effect on neither proliferating nor differentiating cells. Previous findings suggested that a reduction of QPRT, the only enzyme catabolizing quinolinic acid (QUIN), leads to an accumulation of QUIN, which in turn may induce neuronal cell death by over-activating NMDA-R and increase nitric oxide (NO) production [46]. Altered QUIN levels could also lead to a change in NAD$^+$ production which in turn could change poly (ADP-ribose) polymerase (PARP) activity [60]. In *QPRT-KO* mice, the striatum showed an accumulation of QUIN leading to neurodegeneration [30] as well as altered expression of enzymes of the kynurenine pathway and of NMDA-receptors. No ASD-like behaviors were studied in these mice, but the animals showed no growth or developmental abnormalities. As the kynurenine pathway was associated with Parkinson's disease [61], the authors performed a behavioral test measuring the stride length of WT and KO mice. Indeed, they reported shorter stride lengths in aged but not middle-aged *QPRT-KO* mice as usually seen in mouse models of Parkinson's disease [30]. In another study, no differences of histological features of the cerebrum of *QPRT-KO* mice were observed [31]. Although we were not able to mimic QPRT loss in WT cells by application of increased QUIN levels, we tried to rescue differentiating QPRT-KO cells from cell death during differentiation by modulation of QUIN-related metabolism and signaling. Inhibition of NMDA-receptors was expected to protect *QPRT-KO* cells from the possible QUIN-induced excitotoxicity. However, the application of different concentrations of an NMDA-R inhibitor did not prevent cell death. Similarly, inhibition of NOS1 with the aim to reduce the production of NO did not affect viability. Finally, we tried to increase the viability of differentiating cells via the application of NAD$^+$ to rescue PARP activity. Again, *QPRT-KO* cells could not be rescued from cell death during differentiation. In accordance with these observations, *QPRT-KO* cells did not show changes in the expression levels of any genes coding for PARP enzymes. In addition, QUIN could not be detected in any of our samples, and none of the metabolites of tryptophan catabolism was significantly changed upon KO of *QPRT* in the performed metabolite assays. Taken together, we conclude that the detrimental effect of QPRT loss on viability during SH-SY5Y differentiation is independent of QUIN levels as well as of QUIN-induced metabolic changes or the kynurenine pathway in general.

To elucidate the underlying mechanisms of *QPRT-KO*-induced cell death during SH-SY5Y neuronal differentiation, we performed a hypothesis-free transcriptomic approach. These findings suggest that loss of *QPRT* may lead to an increased negative regulation of cytoskeleton organization and to an inhibition of neuronal differentiation and dendritic spine development. In our KD model, we observed an alteration of neuritic complexity, which strongly supports the functional role of *QPRT* in these processes.

The functional association of *QPRT* with ASD is supported by the following results of our study: *QPRT-KO* led to inhibition of *GABRB3*, which has been well established as an ASD risk gene [62]. *GABRB3* codes for a subunit of an inhibitory GABA receptor. It is located on Chr15q11-13, a region strongly implicated in ASD [63]. Similarly, the gene *SNTG2* also downregulated in *QPRT-KO* cells, codes for a synaptic scaffolding protein involved in actin and PDZ domain binding. *SNTG2* is located in 2p25.3, a region linked to intellectual disability [64] and associated with ASD [65]. Furthermore, SNTG2 protein interacts with *neuroligins* (*NLGN*), and this interaction is altered by ASD associated mutations in the *NLGN* genes [66]. QPRT was also found to physically interact with NLGN3 (neuroligin 3; [33]). Although the function of this interaction is still unclear, it is likely that QPRT is involved in the formation of the postsynaptic density of GABAergic neurons. *KCNQ3*, another ASD candidate gene, downregulated upon *QPRT-KO*, encodes a protein regulating neuronal excitability. Variants of this gene were found to be implicated in the development of ASD and epilepsies [67]. Finally, we also found *CNTNAP2*, a well-replicated risk gene for ASD [68] located in 7q22-q36, to be downregulated in *QPRT-KO* cells. In a previous study, we reported *CNTNAP2* promoter variants reducing transcription to be risk factors for ASD [69].

Besides ASD-associated differentially regulated genes, we report six novel candidates (i.e., *COX17*, *GUCA1A*, *COX17P1*, *VSTM2A*, *LINC01760*, and *ARHGAP20*). At this stage, we cannot find any link to neuronal development for the photoreceptor-associated *guanylate cyclase activator 1A GUCA1A*, the preadipocyte development implicated *V-set and transmembrane domain containing 2A VSTM2A* gene, and the long intergenic non-coding RNA *LINC01760*. However, the *cytochrome c oxidase copper chaperone COX17* (and its pseudogene *COX17P1*) and the *Rho GTPase-activating protein 20 ARHGAP20* are functionally related to neuronal development: COX17 is part of the terminal component of the mitochondrial respiratory chain, catalyzing the electron transfer from reduced cytochrome c to oxygen, and might thus be involved in the regulation of oxidative stress and energy metabolism, both processes that have previously been associated with ASD [36]. The ARHGAP20 enzyme is implicated in neurite outgrowth and thus potentially associated with the here observed neuromorphological phenotypes [70].

Translating the in vitro transcriptomic effect of *QPRT-KO* in SH-SY5Y cells to the gene networks active during human brain development [34], we observed differentially regulated genes to be enriched in modules previously associated with cell cycle regulation (Kang-Module 1), transcription factors regulating progenitor cell fate (Kang Module 20), neuronal development (Kang-Module 10 and 20), morphogenesis (Kang Modules 17 and 2), and synaptic transmission (Kang-Module 2 and 15). In addition, the Kang-Modules identified to be affected by *QPRT-KO* were also reported to be highly co-expressed ($\rho \geq 0.68$) with markers for glutamatergic (Kang-Module 10) and GABAergic neurons (Kang-Modules 2 and 15) or astrocytes (Kang-Module 2). In addition, Kang-Module 1 is implicated in the early development of the hippocampus and amygdala, two regions significantly associated with ASD after meta-analysis [71, 72]. These associations identified in the translational approach suggest that *QPRT* loss might trigger alterations in the development of excitatory/inhibitory neuronal networks, a pathomechanism postulated to underlie the etiology of ASD [73, 74].

In summary, our findings allow us to conclude that in the neuroblastoma model SH-SY5Y a loss of *QPRT* impairs neuronal development in vitro by changing genetic networks previously implicated in the etiology of ASD. To confirm these results and the role of *QPRT* in the etiology of ASD in general, further studies in other neuronal or animal models are needed. In particular, analyzing the above described *QPRT-KO* mouse model [30, 31] could elucidate the effect of QPRT loss at systems level.

Conclusions

Here, we report *QPRT*, a gene within the ASD-associated 16p11.2 CNV region, to be essential for and causally related to SH-SY5Y neuronal differentiation in vitro. This corroborates postmortem findings of a disturbed

neuronal development in ASD. The functional mechanism is still elusive; however, based on our results, we can exclude alterations of QUIN levels or other products of the kynurenine pathway in the here described SH-SY5Y model. Further, the transcriptomic approach suggests that a reduced availability of *QPRT* impacts on genes and networks associated with ASD, such as neuron differentiation, synapse organization, or the development of excitatory/inhibitory neurons. Overall this study suggests an alteration of *QPRT* expression or of *QPRT* related genes to be underlying the etiology of ASD in 16p11.2 CNV carriers. Further studies are needed to confirm our findings in more mature neuronal systems or animal models.

Additional files

Additional file 1: Supplementary information: Supplementary methods, supplementary results, supplementary table S1, supplementary figures S1-S6. (DOCX 555 kb)

Additional file 2: Supplementary table S2. Results from DESeq2 analysis and count data from RNA-Seq (MACE analysis). (XLSX 5308 kb)

Additional file 3: Supplementary table S3. Results from GO term enrichment analysis. (XLSX 36 kb)

Abbreviations

3HAA: 3-Hydroxyanthranilic acid; 3HK: 3-Hydroxykynurenine; A1: Primary auditory; A1C: Primary auditory (A1) cortex; AA: Anthranilic acid; ACTB: β-Actin; ADI-R: Autism Diagnostic Interview-Revised; ADORA2A: Adenosine receptor 2A; ADOS: Autism Observation Schedule; AMY: Amygdala; ARHGAP20: Rho GTPase-activating protein 20; ASD: Autism spectrum disorder; BAK1: BCL2-antagonist/killer 1; BDNF: Brain-derived neurotrophic factor; BRINP1: BMP/retinoic acid-inducible neural specific 1; CBC: Cerebellar cortex; CCK: Cholecystokinin; CNTNAP2: Contactin-associated protein-like 2; CNV: Copy number variation; COX17: COX17, cytochrome c oxidase copper chaperone; COX17P1: COX17, cytochrome c oxidase copper chaperone pseudogene 1; del268T: QPRT NM_014298 del268T; Ex2.1; DFC: Dorsolateral prefrontal cortex; DMEM: Dulbecco's modified Eagle medium; DOC2A: Double C2 domain alpha; DPBS: Dulbecco's phosphate buffered saline; DRD2: Dopamine receptor D2; eCtrl: Empty control vector; ERK/MAPK: Extracellular signaling-related kinase; FAM57BA: Family with sequence similarity 57, member Ba; FBS: Fetal bovine serum; FC: Fold change; GABRB3: Gamma-aminobutyric acid type A receptor beta3 subunit; GAPDH: Glyceraldehyde-3-phosphate dehydrogenase; GC/MS: Gas chromatography-mass spectrometry; GUCA1A: Guanylate cyclase activator 1A; GUSB: Glucuronidase beta; HIP: Hippocampus; HSD: Honest significance difference; ins395A: QPRT NM_014298 ins395A; Ex2.2; IPC: Posterior inferior parietal cortex; ITC: Inferior temporal cortex; KA: Kynurenic acid; KCNQ3: Potassium voltage-gated channel subfamily Q member 3; KCTD13: Potassium channel tetramerization domain containing 13; KD: Knockdown; KIF22: Kinesin family member 22; KO: Knock out; KYN: Kynurenine; LCL: Lymphoblastoid cell line; LINC01760: Long intergenic non-protein coding RNA 1760; MACE: Massive analysis of cDNA ends; MAPK3: Mitogen-activated protein kinase 3; MFC: Medial prefrontal cortex; NAD: Nicotinamide adenine dinucleotide; NLGN: Neuroligins; NLGN3: Neuroligin 3; NMDA-R: N-methyl-D-aspartate receptor; NMNAT2: Nicotinamide nucleotide adenylyltransferase 2; NO: Nitric oxide; NOS1: Nitric oxide synthase 1; OFC: Orbitofrontal cortex; PA: Phthalic acid; PARP: Poly (ADP-ribose) polymerase; PI: Propidium iode; PIC: Picolinic acid; PSMD7: Proteasome 26S subunit, non-ATPase 7; QPRT: Quinolinate phosphoribosyltransferase; QUIN: Quinolinic acid; RA: Retinoic acid; RIN: RNA integrity number; SCRIB: Scribbled planar cell polarity protein; siCtrl: Non-targeting siRNA control; siQ1-siQ3: QPRT targeting siRNA1-3; SNTG2: Syntrophin gamma 2; SRRM4: Serine/arginine repetitive matrix 4;

STR: Striatum; TAOK2: TAO kinase 2; TBX6: T-box 6; TRP: Tryptophan; UHPLC: Ultra-high-performance liquid chromatography; UPL: Universal probe library; V1: Primary visual; V1C: Primary visual (V1) cortex; VFC: Ventrolateral prefrontal cortex; VSTM2A: V-set and transmembrane domain containing 2A; WGCNA: Weighted gene co-expression network analysis; WT: Wild type

Acknowledgements
We thank J Heine for technical support and J Ludwig and M Jones for fruitful discussions.

Funding
The study has been funded by Dr. Paul and Cilli Weill Price for excellent early career researchers in medical sciences at the Goethe University awarded to AGC.

Authors' contributions
AGC and DH designed the study and wrote the manuscript. DH, SL, and IS performed the experiments. CMF, RW, and AY supported the manuscript preparation. AGC, DH, NK, BR, and AY performed the statistical analyses. TA, BKG, and MMT shared their experience and protocols for CRISPR/Cas9 experiments. GJG and CKL shared expertise on tryptophan metabolism and performed the metabolite analysis. SF and IS helped in designing and performing siRNA experiments, as well as imaging of transfected cells in a high throughput manner, and shared their expertise and equipment. AGC, CMF, and AAP hosted fruitful discussions for project planning and strongly supported the project. All authors read and approved the final manuscript.

Competing interests
All authors declare that they have no competing interests.

Author details
[1]Department of Child and Adolescent Psychiatry, Psychosomatics and Psychotherapy, University Hospital Frankfurt, JW Goethe University Frankfurt, Frankfurt am Main, Germany. [2]Institute of Experimental Cancer Research in Pediatrics, Frankfurt am Main, Germany. [3]Faculty of Medicine and Health Sciences, Macquarie University, Sydney, New South Wales, Australia. [4]Neuropathology, University of Giessen, Giessen, Germany. [5]Department of Microvascular Biology and Pathobiology, European Center for Angioscience (ECAS), Medical Faculty Mannheim, University of Heidelberg, Heidelberg, Germany. [6]Institute of Cell Biology and Neuroscience and Buchmann Institute for Molecular Life Sciences (BMLS), JW Goethe University of Frankfurt, Frankfurt am Main, Germany. [7]GenXPro GmbH, Frankfurt am Main, Germany.

References
1. Raymond GV, Bauman ML, Kemper TL. Hippocampus in autism: a Golgi analysis. Acta Neuropathol. 1996;91:117–9.
2. Jacot-Descombes S, Uppal N, Wicinski B, Santos M, Schmeidler J, Giannakopoulos P, et al. Decreased pyramidal neuron size in Brodmann areas 44 and 45 in patients with autism. Acta Neuropathol. 2012;124:67–79. https://doi.org/10.1007/s00401-012-0976-6.
3. Casanova MF, Kooten v, Imke AJ, Switala AE, van Engeland H, Heinsen H, Steinbusch HWM, et al. Minicolumnar abnormalities in autism. Acta Neuropathol. 2006;112:287–303. https://doi.org/10.1007/s00401-006-0085-5.
4. Stoner R, Chow ML, Boyle MP, Sunkin SM, Mouton PR, Roy S, et al. Patches of disorganization in the neocortex of children with autism. N Engl J Med. 2014;370:1209–19. https://doi.org/10.1056/NEJMoa1307491.
5. Sanders SJ, He X, Willsey AJ, Ercan-Sencicek AG, Samocha KE, Cicek AE, et al. Insights into autism spectrum disorder genomic architecture and biology from 71 risk loci. Neuron. 2015;87:1215–33. https://doi.org/10.1016/j.neuron.2015.09.016.
6. Pinto D, Delaby E, Merico D, Barbosa M, Merikangas A, Klei L, et al. Convergence of genes and cellular pathways dysregulated in autism spectrum disorders. Am J Hum Genet. 2014;94:677–94. https://doi.org/10.1016/j.ajhg.2014.03.018.
7. Woodbury-Smith M, Scherer SW. Progress in the genetics of autism spectrum disorder. Dev Med Child Neurol. 2018. https://doi.org/10.1111/dmcn.13717.
8. Stein JL. Copy number variation and brain structure: lessons learned from chromosome 16p11.2. Genome Med. 2015;7:13. https://doi.org/10.1186/s13073-015-0140-8.
9. NIH Genetics Home Reference. https://ghr.nlm.nih.gov/condition/16p112-deletion-syndrome. Accessed 30 Apr 2018.
10. NIH Genetics Home Reference. https://ghr.nlm.nih.gov/condition/16p112-duplication. Accessed 30 Apr 2018.
11. Blumenthal I, Ragavendran A, Erdin S, Klei L, Sugathan A, Guide JR, et al. Transcriptional consequences of 16p11.2 deletion and duplication in mouse cortex and multiplex autism families. Am J Hum Genet. 2014;94:870–83. https://doi.org/10.1016/j.ajhg.2014.05.004.
12. Blaker-Lee A, Gupta S, McCammon JM, de RG, Sive H. Zebrafish homologs of genes within 16p11.2, a genomic region associated with brain disorders, are active during brain development, and include two deletion dosage sensor genes. Dis Model Mech. 2012;5:834–51. https://doi.org/10.1242/dmm.009944.
13. McCammon JM, Blaker-Lee A, Chen X, Sive H. The 16p11.2 homologs fam57ba and doc2a generate certain brain and body phenotypes. Hum Mol Genet. 2017;26:3699–712. https://doi.org/10.1093/hmg/ddx255.
14. Arbogast T, Ouagazzal A-M, Chevalier C, Kopanitsa M, Afinowi N, Migliavacca E, et al. Reciprocal effects on neurocognitive and metabolic phenotypes in mouse models of 16p11.2 deletion and duplication syndromes. PLoS Genet. 2016;12:e1005709. https://doi.org/10.1371/journal.pgen.1005709.
15. Pucilowska J, Vithayathil J, Tavares EJ, Kelly C, Karlo JC, Landreth GE. The 16p11.2 deletion mouse model of autism exhibits altered cortical progenitor proliferation and brain cytoarchitecture linked to the ERK MAPK pathway. J Neurosci. 2015;35:3190–200. https://doi.org/10.1523/JNEUROSCI.4864-13.2015.
16. Horev G, Ellegood J, Lerch JP, Son Y-EE, Muthuswamy L, Vogel H, et al. Dosage-dependent phenotypes in models of 16p11.2 lesions found in autism. Proc Natl Acad Sci U S A. 2011;108:17076–81. https://doi.org/10.1073/pnas.1114042108.
17. Blizinsky KD, Diaz-Castro B, Forrest MP, Schurmann B, Bach AP, Martin-de-Saavedra MD, et al. Reversal of dendritic phenotypes in 16p11.2 microduplication mouse model neurons by pharmacological targeting of a network hub. Proc Natl Acad Sci U S A. 2016;113:8520–5. https://doi.org/10.1073/pnas.1607014113.
18. Grissom NM, McKee SE, Schoch H, Bowman N, Havekes R, O'Brien WT, et al. Male-specific deficits in natural reward learning in a mouse model of neurodevelopmental disorders. Mol Psychiatry. 2017. https://doi.org/10.1038/mp.2017.184.
19. Toma C, Hervás A, Balmaña N, Salgado M, Maristany M, Vilella E, et al. Neurotransmitter systems and neurotrophic factors in autism: association study of 37 genes suggests involvement of DDC. World J Biol Psychiatry. 2013;14:516–27. https://doi.org/10.3109/15622975.2011.602719.
20. Freitag CM, Agelopoulos K, Huy E, Rothermundt M, Krakowitzky P, Meyer J, et al. Adenosine A(2A) receptor gene (ADORA2A) variants may increase autistic symptoms and anxiety in autism spectrum disorder. Eur Child Adolesc Psychiatry. 2010;19:67–74. https://doi.org/10.1007/s00787-009-0043-6.
21. Golzio C, Willer J, Talkowski ME, Oh EC, Taniguchi Y, Jacquemont S, et al. KCTD13 is a major driver of mirrored neuroanatomical phenotypes of the

16p11.2 copy number variant. Nature. 2012;485:363–7. https://doi.org/10.1038/nature11091.

22. Ip JPK, Nagakura I, Petravicz J, Li K, Wiemer EAC, Sur M. Major vault protein, a candidate gene in 16p11.2 microdeletion syndrome, is required for the homeostatic regulation of visual cortical plasticity. J Neurosci. 2018. https://doi.org/10.1523/JNEUROSCI.2034-17.2018.

23. Calderon de Anda F, Rosario AL, Durak O, Tran T, Gräff J, Meletis K, et al. Autism spectrum disorder susceptibility gene TAOK2 affects basal dendrite formation in the neocortex. Nat Neurosci. 2012;15:1022–31. https://doi.org/10.1038/nn.3141.

24. Li Z, He X, Feng J. 16p11.2 is required for neuronal polarity. WJNS. 2013;03: 221–7. https://doi.org/10.4236/wjns.2013.34029.

25. Qureshi AY, Mueller S, Snyder AZ, Mukherjee P, Berman JI, Roberts TPL, et al. Opposing brain differences in 16p11.2 deletion and duplication carriers. J Neurosci. 2014;34:11199–211. https://doi.org/10.1523/JNEUROSCI.1366-14.2014.

26. Subramanian M, Timmerman CK, Schwartz JL, Pham DL, Meffert MK. Characterizing autism spectrum disorders by key biochemical pathways. Front Neurosci. 2015;9:313. https://doi.org/10.3389/fnins.2015.00313.

27. Lin GN, Corominas R, Lemmens I, Yang X, Tavernier J, Hill DE, et al. Spatiotemporal 16p11.2 protein network implicates cortical late mid-fetal brain development and KCTD13-Cul3-RhoA pathway in psychiatric diseases. Neuron. 2015;85:742–54. https://doi.org/10.1016/j.neuron.2015.01.010.

28. Chiocchetti AG, Haslinger D, Stein JL, de La T-UL, Cocchi E, Rothamel T, et al. Transcriptomic signatures of neuronal differentiation and their association with risk genes for autism spectrum and related neuropsychiatric disorders. Transl Psychiatry. 2016;6:e864. https://doi.org/10.1038/tp.2016.119.

29. Ting KK, Brew BJ, Guillemin GJ. Effect of quinolinic acid on human astrocytes morphology and functions: implications in Alzheimer's disease. J Neuroinflammation. 2009;6:36. https://doi.org/10.1186/1742-2094-6-36.

30. Fukuoka S-I, Kawashima R, Asuma R, Shibata K, Fukuwatari T. Quinolinate accumulation in the brains of the quinolinate phosphoribosyltransferase (qprt) knockout mice; 2012. https://doi.org/10.5772/31749.

31. Terakata M, Fukuwatari T, Sano M, Nakao N, Sasaki R, Fukuoka S-I, Shibata K. Establishment of true niacin deficiency in quinolinic acid phosphoribosyltransferase knockout mice. J Nutr. 2012;142:2148–53. https://doi.org/10.3945/jn.112.167569.

32. Lim CK, Essa MM, de PMR, Lovejoy DB, Bilgin AA, Waly MI, et al. Altered kynurenine pathway metabolism in autism: implication for immune-induced glutamatergic activity. Autism Res. 2015. https://doi.org/10.1002/aur.1565.

33. Shen C, L-r H, X-l Z, P-r W, Zhong N. Novel interactive partners of neuroligin 3: new aspects for pathogenesis of autism. J Mol Neurosci. 2015;56:89–101. https://doi.org/10.1007/s12031-014-0470-9.

34. Kang HJ, Kawasawa YI, Cheng F, Zhu Y, Xu X, Li M, et al. Spatio-temporal transcriptome of the human brain. Nature. 2011;478:483–9. https://doi.org/10.1038/nature10523.

35. Neitzel H. A routine method for the establishment of permanent growing lymphoblastoid cell lines. Hum Genet. 1986;73:320–6.

36. Chiocchetti AG, Haslinger D, Boesch M, Karl T, Wiemann S, Freitag CM, et al. Protein signatures of oxidative stress response in a patient specific cell line model for autism. Mol Autism. 2014;5:10. https://doi.org/10.1186/2040-2392-5-10.

37. Poustka F, Lisch S, Rühl D, Sacher A, Schmötzer G, Werner K. The standardized diagnosis of autism, autism diagnostic interview-revised: interrater reliability of the German form of the interview. Psychopathology. 1996;29:145–53.

38. Lord C, Rutter M, Le Couteur A. Autism diagnostic interview-revised: a revised version of a diagnostic interview for caregivers of individuals with possible pervasive developmental disorders. J Autism Dev Disord. 1994;24:659–85.

39. Bölte S, Poustka F. Diagnostische Beobachtungsskala für Autistische Störungen (ADOS): Erste Ergebnisse zur Zuverlässigkeit und Gültigkeit. Z Kinder Jugendpsychiatr Psychother. 2004;32:45–50. https://doi.org/10.1024/1422-4917.32.1.45.

40. Schindelin J, Rueden CT, Hiner MC, Eliceiri KW. The ImageJ ecosystem: an open platform for biomedical image analysis. Mol Reprod Dev. 2015;82:518–29. https://doi.org/10.1002/mrd.22489.

41. Ristanović D, Milosević NT, Stulić V. Application of modified Sholl analysis to neuronal dendritic arborization of the cat spinal cord. J Neurosci Methods. 2006;158:212–8. https://doi.org/10.1016/j.jneumeth.2006.05.030.

42. ImageJ Sholl Analysis. http://imagej.net/Sholl_Analysis. Accessed 30 Apr 2018.

43. Ran FA, Hsu PD, Wright J, Agarwala V, Scott DA, Zhang F. Genome engineering using the CRISPR-Cas9 system. Nat Protoc. 2013;8:2281–308. https://doi.org/10.1038/nprot.2013.143.

44. CRISPR design. http://crispr.mit.edu/. Accessed 30 Apr 2018.

45. Braidy N, Guillemin GJ, Grant R. Effects of kynurenine pathway inhibition on NAD metabolism and cell viability in human primary astrocytes and neurons. Int J Tryptophan Res. 2011;4:29–37. https://doi.org/10.4137/IJTR.S7052.

46. Braidy N, Grant R, Adams S, Brew BJ, Guillemin GJ. Mechanism for quinolinic acid cytotoxicity in human astrocytes and neurons. Neurotox Res. 2009;16: 77–86. https://doi.org/10.1007/s12640-009-9051-z.

47. Petroni D, Tsai J, Mondal D, George W. Attenuation of low dose methylmercury and glutamate induced-cytotoxicity and tau phosphorylation by an N-methyl-D-aspartate antagonist in human neuroblastoma (SHSY5Y) cells. Environ Toxicol. 2013;28:700–6. https://doi.org/10.1002/tox.20765.

48. Candemir E, Kollert L, Weissflog L, Geis M, Muller A, Post AM, et al. Interaction of NOS1AP with the NOS-I PDZ domain: implications for schizophrenia-related alterations in dendritic morphology. Eur Neuropsychopharmacol. 2016;26:741–55. https://doi.org/10.1016/j.euroneuro.2016.01.008.

49. Zheng T, Xu SY, Zhou SQ, Lai LY, Li L. Nicotinamide adenine dinucleotide (NAD+) repletion attenuates bupivacaine-induced neurotoxicity. Neurochem Res. 2013;38:1880–94. https://doi.org/10.1007/s11064-013-1094-0.

50. Lim CK, Bilgin A, Lovejoy DB, Tan V, Bustamante S, Taylor BV, et al. Kynurenine pathway metabolomics predicts and provides mechanistic insight into multiple sclerosis progression. Sci Rep. 2017;7:41473. https://doi.org/10.1038/srep41473.

51. Zhernakov A, Rotter B, Winter P, Borisov A, Tikhonovich I, Zhukov V. Massive Analysis of cDNA Ends (MACE) for transcript-based marker design in pea (Pisum sativum L.). Genom Data. 2017;11:75–6. https://doi.org/10.1016/j.gdata.2016.12.004.

52. Müller S, Rycak L, Afonso-Grunz F, Winter P, Zawada AM, Damrath E, et al. APADB: a database for alternative polyadenylation and microRNA regulation events. Database (Oxford). 2014. https://doi.org/10.1093/database/bau076.

53. Nold-Petry CA, Lo CY, Rudloff I, Elgass KD, Li S, Gantier MP, et al. IL-37 requires the receptors IL-18Rα and IL-1R8 (SIGIRR) to carry out its multifaceted anti-inflammatory program upon innate signal transduction. Nat Immunol. 2015;16:354–65. https://doi.org/10.1038/ni.3103.

54. Langmead B, Salzberg SL. Fast gapped-read alignment with Bowtie 2. Nat Methods. 2012;9:357–9. https://doi.org/10.1038/nmeth.1923.

55. Livak KJ, Schmittgen TD. Analysis of relative gene expression data using real-time quantitative PCR and the 2(-delta delta C(T)) method. Methods. 2001;25:402–8. https://doi.org/10.1006/meth.2001.1262.

56. Love MI, Huber W, Anders S. Moderated estimation of fold change and dispersion for RNA-seq data with DESeq2. Genome Biol. 2014;15:550. https://doi.org/10.1186/s13059-014-0550-8.

57. Yousaf A, Duketis E, Jarczok T, Sachse M, Biscaldi M, Degenhardt F, et al. Mapping the genetics of neuropsychological traits to the molecular network of the human brain using a data integrative approach. bioRxiv. 2018. https://doi.org/10.1101/336776.

58. SFARI Gene. https://gene.sfari.org/database/human-gene/. Accessed 30 Apr 2018.

59. Deshpande A, Yadav S, Dao DQ, Wu Z-Y, Hokanson KC, Cahill MK, et al. Cellular phenotypes in human iPSC-derived neurons from a genetic model of autism spectrum disorder. Cell Rep. 2017;21:2678–87. https://doi.org/10.1016/j.celrep.2017.11.037.

60. Sahm F, Oezen I, Opitz CA, Radlwimmer B, von Deimling A, Ahrendt T, et al. The endogenous tryptophan metabolite and NAD+ precursor quinolinic acid confers resistance of gliomas to oxidative stress. Cancer Res. 2013;73: 3225–34. https://doi.org/10.1158/0008-5472.CAN-12-3831.

61. Campbell BM, Charych E, Lee AW, Möller T. Kynurenines in CNS disease: regulation by inflammatory cytokines. Front Neurosci. 2014;8:12. https://doi.org/10.3389/fnins.2014.00012.

62. Buxbaum JD, Silverman JM, Smith CJ, Greenberg DA, Kilifarski M, Reichert J, et al. Association between a GABRB3 polymorphism and autism. Mol Psychiatry. 2002;7:311–6. https://doi.org/10.1038/sj.mp.4001011.

63. de La Torre-Ubieta L, Won H, Stein JL, Geschwind DH. Advancing the understanding of autism disease mechanisms through genetics. Nat Med. 2016;22:345–61. https://doi.org/10.1038/nm.4071.

64. Bulayeva K, Lesch K-P, Bulayev O, Walsh C, Glatt S, Gurgenova F, et al. Genomic structural variants are linked with intellectual disability. J Neural Transm (Vienna). 2015;122:1289–301. https://doi.org/10.1007/s00702-015-1366-8.

65. Rosenfeld JA, Ballif BC, Torchia BS, Sahoo T, Ravnan JB, Schultz R, et al. Copy number variations associated with autism spectrum disorders contribute to a spectrum of neurodevelopmental disorders. Genet Med. 2010;12:694–702. https://doi.org/10.1097/GIM.0b013e3181f0c5f3.

66. Yamakawa H, Oyama S, Mitsuhashi H, Sasagawa N, Uchino S, Kohsaka S, Ishiura S. Neuroligins 3 and 4X interact with syntrophin-gamma2, and the interactions are affected by autism-related mutations. Biochem Biophys Res Commun. 2007;355:41–6. https://doi.org/10.1016/j.bbrc.2007.01.127.

67. Gilling M, Rasmussen HB, Calloe K, Sequeira AF, Baretto M, Oliveira G, et al. Dysfunction of the heteromeric KV7.3/KV7.5 potassium channel is associated with autism spectrum disorders. Front Genet. 2013;4:54. https://doi.org/10.3389/fgene.2013.00054.

68. Peñagarikano O, Geschwind DH. What does CNTNAP2 reveal about autism spectrum disorder? Trends Mol Med. 2012;18:156–63. https://doi.org/10.1016/j.molmed.2012.01.003.

69. Chiocchetti AG, Kopp M, Waltes R, Haslinger D, Duketis E, Jarczok TA, et al. Variants of the CNTNAP2 5' promoter as risk factors for autism spectrum disorders: a genetic and functional approach. Mol Psychiatry. 2015;20:839–49. https://doi.org/10.1038/mp.2014.103.

70. Yamada T, Sakisaka T, Hisata S, Baba T, Takai Y. RA-RhoGAP, Rap-activated Rho GTPase-activating protein implicated in neurite outgrowth through Rho. J Biol Chem. 2005;280:33026–34.

71. Amaral DG, Schumann CM, Nordahl CW. Neuroanatomy of autism. Trends Neurosci. 2008;31:137–45. https://doi.org/10.1016/j.tins.2007.12.005.

72. Patriquin MA, DeRamus T, Libero LE, Laird A, Kana RK. Neuroanatomical and neurofunctional markers of social cognition in autism spectrum disorder. Hum Brain Mapp. 2016;37:3957–78. https://doi.org/10.1002/hbm.23288.

73. Dickinson A, Jones M, Milne E. Measuring neural excitation and inhibition in autism: different approaches, different findings and different interpretations. Brain Res. 2016;1648:277–89. https://doi.org/10.1016/j.brainres.2016.07.011.

74. Bozzi Y, Provenzano G, Casarosa S. Neurobiological bases of autism-epilepsy comorbidity: a focus on excitation/inhibition imbalance. Eur J Neurosci. 2017. https://doi.org/10.1111/ejn.13595.

75. Guglielmi L, Servettini I, Caramia M, Catacuzzeno L, Franciolini F, D'Adamo MC, Pessia M. Update on the implication of potassium channels in autism: K(+) channelautism spectrum disorder. Front Cell Neurosci. 2015;9:34. https://doi.org/10.3389/fncel.2015.00034.

76. Iourov IY, Vorsanova SG, Voinova VY, Yurov YB. 3p22.1p21.31 microdeletion identifies CCK as Asperger syndrome candidate gene and shows the way for therapeutic strategies in chromosome imbalances. Mol Cytogenet. 2015;8:82. https://doi.org/10.1186/s13039-015-0185-9.

77. Varghese M, Keshav N, Jacot-Descombes S, Warda T, Wicinski B, Dickstein DL, et al. Autism spectrum disorder: neuropathology and animal models. Acta Neuropathol. 2017. https://doi.org/10.1007/s00401-017-1736-4.

78. Berkowicz SR, Featherby TJ, Qu Z, Giousoh A, Borg NA, Heng JI, et al. Brinp1(−/−) mice exhibit autism-like behaviour, altered memory, hyperactivity and increased parvalbumin-positive cortical interneuron density. Mol Autism. 2016;7:22. https://doi.org/10.1186/s13229-016-0079-7.

79. Quesnel-Vallières M, Dargaei Z, Irimia M, Gonatopoulos-Pournatzis T, Ip JY, Wu M, et al. Misregulation of an activity-dependent splicing network as a common mechanism underlying autism spectrum disorders. Mol Cell. 2016;64:1023–34. https://doi.org/10.1016/j.molcel.2016.11.033.

13

Sociability deficits after prenatal exposure to valproic acid are rescued by early social enrichment

Marcos Campolongo[1,2], Nadia Kazlauskas[1,2], German Falasco[3], Leandro Urrutia[3], Natalí Salgueiro[1,2], Christian Höcht[4] and Amaicha Mara Depino[1,2,5]*

Abstract

Background: Autism spectrum disorder (ASD) is characterized by impaired social interactions and repetitive patterns of behavior. Symptoms appear in early life and persist throughout adulthood. Early social stimulation can help reverse some of the symptoms, but the biological mechanisms of these therapies are unknown. By analyzing the effects of early social stimulation on ASD-related behavior in the mouse, we aimed to identify brain structures that contribute to these behaviors.

Methods: We injected pregnant mice with 600-mg/kg valproic acid (VPA) or saline (SAL) at gestational day 12.5 and evaluated the effect of weaning their offspring in cages containing only VPA animals, only SAL animals, or mixed. We analyzed juvenile play at PD21 and performed a battery of behavioral tests in adulthood. We then used preclinical PET imaging for an unbiased analysis of the whole brain of these mice and studied the function of the piriform cortex by c-Fos immunoreactivity and HPLC.

Results: Compared to control animals, VPA-exposed animals play less as juveniles and exhibit a lower frequency of social interaction in adulthood when reared with other VPA mice. In addition, these animals were less likely to investigate social odors in the habituation/dishabituation olfactory test. However, when VPA animals were weaned with control animals, these behavioral alterations were not observed. Interestingly, repetitive behaviors and depression-related behaviors were not affected by social enrichment. We also found that VPA animals present high levels of glucose metabolism bilaterally in the piriform cortex (Pir), a region known to be involved in social behaviors. Moreover, we found alterations in the somatosensory, motor, and insular cortices. Remarkably, these effects were mostly reversed after social stimulation. To evaluate if changes in glucose metabolism in the Pir correlated with changes in neuronal activity, we measured c-Fos immunoreactivity in the Pir and found it increased in animals prenatally exposed to VPA. We further found increased dopamine turnover in the Pir. Both alterations were largely reversed by social enrichment.

Conclusions: We show that early social enrichment can specifically rescue social deficits in a mouse model of ASD. Our results identified the Pir as a structure affected by VPA-exposure and social enrichment, suggesting that it could be a key component of the social brain circuitry.

Keywords: Autism spectrum disorder, Sociability, Piriform cortex, Dopamine

* Correspondence: adepino@conicet.gov.ar
[1]Universidad de Buenos Aires, Facultad de Ciencias Exactas y Naturales, Departamento de Fisiología, Biología Molecular y Celular, Buenos Aires, Argentina
[2]CONICET-Universidad de Buenos Aires, Instituto de Fisiología, Biología Molecular y Neurociencias (IFIBYNE), Buenos Aires, Argentina
Full list of author information is available at the end of the article

Background

Autism spectrum disorder (ASD) is a group of neurodevelopmental pathologies characterized by persistent deficits in social communication and restricted, repetitive behaviors and interests [1]. Symptoms appear in early childhood and persist throughout adulthood. Although both genetic and environmental causes have been proposed and tested [2], their etiology remains unknown. There is currently no consensus on the underlying neuropathology, and many brain structures have been claimed to play a relevant role in ASD symptoms, e.g., hippocampus [3, 4], prefrontal cortex [5], and cerebellum [3, 6].

While great strides have been made in the treatment of ASD, its effectiveness varies greatly depending on the case, and the underlying mechanisms of partially successful therapies are unknown [7]. In particular, clinical studies suggest that early social stimulation is the most effective treatment for autistic children, who show significant improvements in social behavior (e.g. [8–10]). Early social stimulation could counteract genetic and/or environmental risk factors, helping children to interact better with others [11].

There is extensive evidence on the effects of early environmental enrichment on brain development in animal models. Enrichment has been demonstrated to diminish the effects of genetic risk and injury on brain malfunction [12, 13], and environmental enrichment can revert many of the ASD-related behaviors in rodent models of autism [14, 15]. Our aim is to analyze the effects of early social stimulation (a specific component of environmental enrichment) on ASD-related behavior in a mouse model of ASD and to assess its consequences on brain function.

It has been extensively shown that prenatal exposure of mice to valproic acid (VPA) at gestational day 12.5 results in reduced social interaction in the adult male offspring [16] and increased stereotyped behaviors [17], and that these animals present several cellular and molecular alterations also observed in autistic individuals [16, 18]. In these studies, experimental mice exposed to VPA were weaned with other VPA-exposed mice.

To evaluate the contribution of the early social environment to the levels of sociability in adulthood, we weaned VPA mice in VPA only cages (VPA-VPA mice), or mixed them in cages containing animals prenatally exposed to VPA (VPA-SAL mice) and saline-treated animals (SAL-VPA mice) in 2:3 or 3:2 ratio. Mice interacted from postnatal day (PD) 21 to PD60 in their homecage. Given that we assume that social interactions are reciprocal after weaning, VPA-SAL animals, i.e., mice prenatally exposed to VPA who lived with control animals since PD21, received social stimulation from control animals, while VPA-VPA mice did not. These differences in social stimulation in the home cage could affect sociability in adulthood.

We next performed a battery of adult behavioral tests in order to compare VPA-VPA mice with VPA-SAL animals, to reveal if peers could rescue the behavioral phenotype caused by prenatal VPA exposure. In particular, we evaluated ASD-related behaviors and found that early social stimulation can revert the reduction in sociability observed in VPA-VPA mice in the social interaction test, but repetitive behaviors are increased in all VPA-exposed mice (evaluated in self-grooming and spontaneous alternation in the Y maze). The olfactory habituation/dishabituation test was performed to evaluate olfactory function and response to social odors, and VPA-VPA mice showed a specific deficit in social odors investigation. The novel object recognition test was performed to evaluate short-term memory and neophobia, two confounders in the social interaction test, and showed no differences between groups. We then analyzed anxiety- and depression-related behaviors since mood disorders have a high comorbidity with ASD [19] and can be affected by changes in social stimuli early in life, and found that VPA-exposed animals show less exploratory behaviors and increased depression-related behaviors.

After characterizing the behavioral alterations in our experimental groups, we analyzed brain glucose metabolism in an attempt to identify brain structures involved in these behavioral phenotypes. As our unbiased preclinical PET study pointed to altered function of the piriform cortex, we further analyzed this area and found changes in neuronal activity and dopaminergic function that are comparable to the alterations in sociability observed in VPA-VPA mice.

Methods

Animals and treatments

Outbred CrlFcen:CF1 female and male adult mice were obtained from the animal house at the Facultad de Ciencias Exactas y Naturales, University of Buenos Aires (Buenos Aires, Argentina). We chose this outbred strain because (1) it shows reliable intermediate levels of the behaviors analyzed, allowing the detection of increases and decreases in the behavioral parameters evaluated; (2) it has better breeding performance than inbred strains; and (3) it shows no VPA toxicity during pregnancy (neither litter size nor gestation time are affected). All animals were housed in the animal house on a 12:12 light to dark cycle and 18–22 °C temperature, with food and water ad libitum. All animal procedures were performed according to the regulations for the use of laboratory animals of the National Institute of Health (Washington, DC, USA) and approved by the institutional animal care and use committee of the Facultad de Ciencias Exactas y Naturales, University of Buenos Aires (CICUAL Protocol Nr. 6/2). Eight- to 10-week-old male mice were mated with nulliparous 8–10-week-old female mice. Females were controlled every morning, and the day when a vaginal plug was detected was considered the gestational day (GD) 0.5.

Prenatal treatment

On GD12.5, pregnant female mice were injected subcutaneously with either 600 mg/kg of valproic acid sodium salt (VPA; Sigma, St. Louis, MO, USA) in saline solution or with saline solution (SAL), and housed individually. The parturition day was registered as postnatal day 0 (PD0), and the cage bedding was not changed during the first postnatal week to avoid nest and maternal care alterations.

Postnatal treatment

On PD21, male pups prenatally exposed to VPA were weaned in cages containing four-five animals of the same treatment (VPA-VPA animals), or with control male pups (VPA-SAL animals) in cages containing two-three VPA-treated mice with three-two saline-treated mice (SAL-VPA animals). Control animals weaned with other control animals were denominated SAL-SAL animals (Fig. 2a). Mice interacted from PD21 to PD60 in their homecage. Littermates were assigned to different postnatal treatments (X-SAL and X-VPA), and offspring belonging to the same prenatal treatment group from different mothers were mixed at weaning. We performed all the studies on males because female offspring of VPA-injected dams does not show ASD-related behaviors (unpublished data; [17, 20]).

Juvenile play

To evaluate sociability at weaning, an independent cohort of 16 VPA and 16 SAL animals was tested for juvenile play at PD21. We used an independent group to avoid interfering with the social enrichment process (postnatal treatment). Non-sibling mice from the same prenatal treatment were matched for similar body weights within 1-g difference. On PD20, one mouse in each pair was marked on its back with black marker to distinguish between animals during testing. On PD21, mice were isolated for 30 min and allowed to habituate to the testing room (10 lx). Each animal was then placed for a 10-min habituation period in the testing arena (floor: 30 cm × 30 cm of black PVC; walls: 30 cm high of black formic). Afterward, the pair of animals was placed again in the testing arena for 30 min, allowing them to interact freely while they were filmed. Testing was performed during the 2 h prior to the start of the dark phase (18:00 to 20:00 h) to maximize activity.

Behaviors were scored separately for each mouse in the pair. All behaviors were scored manually using keys and the video-tracking system ANY-maze (Stoelting, IL,

USA) by an experimenter (M.C.) blind to treatment. We evaluated play solicitation (crawling and approaching events), investigative behaviors (events of anogenital sniffing, nose to nose sniffing or following), affiliative behaviors (time spent sitting side by side or in social grooming), and non-social behaviors (time spent exploring, self-grooming or sitting alone) as previously reported [21, 22].

Adult behavioral testing

All adult behavioral tests were performed during the light period (between 10:00 and 17:00 h), with the exception of the Y-maze test that was performed during the 2 h before the start of the dark phase (18:00 to 20:00 h) to maximize exploration. For adult behavior, data from three independent cohorts are presented. Each cohort consisted of five or six litters per prenatal treatment. Mice were 8 weeks old at the beginning of testing, and all tests were separated by 1-week intervals to reduce any inter-test effect. Tests were performed in the order listed below (Fig. 2b). Mice were tested in a room next to the holding room. Previous to the beginning of each test, all animals were habituated to the illumination in the testing room for 30 min. After testing, each mouse was identified and placed in a holding cage until all animals from a cage had been tested. All the behavioral testing and manual scoring were performed by two experimenters (M.C. and N.K.) blind to treatment groups.

Social interaction test

The social interaction test was performed as previously described [4]. Briefly, animals were exposed to a 40 cm × 15 cm black rectangular arena divided in three interconnected chambers and placed under dim light (10 lx). A clear Plexiglass cylinder (7.5 cm of diameter, with several holes to allow for auditory, visual, and olfactory investigation between a test and stimulus mouse) was placed in each side of the compartment at the beginning of the test. Prior to the start of each test, one of the end chambers was randomly designated as the "non-social side" and the other as the "social side". Animals were placed in the central compartment and allowed to explore for 5 min (habituation). Then, an unfamiliar, young (3 weeks of age) CF1 male mouse (social stimulus) was placed in one of the cylinders (social side), and an object (white, plastic 3-cm-tall cylinder) was placed in the other cylinder (non-social side). Social interaction was evaluated during a 10-min period. The time the subject spent sniffing the social stimulus or the non-social stimulus (nose inside a hole of the cylinder) was recorded manually using a key in the video-tracking system ANY-maze (Stoelting, IL, USA). The entire apparatus, including the cylinders, was cleaned with a 20% ethanol solution between tests to eliminate odors. The apparatus floor was covered with bedding to reduce the stress and was replaced after each test.

Elevated plus maze test

The elevated plus maze test (EPM) was performed as previously described [23]. The apparatus consisted of two open and two closed arms (open arms: 30 cm × 5 cm, 100 lx, surrounded by a 0.5-cm high border; closed arms: 30 cm × 5 cm, 43 lx, surrounded by 19 cm high walls), both elevated 50 cm above the floor. The walls and the floor were made of black PVC. Mice were placed into the central platform of the maze (5 cm × 5 cm, 100 lx) facing towards an open arm and allowed to explore the maze for 5 min. Locomotion data were collected by a video-tracking system (ANY-maze, Stoelting). Measured locomotor parameters were time spent in open arms, time in closed arms, time in the central platform, traveled distance in both open and closed arms, % distance in the open arms, and total traveled distance. Ethological parameters were scored manually during each session: number of rearings, grooming time, number of head dippings, and number of protected head dippings—which consisted in head dippings specifically performed in the center of the maze. The entire apparatus was cleaned with a 20% ethanol solution between tests to eliminate odors. For statistical analysis of this test, we selected uncorrelated variables ($|r| < 0.7$): the time spent in the open arms, the time spent in the closed arms, the time spent in the central platform, the distance traveled in closed arms, number of rearings, grooming time and number of both head dippings and protected head dippings.

Open field test

The open field test (OF) was performed as previously described [23]. Mice were placed in the arena (floor: 45 cm × 45 cm of black PVC; walls: 30 cm high of black formic; 100 lx) for 30 min. Animals were initially placed along one side of the arena, and the center region was defined as the central 23 cm × 23 cm area. Locomotion data were collected by a video-tracking system (ANY-maze, Stoelting). Measured behavioral parameters were time spent in the center, time spent in the border, distance traveled in the center, distance traveled in the border, % distance in the center, and total distance traveled. Grooming time and the number of rearings were scored manually during each session. For statistical analysis of this test, we selected uncorrelated variables ($|r| < 0.7$): total distance traveled, time spent in the center, time grooming, and number of rearings.

The olfactory habituation/dishabituation test

Olfactory discrimination was investigated using a slightly modified habituation/dishabituation protocol [24]. Each

mouse was isolated in the testing cage (floor: 27 cm × 16 cm, height 12 cm) and habituated to a non-odorant cotton tip for 30 min. Then, animals were given three 2-min presentations of each odor: water, two non-social odors, and two social odors. Non-social odors were imitation vanilla and banana extracts, and social odors were male and female cage swipes. Odors were presented using a cotton tip with a 1-min inter-trial interval, which is the amount of time needed to change the cotton tip. The testing room was illuminated with 50 lx. The time spent sniffing the cotton tip was recorded manually using a key of the ANY-maze software (Stoelting). Animals that did not explore any of the presentations of an odor were excluded from the analysis (3 SAL-VPA, 2 VPA-SAL, 3 VPA-VPA).

Novel object recognition test

The novel object recognition test (NOR) was modified from a previous study [25]. Animals were first habituated to the experimental box (floor: 30 cm × 30 cm of black PVC; walls: 30-cm high of black formic; 10 lx) during 5 min and then placed individually in a holding cage during 5 min. After that, animals were placed again in the experimental box containing two identical objects, allowing them to explore the objects during a 5-min trial (training session). Animals were placed again in their cage for a 5-min period, to generate new short-term memories. Finally, animals were placed again in the experimental box, allowing them to explore two different objects (testing session) for 5 min. One of the objects was identical to those explored during the training session (familiar object), and the other was a different object (novel object). The objects were presented in the same locations as in the training session. The location of the novel object was randomly assigned (left or right) for each animal to avoid place preference during the testing session. The objects used were a small transparent glass Erlenmeyer or a 1.5-ml Eppendorf tube of similar size. The time spent sniffing each object was scored manually using keys in the ANY-maze software (Stoelting). The objects and the experimental box were cleaned with 20% ethanol solution between animals to eliminate olfactory cues. One VPA-SAL animal was removed from the analysis because it did not explore any of the objects during the test.

Self-grooming test

Mice were scored for spontaneous grooming behaviors as described earlier [4, 21]. Each mouse was placed individually into a clear Plexiglass cylinder (20 cm high, 5.5 cm wide), illuminated at 10 lx. Before testing, animals were habituated to the test cylinder in the testing room, for 1 h in two consecutive days. On the testing day, each mouse was scored during 10 min for cumulative time spent grooming all body regions, using a key of the ANY-maze software (Stoelting).

Light-dark box test

The light-dark (LD) test was performed as previously described [26]. A 45 cm × 45 cm arena was divided in half with an inverted black box (lit side: 100 lx; dark side: 1 lx). Animals were able to cross from one compartment to the other through a small hole in the wall (12-cm height, 8-cm width). Each mouse was placed under the hole facing the illuminated side of the box and tracked for 5 min using the ANY-maze software (Stoelting). Behavioral parameters analyzed were time spent in the lit compartment and distance traveled in the lit compartment.

Tail suspension test

The tail suspension test (TST) was performed as previously described [26]. Animals were suspended in the air using adhesive tape wrapped around the subject's tail (about 4/5 from the base) and fixed to a wire at 25 cm of height from a wooden surface. This test was performed under 50 lx. The immobility time was scored during 5 min, using a key of the ANY-maze software (Stoelting). One animal was removed from this test because it learned to climb its tail.

Forced swimming test

The forced swimming test (FST) was performed as previously described [26]. Animals were gently placed in a beaker glass (15 cm in diameter and 25 cm in height), filled with 14 cm of water at 25 °C and illuminated with 50 lx. Immobility time was scored during 6 min using a key in the ANY-maze software (Stoelting). At the end of the test, animals were dried with a paper towel and placed into a holding cage.

Y maze test

The Y-maze was constructed of Plexiglas with three identical arms (42-cm long, 12-cm tall walls, 30 lx), and visual cues were located on the walls outside the maze. The maze floor was made of black PVC. One of the three arms was arbitrarily designated as the start and exploration was recorded using the ANY-maze software (Stoelting). Total locomotion and percentage of alternation are reported. Percentage of alternation was calculated as (alternations × 100)/(Total arm visits− 2), where an alternation was considered as consecutively visiting the three arms. One VPA-SAL animal was excluded because it performed less than fifteen alternations.

Pre-clinical PET imaging
Imaging system

Images were acquired using a preclinical PET TriFoil Lab-PET 4 with LYSO and GYSO crystals and 1536 APD detectors groups. Approximated spatial resolution FWHM = 1.2 mm (*full width at half maximum*), 3.7 cm axial and 11 cm trans-axial FOV (*field of view*).

Animal handling

Pre-clinical PET imaging was performed on 15–17 animals for each experimental group, from two independent cohorts. Animals were starved during 18 h and then injected with 25 μCi/gr of [18F]-FDG i.p. and left undisturbed in an individual temperature-controlled (29 °C) cage for 30 min during radiopharmaceutical incorporation. Mice were then anesthetized using a mixture of isoflurane and O_2 (inhalation, 4.5% induction and 1.5% maintenance dose) and maintained in a warm table (35 °C) during the acquisition.

Acquisition and reconstruction setup

Each subject was acquired for 12 min using list-mode acquisition. Images were reconstructed using an OSEM 3D algorithm with 30 iterations, to maximize SNR (*signal-to-noise ratio*). If motion was detected during acquisition, a dynamic reconstruction was performed in order to correct it using SPM5 on MATLAB® realign algorithm.

Image spatial processing

The images were confined to a bounding-box that only includes the brain. A normal subject-based template was created in order to have an anatomic reference for realignment and normalization. All subjects were smoothed using an isotropic Gaussian kernel with 1 mm FWHM. All images were co-registered and normalized to this template using SPM5 on MATLAB®, according to these parameters: Normalized mutual information as objective function and 7-mm smoothing histogram for rigid co-registration; and affine regularization to the averaged template size, no-smooth and 2–0.1 mm of separation for the non-rigid normalization. Previous to intensity normalization and statistical analysis, a brain masking avoiding Harderiand glands was applied to all subjects since the uptake in these glands can significantly modify the intensity normalization values.

Image statistical analysis

All subject groups were analyzed as a full-factorial ANOVA test using SPM5 on MATLAB®. Intensity normalization was considered as a regressor variable for each factor using grand mean scaling (ANCOVA). Global calculation of individual means was calculated over each masked brain. Parametric statistical images were calculated for all possible experimental group contrasts. In order to correct for multiple comparisons, false discovery rate (FDR) approach was applied using SPM5 (*p* value FDR: 0.05). In order to have an accurate anatomical reference, all results of statistical differences where co-registered with an MRI atlas [27].

Spatial transformation was applied to the MRI atlas to correct for the differences between mice strains and methodological animal handling.

Catecholamine determination

An independent group of animals ($N = 4-5$ animals per group) was used for catecholamine determination as previously described [28]. Mice were sacrificed via cervical dislocation and punches of piriform cortex were taken and quickly frozen and kept at -80 °C. Tissue was homogenized in 1 ml of 0.3 M perchloric acid, centrifuged for 15 min at 3000 g at 4 °C and then frozen at 80 °C. Levels of DA, DOPAC, 5-HT, and 5-HIAA were measured by high pressure liquid chromatography coupled to electrochemical detection (HPLC-EC) using a Phenomenex Luna 5 µm, C18, 250 mm × 4.60 mm column (Phenomenex, Torrance, CA, USA) and LC-4C electrochemical detector with glassy carbon electrode (BAS). The working electrode was set at $+0.65$ V versus an Ag/AgCl reference electrode. The mobile phase contained 0.76 M NaH2PO4·H2O, 0.5 mM EDTA, 1.2 mM 1-octane sulfonic acid, and 5% acetonitrile; pH was adjusted to 3.0. Catecholamine quantification was referred to total protein content, measured using the NanoDrop 1000 Spectrophotometer (Thermo Scientific).

cFos immunohistochemistry

Animals from the second cohort of behavioral testing were randomly selected (7 SAL-SAL, 6 SAL-VPA, 5 VPA-SAL, and 6 VPA-VPA). Two weeks after the last behavioral test, mice were deeply anesthetized with ketamine/xilacine and transcardially perfused with 4% paraformaldehyde (PFA). Brains were post-fixed for 4 h in 4% PFA and criopreserved in 30% sucrose. 0.035-mm thick coronal sections were prepared on a cryostat (Leica, Wetzlar, Germany), and cFos immunohistochemistry was performed as previously described [29]. We used the primary antibody rabbit anti-c-Fos (1:1000 in blocking solution; EMD Millipore, Burlington, MA, USA), the secondary antibody biotin-SP-conjugated donkey anti-rabbit (Jackson ImmunoResearch, West Grove, PA, USA) and the ABC kit (Vector Laboratories, Burlingame, CA, USA). Sections were then stained with cresyl violet (5 mg/ml in 0.6% acetic acid). Positive cells in the layer 2 of the piriform cortex were counted on × 400 magnification in a light-field microscope (CX31: Olympus, Buenos Aires, Argentina) by a researcher (N.S.) blinded to treatments. Total c-Fos-positive nuclei are presented normalized by the volume of the layer 2. To this end, each counted section was photographed under × 40 magnification using a digital camera (Infinity 1; Lumera Corporation, Ottawa, ON, Canada) attached to the microscope. The volume of layer 2 in each image was determined using ImageJ [30]: the area in pixels was transformed to square millimeters and multiplied by the thickness of the section (0.035 mm). The limit between the anterior and posterior parts of the piriform cortex was determined with the aid of the mouse brain atlas [31] and set to the bregma position when the posterior branch of the anterior commissure is visible (AP − 0.26 mm).

Statistical analyses

Sample sizes were estimated based on similar, previously conducted studies. No statistical methods were used to predetermine sample size. Group comparisons were done using unpaired Student's t test, or two- or three-way ANOVAs for normally distributed data (confirmed by the D'Agostino & Pearson omnibus normality test), with litter as a nested factor. The statistical designs and outcomes are outlined in Additional file 1: Tables S1-S4. Whenever appropriate, Tukey's multiple comparisons test was used for post hoc comparisons. All tests were performed with the Statistica software (version 8, StatSoft Inc., Tulsa, OK, USA), and statistical significance was assumed where $p < 0.05$. We only used statistical methods to correct for multiple testing in the PET studies. Animal exclusions in behavioral tests are specified in each behavioral test description.

Results

Social stimulation between PD21 and PD60 reverts the sociability alterations observed after prenatal exposure to VPA

To evaluate if social deficiencies were already present in VPA animals at weaning, we evaluated juvenile play at PD21 (Fig. 1a). VPA mice solicited play less frequently (unpaired Student's t test, $t_{30} = 2.070$, $p = 0.047$; Fig. 1b), displayed less anogenital sniffing (unpaired Student's t test, $t_{30} = 2.281$, $p = 0.047$; Fig. 1c) and showed a tendency to follow less their partners (unpaired Student's t test with Welch's correction, $t_{24} = 2.035$, $p = 0.053$; Fig. 1d). SAL and VPA animals did not show differences in the time spent performing affiliative behaviors (unpaired Student's t test, $t_{30} = 0.399$, $p = 0.692$; Fig. 1e, left) or non-social behaviors (unpaired Student's t test, $t_{30} = 1.073$, $p = 0.292$; Fig. 1e, right). These results show that VPA-exposed animals already show alterations in social behaviors at weaning.

To assess the effects of social stimulation on VPA-exposed animals, we weaned VPA animals either with other VPA mice (VPA-VPA animals) or with SAL mice (VPA-SAL animals) (Fig. 2a) and evaluated their adult behavior along a battery of behavioral tests (Fig. 2b). At PD60, these experimental groups were evaluated in the social interaction test and compared with SAL-SAL and SAL-VPA mice. A two-way ANOVA showed a prenatal treatment effect ($F_{1, 75} = 6.656$, $p = 0.012$) and a postnatal

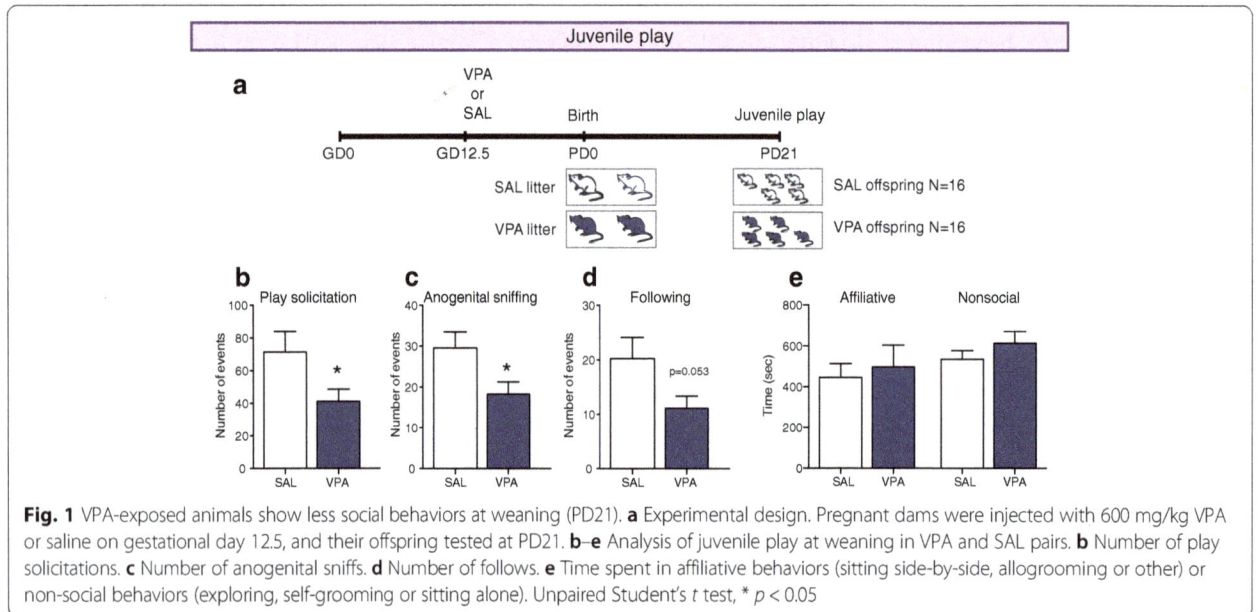

Fig. 1 VPA-exposed animals show less social behaviors at weaning (PD21). **a** Experimental design. Pregnant dams were injected with 600 mg/kg VPA or saline on gestational day 12.5, and their offspring tested at PD21. **b–e** Analysis of juvenile play at weaning in VPA and SAL pairs. **b** Number of play solicitations. **c** Number of anogenital sniffs. **d** Number of follows. **e** Time spent in affiliative behaviors (sitting side-by-side, allogrooming or other) or non-social behaviors (exploring, self-grooming or sitting alone). Unpaired Student's t test, * $p < 0.05$

treatment effect ($F_{1, 75} = 9.099$, $p = 0.003$) in the time spent sniffing the stimulus mouse, with no interaction between factors ($F_{1, 75} = 1.315$, $p = 0.255$). VPA-VPA animals spent less time interacting with the social stimulus than any other group (Fig. 2c). These results confirm previous reports showing an effect of prenatal VPA exposure on adult sociability [16]. In addition, the observation that VPA-SAL animals spent more time in social interaction that VPA-VPA mice, and that their interaction time was similar to that observed in the control groups, indicate that social interactions between PD21 and PD60 can rescue alterations on social behavior due to prenatal exposure to VPA.

We were able to rule out neophobia as the cause of the decrease in social interaction since (a) all groups showed similar investigation times of the novel cylinders in the habituation phase of the social interaction test (Additional file 1: Figure S1a); (b) all groups spent a similar amount of time exploring the two identical objects in the training session of the novel object recognition test (Additional file 1: Figure S1b); and (c) all groups responded similarly to a novel object, spending around 65–70% of the total time exploring it during the testing session (two-way ANOVA, prenatal treatment: $F_{1, 74} = 0.040$, $p = 0.842$; postnatal treatment: $F_{1, 74} = 0.009$, $p = 0.926$; interaction: $F_{1, 74} = 0.730$, $p = 0.396$; Fig. 2d).

VPA-VPA mice could have alterations in olfactory function, which would likely result in altered responses to novel social stimuli. To test this, we performed the olfactory habituation/dishabituation test. We found no differences between groups in the habituation to non-social odors or male urine, with all animals showing significant

habituation (Fig. 2e and Additional file 1: Table S1). However, we found a significant interaction between trial and postnatal treatment for the female odor (Three-way repeated-measure ANOVA, $F_{2, 134} = 4.094$, $p = 0.019$), with VPA-VPA mice only showing habituation to this odor in the third trial. The amount of time spent investigating novel odors can be an indicator of arousal/motivation, so we pooled all novel (trial 1) odor investigation durations across non-social (vanilla and banana) and social (male and female) odors (Fig. 2f). All groups show similar levels of investigation of non-social odors (two-way ANOVA, prenatal treatment: $F_{1, 66} = 3.40$, $p = 0.070$; postnatal treatment: $F_{1, 66} = 0.505$, $p = 0.480$; interaction: $F_{1, 66} = 0.014$, $p = 0.906$). We found a significant interaction between prenatal and postnatal treatments in the time investigating the first presentation of social odors ($F_{1, 66} = 4.141$, $p = 0.046$), with VPA-VPA mice investigating the stick less time than the other three groups (Fig. 2f). These results show that the behavioral phenotype of VPA-VPA mice is specific to social odors.

Prenatal exposure to VPA results in repetitive patterns of behavior, which are not rescued by early social stimulation

Repetitive, stereotyped behaviors are a common behavioral phenotype observed in ASD patients. To evaluate if VPA-exposed mice exhibit repetitive or stereotyped patterns of behavior, we performed two behavioral tests: the self-grooming and the Y maze tests. We found an effect of prenatal treatment on the time spent grooming ($F_{1, 73} = 4.215$, $p = 0.044$), with VPA-exposed mice spending significantly more time in self-grooming than the offspring of SAL-injected dams (Fig. 2g). In addition, we found an

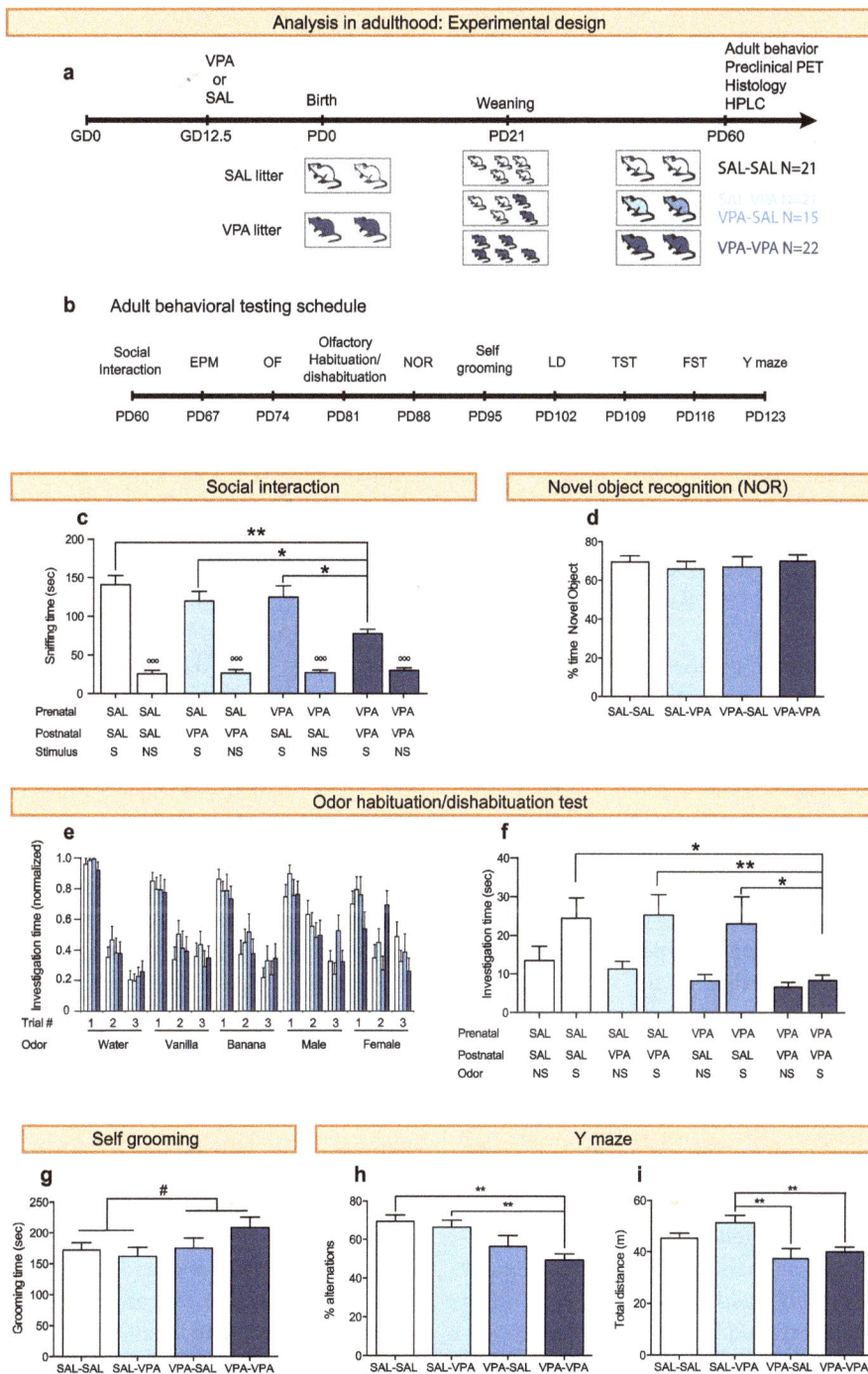

Fig. 2 (See legend on next page.)

effect of prenatal treatment on the percentage of alternations in the Y maze ($F_{1,\ 74} = 15.501$, $p < 0.001$). Post hoc analysis revealed that VPA-VPA animals alternate less than SAL-SAL or SAL-VPA animals, while VPA-SAL mice showed an intermediate performance (Fig. 2h). We also observed an effect of prenatal treatment on the total distance traveled in the

Y maze ($F_{1,\ 74} = 13.582$, $p < 0.001$], with animals prenatally exposed to VPA showing less exploratory behavior (Fig. 2i).

These data show that the increment in repetitive behaviors observed in VPA-exposed mice is not reversed, but only partially ameliorated, by early social stimulation. Although we cannot rule it out, the similar results

(See figure on previous page.)

Fig. 2 Peers can rescue the reduction in sociability observed in mice prenatally exposed to VPA, but not the increase in repetitive patterns of behavior. **a** Experimental design. Pregnant dams were injected with 600 mg/kg VPA or saline on gestational day 12.5. Offspring exposed to VPA (dark blue mice on PD21) and SAL (white mice on PD21) were weaned on PD21 in three type of cages. Due to interaction in the home cage until PD60, four experimental groups were generated: VPA animals weaned with other VPA animals (VPA-VPA group; dark blue); VPA animals weaned with saline mice (VPA-SAL group; blue); saline animals weaned with VPA animals (SAL-VPA group; light blue); and saline animals weaned with other saline animals (SAL-SAL group; white). **b** Adult behavioral analysis. Starting at PD60, all animals were subjected to a battery of behavioral tests performed in the order depicted. Tests were separated by 1-week intervals to reduce any inter-test effect. EPM, elevated plus maze; FST, forced swimming test; LD, light-dark box; NOR, novel object recognition; OF, open field; TST, tail suspension test. **c** Time spent sniffing the social (S) or non-social (NS) stimulus in the social interaction test. **d** Percentage of time exploring a novel object in the NOR test. **e, f** Odor habituation/dishabituation test: (E) Normalized time spent investigating each odor presentation, during three consecutive trials; (F) Time spent investigating the first presentation of non-social (NS) or social (S) odors. **g** Self-grooming test. **h** Spontaneous alternations in the Y maze. **i** Total distance traveled in the Y maze. Paired Student's t test, $^{ooo}p < 0.001$. Two-way ANOVA prenatal factor effect, $^{#}p < 0.05$. Tukey's post hoc test, $^{*}p < 0.05$, $^{**}p < 0.01$, $^{***}p < 0.001$. Graphs indicate means + s.e.m. Detailed statistical information is available in Additional file 1: Table S1

obtained in the self-grooming and Y maze tests suggest that they are not be affected by previous testing.

Prenatal exposure to VPA results in reduced exploration and increased depression-related behaviors in adult mice

Anxiety shows a high comorbidity with ASD [32]. To assess anxiety-related behavior, we performed the EPM, the OF, and the LD tests in the four experimental groups. We did not find evidence of anxiety-related behavior in the EPM, as all animals spent a similar amount of time in open and closed arms (Additional file 1: Table S2). However, VPA-exposed mice explored less the maze, walking less in the closed arms (two-way ANOVA prenatal effect: $F_{1, 75} = 4.936$, $p = 0.029$; Fig. 3a), and showing a tendency to perform less rearings (two-way ANOVA prenatal effect: $F_{1, 75} = 3.835$, $p = 0.054$; Fig. 3b). In addition, we observed an effect of postnatal treatment on the time spent in the center of the maze ($F_{1, 75} = 7.079$, $p = 0.009$), a zone were animals can assess risk, suggesting that early social stimulation can generate changes in the risk assessment strategy independently of the prenatal treatment. Finally, we did not observe differences between groups with regard to the number of head dippings and protected head dippings, or grooming time (Additional file 1: Table S2).

Again, we did not find evidence of anxiety-related behavior in the OF, as all animals spent a similar amount of time in the center of the field (Additional file 1: Table S2). However, animals exposed to VPA walk less (two-way ANOVA prenatal effect: $F_{1, 74} = 7.911$, $p = 0.006$; Fig. 3c) and spend more time in grooming (two-way ANOVA prenatal effect: $F_{1, 74} = 4.872$, $p = 0.030$; Fig. 3d). This last result goes in line with the evidence observed in the self-grooming test for repetitive patterns of behavior. We also observed prenatal ($F_{1, 74} = 12.319$, $p < 0.001$) and postnatal effects ($F_{1, 74} = 4.690$, $p = 0.034$) on the number of rearings in the OF, with rescued mice performing less vertical explorations than SAL animals.

In agreement with the previous results, we did not observe differences between the experimental groups in

the LD test. Animals walked similar distances in the lit compartment (Fig. 3e) and spent a similar amount of time in the lit compartment (Fig. 3f) (Additional file 1: Table S2).

We also evaluated immobility in the TST and FST, a variable that is affected by the treatment with anti-depressant drugs and has been interpreted as "behavioral despair". For the TST, a three-way ANOVA with repeated measures showed only a significant effect of prenatal treatment ($F_{1, 74} = 17.713$, $p < 0.001$; Fig. 3g), with VPA-exposed animals spending more time immobile (Fig. 3g, h). Similarly, a three-way ANOVA with repeated measures showed a significant effect of prenatal treatment on the time spent immobile in the FST ($F_{1, 75} = 6.638$, $p = 0.012$; Fig. 3i) and a prenatal effect for the cumulative immobility time between 3 and 6 min (two-way ANOVA, $F_{1, 75} = 5.981$, $p = 0.017$; Fig. 3j), with VPA-exposed animals spending more time immobile.

These results collectively show that prenatal VPA exposure results in animals with reduced exploration and increased depression-related behaviors but does not impact anxiety-related behaviors. We did not observe any effects of the postnatal treatment.

A preclinical PET analysis shows that prenatal VPA exposure results in altered patterns of brain glucose metabolism that are reversed by early social stimulation

To gain insight into the physiological changes that accompany the behavioral alterations observed after prenatal exposure to VPA and early social stimulation, we injected animals with [18F]-FDG and evaluated basal glucose metabolism 30 min after injection. We found evidence of increased glucose metabolism in the piriform cortex (Pir) of VPA-VPA animals when compared to either SAL-SAL or VPA-SAL mice (Fig. 4). This increase was bilateral and circumscribed to the anterior part of the Pir, and it was more significative when VPA-VPA animals were compared to rescued animals. We also observed increased glucose metabolism in the frontal motor cortex (M1) and reduced metabolism in

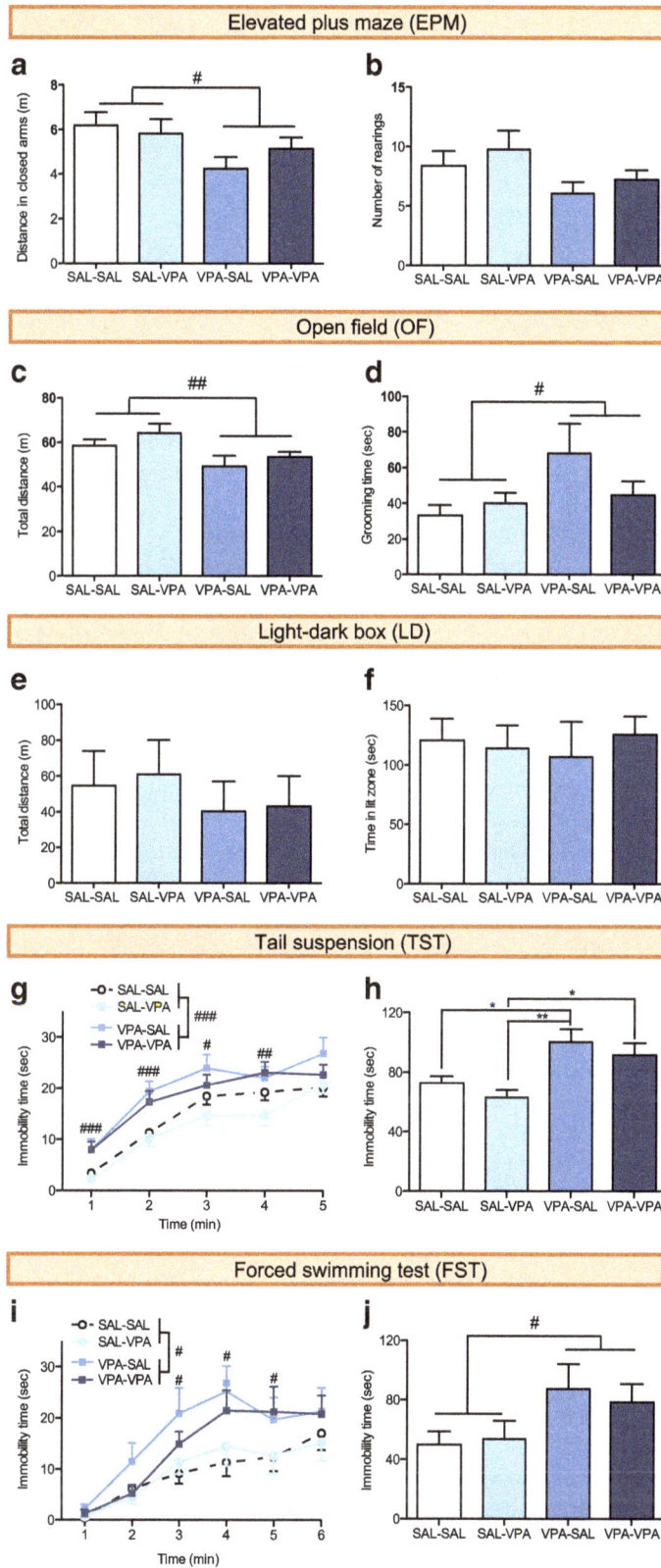

Fig. 3 (See legend on next page.)

(See figure on previous page.)
Fig. 3 Mice prenatally exposed to VPA show reduced exploration and increased levels of depression-related behavior. **a**, **b** Distance traveled in the closed arms (**a**) and number of rearings (**b**) in the EPM. **c**, **d** Total distance traveled (**c**) and time spent grooming (**d**) in the OF. **e**, **f** Total distance traveled (**e**) and time spent (**f**) in the lit compartment in the LD box. **g**, **h** Time spent immobile in 1-min bins (**g**) and accumulated time (**h**) in the TST. **i**, **j** Time spent immobile in 1-min bins (**i**) and cumulative time between 3 and 6 min (**j**) in the FST. Two-way or repeated measures ANOVA prenatal effect, $^{#}p < 0.05$, $^{##}p < 0.01$, $^{###}p < 0.001$. Tukey's post hoc test, $^{*}p < 0.05$, $^{**}p < 0.01$. Graphs indicate means + s.e.m. Detailed statistical information is available in Additional file 1: Table S2

the caudal part of the motor cortex (M1/M2) of VPA-VPA animals when compared with VPA-SAL mice. In addition, we observed increased glucose metabolism in the insular cortex (Ins) in VPA-VPA mice when compared with either SAL-SAL or VPA-SAL mice. Finally, we observed reduced glucose metabolism in the primary somatosensory cortex, barrel field (S1BF) in VPA-VPA mice.

Interestingly, VPA-SAL animals showed patterns of glucose metabolism more similar to SAL-SAL animals than VPA-VPA mice, suggesting that early social stimulation can revert the brain alterations caused by prenatal VPA exposure.

c-Fos immunoreactivity and neurotransmitters alterations in the piriform cortex of VPA-VPA mice are alleviated by early social stimulation

The increase in glucose metabolism in the Pir of VPA-VPA mice observed with the preclinical PET could be due to increased cellular activity. c-Fos is an immediate early gene whose expression is stimulated by neuronal depolarization and has been previously used to map changes in neuronal activity due to altered excitation/inhibition balance [33, 34]. We counted the number of c-Fos-positive nuclei in the layer 2 of the Pir and found it increased in VPA-VPA mice compared to SAL-SAL mice (Fig. 5a). To further characterize this increment, we analyzed the anterior and posterior parts of the Pir (Fig. 5b), and found it particularly significant in the aPir (Fig. 5c, d, Additional file 1: Figure S2a-d). Interestingly, both SAL-VPA and VPA-SAL mice exhibit an intermediate phenotype. Differences in the density of c-Fos-positive cells in the pPir were not statistically significant (Fig. 5e, f, and Additional file 1: Figure S2e–h). We found no c-Fos-positive cells in the layer 1 of the Pir, and only few c-Fos-positive cells in the layer 3 (Additional file 1: Figure S2), where we found no differences between groups (Additional file 1: Table S3).

The Pir is highly innervated by serotoninergic neurons of the raphe nucleus [35] and midbrain dopaminergic neurons [36], neurotransmitters that can modulate the activity of principal cells and interneurons [37, 38]. To evaluate dopaminergic and serotoninergic function in the Pir, we measured the levels of these neurotransmitters and their metabolites by HPLC-ED. We found no differences between groups neither in the levels of dopamine (DA; Fig. 5g) or its metabolite DOPAC (Fig. 5h),

serotonin (5-HT; Fig. 5j) or its metabolite 5-HIAA (Fig. 5k) nor the 5-HIAA/5-HT ratio (Fig. 5l). However, we found an increased dopaminergic turnover in the Pir of VPA-VPA mice when compared with mice prenatally exposed to SAL (Fig. 5i).

These results show that VPA-VPA mice have altered neuronal function in the Pir, and early social stimulation at least partially reverts these alterations.

Discussion

Taken together, our results show that early social stimulation can revert the decrease in sociability observed in VPA-exposed mice, while other behaviors are not affected by this postnatal treatment. In addition, preclinical PET analysis identified specific brain regions whose metabolism is altered by prenatal VPA treatment. Interestingly, most of these regions regain the control levels when VPA animals are reared with SAL mice. Among these brain structures, the piriform cortex (Pir) shows a bilaterally increased metabolism in VPA-VPA animals when compared with SAL-SAL or VPA-SAL mice. We also observed that VPA-VPA mice have more cFos-positive cells in the aPir and increased dopamine turnover in the Pir.

Performing a battery of behavioral tests and measuring a significant number of physiological variables leads to the problem of multiple testing when performing statistical analyses of the results. We reasoned that methods that provide more strict p values (e.g., Bonferroni correction or FDR) could contribute to avoiding false positives, but because of the extensive nature of our analysis, they could also lead to false negatives. VPA treatment, social enrichment, and the use of an outbred strain, all contribute to biological variability, making it difficult to detect meaningful differences. As an alternative, we have employed different strategies in order to minimize the effect of multiple testing on our results. On one hand, we used independent cohorts for juvenile play, PET studies (two cohorts), and HPLC analysis. In addition, adult behavioral testing was performed in three different cohorts, and each behavioral domain was evaluated in more than one test and variable. Moreover, animals employed for c-Fos expression analysis were randomly selected from a behavioral cohort, and a FDR approach was used in PET studies. All these approaches contribute to reducing type 1 error without significantly increasing

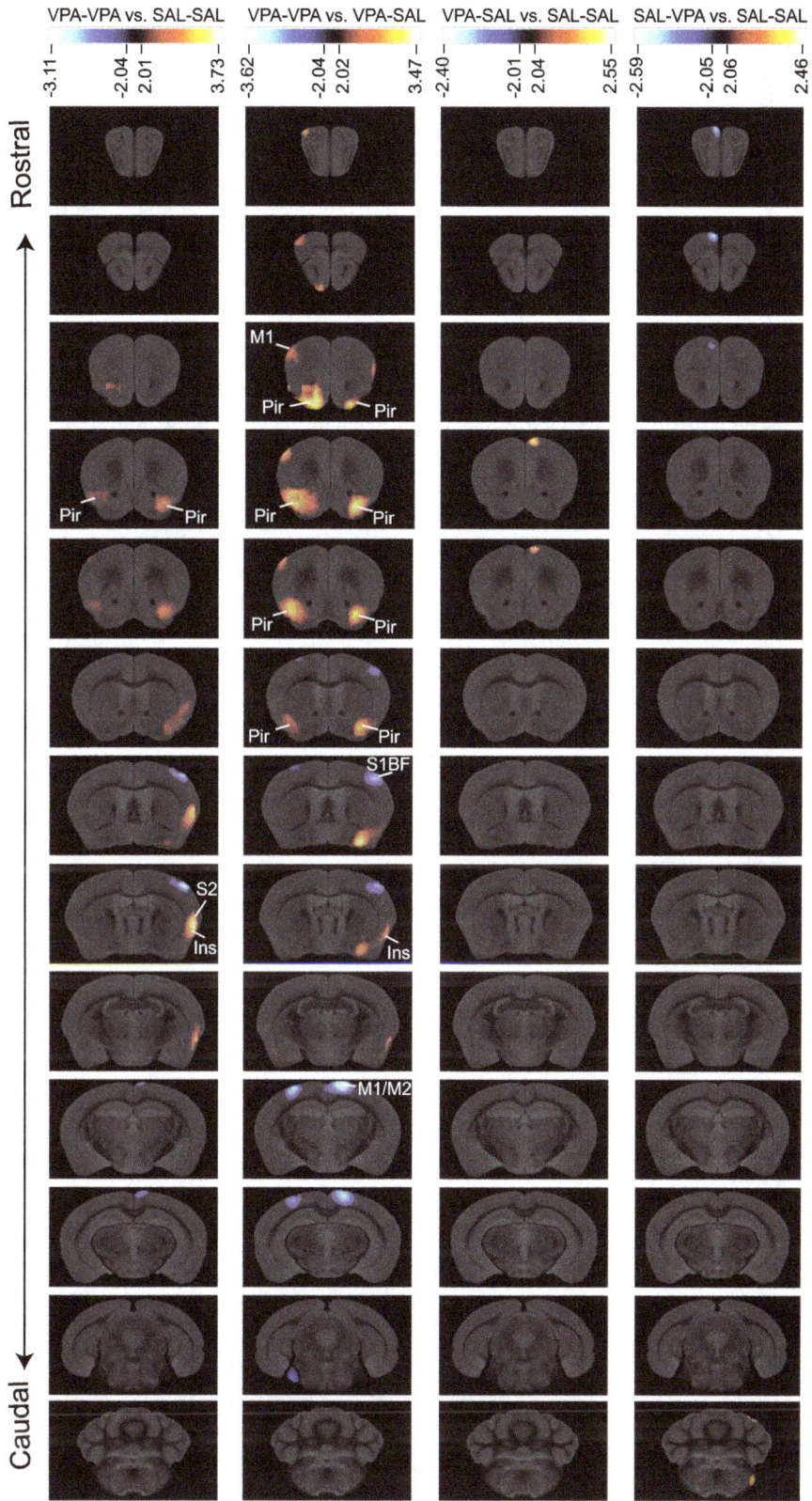

Fig. 4 (See legend on next page.)

(See figure on previous page.)
Fig. 4 Brain areas showing significant changes in glucose metabolism induced by prenatal and postnatal treatments. Rostral-caudal coronal sections (lines) showing the comparison between the different experimental groups (columns). Significant decreases are shown blue and increases red-yellow, t values for $p < 0.05$ are specified for each comparison. Ins, insular cortex; M1, primary motor cortex; M2, secondary motor cortex; Pir, piriform cortex; S1BF, primary somatosensory cortex, barrel field; S2, secondary somatosensory cortex

type 2 error and the number of animals used for experiments.

The development, organization, and function of the social brain circuitry result from the interaction between the child and his/her social environment [11]. Reciprocal social interactions are required for the integration of social stimuli to engage brain regions involved in reward, motor control, and attention [39]. In mammals, social interactions take place first with the parents and subsequently with the peers. Altered social environments can worsen genetic or prenatal factors affecting sociability, and we reasoned that, conversely, a rich social environment could counteract prenatal factors affecting sociability. Indeed, most early behavioral interventions employed in treating ASD target social aspects of behavior (e.g., language, social interaction) [40].

We have previously shown that maternal behavior is not affected by injecting VPA to the dams at GD12.5 [41], suggesting that maternal care is not contributing to the social deficits observed at weaning (Fig. 2a–c). After weaning, animals only interact with peers in the home cage. We hypothesized that the poor social environment experienced by VPA-exposed mice reared with other VPA-exposed mice could contribute to the reduction in sociability observed in adulthood. In addition, we hypothesized that VPA-exposed animals reared with animals showing more sociability could reverse their phenotype. Our design allowed us to specifically test the role of reciprocal interactions, without the confounding effect of the mother that could emerge from earlier interventions. Moreover, the developmental processes taking place in the rodent brain from PD20-PD25 are

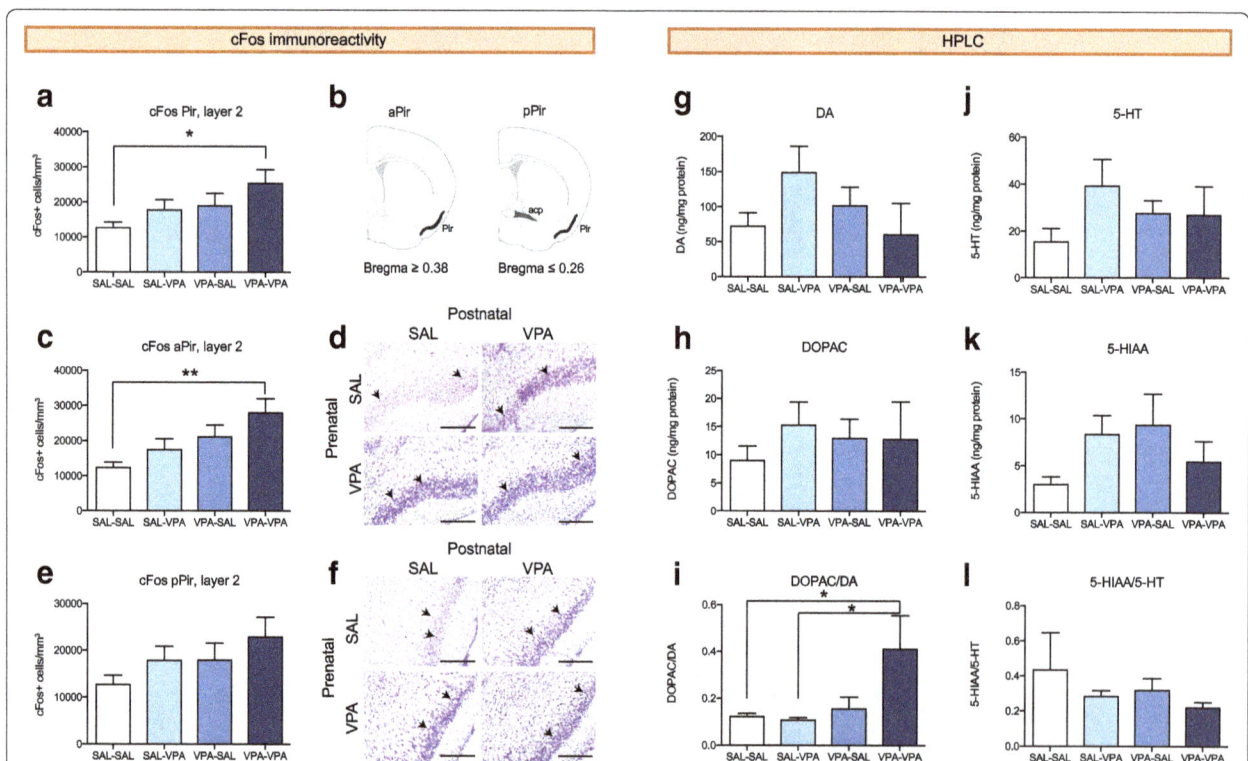

Fig. 5 VPA-VPA mice show increased c-Fos immunoreactivity and dopaminergic turnover in the piriform cortex. **a–f** Density of c-Fos-positive nuclei was measured in the whole Pir (**a**). Schemes in **b** show the posterior limit of the aPir and the anterior limit of the pPir, where the posterior part of the anterior commissure (acp, dark gray) is visible. Data is also presented discriminating between the anterior part of the Pir (**c**, aPir) and the posterior part of the Pir (**e**, pPir). $n = 5$–7 mice/group. Representative images of the aPir (**d**) and pPir (**f**) for the four experimental groups are shown. c-Fos-positive nuclei (black, arrows show examples) in Nissl stained slices. Bars, 200 μm. **g–l** Monoamine levels in the Pir were measured by HPLC-ED. **g** DA, **h** DOPAC, **i** DA turnover (DOPAC/DA), **j** 5-HT, **k** 5-HIAA, and **l** 5-HT turnover (5-HIAA/5-HT). $n = 4$–5 mice/group. Two-way ANOVA followed by Tukey's post hoc tests, *$p < 0.05$, **$p < 0.01$. Graphs indicate means + s.e.m. Detailed statistical information is available in Additional file 1: Table S3

similar to those occurring in the 2–5-year-old human brain [42], when usually ASD symptoms are detected.

We found that post-weaning social enrichment can reverse the altered sociability observed in young VPA-exposed mice, resulting in adult animals showing more social interaction that VPA-exposed animals reared with other VPA mice. Particularly, we show that VPA-VPA animals spend less time sniffing a novel mouse than any of the other groups (SAL-SAL, SAL-VPA, or VPA-SAL). The maze that we have employed in this work, originally described in [43], consists of small chambers. As a consequence, when animals are located in the lateral chambers they are mostly exploring the cylinder, rarely exploring the maze. Therefore, "sniffing" is the most reliable parameter of sociability since it involves the actual investigation of the social stimulus or the exploration of the control tube. However, it also implies a limitation because we can only provide one measure of social interaction. To evaluate the specificity of this effect, we analyzed other behaviors that are altered by prenatal VPA-exposure. We found that the VPA effects on repetitive behaviors, exploration, and depression-related behavior are not reversed by early social enrichment (Figs. 3 and 4). These results suggest that the previous reported effects of enriched environments on these behaviors [14, 44, 45] are due to the opportunity to explore a richer physical environment and not to the social stimulation available in such environments.

Alterations in juvenile play are observable at PD21 in mice prenatally exposed to VPA. Our results suggest that there is an additional critical period starting around PD21, when the interactions with peers can set the level of sociability in mice. Although we cannot claim a specific critical period of development for this effect, previous work suggests adolescence (approximately from PD21 to PD42) as a critical period for the establishment of social behaviors [reviewed in [46]]. Future work could narrow this critical period of postnatal development and identify the mechanisms through which they act. Although VPA and SAL animals show different levels of sociability at PD21 and the only variable we modified was the composition of the cages from PD21 to PD60, we did not specifically evaluate the levels of social stimulation on VPA-exposed animals in VPA-VPA and VPA-SAL groups. Therefore, we cannot rule out the contribution of additional unknown parameters (e.g., microbiota in the fecal matter [47]) that might affect the development and consolidation of sociability.

Here, we report the effects of VPA and early social stimulation on male offspring. We circumscribed our analysis to males since we did not observe any effects of prenatal VPA on social interactions in female offspring compared with the controls (unpublished results). This is consistent with the reports in CD1 mice [48], Sprague-Dawley rats [20], and Wistar rats [17]. This differential impact of VPA on male and female offspring adds face validity to this ASD model, as this disorder is four times more common in males than in females [49]. However, the prevalence of autism in children prenatally exposed to VPA is characterized by a 1:1 male to female ratio [50], and in the VPA model, there is an even effect on both sexes in other ASD-related phenotypes such as anxiety-related behaviors and repetitive behaviors [17, 48]. Moreover, female VPA offspring exhibit physiological and cellular changes that are consistent with the alterations observed in ASD children [17, 41, 51]. However, to date, sociability defects in female mice as a result of VPA exposure have not been found. The effects of social enrichment on females prenatally exposed to VPA needs to be further analyzed, as it can contribute to the treatment of girls diagnosed with ASD.

Most of our knowledge on brain circuit abnormalities in ASD individuals comes from functional MRI studies [5, 52]. However, these reports show numerous inconsistencies on the brain areas involved. We reasoned that our rescued group of animals would be a valuable tool to validate alterations observed in the VPA model. Using [18F]-FDG preclinical PET, we found that brain activity of VPA-SAL animals is more similar to SAL-SAL brains than VPA-VPA brains, as we found alterations in metabolism in the VPA-VPA brain that are not present in rescued animals. These structures appear then as candidate components of the social brain circuitry of the mouse. Interestingly, our results show differences in glucose metabolism in the resting state, similar to studies describing altered connectivity in people with ASD [5].

The circuitry that regulates social behavior involves many brain structures. In rodents, these structures are mainly components of the olfactory system, such as the anterior olfactory nucleus (AON) and the Pir. Indeed, the Pir controls olfactory perception and is activated by social stimuli [53], and during the discrimination between familiar and non-familiar social stimuli [54, 55]. Moreover, the oxytocin receptor-expressing neurons in the Pir mediate odor-driven social learning [56]. In line with this, we found a bilateral hyperactivation of the Pir in adult VPA-VPA mice, when compared to either control or rescued mice (Fig. 4). Moreover, we found increased cFos immunoreactivity in the layer 2 of the aPir (Fig. 5c), suggesting increased basal neuronal activity in VPA-VPA mice. Although we did not identify the type of neurons expressing c-Fos, the fact that they are localized for the most part in the layer 2 together with their morphology suggest that they are mostly glutamatergic principal neurons.

The Pir projects to the amygdala, basal ganglia, and hippocampus, areas implicated in behavioral output, with the aPir particularly projecting to the anterior part of the amygdala and the mediodorsal thalamus [57]. Alterations in the aPir function could then result in alterations in the circuitry engaged during social interactions. The Pir shows increased cFos immunoreactivity after exposure to a juvenile conspecific, but it is reduced after a neutral odor [55]. The increased basal neuronal activity observed in VPA-VPA mice could then preclude the circuitry to respond normally to a social stimulus, leaving the response to non-social odors unaffected (Fig. 2e, f).

In addition, we found increased dopaminergic turnover in the Pir of VPA-VPA mice (Fig. 5i). Cells in the Pir receive input from midbrain dopaminergic neurons [36], express dopamine receptors [58], and exhibit dose-dependent responses to dopamine [59]. Rodent dopaminergic projections and dopamine receptor expression in the brain undergo profound changes during the juvenile (PD21-PD28) and adolescent (PD34-PD49) stages [60, 61]. Social enrichment could modify a VPA-induced aberrant pattern of maturation of dopaminergic innervations, restoring normal dopaminergic function. Coactivation of dopamine D1 and D2 receptors results in reduced social interaction [62], suggesting a possible mechanism by which increased dopaminergic function in the Pir could result in diminished sociability in VPA-VPA mice.

In summary, VPA-VPA mice show reduced sociability and increases in glucose metabolism, neuronal activity, and dopaminergic turnover. In turn, VPA-SAL mice show no significant differences in any of these parameters when compared with SAL-SAL mice, displaying a phenotype that was indistinguishable from that of control animals. In addition, VPA-SAL sociability levels are significantly higher and glucose metabolism in the Pir is significantly lower when compared with VPA-VPA mice. These differences are partially explained by the reduction in neuronal activity and dopaminergic turnover observed in VPA-SAL mice, but additional neuronal changes in the Pir may be involved, as it is suggested by the larger differences observed in the PET between both VPA-exposed groups than in the VPA-VPA vs SAL-SAL comparison.

Our preclinical PET results also show alterations in glucose metabolism in other brain structures, the motor cortex (M1/M2), the somatosensory cortex (S2 and S1BF) and the insular cortex. We need to further study these structures to elucidate if they play a role in modulating the behaviors altered in animals prenatally exposed to VPA. It was recently shown that maternal immune activation (MIA) results in cortical patches of reduced cellular activity (cFos-positive cells) in the primary somatosensory cortex (S1) and secondary motor cortex (M2) [34]. Interestingly, these patches were often present unilaterally, similar to the pattern that we

observed (Fig. 4). MIA offspring show behavioral alterations comparable to those observed in VPA-exposed mice, and the specific manipulation of neuronal activity on the S1 can modulate social interaction and repetitive behaviors in MIA offspring [34]. These results demonstrate a role of the S1 in modulating these behaviors and suggest that the reduction in glucose metabolism observed unilaterally in S1 and M2 in VPA-VPA mice could also contribute to the abnormal behavior of these animals.

Our unbiased analysis of brain activity in a mouse model of ASD adds to previous fMRI studies on brain connectivity and neuronal activity in the acallosal and socially impaired BTBR strain [63, 64]. BTBR mice showed reduced basal neuronal activity and metabolism in the somatosensory and piriform cortex, when compared with C57BL/6J mice. In addition, brain activity mapping was previously performed in a mouse model of Rett syndrome (the Mecp2 null mice), using a histological technique (Fos labeling) [33]. Interestingly, that analysis reports reduced neuronal activity in the Pir, somatosensory, and motor cortices. As Mecp2 null mice [65] and BTBR mice [66] show deficits in social behavior, our results add to those reports in suggesting that these structures could be central to its regulation.

Conclusions

In conclusion, this study demonstrates that social enrichment after weaning can reverse the detrimental effects of prenatal VPA exposure on sociability. Our model of rescued mice can then be valuable to test whether molecular and cellular alterations can be reversed in the VPA model when social deficits are reversed. As other ASD-related behaviors are not affected by the rearing protocol, this model can also be used to disentangle the circuits that are engaged in social and repetitive behaviors. Finally, our results highlight the relevance of studying the role of the Pir in modulating social behavior.

Additional file

Additional file 1: Table S1. Summary of ANOVA results for the behavioral analyses conducted on adult offspring in the four experimental groups (data corresponding to main Fig. 2). **Table S2.** Summary of ANOVA results for the behavioral analyses conducted on adult offspring in the four experimental groups (data corresponding to main Fig. 3). **Table S3.** Summary of ANOVA results for the histological analyses and HPLC conducted on adult offspring in the four experimental groups (data corresponding to main Fig. 5). **Figure S1.** Animals show normal responses to novel objects. **Figure S2.** Animals show similar numbers of cFos-positive cells in the layer 3 of the piriform cortex. **Figure S3.** Representative images of sections processed for c-Fos immunoreativity and Nissl staining (DOCX 729 kb)

Abbreviations
ASD: Autism spectrum disorder; EPM: Elevated plus maze test; FST: Forced swimming test; LD: Light-dark box test; NOR: Novel object recognition test;

OF: Open field test; Pir: Piriform cortex; TST: Tail suspension test; VPA: Valproic acid

Acknowledgements
We want to thank the staff of the Laboratory of Preclinical Imaging, especially to Ms. Nadia Levanovich for the contribution in image acquisitions and animal care. Also, we extend our gratitude to the group Cyclotron-Radiopharmacty of the Centro de Imágenes Moleculares of FLENI. We want to thank Dr. Patricia Agostino and Julieta Acosta for preparing the samples for HPLC analysis and Dr. Maria de la Paz Fernandez for critically reading the manuscript.

Funding
This work was supported by a National Agency of Promotion of Science and Technology (ANPCyT) Grant (PICT2013-1362) and a University of Buenos Aires grant (UBACYT2016-20020150100120BA). A.M.D. is a member of the Research Career of the National Council of Scientific and Technological Research (CONICET), Argentina, and a full-time researcher at the Faculty of Exact and Natural Sciences, University of Buenos Aires, Argentina. M.C. and N.K. are fellows of the CONICET. N. S. is a fellow of the University of Buenos Aires.

Authors' contributions
MC, NK, GF, LU, NS, CH, and AMD performed the experiments. MC, GF, LU, and AMD designed the experiments, analyzed the data, and interpreted the results. AMD supervised the studies and drafted the manuscript. All the authors approved the final version of the manuscript.

Competing interests
The authors declare that they have no competing interests.

Author details
[1]Universidad de Buenos Aires, Facultad de Ciencias Exactas y Naturales, Departamento de Fisiología, Biología Molecular y Celular, Buenos Aires, Argentina. [2]CONICET-Universidad de Buenos Aires, Instituto de Fisiología, Biología Molecular y Neurociencias (IFIBYNE), Buenos Aires, Argentina. [3]FLENI, Centro de Imágenes Moleculares, Laboratorio de Imágenes Preclínicas, Buenos Aires, Argentina. [4]Facultad de Farmacia y Bioquímica, Cátedra de Farmacología, Universidad de Buenos Aires, Buenos Aires, Argentina. [5]UBA-CONICET, Ciudad Universitaria, Int. Guiraldes 2160, Pabellon 2, Ciudad de Buenos Aires, Argentina.

References
1. American Psychiatric Association. Diagnostic and statistical manual of mental disorders. 5th ed; 2013.
2. Betancur C. Etiological heterogeneity in autism spectrum disorders: more than 100 genetic and genomic disorders and still counting. Brain Res. 2011; 1380:42–77.
3. Sussman D, Leung RC, Vogan VM, Lee W, Trelle S, Lin S, Cassel DB, Chakravarty MM, Lerch JP, Anagnostou E, Taylor MJ. The autism puzzle: diffuse but not pervasive neuroanatomical abnormalities in children with ASD. Neuroimage Clin. 2015;8:170–9.
4. Depino AM, Lucchina L, Pitossi F. Early and adult hippocampal TGF-beta1 overexpression have opposite effects on behavior. Brain Behav Immun. 2011;25:1582–91.
5. Cheng W, Rolls ET, Gu H, Zhang J, Feng J. Autism: reduced connectivity between cortical areas involved in face expression, theory of mind, and the sense of self. Brain. 2015;138:1382–93.
6. Fatemi SH, Aldinger KA, Ashwood P, Bauman ML, Blaha CD, Blatt GJ, Chauhan A, Chauhan V, Dager SR, Dickson PE, et al. Consensus paper: pathological role of the cerebellum in autism. Cerebellum. 2012;11:777–807.
7. Rossignol DA. Novel and emerging treatments for autism spectrum disorders: a systematic review. Ann Clin Psychiatry. 2009;21:213–36.
8. Cohen H, Amerine-Dickens M, Smith T. Early intensive behavioral treatment: replication of the UCLA model in a community setting. J Dev Behav Pediatr. 2006;27:S145–55.
9. Dawson G, Rogers S, Munson J, Smith M, Winter J, Greenson J, Donaldson A, Varley J. Randomized, controlled trial of an intervention for toddlers with autism: the Early Start Denver Model. Pediatrics. 2010;125:e17–23.
10. Smith T, Groen AD, Wynn JW. Randomized trial of intensive early intervention for children with pervasive developmental disorder. Am J Ment Retard. 2000;105:269–85.
11. Dawson G. Early behavioral intervention, brain plasticity, and the prevention of autism spectrum disorder. Dev Psychopathol. 2008;20:775–803.
12. Francis DD, Diorio J, Plotsky PM, Meaney MJ. Environmental enrichment reverses the effects of maternal separation on stress reactivity. J Neurosci. 2002;22:7840–3.
13. Faverjon S, Silveira DC, Fu DD, Cha BH, Akman C, Hu Y, Holmes GL. Beneficial effects of enriched environment following status epilepticus in immature rats. Neurology. 2002;59:1356–64.
14. Schneider T, Turczak J, Przewlocki R. Environmental enrichment reverses behavioral alterations in rats prenatally exposed to valproic acid: issues for a therapeutic approach in autism. Neuropsychopharmacology. 2006;31:36–46.
15. Yamaguchi H, Hara Y, Ago Y, Takano E, Hasebe S, Nakazawa T, Hashimoto H, Matsuda T, Takuma K. Environmental enrichment attenuates behavioral abnormalities in valproic acid-exposed autism model mice. Behav Brain Res. 2017;333:67–73.
16. Lucchina L, Depino AM. Altered peripheral and central inflammatory responses in a mouse model of autism. Autism Res. 2014;7:273–89.
17. Schneider T, Roman A, Basta-Kaim A, Kubera M, Budziszewska B, Schneider K, Przewlocki R. Gender-specific behavioral and immunological alterations in an animal model of autism induced by prenatal exposure to valproic acid. Psychoneuroendocrinology. 2008;33:728–40.
18. de Theije CG, Wopereis H, Ramadan M, van Eijndthoven T, Lambert J, Knol J, Garssen J, Kraneveld AD, Oozeer R. Altered gut microbiota and activity in a murine model of autism spectrum disorders. Brain Behav Immun. 2014;37:197–206.
19. Hofvander B, Delorme R, Chaste P, Nyden A, Wentz E, Stahlberg O, Herbrecht E, Stopin A, Anckarsater H, Gillberg C, et al. Psychiatric and psychosocial problems in adults with normal-intelligence autism spectrum disorders. BMC Psychiatry. 2009;9:35.
20. Kim KC, Kim P, Go HS, Choi CS, Park JH, Kim HJ, Jeon SJ, Dela Pena IC, Han SH, Cheong JH, et al. Male-specific alteration in excitatory post-synaptic development and social interaction in pre-natal valproic acid exposure model of autism spectrum disorder. J Neurochem. 2013;124: 832–43.
21. McFarlane HG, Kusek GK, Yang M, Phoenix JL, Bolivar VJ, Crawley JN. Autism-like behavioral phenotypes in BTBR T+tf/J mice. Genes Brain Behav. 2008;7:152–63.
22. Cox KH, Rissman EF. Sex differences in juvenile mouse social behavior are influenced by sex chromosomes and social context. Genes Brain Behav. 2011;10:465–72.
23. Depino AM, Tsetsenis T, Gross C. GABA homeostasis contributes to the developmental programming of anxiety-related behavior. Brain Res. 2008; 1210:189–99.
24. Yang M, Crawley JN: Simple behavioral assessment of mouse olfaction. Curr Protoc Neurosci 2009, Chapter 8:Unit 8 24.
25. Federman N, de la Fuente V, Zalcman G, Corbi N, Onori A, Passananti C, Romano A. Nuclear factor kappaB-dependent histone acetylation is specifically involved in persistent forms of memory. J Neurosci. 2013;33: 7603–14.
26. Depino AM. Early prenatal exposure to LPS results in anxiety- and depression-related behaviors in adulthood. Neuroscience. 2015;299:56–65.

27. Ullmann JF, Watson C, Janke AL, Kurniawan ND, Reutens DC. A segmentation protocol and MRI atlas of the C57BL/6J mouse neocortex. Neuroimage. 2013;78:196–203.

28. Acosta J, Campolongo MA, Hocht C, Depino AM, Golombek DA, Agostino PV. Deficits in temporal processing in mice prenatally exposed to valproic acid. Eur J Neurosci. 2018;47:619–30.

29. Campolongo M, Benedetti L, Podhajcer OL, Pitossi F, Depino AM. Hippocampal SPARC regulates depression-related behavior. Genes Brain Behav. 2012;11:966–76.

30. Schneider CA, Rasband WS, Eliceiri KW. NIH Image to ImageJ: 25 years of image analysis. Nat Methods. 2012;9:671–675.

31. Paxinos G, Franklin K. The mouse brain in stereotaxic coordinates. 2nd ed. San Diego: Academic Press; 2001.

32. van Steensel FJ, Bogels SM, Perrin S. Anxiety disorders in children and adolescents with autistic spectrum disorders: a meta-analysis. Clin Child Fam Psychol Rev. 2011;14:302–17.

33. Kron M, Howell CJ, Adams IT, Ransbottom M, Christian D, Ogier M, Katz DM. Brain activity mapping in Mecp2 mutant mice reveals functional deficits in forebrain circuits, including key nodes in the default mode network, that are reversed with ketamine treatment. J Neurosci. 2012;32:13860–72.

34. Shin Yim Y, Park A, Berrios J, Lafourcade M, Pascual LM, Soares N, Yeon Kim J, Kim S, Kim H, Waisman A, et al. Reversing behavioural abnormalities in mice exposed to maternal inflammation. Nature. 2017;549:482–7.

35. Datiche F, Luppi PH, Cattarelli M. Serotonergic and non-serotonergic projections from the raphe nuclei to the piriform cortex in the rat: a cholera toxin B subunit (CTb) and 5-HT immunohistochemical study. Brain Res. 1995;671:27–37.

36. Haberly LB, Price JL. Association and commissural fiber systems of the olfactory cortex of the rat. J Comp Neurol. 1978;178:711–40.

37. Sheldon PW, Aghajanian GK. Excitatory responses to serotonin (5-HT) in neurons of the rat piriform cortex: evidence for mediation by 5-HT1C receptors in pyramidal cells and 5-HT2 receptors in interneurons. Synapse. 1991;9:208–18.

38. Narla C, Dunn HA, Ferguson SS, Poulter MO. Suppression of piriform cortex activity in rat by corticotropin-releasing factor 1 and serotonin 2A/C receptors. Front Cell Neurosci. 2015;9:200.

39. Kuhl PK. Is speech learning 'gated' by the social brain? Dev Sci. 2007;10:110–20.

40. National Research Council. Educating children with autism. Washington, DC: National Academy Press; 2001.

41. Kazlauskas N, Campolongo M, Lucchina L, Zappala C, Depino AM. Postnatal behavioral and inflammatory alterations in female pups prenatally exposed to valproic acid. Psychoneuroendocrinology. 2016;72:11–21.

42. Semple BD, Blomgren K, Gimlin K, Ferriero DM, Noble-Haeusslein LJ. Brain development in rodents and humans: identifying benchmarks of maturation and vulnerability to injury across species. Prog Neurobiol. 2013;106-107:1–16.

43. Brodkin ES, Hagemann A, Nemetski SM, Silver LM. Social approach-avoidance behavior of inbred mouse strains towards DBA/2 mice. Brain Res. 2004;1002:151–7.

44. Powell SB, Newman HA, McDonald TA, Bugenhagen P, Lewis MH. Development of spontaneous stereotyped behavior in deer mice: effects of early and late exposure to a more complex environment. Dev Psychobiol. 2000;37:100–8.

45. Turner CA, Yang MC, Lewis MH. Environmental enrichment: effects on stereotyped behavior and regional neuronal metabolic activity. Brain Res. 2002;938:15–21.

46. Spear LP. The adolescent brain and age-related behavioral manifestations. Neurosci Biobehav Rev. 2000;24:417–63.

47. Buffington SA, Di Prisco GV, Auchtung TA, Ajami NJ, Petrosino JF, Costa-Mattioli M. Microbial reconstitution reverses maternal diet-induced social and synaptic deficits in offspring. Cell. 2016;165:1762–75.

48. Kataoka S, Takuma K, Hara Y, Maeda Y, Ago Y, Matsuda T. Autism-like behaviours with transient histone hyperacetylation in mice treated prenatally with valproic acid. Int J Neuropsychopharmacol. 2013;16:91–103.

49. Fombonne E. Epidemiological trends in rates of autism. Mol Psychiatry. 2002;7(Suppl 2):S4–6.

50. Rasalam AD, Hailey H, Williams JH, Moore SJ, Turnpenny PD, Lloyd DJ, Dean JC. Characteristics of fetal anticonvulsant syndrome associated autistic disorder. Dev Med Child Neurol. 2005;47:551–5.

51. Hara Y, Maeda Y, Kataoka S, Ago Y, Takuma K, Matsuda T. Effect of prenatal valproic acid exposure on cortical morphology in female mice. J Pharmacol Sci. 2012;118:543–6.

52. Maximo JO, Cadena EJ, Kana RK. The implications of brain connectivity in the neuropsychology of autism. Neuropsychol Rev. 2014;24:16–31.

53. Ferguson JN, Aldag JM, Insel TR, Young LJ. Oxytocin in the medial amygdala is essential for social recognition in the mouse. J Neurosci. 2001; 21:8278–85.

54. Borelli KG, Blanchard DC, Javier LK, Defensor EB, Brandao ML, Blanchard RJ. Neural correlates of scent marking behavior in C57BL/6J mice: detection and recognition of a social stimulus. Neuroscience. 2009;162:914–23.

55. Richter K, Wolf G, Engelmann M. Social recognition memory requires two stages of protein synthesis in mice. Learn Mem. 2005;12:407–13.

56. Choe HK, Reed MD, Benavidez N, Montgomery D, Soares N, Yim YS, Choi GB. Oxytocin mediates entrainment of sensory stimuli to social cues of opposing valence. Neuron. 2015;87:152–63.

57. Schwabe K, Ebert U, Loscher W. The central piriform cortex: anatomical connections and anticonvulsant effect of GABA elevation in the kindling model. Neuroscience. 2004;126:727–41.

58. Campbell KM, de Lecea L, Severynse DM, Caron MG, McGrath MJ, Sparber SB, Sun LY, Burton FH. OCD-like behaviors caused by a neuropotentiating transgene targeted to cortical and limbic D1+ neurons. J Neurosci. 1999;19: 5044–53.

59. Gellman RL, Aghajanian GK. Pyramidal cells in piriform cortex receive a convergence of inputs from monoamine activated GABAergic interneurons. Brain Res. 1993;600:63–73.

60. Kalsbeek A, Voorn P, Buijs RM, Pool CW, Uylings HB. Development of the dopaminergic innervation in the prefrontal cortex of the rat. J Comp Neurol. 1988;269:58–72.

61. Garske AK, Lawyer CR, Peterson BM, Illig KR. Adolescent changes in dopamine D1 receptor expression in orbitofrontal cortex and piriform cortex accompany an associative learning deficit. PLoS One. 2013;8:e56191.

62. Zenko M, Zhu Y, Dremencov E, Ren W, Xu L, Zhang X. Requirement for the endocannabinoid system in social interaction impairment induced by coactivation of dopamine D1 and D2 receptors in the piriform cortex. J Neurosci Res. 2011;89:1245–58.

63. Sforazzini F, Bertero A, Dodero L, David G, Galbusera A, Scattoni ML, Pasqualetti M, Gozzi A. Altered functional connectivity networks in acallosal and socially impaired BTBR mice. Brain Struct Funct. 2016;221:941–54.

64. Dodero L, Damiano M, Galbusera A, Bifone A, Tsaftsaris SA, Scattoni ML, Gozzi A. Neuroimaging evidence of major morpho-anatomical and functional abnormalities in the BTBR T+TF/J mouse model of autism. PLoS One. 2013;8:e76655.

65. Kerr B, Alvarez-Saavedra M, Saez MA, Saona A, Young JI. Defective body-weight regulation, motor control and abnormal social interactions in Mecp2 hypomorphic mice. Hum Mol Genet. 2008;17:1707–17.

66. Moy SS, Nadler JJ, Young NB, Perez A, Holloway LP, Barbaro RP, Barbaro JR, Wilson LM, Threadgill DW, Lauder JM, et al. Mouse behavioral tasks relevant to autism: phenotypes of 10 inbred strains. Behav Brain Res. 2007;176:4–20.

14

Delineation of the genetic and clinical spectrum of Phelan-McDermid syndrome caused by *SHANK3* point mutations

Silvia De Rubeis[1,2†], Paige M. Siper[1,2†], Allison Durkin[1], Jordana Weissman[1], François Muratet[1,2], Danielle Halpern[1,2], Maria del Pilar Trelles[1,2], Yitzchak Frank[1,3], Reymundo Lozano[1,2,4,5], A. Ting Wang[1,2], J. Lloyd Holder Jr[6], Catalina Betancur[7*], Joseph D. Buxbaum[1,2,5,8,9,10*] and Alexander Kolevzon[1,2,4,10*]

Abstract

Background: Phelan-McDermid syndrome (PMS) is a neurodevelopmental disorder characterized by psychiatric and neurological features. Most reported cases are caused by 22q13.3 deletions, leading to *SHANK3* haploinsufficiency, but also usually encompassing many other genes. While the number of point mutations identified in *SHANK3* has increased in recent years due to large-scale sequencing studies, systematic studies describing the phenotype of individuals harboring such mutations are lacking.

Methods: We provide detailed clinical and genetic data on 17 individuals carrying mutations in *SHANK3*. We also review 60 previously reported patients with pathogenic or likely pathogenic *SHANK3* variants, often lacking detailed phenotypic information.

Results: *SHANK3* mutations in our cohort and in previously reported cases were distributed throughout the protein; the majority were truncating and all were compatible with de novo inheritance. Despite substantial allelic heterogeneity, four variants were recurrent (p.Leu1142Valfs*153, p.Ala1227Glyfs*69, p.Arg1255Leufs*25, and c.2265+1G>A), suggesting that these are hotspots for de novo mutations. All individuals studied had intellectual disability, and autism spectrum disorder was prevalent (73%). Severe speech deficits were common, but in contrast to individuals with 22q13.3 deletions, the majority developed single words, including 41% with at least phrase speech. Other common findings were consistent with reports among individuals with 22q13.3 deletions, including hypotonia, motor skill deficits, regression, seizures, brain abnormalities, mild dysmorphic features, and feeding and gastrointestinal problems.

Conclusions: Haploinsufficiency of *SHANK3* resulting from point mutations is sufficient to cause a broad range of features associated with PMS. Our findings expand the molecular and phenotypic spectrum of PMS caused by *SHANK3* point mutations and suggest that, in general, speech impairment and motor deficits are more severe in the case of deletions. In contrast, renal abnormalities associated with 22q13.3 deletions do not appear to be related to the loss of *SHANK3*.

Keywords: *SHANK3*, Phelan-McDermid syndrome, 22q13 deletion syndrome, Sequence variants, Phenotype, Autism spectrum disorder, Intellectual disability

* Correspondence: catalina.betancur@inserm.fr; joseph.buxbaum@mssm.edu; alexander.kolevzon@mssm.edu
Catalina Betancur, Joseph D. Buxbaum, and Alexander Kolevzon are co-senior authors.
†Equal contributors
[7]Sorbonne Université, INSERM, CNRS, Neuroscience Paris Seine, Institut de Biologie Paris Seine, 75005 Paris, France
[1]Seaver Autism Center, Icahn School of Medicine at Mount Sinai, New York, NY 10029, USA
Full list of author information is available at the end of the article

Background

Phelan-McDermid syndrome (PMS, OMIM 606232) is a rare neurodevelopmental disorder characterized by neonatal hypotonia, global developmental delay, intellectual disability (ID), severely delayed or absent speech, and frequent autism spectrum disorder (ASD) [1]. The neurobehavioral phenotype of PMS is usually severe. In a prospective study of 32 PMS individuals, 77% manifested severe-to-profound ID and 84% met criteria for ASD using gold standard diagnostic tools [2]. Dysmorphic features are usually mild and include long eyelashes, large or prominent ears, bulbous nose, pointed chin, fleshy hands, and dysplastic toenails [1]. Additional features include gastrointestinal problems, seizures, motor deficits, structural brain abnormalities, renal malformations, lymphedema, and recurrent infections [1].

The major neurodevelopmental features of PMS are caused by deletions or mutations of the *SHANK3* gene, which encodes a scaffolding protein of the postsynaptic density of glutamatergic synapses. Most reported cases of PMS are caused by 22q13.3 deletions, which usually encompass many genes and can extend up to 9.2 Mb [2–4]. Genotype-phenotype analyses indicate that the size of the deletion and the number and/or severity of clinical manifestations are positively correlated [2, 4–7]. Specifically, correlations have been reported between deletion size and hypotonia [5–7], developmental delay [5–7], dysmorphic features [2, 7], speech abilities [4], social communication deficits related to ASD [2], and other medical conditions [2]. Furthermore, individuals with small terminal deletions may have more favorable developmental trajectories than those with larger deletions [8].

De novo truncating and missense mutations in *SHANK3* have been identified in cohorts ascertained for ASD [9–16] or ID [17–21]. In addition, there is a single report of two families ascertained for schizophrenia with mutations in *SHANK3*; affected individuals also had ID [22]. Despite the increasing number of mutations in *SHANK3*, their prevalence in PMS and more broadly in ASD is underestimated because clinical sequencing is still uncommon compared to chromosomal microarray. In addition, *SHANK3* has been poorly covered by whole exome sequencing due to high GC content [13, 23], and there is little in the PMS phenotype that would prompt a clinician to specifically target *SHANK3* for optimized Sanger sequencing. We and others estimate that *SHANK3* haploinsufficiency might account for up to 1% of more severely affected ASD cases [13, 23].

Given the dearth of identified cases with *SHANK3* mutations, analyses of PMS cohorts have largely focused on individuals with 22q13.3 deletions [2–8, 24]. Only two studies on PMS have included a few individuals carrying *SHANK3* mutations [2, 24]. These observations have been complemented by the description of a small number of individuals identified through *SHANK3* targeted sequencing in ASD cohorts [9–13]. Large-scale sequencing studies have been instrumental in revealing additional *SHANK3* mutations but have not provided detailed phenotypic information [14–16, 19–21].

The limited number of subjects with *SHANK3* mutations examined thus far, and the lack of systematic clinical evaluation have hindered the characterization of the phenotypic spectrum associated with *SHANK3* mutations. Here, we aimed to delineate the genetic spectrum of *SHANK3* mutations and their associated phenotype in relationship to PMS features.

Methods

Participants

The study includes 14 participants (S1–S14) enrolled at the Seaver Autism Center for Research and Treatment at the Icahn School of Medicine at Mount Sinai, and three individuals (B1–B3) evaluated at Baylor College of Medicine. Individuals were referred through the Phelan-McDermid Syndrome Foundation, ongoing research studies, and communication between families. The study was approved by the Program for the Protection of Human Subjects at the Icahn School of Medicine at Mount Sinai and the Baylor College of Medicine Institutional Review Board. Parents or legal guardians provided informed consent for participation and publication. Consent was also obtained to publish the photos shown in Fig. 1.

Genetic testing

All mutations were identified and/or validated by Clinical Laboratory Improvement Amendments (CLIA)-certified laboratories. The mutation in individual S1 was identified by whole exome sequencing (WES) and then validated by Sanger sequencing at the Seaver Autism Center [2] and by GeneDx. The mutation in S2 was identified by panel sequencing at the Michigan Medical Genetics Laboratories. The mutation in S3 was identified and validated at Seaver as previously reported [2] and further confirmed by Athena Diagnostics. The mutation in S4 was identified through clinical WES by the Columbia University Laboratory of Personalized Medicine. The mutations in S5, S11, and B1 were identified through clinical WES by the Medical Genetics Laboratory at the Baylor College of Medicine. The mutations in S6, S7, S9, S10, S12, and S14 were identified through clinical WES by GeneDx. The mutation in S8 was identified through clinical WES by AmbryGenetics. The variants in S13 were identified at the Seaver Autism Center and confirmed by GeneDx. The mutation in B2 and B3 was identified through clinical WES by Transgenomic.

Variants were described according to the Human Genome Variation Society guidelines. As previously

Delineation of the genetic and clinical spectrum of Phelan-McDermid syndrome caused by SHANK3...

181

[2], the human genome reference assembly (GRCh37/hg19 and GRCh38/hg38) is missing the beginning of exon 11 (NM_033517.1:c.1305_1346, 5′-cccgagcgggcccg gcggccccggccccgcgcccggccccgg-3′, coding for 436-PSG PGGPGPAPGPG-449). We numbered nucleotide and amino acid positions according to the *SHANK3* RefSeq mRNA (NM_033517.1) and protein (NP_277052.1) sequence, in which this mistake has been corrected. Variants were interpreted according to the American College of Medical Genetics and Genomics (ACMG) guidelines [25].

Review of previously reported *SHANK3* mutations

We searched the literature for pathogenic or likely pathogenic mutations in *SHANK3* and retrieved the molecular and clinical information (Additional file 1: Tables S1–S3). We also included mutations reported in ClinVar (http://www.ncbi.nlm.nih.gov/clinvar/). To avoid duplicate counting of affected individuals, we reviewed all available information (including gender, country of origin, and phenotype) and contacted the authors when doubts persisted. Individuals reported more than once are indicated in Additional file 1: Table S1.

Clinical evaluation

Prospective clinical and psychological characterization was completed for 12 individuals seen at the Seaver Autism Center (S1–S4, S6–S8, S10–S14), including three previously reported (S1 and S3 [2] and S13 [26]). A battery of standardized assessments was used to examine ASD, intellectual functioning, adaptive behavior, language, motor skills, and sensory processing (see below). The medical evaluation included psychiatric, neurological, and clinical genetics examinations and medical record review. The evaluation of the individuals seen at Baylor College of Medicine (B1–B3) included parent interview, neurological examination, and medical record review. Their seizure phenotype and brain magnetic resonance imaging (MRI) findings were reported previously [24]. Two additional individuals (S5 and S9) received genetic testing through the Seaver Autism Center but were not evaluated clinically. Their caregivers completed surveys to capture developmental, medical, and behavioral health issues and were interviewed by phone.

ASD phenotype

Gold-standard ASD diagnostic testing included the Autism Diagnostic Observation Schedule, Second Edition (ADOS-2) [27], the Autism Diagnostic Interview-Revised (ADI-R) [28], and a clinical evaluation to assess Diagnostic and Statistical Manual for Mental Disorders, Fifth Edition (DSM-5) criteria for ASD [29]. The ADOS-2 and ADI-R were administered and scored by research reliable raters, and the psychiatric evaluation was completed by a board-certified child and adolescent psychiatrist. The ADOS-2 is a semi-structured observational assessment that provides scores in the domains of social affect, restricted and repetitive behavior, and a total score. A comparison score ranging from 1 to 10, with higher scores reflecting a greater number of symptoms, was calculated to examine symptom severity within each ADOS-2 domain and in total [30]. Nine individuals (S1–S4, S6, S8, S11, S13, S14) received module 1 of the ADOS, for children who are nonverbal or communicate using single words. Two individuals (S7, S10) received module 3, for children who are verbally fluent. The ADI-R is a structured caregiver interview that assesses ASD symptomatology within the domains of socialization, communication, and repetitive and restricted interests and behavior. A consensus diagnosis was determined for each participant based on results from the ADOS-2, ADI-R, and clinical evaluation using DSM-5.

Intellectual functioning

Global cognitive ability was measured using the Mullen Scales of Early Learning [31] ($n = 10$), the Stanford Binet Intelligence Scales, Fifth Edition [32] ($n = 1$), and the Differential Ability Scales, Second Edition (DAS-II) [33] ($n = 1$), depending on age and verbal ability. The Mullen is validated for children from birth to 68 months but is commonly used for older individuals with ID [34]. Developmental quotients were calculated using age equivalents divided by chronological age as has been done in previous studies [35]. For example, a nonverbal developmental quotient was computed by dividing the mean age equivalents on the visual reception and fine motor scales by the child's chronological age and then multiplying by 100. The DAS-II is a measure of cognitive functioning that assesses a child's verbal reasoning, nonverbal reasoning, and spatial abilities. A general conceptual ability can be calculated to assess overall intellectual functioning. The Stanford-Binet Intelligence Scales, Fifth Edition is an intelligence test that produces a nonverbal intellectual quotient (IQ), verbal IQ, and full scale IQ based on performance across five scales: fluid reasoning, knowledge, quantitative reasoning, visual-spatial, and working memory.

Adaptive behavior

The Vineland Adaptive Behavior Scales, Second Edition, Survey Interview Form (Vineland-II) [36] is a clinician-administered interview that assesses adaptive behavior in the domains of communication, daily living, socialization, and motor skills. The Vineland-II was completed for 11 individuals. The motor domain is intended for children ages 6 years and under but was assessed in all individuals given significant motor delays in this population. The

Vineland-II was also used in conjunction with cognitive testing to identify the presence and severity of ID.

Language skills
Language milestones were assessed during the ADI-R ($n = 11$) and the psychiatric evaluation. Current expressive and receptive language abilities were assessed using the Mullen ($n = 10$), Vineland-II ($n = 11$), MacArthur-Bates Communicative Development Inventories [37] ($n = 10$), Peabody Picture Vocabulary Test, Fourth Edition [38] ($n = 3$), and Expressive Vocabulary Test [39] ($n = 2$).

Motor skills
Motor milestones were assessed during the ADI-R ($n = 11$) and the psychiatric evaluation ($n = 12$). Current motor skills were assessed using the Vineland-II ($n = 11$) and Mullen ($n = 10$) fine and gross motor skills domains. The Beery Visual-Motor Integration Test, 6th Edition [40] was completed when appropriate ($n = 2$).

Sensory processing
Sensory processing was assessed using the Short Sensory Profile [41] and the Sensory Assessment for Neurodevelopmental Disorders (SAND) [42]. The Short Sensory Profile is a 38-item caregiver report form that investigates daily life sensory experiences. The SAND is a standardized assessment that includes a clinician-administered observation and a 36-item corresponding caregiver interview. The scoring algorithm measures sensory hyperreactivity, hyporeactivity, and seeking behavior across visual, tactile, and auditory domains.

Results
SHANK3 mutations
We report 17 individuals (including two monozygotic twins) with SHANK3 mutations identified through WES or panel sequencing. The variants were distributed throughout the protein and included 13 frameshift, two nonsense, and one missense mutation (Table 1, Fig. 1a). Notably, we observed an identical frameshift mutation, c.3679dupG (p.Ala1227Glyfs*69), in three unrelated individuals. Mutations were confirmed to be de novo in 15 individuals and non-paternal or non-maternal in two (no DNA was available from the other two parents). In addition to a nonsense mutation, individual S13 carries a missense variant (p.Ser1291Leu) absent in the mother but present in the unaffected sister and in four individuals in the Genome Aggregation Database (gnomAD), suggesting it is likely benign, despite being predicted as damaging by several in silico tools (Additional file 1: Table S3). All other mutations are absent from the Exome Variant Server (EVS) and gnomAD. The

missense mutation in S14 (p.Asp1672Tyr) affects a highly conserved residue and is predicted to be damaging by all algorithms used, including Polyphen-2, SIFT, PANTHER, MutPred2, Condel2, CADD, and M-CAP (Additional file 1: Table S3).

We also searched the literature and ClinVar for SHANK3 mutations and assessed their pathogenicity. Variants listed in Additional file 1: Table S1 meet the following criteria: (1) loss-of-function variants (frameshift, nonsense, and splice site), or de novo missense variants predicted to be deleterious by several bioinformatics predictors, and (2) absent from control databases (EVS and gnomAD). After removing cases ascertained or reported multiple times, we identified 60 additional individuals from 55 families with SHANK3 mutations classified as pathogenic or likely pathogenic according to ACMG [25]. All the mutations with parental samples available were de novo. Three families had multiple affected siblings, consistent with germline mosaicism [9, 22, 43]. Four de novo missense variants reported in children with ASD, ID, or infantile spasms (p.Thr337Ser, p.Ser1197Gly, p.Ala1214Pro, and p.Arg1255Gly) [15, 44–46] were classified as variants of uncertain significance because, although not present in controls, in silico predictions did not provide consistent evidence for pathogenicity (Additional file 1: Tables S1, S3). Given that SHANK3 is highly constrained against missense variation (Exome Aggregation Consortium Z score 4.92) [47], further studies are needed to determine the pathogenicity of these and other missense variants.

Three of the mutations in our cohort are recurrent, having been previously observed in unrelated individuals (Fig. 1a, Additional file 1: Table S1). The mutation in S6, p.Leu1142Valfs*153, was reported in a boy with ASD [13]. The mutation c.3679dupG (p.Ala1227Glyfs*69), shared by three of our patients (S7, S8, B1), is within a stretch of eight guanines and has been identified in three independent cases [9, 15, 20]. p.Arg1255Leufs*25, present in S9, has been reported in three unrelated patients [13, 21]. The donor splice site at position c.2265+1 is another hotspot: there are three individuals with a G>A substitution [16, 24, 48], and one with a deletion of the same G (c.2265+1delG), shown to result in a frameshift (p.Ser755Serfs*1) [11]. Overall, there were four recurrent and 56 private pathogenic/likely pathogenic mutations in SHANK3 (Fig. 1a, Additional file 1: Table S1).

We also searched for potentially deleterious variants inherited from unaffected parents or present in population controls (Additional file 1: Table S4). An inherited frameshift variant reported as pathogenic in two unrelated children with ASD [12, 49], and classified as damaging in the Human Gene Mutation Database, is in fact intronic when annotated in the correct reference sequence, NM_033517.1 [49], and is present 173 times

Table 1 SHANK3 point mutations in 17 individuals described in this study

ID	Coding DNA change[a]	Protein change[b]	Genomic change (hg19)	Location	Effect	Inheritance	Variant classification [25]
S1[c]	c.1527G>A	p.Trp509*	chr22:g.51137146G>A	Exon 12	Nonsense	De novo	Pathogenic
S2	c.2471delC	p.Pro824Argfs*69	chr22:g.51158732delC	Exon 21	Frameshift	De novo	Pathogenic
S3[d]	c.2499delG	p.Pro834Argfs*59	chr22:g.51158760delG	Exon 21	Frameshift	De novo	Pathogenic
S4	c.2946_2949delCCGC	p.Arg983Serfs*94	chr22:g.51159207_51159210delCCGC	Exon 21	Frameshift	De novo	Pathogenic
S5	c.3095_3107delTGGGGGCCATCGA	p.Val1032Glyfs*42	chr22:g.51159356_51159368delTGGGGGCCATCGA	Exon 21	Frameshift	De novo	Pathogenic
S6	c.3424_3425delCT	p.Leu1142Valfs*153	chr22:g.51159685_51159686delCT	Exon 21	Frameshift	De novo	Pathogenic
S7	c.3679dupG	p.Ala1227Glyfs*69	chr22:g.51159940dupG	Exon 21	Frameshift	Non-paternal	Pathogenic
S8	c.3679dupG	p.Ala1227Glyfs*69	chr22:g.51159940dupG	Exon 21	Frameshift	De novo	Pathogenic
B1[e]	c.3679dupG	p.Ala1227Glyfs*69	chr22:g.51159940dupG	Exon 21	Frameshift	De novo	Pathogenic
S9	c.3764_3776delGGGCGCCAGCCCC	p.Arg1255Leufs*25	chr22:g.51160025_51160037delGGGCGCCAGCCCC	Exon 21	Frameshift	De novo	Pathogenic
B2, B3[e,f]	c.4065_4066delTG	p.Val1357Glyfs*4	chr22:g.51160326_51160327delTG	Exon 21	Frameshift	De novo	Pathogenic
S10	c.4229delC	p.Pro1410Hisfs*18	chr22:g.51160490delC	Exon 21	Frameshift	De novo	Pathogenic
S11	c.4577_4578delCC	p.Ala1526Glufs*16	chr22:g.51160838_51160839delCC	Exon 22	Frameshift	De novo	Pathogenic
S12	c.4906_4921dupTCCCCCTCGCCGTCGC	p.Pro1641Leufs*58	chr22:g.51169450_51169465dupTCCCCCTCGCCGTCGC	Exon 22	Frameshift	De novo	Pathogenic
S13[g]	c.5008A>T	p.Lys1670*	chr22:g.51169552A>T	Exon 22	Nonsense	Non-maternal	Likely pathogenic
	c.3872C>T	p.Ser1291Leu	chr22:g.51160133C>T	Exon 21	Missense	Non-maternal	Likely benign
S14	c.5014G>T	p.Asp1672Tyr	chr22:g.51169558G>T	Exon 22	Missense	De novo	Likely pathogenic

[a]NM_033517.1

[b]NP_277052.1 (Q9BYB0-1)

[c]S1 also has a de novo pathogenic 17q12 microduplication [62]. Reported previously [2, 26]

[d]Reported previously [2, 26]

[e]Reported previously [24]

[f]Monozygotic twins

[g]Reported previously [26]. This individual has two variants in SHANK3; the missense variant is likely benign and is not shown in Fig. 1a

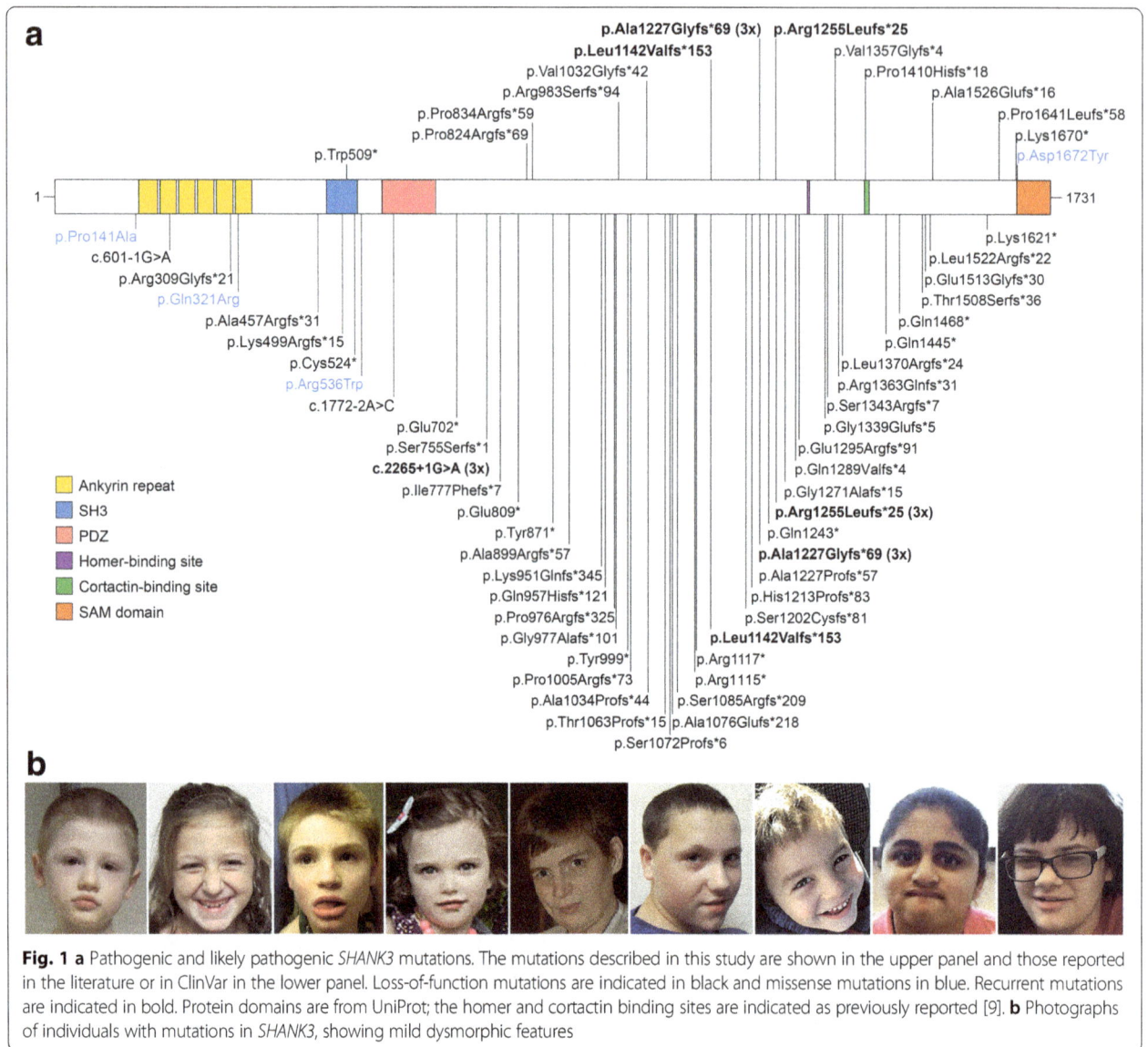

Fig. 1 a Pathogenic and likely pathogenic *SHANK3* mutations. The mutations described in this study are shown in the upper panel and those reported in the literature or in ClinVar in the lower panel. Loss-of-function mutations are indicated in black and missense mutations in blue. Recurrent mutations are indicated in bold. Protein domains are from UniProt; the homer and cortactin binding sites are indicated as previously reported [9]. **b** Photographs of individuals with mutations in *SHANK3*, showing mild dysmorphic features

in gnomAD (chr22:g.51135705dupG, hg19). An inherited substitution in a splice region (c.1772-4G>A) reported in ASD [12] is present seven times in gnomAD and is thus unlikely to be deleterious. gnomAD contains 21 variants predicted to be loss-of-function when annotated in the Ensembl canonical transcript ENST00000262795 (which is missing the beginning of exon 11 and contains three extra, unvalidated exons). When annotated in NM_033517.1, many of these variants are in fact intronic. The remaining 10 loss-of-function variants are all singletons; seven are flagged because they were found in sites covered in a limited number of individuals, which may indicate low-quality sites, one is located at the extreme 3′ end, and one has an abnormal allele balance. These findings confirm that truncating variants in *SHANK3* are highly penetrant and unlikely to be present in unaffected individuals.

Four in-frame deletions [10, 13, 19, 50] and one in-frame insertion [50] in *SHANK3* have been reported in ASD/ID (Additional file 1: Table S4). Three of these variants were inherited [10, 13, 50], and one was found in two controls [50], suggesting that some short in-frame deletions or insertions may be tolerated. An in-frame deletion of five amino acids (p.Gly1453_Ala1457del) reported in an ASD proband and his unaffected mother [10] was detected in six individuals in the gnomAD database. gnomAD lists 15 in-frame deletions or insertions (after annotation in NM_033517.1); six are on multiallelic sites, and four others are flagged because of low coverage. Among the remaining in-frame variants, p.Glu1230del was observed in five individuals and p.Gly1518del in four (Additional file 1: Table S4). These findings indicate that at least some in-frame variants in *SHANK3* can be present in seemingly unaffected individuals.

Clinical phenotype of *SHANK3* haploinsufficiency
Phenotypic spectrum in the individuals from our cohort

Detailed clinical information of the 17 individuals (9 males and 8 females, 3–42 years old at evaluation) is summarized in Tables 2 and 3 and Additional file 2: Table S5.

ASD Findings of ASD were widespread, with 69% (11/16) receiving a diagnosis of ASD. Among the 11 individuals of the Seaver cohort who received ASD diagnostic testing and a psychiatric evaluation, 82% (9/11) met criteria for ASD on the ADOS and 73% (8/11) met criteria for ASD on the ADI-R. A consensus diagnosis of ASD, accounting for both standardized assessments and clinical impression based on DSM-5 criteria, was reached in 73% (8/11) (Additional file 2: Tables S5, S6). All three children who did not receive an ASD diagnosis (S3, S7, S10) showed relevant features, including two with scores above the ASD cutoff on the ADOS-2 or the ADI-R but not both. It is notable that two of these three individuals (S7 and S10) were verbally fluent with cognitive functioning on the cusp of mild ID/borderline cognitive functioning.

Additional behavioral findings All participants from the Seaver cohort had significant repetitive behaviors ($n = 14$), including hand flapping and stereotypic motor movements (11/14, 79%), chewing and teeth grinding (7/14, 50%), pica and mouthing of objects (8/14, 57%), and stereotypic vocalizations (5/14, 36%). The majority of participants were described as hyperactive (11/17, 65%), although the extent and severity of hyperactivity varied widely as did the extent of impulsivity and inattention. Participants were also prone to aggression (8/17, 47%) and self-injury (3/15, 20%), particularly when frustrated. Sleep disturbance was common (10/17, 59%).

Intellectual functioning ID was observed in all cases that received standardized testing ($n = 13$), with 10 cases falling in the range of a severe-to-profound ID and three cases in the mild range. Two individuals (B2, B3) who did not receive standardized testing were characterized as mildly intellectually disabled based on the extent of language and developmental delay. All individuals within the normed range of up to 68 months (S2, S4, S6, S14) achieved the lowest possible standard score on the Mullen Early Learning Composite (< 49, < 1st percentile), indicating that the instrument reached its lower limit for reliable data collection ("floor" effect). Developmental quotients (DQ) were calculated for all individuals (excluding the 42-year-old individual) and ranged from 6.7 to 30 (mean ± SD, 15.6 ± 8.0). Verbal DQ ranged from 9.2 to 35 (19.9 ± 9.2), and nonverbal DQ ranged

from 3.1 to 25.8 (11.39 ± 7.16) (Additional file 2: Table S6). Results from three additional cases who received other cognitive measures (S7, S10, and B1) indicated the presence of mild-to-moderate ID (Table 2).

Adaptive behavior Results from the Vineland-II indicated that adaptive functioning was consistent with cognitive functioning (Additional file 2: Table S5). Overall, motor skills and socialization skills were better developed than communication and daily living skills. Two children (S7, S10) fell within the borderline range; all others fell below the first percentile.

Language skills Language impairment was prominent (17/17, 100%); results are summarized in Table 2. All subjects were delayed in achieving language milestones. With regard to current language abilities, the ADOS-2 ($n = 11$) indicated that five individuals used no words, three used < 5 recognizable words or word approximations, one used mostly single words, and two used complex speech with frequent grammatical errors. Receptive and expressive language were equally delayed (Additional file 2: Table S7). Three individuals (S7, S10, S14) were administered the Peabody Picture Vocabulary Test and achieved scores between < 1st and 7th percentiles. Two of these individuals (S7, S10) achieved scores of 70 (2nd percentile) on the Expressive Vocabulary Test, indicating that despite fluent speech, expressive language abilities were significantly delayed relative to same-aged peers. Two of the Baylor participants were also reported to speak in sentences, but one was mostly echolalic.

Motor skills Most individuals achieved motor milestones on time, despite significant fine and gross motor delays in all participants at the time of evaluation. Hypotonia (16/17, 94%) and gait abnormalities (14/17, 82%) were present in the majority of individuals. Gross motor skills were significantly better developed than fine motor skills ($n = 9$, $p = 0.02$ for both the Mullen and the Vineland-II, Wilcoxon signed-rank test; Additional file 2: Table S7). Two individuals (S7, S10) were administered the Beery Visual-Motor Integration Test and received standard scores of 45 and 65, respectively, which is indicative of visual-motor deficits.

Sensory processing According to parent report, 16 of 17 participants had increased pain tolerance (94%). Results from the Sensory Assessment for Neurodevelopmental Disorders ($n = 10$) and clinical observation indicated that sensory hyporeactivity (i.e., underresponsiveness to stimuli) was prominent. These findings are consistent with the results from the Short Sensory Profile ($n = 11$), indicating high scores in the

Table 2 Main clinical features of individuals with *SHANK3* mutations

	S1	S2	S3	S4	S5[a]	S6	S7	S8	S9[a]	S10
Gender	M	M	M	F	F	M	F	M	M	M
Gestational age (wks)	36	39	40	Term	38	Term	33	40	39	Term
Birth weight (g)	2863	3400	3657	4000	3175	2948	1940	4111	4630	3230
Birth length (cm)	47	55	NK	53	NK	50	46	58	55	50
Postnatal growth										
Age at examination (y)	12	5	7	3	9	5	7	9	12	9
Height (cm, percentile)	131 (<1)	110 (27)	108 (27)	103 (93)	NK	109 (50)	125 (45)	148 (95)	142 (17)	135 (56)
Weight (kg, percentile)	32.6 (11)	20 (53)	18.8 (5)	17.2 (88)	NK	17.3 (50)	35 (96)	36 (78)	29.5 (3)	29.5 (55)
OFC (cm, percentile)	56 (95)	50.8 (36)	52.7 (70)	50 (75)	NK	NK	51.2 (40)	54 (82)	NK	53 (64)
Psychomotor development										
Sat independently (mo)	12	5–6	9–10	6	12	9	8–11	6	8–9	6
Walked independently (mo)	24	16	14	15	16	14	18	14	14–15	12
First words and current language ability	3 y; now non-verbal	No speech; vowel sounds and sounds of pleasure present	No speech; previously had 10 signs but regressed to 3–4, babbling present, apraxic	No speech; uses about 5 signs with word approximations	Non-verbal	36 mo; 2-word phrases at 3.5 y; primarily single words with some phrase speech, stereotyped speech and echolalia	14 mo; first phrases at 24 mo, verbally fluent, complex speech	15 mo; never developed 2-word phrases, eventually lost all words	Non-verbal	8 mo; 2-word phrases by 24 mo, now verbally fluent
Intellectual disability (IQ or DQ)	Profound ID (Mullen: DQ 6.7, NVDQ 10.3, VDQ 3.1)	Profound ID (Mullen: DQ 21.3, NVDQ 30.1, VDQ 12.5)	Profound ID (Mullen: DQ 14.7, NVDQ 18.8, VDQ 10.6)	Profound ID (Mullen: DQ 16.5, NVDQ 19.5, VDQ 13.4)	ID (no testing available)	Severe ID (Mullen: CSS <49, DQ 30.4, NVDQ 35, VDQ 25.8)	Mild ID (DAS-II: GCA 50, Verbal 52, NV reasoning 74, spatial 32, special NV 49)	Profound ID (Mullen: DQ 11.5, NVDQ 14.5, VDQ 8.5)	Severe ID (no testing available)	Mild ID (Stanford Binet: FSIQ 56, NVIQ 60, VIQ 56)
Feeding difficulties	+ (chewing problems)	–	+ (regurgitation, oral motor dysfunction, difficulty consuming solid foods, PEG tube)	+ (oral motor dysfunction since birth, dysphagia, drooling, overeating, chewing problems)	+ (failure to thrive, g-tube)	–	– (drooling)	+ (dysphagia, drooling, may induce vomiting when over-eats)	+ (difficulty chewing, dysphagia)	+ (history of oral motor dysfunction, drooling)
Hypotonia	+	+	+	+	+	+	+	+	+	+

Table 2 Main clinical features of individuals with *SHANK3* mutations (*Continued*)

	S1	S2	S3	S4	S5[a]	S6	S7	S8	S9[a]	S10
Gait abnormalities	+ (apraxic, hypotonic, toe-walking)	+ (toe-walking, unsteady, needs assistance)	+	+	+ (slow pace)	+ (toe walking)	+ (mildly hypotonic)	+	+	+
Behavioral abnormalities										
ASD	+	+	–	+	+	+	–	+	+	–
Hyperactivity	+	+	+	+	+	+	+	–	+	+
Aggression	–	–	+	+	–	–	+	–	–	+
Self-injury	–	–	+	–	–	–	–	+	–	+
Sleep disturbance	–	+	+	+	+	–	–	–	+	–
Pica	+	+	+	+	+	+	–	+	+	–
Repetitive behaviors (type)	+ (stereotypic motor movements in upper and lower extremities, forced exhalations)	+ (spinning, hand-flapping, teeth grinding)	+ (repetitive motor mannerisms, stereotypic vocalizations)	+ (bouncing, tapping, upper extremity motor stereotypies)	+ (chewing, teeth grinding, breath holding)	+ (chewing, teeth grinding, hand flapping, stereotypic vocalizations)	+ (self-stimulation, insistence on routines)	+ (hand-flapping, chewing)	+ (hand-flapping)	+ (restricted interests, perseveration)
Psychosis	–	–	–	–	–	–	–	–	–	–
Regression (age and details)	+ (5 y; some language loss)	–	+ (6 y; motor regression and lost some sign language, at one point stopped walking for 6 weeks, slowly regained ambulatory skills; at 5 y, some language loss)	+ (15 mo; stopped babbling, loses motor skills when sick)	–	–	–	+ (3.5 y; language and motor skills, stopped walking, socially withdrawn and less responsive)	+ (3–4 y; loss of fine motor skills)	–
Neurological findings										
Brain MRI (age)	Diffuse ventricular enlargement, colpocephaly, communicating hydrocephalus, thinning of parieto-occipital white matter and corpus callosum (8 y)	No MRI	Leukodystrophy (5 y)	Grossly normal but scattered areas of subtle FLAIR hyperintensity (2 y)	NK	Grossly normal but hyper-intensity in the left inferior parietal subcortical white matter possibly related to gliosis (4 y)	Normal (5 y)	Normal (3 y)	Normal (5, 9, and 11 y)	Normal (7 y)
Seizures (age of onset, type)	–	–	+ (5 y, Landau-Kleffner variant; 6 y epileptic encephalopathy)	–	–	–	–	–	– (10 y, suspected complex partial seizures)	–

Table 2 Main clinical features of individuals with SHANK3 mutations (Continued)

	S1	S2	S3	S4	S5[a]	S6	S7	S8	S9[a]	S10
Abnormal EEG	–	–	+ (localized sleep potentiated epileptiform discharges mainly in the midline and central regions during slow wave sleep)	+ (increased theta wave activity; bilateral K-complexes, and spindles and vertex waves during sleep. Left frontal spike and wave activity)	+ (spikes)	+ (spike and wave activity in frontotemporal lobes; no seizures)	–	–	+ (right frontal lobe spikes, slowing)	–
Gastrointestinal problems										
Gastroesophageal reflux	–	+	+	–	–	–	–	+	+	–
Constipation	+	–	+	+	+	+	–	–	+	–
Diarrhea	–	–	+	–	+	–	–	+	–	–
Additional features										
Increased pain tolerance	+	+	+	+	+	–	+	+	+	+
Decreased perspiration/heat intolerance	–	–	+	NK	–	NK	–	NK	+	–
Recurrent infections	–	+ (otitis, MT)	+ (otitis)	–	–	+ (otitis, upper respiratory tract)	–	+ (otitis, MT)	–	+ (otitis, tonsillitis)
Visual problems	–	+ (strabismus, corrective surgery)	+ (mild hyperopic astigmatism)	–	–	+ (strabismus)	–	–	–	–
Congenital heart defect	–	–	–	–	–	–	+ (coronary artery fistula)	–	–	–
Renal abnormalities	–	–[c]	–	–	–	–	–[c]	–	–	–
Allergies	+ (penicillin)	+ (food, seasonal)	–	–	+ (food)	+ (penicillin, seasonal)	+ (seasonal)	+ (food)	+ (seasonal)	+ (penicillin)
Asthma	–	–	–	–	–	+	+ (allergy induced)	–	–	–
Eczema	–	+	–	–	–	–	–	+	+	+
Other							Birth by in vitro fertilization		Sleep apnea	

+ present, – absent, ASD autism spectrum disorder, BDI Battelle Developmental Inventory, CSS Composite Standard Score, DAS-II Differential Ability Scales, Second Edition, DQ developmental quotient, EEG electroencephalography, F female, FSIQ full scale intelligence quotient, GCA general conceptual ability, ID intellectual disability, M male, MRI magnetic resonance imaging, MT myringotomy tubes, NA not applicable, NK not known, NV non-verbal, NVDQ non-verbal developmental quotient, NVIQ non-verbal intelligence quotient, PEG percutaneous endoscopic gastrostomy, SS standard score, VDQ verbal developmental quotient, VIQ verbal intelligence quotient

[a]Individuals not directly evaluated
[b]Monozygotic twins
[c]Normal renal evaluation (ultrasound or computed tomography)

Table 2 Main clinical features of individuals with SHANK3 mutations (Continued)

	S11	S12	S13	S14	B1	B2[b]	B3[b]	Total (%)
Gender	F	F	M	M	F	F	F	9 M, 8 F
Gestational age (wks)	36.5	Term	40	41	40	36	36	
Birth weight (g)	3000	3728	2700	3090	2438	2551	2523	
Birth length (cm)	53	NK	48	51	48	NK	NK	
Postnatal growth								
Age at examination (y)	6	42	15	4	14	14	14	3–42
Height (cm, percentile)	111 (4)	170 (85)	149 (<1)	97 (4)	151 (25–50)	145 (<1)	145 (<1)	5/16 (31%) short
Weight (kg, percentile)	18.2 (7)	69.4 (82)	48.1 (18)	15.4 (19)	55.1 (75)	59.1 (75)	40.5 (12)	
OFC (cm, percentile)	50.5 (27)	57 (99)	54.5 (40)	46 (<1)	52.7 (30)	57 (98)	57 (98)	3/14 (21%) macrocephaly; 1 (7%) microcephaly
Psychomotor development								
Sat independently (mo)	Normal	8	NK	5	8	6	6	
Walked independently (mo)	24	20	14	13	14	19	19	
First words and current language ability	4 y; had approximately 10 words; currently uses no words	15 mo; phrase speech at 3 y; was verbally fluent until 12–13 y but currently uses no words	10–15 words by 18 mo; understands roughly 40 signs; comprehension and expressive language is limited	10 mo; uses a few word approximations, some signs, apraxic	At 3 y had approximately 200 words but only used 50 routinely; can speak in 2–3 word sentences but mostly echolalia	19 mo; combined words at 3.5 y; currently speaks in full sentences but developed word finding difficulties	19 mo; combined words at 3.5 y; spoke in full sentences but regressed at 9 y to only say 2–3 words, regained some vocabulary but fluctuating language	Currently non-verbal 9/17 (53%), fluent speech 3/17 (18%)
Intellectual disability (IQ or DQ)	Profound ID (Mullen: DQ 105, NVDQ 13.2, VDQ 7.9)	Profound ID (Mullen: DQ 0.63, NVDQ 0.97, VDQ 0.29)	Profound ID (Mullen: DQ 10.4, NVDQ 15.5, VDQ 5.2)	Severe ID (Mullen: CSS < 49, DQ 26.4, NVDQ 33, VDQ 19.8)	Mild ID (BDI at 4 y: adaptive SS 65, cognitive 65, communication 65, fine motor 72, gross motor 69, social 65)	Mild ID (no testing available)	Mild ID (no testing available)	17/17 (100%)
Feeding difficulties	+ (history of dysphagia)	+ (drooling, dysphagia)	+ (difficulty latching, currently gagging and choking behaviors, dysphagia, drooling)	+ (oral motor dysfunction)	–	+ (difficulty latching)	+ (difficulty latching)	13/17 (76%)
Hypotonia	+	+	+	+	–	+	+	16/17 (94%)

Table 2 Main clinical features of individuals with *SHANK3* mutations *(Continued)*

	S11	S12	S13	S14	B1	B2[b]	B3[b]	Total (%)
Gait abnormalities	+ (apraxia)	+ (slow, hesitant and apraxic; previously reported as wide-based gait)	+ (mild but went through 6-month period in early childhood when he was unable to ambulate due to muscle weakness)	+	–	–	–	14/17 (82%)
Behavioral abnormalities								
ASD	+	NK	+	+	+	–	–	11/16 (69%)
Hyperactivity	+	–	–	–	+	–	–	11/17 (65%)
Aggression	+	+	+	–	–	+	+	8/17 (47%)
Self-injury	–	+	–	–	–	NK	NK	3/15 (20%)
Sleep disturbance	+	+	+	+	+	–	–	10/17 (59%)
Pica	–	–	–	–	–	–	–	8/17 (47%)
Repetitive behaviors (type)	+ (teeth grinding, repeatedly taps objects, walks in circles)	+ (pacing, upper extremity motor stereotypies)	+ (hand flapping, chewing, stereotypic vocalizations, teeth grinding)	+ (chewing, hand flapping, repetitive jumping, stereotypic vocalizations)	+ (finger and toe tapping)	–	+ (chewing, tapping teeth with finger)	16/17 (94%)
Psychosis	–	+ (12–13 y)	–	–	–	+ (13 y; "manic-like" behavior)	–	1/17 (6%)
Regression (age and details)	+ (4.5 y; loss of language and motor skills, lost ability to ambulate and eye contact, lethargic, developed unusual motor stereotypies, regression coincided with diagnosis of parasitic infection)	+ (12–13 y; intermittent periods of behavioral, motor, and language regressions sometimes preceded by viral infection, included psychiatric symptoms. Currently non-verbal and unable to walk unsupported)	+ (2 y; lost all words, 7 y; regression in handwriting [can no longer hold a pen], motor regression began roughly around when seizures started)	+ (12–18 mo; loss of babbling, loss of few words, eye contact, and gesturing to request)	–	+ (9–10 y; "manic-like" behavior)	–	11/17 (65%)
Neurological findings								
Brain MRI (age)	Normal (4.5 y)	Normal (14 and 18 y)	Venous angioma (6 y); normal (16 y)	Normal (3 y)	Bilateral T2 hyper-intensities of posterior centrum semiovale (12 y)	Mild cerebellar tonsillar ectopia (14 y)	Normal (14 y)	Abnormal in 5/15 (33%)
Seizures (age of onset, type)	–	–	+ (3 y febrile; 6 y focal; 15 y began 1–10 absence or partial seizures daily)	+ (4 y, generalized myoclonic seizures)	–	+ (14 y, atypical absence)	+ (7 y, atypical absence and tonic)	5/17 (29%)

Table 2 Main clinical features of individuals with *SHANK3* mutations *(Continued)*

	S11	S12	S13	S14	B1	B2[b]	B3[b]	Total (%)
Abnormal EEG	+ (left frontal spikes/ polyspikes, intermittent polymorphic slowing [L>R] in the temporal region, and background slowing during sleep)	–	+ (high-voltage spike and sharp activity in frontal regions)	+ (occasional generalized polyspikes or polyspike-wave with shifting hemispheric predominance during sleep)	–	+ (no occipital dominant rhythm)	–	9/17 (53%)
Gastrointestinal problems								
Gastroesophageal reflux	–	+	–	–	–	–	–	5/17 (29%)
Constipation	–	+	+	–	+	–	–	9/17 (53%)
Diarrhea	+	–	+	–	–	–	–	5/17 (29%)
Additional features								
Increased pain tolerance	+	+	+	+	+	+	+	16/17 (94%)
Decreased perspiration/heat intolerance	–	NK	–	NK	–	–	–	2/12 (17%)
Recurrent infections	+ (otitis, MT; yeast)	+ (otitis, bronchitis)	+ (otitis, sinusitis)	+ (otitis, MT)	–	–	–	9/17 (53%)
Visual problems	–	–	–	–	–	+ (myopia)	+ (myopia)	5/17 (29%)
Congenital heart defect	–	–	–	–	–	–	–	1/17 (6%)
Renal abnormalities	–	–	–[c]	–[c]	–[c]	–[c]	–	0/17
Allergies	+ (seasonal)	+ (food, dust, pets)	+ (food)	+ (food)	–	–	–	12/17 (71%)
Asthma	–	–	–	+	–	–	–	3/17 (18%)
Eczema	–	–	+	+	–	–	–	6/17 (35%)
Other		Sleep apnea, atrial fibrillation, intermittent hypoglycemia			Left preauricular skin tag, scoliosis	Episode of idiopathic intracranial hypertension at 12 y		

Table 3 Dysmorphic features in individuals with *SHANK3* mutations

	S1[a]	S2	S3	S4		S7	S8	S10		S11	S12		S13	S14		Total (%)
Gender	M	M	M	F		F	M	M		F	F		M	M		7 M, 4 F
Age at examination (years)	12	5	7	3		7	9	9		6	42		15	4		3–42
Craniofacial features																
Microcephaly[b]	−	−	−	−		−	−	−		−	−		−	+		1/11 (9%)
Macrocephaly[c]	−	−	−	−		−	−	−		−	+		−	−		1/11 (9%)
Dolichocephaly	−	−	+	−		−	−	−		−	−		−	−		1/11 (9%)
Synophrys	−	−	−	−		−	−	−		−	−		−	−		0
Sparse eyebrows	−	−	−	+		−	−	−		−	−		+	−		2/11 (18%)
Long eyelashes	+	+	−	+		+	+	−		+	+		+	−		8/11 (73%)
Periorbital fullness	+	+	−	+		−	−	−		−	−		+	−		4/11 (36%)
Deep set eyes	−	+	−	+		−	+	+		+	−		−	−		5/11 (45%)
Ptosis	−	−	−	−		−	−	−		−	−		−	−		0
Epicanthal folds	+	+	−	+		−	−	+		−	−		−	+		5/11 (45%)
Hypertelorism	−	−	−	−		−	−	−		−	−		−	−		0
Wide nasal bridge	+	+	−	+		+	+	−		−	−		−	+		6/11 (55%)
Bulbous nose	−	+	−	+		+	+	−		−	−		+	+		6/11 (55%)
Anteverted nares	−	−	−	−		+	−	−		−	−		−	−		1/11 (9%)
Full cheeks	−	−	−	+		−	−	−		−	−		+	−		2/11 (18%)
Malar hypoplasia	+	+	−	+		−	−	−		−	+		+	−		5/11 (45%)
Thin upper vermillion	−	+	+	−		−	−	−		+	−		−	−		3/11 (27%)
Thick lower vermillion	+	+	+	−		−	−	−		−	−		−	−		3/11 (27%)
Short philtrum	−	−	−	−		−	−	−		−	−		−	−		0
Long philtrum	−	+	−	−		−	−	+		−	+		−	−		3/11 (27%)
Malocclusion	+	+	−	+		+	+	+		−	+		−	−		7/11 (64%)
High arched palate	+	+	−	+		−	−	+		−	NE		+	+		6/10 (60%)
Ear anomalies	−	−	−	+ (low set ears)		−	−	+ (overfolded helix)		−	+ (fleshy ears)		−	+ (prominent ears)		4/11 (36%)
Micrognathia	−	−	−	−		−	−	−		−	−		−	−		0
Macrognathia	+	−	−	−		+	−	−		−	+		−	−		3/11 (27%)
Pointed chin	+	−	−	+		+	−	+		+	+		+	−		7/11 (64%)
Hand and feet anomalies																
Large fleshy hands	−	−	−	+		−	−	−		−	−		+	+		3/11 (27%)
5th finger clinodactyly	+	+	−	+		+	+	+		−	+		+	+		9/11 (82%)
Partial syndactyly of toes 2–3	−	+	−	+		−	−	+		−	−		+	+		5/11 (45%)
Sandal gap	+	+	+	NE		+	+	−		NE	−		+	−		6/9 (67%)
Hypoplasia of distal phalanges of 5th finger	−	−	−	−		−	−	−		−	+		+	−		2/11 (18%)
Ectodermal anomalies																
Hypertrichosis	−	−	−	−		−	−	−		−	−		−	−		0
Abnormal hair whorl	−	−	−	−		−	−	−		+	−		+	−		2/11 (18%)
Hypoplastic/dysplastic toenails	+	−	−	+		−	+	−		+	+		−	+		6/11 (55%)
Hypoplastic/dysplastic fingernails	+	+	−	−		−	−	−		−	−		−	−		2/11 (18%)

Table 3 Dysmorphic features in individuals with *SHANK3* mutations *(Continued)*

	S1[a]	S2	S3	S4	S7	S8	S10	S11	S12	S13	S14	Total (%)
Other features												
Short stature/delayed growth[d]	+	–	+	–	–	–	–	–	–	+	–	3/11 (27%)
Tall stature/accelerated growth[e]	–	–	–	–	–	–	–	–	–	–	–	0
Hyperextensibility	–	–	–	+	+	+	+	–	NE	+	+	6/10 (60%)
Sacral dimple	–	–	NE	–	–	–	–	–	–	–	–	0
Scoliosis	–	–	–	–	–	–	–	–	–	+	–	1/11 (9%)
Total dysmorphic features	15	16	5	18	10	9	10	6	11	17	11	11/11 (100%)

Only individuals that underwent a detailed evaluation by a clinical geneticist are shown

+ present, – absent, *F* female, *M* male, *NE* not evaluated

[a]S1 also has a de novo pathogenic 17q12 microduplication [62]

[b]Head circumference < 3rd percentile

[c]Head circumference > 98th percentile

[d]Height < 3rd percentile

[e]Height > 98th percentile

underresponsive/seeks sensation domain (10/11) and the low energy/weak domain (9/11).

Neurological findings Seizures were reported in five individuals (5/17, 29%), including febrile ($n = 1$), absence ($n = 3$), focal ($n = 1$), and generalized seizures ($n = 2$) (one individual had febrile, absence, and focal seizures) (Table 2). Age of onset ranged from 4 to 14 years (7.2 ± 4). Nine individuals had an abnormal electroencephalography (EEG) (9/17, 53%), including five without clinical seizures. MRI in 15 individuals revealed abnormal findings in five (33%), including white matter abnormalities ($n = 3$), venous angioma ($n = 1$), and mild cerebellar ectopia ($n = 1$).

Regression For the purpose of this manuscript, we only document regression in patients who clearly and consistently acquired skills for a prolonged period of time and then lost these skills, either permanently or for an extended period. Regression, occurring at various stages of development from early childhood to early adolescence, and affecting language, motor, and behavioral domains, was reported in 11 of 17 cases (65%). At least two caregivers noted regression that was triggered by infection and one reported seizures preceding the onset of regression.

Other medical conditions Gastrointestinal problems were common, including gastroesophageal reflux (5/17, 29%), constipation (9/17, 53%), and diarrhea (5/17, 29%). Feeding problems were also common (13/17, 76%), including dysphagia and chewing difficulties; two individuals required placement of a gastrostomy tube. Recurrent infections were reported in 53% (9/17) of individuals, most often affecting the ears. Visual problems, and strabismus in particular, have been described in

carriers of 22q13.3 deletions [2, 4, 51] and were present in 29% (5/17) of patients, including strabismus ($n = 2$), myopia ($n = 2$), and astigmatism ($n = 1$). Renal or urinary tract abnormalities, reported in 26–40% of cases with 22q13 deletions [2, 4], were absent in our cohort. Similarly, congenital heart defects, reported in 3–13% of patients with 22q13 deletions [2, 52], were uncommon; one individual had a coronary artery fistula that did not require surgical intervention. Lymphedema, cellulitis, precocious or delayed puberty, hearing problems, and hypothyroidism have been reported in cases with 22q13 deletions [2, 4] but were not present in individuals with *SHANK3* mutations (Table 4).

Dysmorphic features Dysmorphology examinations were performed on 11 individuals from the Seaver cohort, using a PMS-specific checklist (Table 3, Fig. 1b). All had at least five usually mild dysmorphic features (range 5–18), without a distinctive facial gestalt. In general, findings were consistent with those reported in patients with 22q13 deletions [2, 4–6]. However, some features were more common than previously reported, including fifth finger clinodactyly (9/11, 82%), malocclusion (7/11, 64%), and wide nasal bridge (6/11, 55%) (Table 4). The use of a PMS-specific checklist could account in part for the higher frequency with which certain features were noted. Other features present in over 50% of the individuals were long eyelashes, bulbous nose, high arched palate, pointed chin, hyperextensibility, dysplastic toenails, and sandal gap.

Phenotype of individuals with SHANK3 mutations in the literature

The clinical features of 45 previously published individuals with pathogenic or likely pathogenic *SHANK3*

Table 4 Clinical features in individuals with *SHANK3* mutations as compared to 22q13 deletions including *SHANK3*

Clinical features	Individuals with *SHANK3* mutations (current study)	Individuals with 22q13 deletions [2]
Intellectual disability	17/17 (100%)	29/30 (97%)
ASD	11/16 (69%)	26/30 (87%)
Verbally fluent	3/17 (18%)	0/30
Repetitive behaviors	16/17 (94%)	30/30 (100%)
Hyperactivity	11/17 (65%)	14/30 (47%)
Aggression	8/17 (47%)	13/30 (43%)
Sleep disturbance	10/17 (59%)	12/30 (40%)
Hypotonia	16/17 (94%)	23/30 (77%)
Gait abnormalities	14/17 (82%)	13/14 (93%)
Seizures	5/17 (29%)	12/30 (40%)
Abnormal brain MRI	5/15 (33%)	18/26 (69%)
Short stature[a]	5/16 (31%)	3/30 (10%)
Tall stature[b]	0/16	1/30 (3%)
Microcephaly[c]	1/14 (7%)	2/30 (7%)
Macrocephaly[d]	3/14 (21%)	9/30 (30%)
Dolichocephaly	1/11 (9%)	7/30 (23%)
Sparse hair/abnormal whorl	2/11 (18%)	5/30 (17%)
Long eyelashes	8/11 (73%)	13/30 (43%)
Periorbital fullness	4/11 (36%)	8/30 (27%)
Hypertelorism	0/11	3/30 (10%)
Deep set eyes	5/11 (45%)	2/30 (7%)
Ptosis	0/11	2/30 (7%)
Epicanthal folds	5/11 (45%)	9/30 (30%)
Strabismus	2/17 (12%)	3/30 (10%)
Wide nasal bridge	6/11 (55%)	4/30 (13%)
Bulbous nose	6/11 (55%)	15/30 (50%)
Full cheeks	2/11 (18%)	8/30 (27%)
Malar hypoplasia	5/11 (45%)	3/30 (10%)
Long philtrum	3/11 (27%)	5/30 (17%)
Malocclusion	7/11 (64%)	5/30 (17%)
Widely spaced teeth	0/11	1/30 (3%)
High arched palate	6/10 (60%)	8/30 (27%)
Ear anomalies	4/11 (36%)	13/30 (43%)
Pointed chin	7/11 (64%)	7/30 (23%)
Large fleshy hands	3/11 (27%)	17/30 (57%)
5th finger clinodactyly	9/11 (82%)	3/30 (10%)
Syndactyly of toes 2–3	5/11 (45%)	3/30 (10%)
Hypoplastic/dysplastic nails	7/11 (64%)	11/30 (37%)
Hyperextensibility	6/10 (60%)	8/30 (27%)
Scoliosis	1/11 (9%)	7/30 (23%)
Sacral dimple	0/10	4/30 (13%)

Table 4 Clinical features in individuals with *SHANK3* mutations as compared to 22q13 deletions including *SHANK3* (*Continued*)

Clinical features	Individuals with *SHANK3* mutations (current study)	Individuals with 22q13 deletions [2]
Gastroesophageal reflux	5/17 (29%)	13/30 (43%)
Constipation/diarrhea	11/17 (65%)	11/30 (37%)
Increased pain tolerance	16/17 (94%)	26/30 (87%)
Recurrent infections	9/17 (53%)	16/30 (53%)
Renal abnormalities	0/17	12/30 (40%)
Congenital heart defect	1/17 (6%)	1/30 (3%)
Hypothyroidism	0/17	1/30 (3%)
Lymphedema	0/17	7/30 (23%)

ASD autism spectrum disorder
[a]Height < 3rd percentile
[b]Height > 98th percentile
[c]Head circumference < 3rd percentile
[d]Head circumference > 98th percentile

variants are summarized in Additional file 1: Table S2. (Fifteen individuals reported only in ClinVar are included in Additional file 1: Table S1 where we summarize the allelic spectrum but are not included here because no phenotype information was available for them.) Although only limited information was available for most cases, the phenotype was consistent with that observed in our cohort, including ID (33/33, 100%), severe language impairment (22/23, 96%), ASD (26/34, 76%), hypotonia (8/12, 67%), seizures (17/30, 57%), and dysmorphic features (13/21, 62%). Regression was reported in 11 individuals.

Discussion

This is the first study to comprehensively describe the phenotype in patients with PMS due to *SHANK3* point mutations. Our findings demonstrate that loss of *SHANK3* alone is sufficient to produce the characteristic features of PMS, including ID, ASD, severe speech impairment, hypotonia, epilepsy, motor skills deficits, feeding difficulties, mild dysmorphic features, increased pain tolerance, gastrointestinal problems, and neuroimaging abnormalities. In addition, we advance the understanding of the genetic architecture of PMS and, in so doing, provide information to aid in the interpretation of *SHANK3* variants.

Genetic findings

Findings in our cohort and in previously reported patients indicate that *SHANK3* mutations are fully penetrant. The identification of three families with *SHANK3* mutations in multiple siblings due to germline mosaicism (5%, 3/57) [9, 22, 43] has important implications for genetic counseling. Of note, we identified four recurrent mutations in *SHANK3*, including p.Leu1142Valfs*153, p.Ala1227-Glyfs*69, p.Arg1255Leufs*25, and c.2265+1G>A. The most common mutation, c.3679dupG (p.Ala1227-Glyfs*69), identified in six individuals, is due to the duplication of a guanine in a stretch of eight guanines, indicating that this segment is prone to replication errors. Functional studies on several of the truncating mutations described here (p.Trp509* in S1, p.Pro834Argfs*59 in S3, p.Lys1670* in S13, and p.A1227Gfs*69 in S7, S8, and B1) provide further support for their deleterious effects [9, 26, 53, 54].

Although the majority of pathogenic/likely pathogenic SHANK3 variants identified to date are truncating, the interpretation of missense variants remains difficult. Missense variant assessment relies on inheritance, segregation within families, frequency in population databases, functional studies, and computational predictions of pathogenicity (see ACMG guidelines [25]). In the case of SHANK3, in silico prediction programs often provide contradictory results (Additional file 1: Table S3). Functional studies could help determine the pathogenicity of missense substitutions; however, previous in vitro analyses have identified synaptic defects associated with missense variants in ASD inherited from healthy parents and found in control databases [9, 53, 54]; hence, more discriminatory functional approaches will need to be developed.

ASD, ID, language, and motor skills

Our results demonstrate the high prevalence of ASD in individuals with PMS resulting from SHANK3 mutations, similar to our previous findings in individuals with 22q13 deletions [2]. The ADOS and ADI-R provided important information regarding ASD features, even in individuals with low mental ages; however, clinical evaluation and consensus discussion proved necessary to determine which individuals did not meet criteria for ASD. Negative ASD findings in the two verbally fluent individuals raise questions about the relationship between ASD diagnosis and severe global developmental delay. Interestingly, in spite of severe-to-profound ID, and significant expressive and receptive language delays in the majority of participants, language appears to be more preserved in individuals with SHANK3 mutations compared to those with 22q13 deletions seen at the same centers [2, 24]. Motor skills deficits were also pronounced, although early motor milestones were achieved on time for the majority of individuals. Gross motor skills were better developed than fine motor skills and, in most cases, appear to be less severely affected than in individuals with 22q13 deletions, particularly regarding gait. These results indicate that SHANK3 haploinsufficiency affects cognition, language, and motor functioning.

Regression and psychotic symptoms

Significant cognitive and behavioral regression has been reported in individuals with PMS [2, 3, 9, 51, 55–59].

Over half of our sample reportedly experienced a regression in motor and language skills that occurred during different periods of development (early childhood or adolescence). These results indicate that SHANK3 haploinsufficiency alone is sufficient to increase risk for regression. However, reports of regression must be interpreted with caution based on a lack of well-defined criteria or standardized assessment instruments and potential recall biases in reporting. Further careful study is needed to characterize the regression phenotype in PMS using longitudinal designs and to begin to elucidate the underlying mechanisms.

Possibly related to regression, psychotic symptoms have emerged as an important area of study in PMS as several reports have suggested that as individuals with PMS age, they may be at increased risk for significant psychiatric disturbance, including bipolar disorder [51, 55–57, 59]. Four of the reported patients had truncating mutations in SHANK3 [9, 56], indicating that SHANK3 is responsible for this phenotype. Mutations in SHANK3 have also been found in four individuals from two families with atypical schizophrenia associated with early onset and ID [22]. The monozygotic twins reported here (B2, B3) showed "manic-like" behavior beginning at 13 years of age in one and at 9–10 years of age in the other. Also, one individual (S12) experienced psychotic symptoms characterized by auditory and visual hallucinations beginning around 12–13 years of age. She had episodic periods of mania and depression, insomnia, decreased appetite and weight loss, unsteady gait, and catatonic posturing, similar to previous reports [51, 55, 56, 59]. Importantly, she also had significant regression in language and motor skills with documented cognitive decline from borderline intellectual functioning before puberty to profound ID based on the current assessment at age 42 (see Table 2). The patient was verbally fluent but became non-verbal. She was also walking independently at 20 months and currently is unable to walk more than several steps without support. Pubertal onset appears to be a potential trigger for shifts in the psychiatric phenotype in PMS; hence, it is important to note that only two of the 14 Seaver participants were post-pubertal.

Other medical findings

Common medical features in individuals with SHANK3 mutations were consistent with published literature in subjects with 22q13.3 deletions [1, 2, 4–6]. Epilepsy has been reported in PMS with a mean prevalence of 32% and a wide range of seizure types, frequencies, and severity [24]. The lower frequency of seizures in our study compared to that for previously reported individuals with SHANK3 point mutations (29% versus 57%) might be due to the young age of many of our patients (seizure onset occurred at ≥ 10 years in 41% [7/17] of new and previously reported individuals). In agreement with our findings, no specific EEG abnormalities have been reported in PMS, and EEG abnormalities (61%) are seen in children with and without a history of clinical seizures [24]. Structural brain abnormalities are observed in about a third of cases with 22q13 deletions (including corpus callosum and cerebellar abnormalities, dysmyelination, ventricular dilatation, and arachnoid cysts) [1, 2, 24]; results from patients with mutations are consistent with those with deletions. Overall, loss of *SHANK3* is sufficient to cause seizures and structural brain changes, although findings remain non-specific to PMS.

Gastrointestinal problems, recurrent infections, and increased pain tolerance were common among individuals with *SHANK3* mutations, consistent with previous estimates in 22q13 deletions [2, 4]. In agreement with these findings, studies in mice showed that SHANK3 is expressed in the spinal cord and primary sensory neurons, where it regulates pain sensitivity [60]. SHANK3 has also been shown to be expressed in intestinal epithelial cells, where it regulates barrier function [61]. In contrast, despite reports of renal and urinary tract abnormalities in 26–40% of cases with 22q13 deletions (including vesicoureteral reflux, hydronephrosis, renal agenesis, and dysplastic or polycystic kidneys) [2, 4], no such anomalies were observed in our cohort. While data from ongoing genotype-phenotype studies are still emerging, it is likely that the genetic risk for renal anomalies is not directly associated to *SHANK3* haploinsufficiency and involves other gene(s) in 22q13.

Despite high variability, mild dysmorphic features were prevalent among patients with *SHANK3* mutations and were consistent with the phenotype in patients with 22q13 deletions [1, 2, 4]. It has been previously reported that the number of dysmorphic features is correlated with deletion size [2] and that several dysmorphic features are associated with larger deletion sizes [7]. Our results suggest that some of the more common dysmorphic features associated with PMS are caused by *SHANK3* mutations, but further studies are needed to determine the contribution of other genes involved in 22q13 deletions.

Conclusions

This represents a first detailed report of the genetic and phenotypic spectrum associated with *SHANK3* mutations, which are being identified with greater frequency as clinical sequencing becomes more widespread. Our findings show that *SHANK3* haploinsufficiency due to point mutations alone is sufficient to cause a broad range of phenotypic features associated with PMS. These include hypotonia, global developmental delay, ID, ASD, language deficits, sleep disturbance, increased pain tolerance, regression, motor skills deficits, seizures, abnormal

EEG, brain imaging abnormalities, feeding difficulties, and gastrointestinal problems. We also describe frequent dysmorphic features in individuals with *SHANK3* mutations, including fifth finger clinodactyly, long eyelashes, bulbous nose, wide nasal bridge, malocclusion, high arched palate, pointed chin, sandal gap, and dysplastic toenails. Importantly, we show that language and motor phenotypes appear to be less severe in individuals with point mutations, as compared to 22q13 deletions. These findings extend the role of *SHANK3* dysfunction in human disease beyond its well-known role at the synapse in the central nervous system.

Additional files

Additional file 1: Table S1. Loss of function and de novo missense variants in *SHANK3* reported previously. **Table S2.** Clinical features of individuals with pathogenic or likely pathogenic *SHANK3* variants reported in the literature. **Table S3.** In silico prediction of pathogenicity of missense variants in *SHANK3* identified in this study and in the literature. **Table S4.** Reported truncating and in-frame variants in *SHANK3* unlikely to be pathogenic. (XLSX 84 kb)

Additional file 2: Table S5. Descriptive and diagnostic data by patient. **Table S6.** ASD and intellectual ability classifications in individuals with *SHANK3* mutations. **Table S7.** Language and motor functioning in individuals with *SHANK3* mutations. (PDF 132 kb)

Abbreviations
ACMG: American College of Medical Genetics and Genomics; ADI-R: Autism Diagnostic Interview-Revised; ADOS-2: Autism Diagnostic Observation Schedule: Second Edition; ASD: Autism spectrum disorder; DAS-II: Differential Ability Scales, Second Edition; DSM-5: Diagnostic and Statistical Manual for Mental Disorders: Fifth Edition; EEG: Electroencephalography; EVS: Exome Variant Server; gnomAD: Genome Aggregation Database; ID: Intellectual disability; IQ: Intellectual quotient; MRI: Magnetic resonance imaging; OMIM: Online Mendelian Inheritance in Man; PMS: Phelan-McDermid syndrome

Acknowledgements
We thank the individuals with PMS and their families for their participation.

Funding
This work was supported by grants from the Beatrice and Samuel A. Seaver Foundation, the Phelan-McDermid Syndrome Foundation, NIMH (R34 MH100276-01 to AK and R21 MH107839 to JDB), and NINDS (U54 NS092090-01 to AK and K08 NS091381 to JLH). SDR is a Seaver fellow. JLH is funded by the Robbins Foundation. CB is a Research Director at INSERM. The funding bodies had no role in the design of the study, in the collection, analysis, and interpretation of data, or in the writing of the manuscript.

Authors' contributions

SDR, PMS, CB, AK, and JDB conceived and designed the study. SDR and CB analyzed and interpreted the genetic data. FM contributed to the molecular validation data and helped with the data processing. PMS, DH, and ATW performed the psychological evaluations. PMS, MPT, and AK analyzed and interpreted the data regarding the psychiatric evaluation. AK, MPT, and CB analyzed and interpreted the data regarding the medical evaluation. YF analyzed and interpreted the data regarding the neurological evaluation. RL analyzed and interpreted the data regarding the dysmorphology exam. AD and JW managed the samples and clinical data. JLH conducted the phenotypic data collection for individuals B1–B3. AK and JDB supervised the study. SDR, PMS, CB, AK, and JDB wrote the manuscript. All authors read and approved the final manuscript.

Competing interests

JDB and Mount Sinai hold a shared parent for the use of insulin-like growth factor-1 (IGF-1) in Phelan-McDermid syndrome. JDB is on the scientific advisory board for Coronis Neuroscience and has consulted for the Gerson Lehrman Group. AK is on the advisory board of Vencerx Therapeutics and consults for Ovid Therapeutics. The remaining authors declare that they have no competing interests.

Author details

[1]Seaver Autism Center, Icahn School of Medicine at Mount Sinai, New York, NY 10029, USA. [2]Department of Psychiatry, Icahn School of Medicine at Mount Sinai, New York, NY 10029, USA. [3]Department of Neurology, Icahn School of Medicine at Mount Sinai, New York, NY 10029, USA. [4]Department of Pediatrics, Icahn School of Medicine at Mount Sinai, New York, NY 10029, USA. [5]Department of Genetics and Genomic Sciences, Icahn School of Medicine at Mount Sinai, New York, NY 10029, USA. [6]Division of Neurology and Developmental Neuroscience, Department of Pediatrics, Baylor College of Medicine and Texas Children's Hospital, Houston, TX 77030, USA. [7]Sorbonne Université, INSERM, CNRS, Neuroscience Paris Seine, Institut de Biologie Paris Seine, 75005 Paris, France. [8]Department of Neuroscience, Icahn School of Medicine at Mount Sinai, New York, NY 10029, USA. [9]Friedman Brain Institute, Icahn School of Medicine at Mount Sinai, New York, NY 10029, USA. [10]Mindich Child Health and Development Institute, Icahn School of Medicine at Mount Sinai, New York, NY 10029, USA.

References

1. Kolevzon A, Angarita B, Bush L, Wang AT, Frank Y, Yang A, et al. Phelan-McDermid syndrome: a review of the literature and practice parameters for medical assessment and monitoring. J Neurodev Disord. 2014;6:39.
2. Soorya L, Kolevzon A, Zweifach J, Lim T, Dobry Y, Schwartz L, et al. Prospective investigation of autism and genotype-phenotype correlations in 22q13 deletion syndrome and SHANK3 deficiency. Mol Autism. 2013;4:18.
3. Bonaglia MC, Giorda R, Beri S, De Agostini C, Novara F, Fichera M, et al. Molecular mechanisms generating and stabilizing terminal 22q13 deletions in 44 subjects with Phelan/McDermid syndrome. PLoS Genet. 2011;7:e1002173.
4. Sarasua SM, Boccuto L, Sharp JL, Dwivedi A, Chen CF, Rollins JD, et al. Clinical and genomic evaluation of 201 patients with Phelan-McDermid syndrome. Hum Genet. 2014;133:847–59.
5. Luciani JJ, de Mas P, Depetris D, Mignon-Ravix C, Bottani A, Prieur M, et al. Telomeric 22q13 deletions resulting from rings, simple deletions, and translocations: cytogenetic, molecular, and clinical analyses of 32 new observations. J Med Genet. 2003;40:690–6.
6. Wilson HL, Wong AC, Shaw SR, Tse WY, Stapleton GA, Phelan MC, et al. Molecular characterisation of the 22q13 deletion syndrome supports the role of haploinsufficiency of SHANK3/PROSAP2 in the major neurological symptoms. J Med Genet. 2003;40:575–84.
7. Sarasua SM, Dwivedi A, Boccuto L, Rollins JD, Chen CF, Rogers RC, et al. Association between deletion size and important phenotypes expands the genomic region of interest in Phelan-McDermid syndrome (22q13 deletion syndrome). J Med Genet. 2011;48:761–6.
8. Zwanenburg RJ, Ruiter SA, van den Heuvel ER, Flapper BC, Van Ravenswaaij-Arts CM. Developmental phenotype in Phelan-McDermid (22q13.3 deletion) syndrome: a systematic and prospective study in 34 children. J Neurodev Disord. 2016;8:16.
9. Durand CM, Betancur C, Boeckers TM, Bockmann J, Chaste P, Fauchereau F, et al. Mutations in the gene encoding the synaptic scaffolding protein SHANK3 are associated with autism spectrum disorders. Nat Genet. 2007;39:25–7.
10. Moessner R, Marshall CR, Sutcliffe JS, Skaug J, Pinto D, Vincent J, et al. Contribution of SHANK3 mutations to autism spectrum disorder. Am J Hum Genet. 2007;81:1289–97.
11. Gauthier J, Spiegelman D, Piton A, Lafreniere RG, Laurent S, St-Onge J, et al. Novel de novo SHANK3 mutation in autistic patients. Am J Med Genet B Neuropsychiatr Genet. 2009;150B:421–4.
12. Boccuto L, Lauri M, Sarasua SM, Skinner CD, Buccella D, Dwivedi A, et al. Prevalence of SHANK3 variants in patients with different subtypes of autism spectrum disorders. Eur J Hum Genet. 2013;21:310–6.
13. Leblond CS, Nava C, Polge A, Gauthier J, Huguet G, Lumbroso S, et al. Meta-analysis of SHANK mutations in autism spectrum disorders: a gradient of severity in cognitive impairments. PLoS Genet. 2014;10:e1004580.
14. De Rubeis S, He X, Goldberg AP, Poultney CS, Samocha K, Cicek AE, et al. Synaptic, transcriptional and chromatin genes disrupted in autism. Nature. 2014;515:209–15.
15. O'Roak BJ, Stessman HA, Boyle EA, Witherspoon KT, Martin B, Lee C, et al. Recurrent de novo mutations implicate novel genes underlying simplex autism risk. Nat Commun. 2014;5:5595.
16. Yuen RK, Merico D, Bookman M, Howe JL. Thiruvahindrapuram B, Patel RV, et al. Whole genome sequencing resource identifies 18 new candidate genes for autism spectrum disorder. Nat Neurosci. 2017;20:602–11.
17. Hamdan FF, Gauthier J, Araki Y, Lin DT, Yoshizawa Y, Higashi K, et al. Excess of de novo deleterious mutations in genes associated with glutamatergic systems in nonsyndromic intellectual disability. Am J Hum Genet. 2011;88:306–16.
18. Gong X, Jiang YW, Zhang X, An Y, Zhang J, Wu Y, et al. High proportion of 22q13 deletions and SHANK3 mutations in Chinese patients with intellectual disability. PLoS One. 2012;7:e34739.
19. Redin C, Gerard B, Lauer J, Herenger Y, Muller J, Quartier A, et al. Efficient strategy for the molecular diagnosis of intellectual disability using targeted high-throughput sequencing. J Med Genet. 2014;51:724–36.
20. Lelieveld SH, Reijnders MR, Pfundt R, Yntema HG, Kamsteeg EJ, de Vries P, et al. Meta-analysis of 2,104 trios provides support for 10 new genes for intellectual disability. Nat Neurosci. 2016;19:1194–6.
21. Deciphering Developmental Disorders Study. Prevalence and architecture of de novo mutations in developmental disorders. Nature. 2017;542:433–8.
22. Gauthier J, Champagne N, Lafreniere RG, Xiong L, Spiegelman D, Brustein E, et al. De novo mutations in the gene encoding the synaptic scaffolding protein SHANK3 in patients ascertained for schizophrenia. Proc Natl Acad Sci U S A. 2010;107:7863–8.
23. Betancur C, Buxbaum JD. SHANK3 haploinsufficiency: a "common" but underdiagnosed highly penetrant monogenic cause of autism spectrum disorders. Mol Autism. 2013;4:17.
24. Holder JL Jr, Quach MM. The spectrum of epilepsy and electroencephalographic abnormalities due to SHANK3 loss-of-function mutations. Epilepsia. 2016;57:1651–9.
25. Richards S, Aziz N, Bale S, Bick D, Das S, Gastier-Foster J, et al. Standards and guidelines for the interpretation of sequence variants: a joint consensus recommendation of the American College of Medical Genetics and Genomics and the Association for Molecular Pathology. Genet Med. 2015;17:405–24.
26. Cochoy DM, Kolevzon A, Kajiwara Y, Schoen M, Pascual-Lucas M, Lurie S, et al. Phenotypic and functional analysis of SHANK3 stop mutations identified in individuals with ASD and/or ID. Mol Autism. 2015;6:23.
27. Lord C, Rutter M, DiLavore PS, Risi S, Gotham K, Bishop D. Autism Diagnostic Observation Schedule, 2nd edition (ADOS-2) manual (part I): modules 1–4. Torrance: Western Psychological Services; 2012.
28. Lord C, Rutter M, Le Couteur A. Autism Diagnostic Interview-Revised: a revised version of a diagnostic interview for caregivers of individuals with possible pervasive developmental disorders. J Autism Dev Disord. 1994;24:659–85.
29. American Psychiatric Association. Diagnostic and Statistical Manual of Mental Disorders, 5th edition, text revision. Washington, DC: American Psychiatric Association; 2013.
30. Hus V, Gotham K, Lord C. Standardizing ADOS domain scores: separating severity of social affect and restricted and repetitive behaviors. J Autism Dev Disord. 2014;44:2400–12.

31. Mullen EM. Mullen Scales of Early Learning. Circle Pines: American Guidance Services; 1995.

32. Roid GH. Stanford Binet Intelligence Scales. 5th ed. Itasca: Riverside Publishing; 2003.

33. Elliot CD. Differential Ability Scales—second edition: introductory and technical manual. San Antonio: Harcourt Assessment; 2007.

34. Bishop SL, Guthrie W, Coffing M, Lord C. Convergent validity of the Mullen Scales of Early Learning and the Differential Ability Scales in children with autism spectrum disorders. Am J Intellect Dev Disabil. 2011;116:331–43.

35. Akshoomoff N. Use of the Mullen Scales of Early Learning for the assessment of young children with autism spectrum disorders. Child Neuropsychol. 2006;12:269–77.

36. Sparrow SS, Cicchetti DV, Balla DA. Vineland Adaptive Behavior Scales: second edition (Vineland II), survey interview form/caregiver rating form. Livonia: Pearson Assessments; 2005.

37. Fenson L, Marchman VA, Thal DJ, Dale PS, Reznick JS, Bates E. MacArthur-Bates communicative development inventories: user's guide and technical manual. 2nd ed. Baltimore: Brookes Publishing Co.; 2007.

38. Dunn LM, Dunn DM. PPVT-4: Peabody Picture Vocabulary Test. Bloomington: Pearson Assessments; 2007.

39. Williams KT. The Expressive Vocabulary Test. 2nd ed. Circle Pines: AGS Publishing; 2007.

40. Beery KE, Buktenica NA, Beery NA. Beery-Buktenica Developmental Test of Visual-Motor Integration. 6th ed. Minneapolis: Pearson; 2010.

41. Dunn W, Westman K. The sensory profile: the performance of a national sample of children without disabilities. Am J Occup Ther. 1997;51:25–34.

42. Siper PM, Kolevzon A, Wang AT, Buxbaum JD, Tavassoli T. A clinician-administered observation and corresponding caregiver interview capturing DSM-5 sensory reactivity symptoms in children with ASD. Autism Res. 2017;10:1133–40.

43. Nemirovsky SI, Cordoba M, Zaiat JJ, Completa SP, Vega PA, Gonzalez-Moron D, et al. Whole genome sequencing reveals a de novo SHANK3 mutation in familial autism spectrum disorder. PLoS One. 2015;10:e0116358.

44. Lim ET, Uddin M, De Rubeis S, Chan Y, Kamumbu AS, Zhang X, et al. Rates, distribution and implications of postzygotic mosaic mutations in autism spectrum disorder. Nat Neurosci. 2017;20:1217–24.

45. Zhang Y, Kong W, Gao Y, Liu X, Gao K, Xie H, et al. Gene mutation analysis in 253 Chinese children with unexplained epilepsy and intellectual/developmental disabilities. PLoS One. 2015;10:e0141782.

46. Bowling KM, Thompson ML, Amaral MD, Finnila CR, Hiatt SM, Engel KL, et al. Genomic diagnosis for children with intellectual disability and/or developmental delay. Genome Med. 2017;9:43.

47. Samocha KE, Robinson EB, Sanders SJ, Stevens C, Sabo A, McGrath LM, et al. A framework for the interpretation of de novo mutation in human disease. Nat Genet. 2014;46:944–50.

48. Bramswig NC, Ludecke HJ, Alanay Y, Albrecht B, Barthelmie A, Boduroglu K, et al. Exome sequencing unravels unexpected differential diagnoses in individuals with the tentative diagnosis of Coffin-Siris and Nicolaides-Baraitser syndromes. Hum Genet. 2015;134:553–68.

49. Kolevzon A, Cai G, Soorya L, Takahashi N, Grodberg D, Kajiwara Y, et al. Analysis of a purported SHANK3 mutation in a boy with autism: clinical impact of rare variant research in neurodevelopmental disabilities. Brain Res. 2011;1380:98–105.

50. Waga C, Okamoto N, Ondo Y, Fukumura-Kato R, Goto Y, Kohsaka S, et al. Novel variants of the SHANK3 gene in Japanese autistic patients with severe delayed speech development. Psychiatr Genet. 2011;21:208–11.

51. Denayer A, Van Esch H, de Ravel T, Frijns JP, Van Buggenhout G, Vogels A, et al. Neuropsychopathology in 7 patients with the 22q13 deletion syndrome: presence of bipolar disorder and progressive loss of skills. Mol Syndromol. 2012;3:14–20.

52. Jeffries AR, Curran S, Elmslie F, Sharma A, Wenger S, Hummel M, et al. Molecular and phenotypic characterization of ring chromosome 22. Am J Med Genet A. 2005;137:139–47.

53. Durand CM, Perroy J, Loll F, Perrais D, Fagni L, Bourgeron T, et al. SHANK3 mutations identified in autism lead to modification of dendritic spine morphology via an actin-dependent mechanism. Mol Psychiatry. 2012;17:71–84.

54. Arons MH, Thynne CJ, Grabrucker AM, Li D, Schoen M, Cheyne JE, et al. Autism-associated mutations in ProSAP2/Shank3 impair synaptic transmission and neurexin-neuroligin-mediated transsynaptic signaling. J Neurosci. 2012;32:14966–78.

55. Vucurovic K, Landais E, Delahaigue C, Eutrope J, Schneider A, Leroy C, et al. Bipolar affective disorder and early dementia onset in a male patient with SHANK3 deletion. Eur J Med Genet. 2012;55:625–9.

56. Serret S, Thummler S, Dor E, Vesperini S, Santos A, Askenazy F. Lithium as a rescue therapy for regression and catatonia features in two SHANK3 patients with autism spectrum disorder: case reports. BMC Psychiatry. 2015;15:107.

57. Egger JI, Zwanenburg RJ, van Ravenswaaij-Arts CM, Kleefstra T, Verhoeven WM. Neuropsychological phenotype and psychopathology in seven adult patients with Phelan-McDermid syndrome: implications for treatment strategy. Genes Brain Behav. 2016;15:395–404.

58. Reierson G, Bernstein J, Froehlich-Santino W, Urban A, Purmann C, Berquist S, et al. Characterizing regression in Phelan McDermid syndrome (22q13 deletion syndrome). J Psychiatr Res. 2017;91:139–44.

59. Verhoeven WM, Egger JI, Willemsen MH, de Leijer GJ, Kleefstra T. Phelan-McDermid syndrome in two adult brothers: atypical bipolar disorder as its psychopathological phenotype? Neuropsychiatr Dis Treat. 2012;8:175–9.

60. Han Q, Kim YH, Wang X, Liu D, Zhang ZJ, Bey AL, et al. SHANK3 deficiency impairs heat hyperalgesia and TRPV1 signaling in primary sensory neurons. Neuron. 2016;92:1279–93.

61. Wei SC, Yang-Yen HF, Tsao PN, Weng MT, Tung CC, Yu LCH, et al. SHANK3 regulates intestinal barrier function through modulating ZO-1 expression through the PKCε-dependent pathway. Inflamm Bowel Dis. 2017;23:1730–40.

62. Brandt T, Desai K, Grodberg D, Mehta L, Cohen N, Tryfon A, et al. Complex autism spectrum disorder in a patient with a 17q12 microduplication. Am J Med Genet A. 2012;158A:1170–7.

15

Clustering the autisms using glutamate synapse protein interaction networks from cortical and hippocampal tissue of seven mouse models

Emily A. Brown[1], Jonathan D. Lautz[1], Tessa R. Davis[2,3], Edward P. Gniffke[1], Alison A. W. VanSchoiack[1,4], Steven C. Neier[2,5,6,7], Noah Tashbook[1], Chiara Nicolini[8], Margaret Fahnestock[8], Adam G. Schrum[9] and Stephen E. P. Smith[1,10]* (iD)

Abstract

Background: Autism spectrum disorders (ASDs) are a heterogeneous group of behaviorally defined disorders and are associated with hundreds of rare genetic mutations and several environmental risk factors. Mouse models of specific risk factors have been successful in identifying molecular mechanisms associated with a given factor. However, comparisons among different models to elucidate underlying common pathways or to define clusters of biologically relevant disease subtypes have been complicated by different methodological approaches or different brain regions examined by the labs that developed each model. Here, we use a novel proteomic technique, quantitative multiplex co-immunoprecipitation or QMI, to make a series of identical measurements of a synaptic protein interaction network in seven different animal models. We aim to identify molecular disruptions that are common to multiple models.

Methods: QMI was performed on 92 hippocampal and cortical samples taken from seven mouse models of ASD: Shank3B, Shank3Δex4-9, Ube3a^{2xTG}, TSC2, FMR1, and CNTNAP2 mutants, as well as E12.5 VPA (maternal valproic acid injection on day 12.5 post-conception). The QMI panel targeted a network of 16 interacting, ASD-linked, synaptic proteins, probing 240 potential co-associations. A custom non-parametric statistical test was used to call significant differences between ASD models and littermate controls, and Hierarchical Clustering by Principal Components was used to cluster the models using mean $\log_2$ fold change values.

Results: Each model displayed a unique set of disrupted interactions, but some interactions were disrupted in multiple models. These tended to be interactions that are known to change with synaptic activity. Clustering revealed potential relationships among models and suggested deficits in AKT signaling in Ube3a^{2xTG} mice, which were confirmed by phospho-western blots.

Conclusions: These data highlight the great heterogeneity among models, but suggest that high-dimensional measures of a synaptic protein network may allow differentiation of subtypes of ASD with shared molecular pathology.

* Correspondence: seps@uw.edu
[1]Center for Integrative Brain Research, Seattle Children's Research Institute, Seattle, WA, USA
[10]Department of Pediatrics and Graduate Program in Neuroscience, University of Washington, Seattle, WA, USA
Full list of author information is available at the end of the article

Background

As the incidence of autism spectrum disorder (ASD) has climbed over the past decades to 1 in 59 children [1], next-generation sequencing studies have described likely causative mutations in hundreds of genes, each accounting for < 0.1–1% of the total autistic population [2–4]. Additional factors such as maternal immune activation [5], maternal anti-brain antibodies [6], chemical exposures [7], and polygenetic inheritance of a susceptible genetic background [8] all likely contribute to the development of ASD on an individual-by-individual basis. Thus, much like cancer, ASD is an individually rare, collectively common disorder with a shared diagnostic phenotype: reduced interest in social interaction, reduced communication, and increased stereotyped or repetitive interests and behaviors [9].

The fact that ASD is a diagnostic entity, with a common set of behavioral impairments shared among patients, has led to the widespread hypothesis that other disease mechanisms must also be shared among patients at the level of anatomy [10], neural circuits [11], genetic networks [12, 13], or molecular pathways [14]. Along these lines, a few clear themes have emerged from combining diverse lines of evidence: the immune system is likely involved, with immune-mediated risk factors (reviewed in [15]), and abnormal peripheral [16] and central ([17, 18], but see [19]) inflammatory phenotypes present. Gene regulatory pathways are clearly implicated by genetic studies, as a large percentage of ASD-linked genes are transcription factors, chromatin remodelers, or translational regulators [4, 12]. Synaptic proteins have also been implicated by genetic studies, and by the fact that one unifying feature of animal models of ASD has been disrupted synaptic transmission [20] (although note that the specific nature of the disruption varies greatly between models, or even between brain regions in the same model, discussed below). Recently, unifying theories of ASD have proposed that disruptions to activity-dependent, homeostatic neuronal processes are an underlying characteristic of ASDs [21, 22]. Indeed, diverse ASD-linked genes can disrupt the complex molecular circuitry that translates synaptic ion currents into intracellular signal transduction cascades, traffics those messages to sites of translation and transcription, and converts protein-level modifications into long-term changes in gene expression.

Despite these hints at convergent mechanisms, heterogeneity is still the dominant theme when comparing different autism types [23], or even when comparing genetically similar autisms. The prototypical example is the gene Shank3, responsible for Phelan-McDermid syndrome-associated autism and implicated in ~ 1% of total ASD cases [24]. Shank3 encodes multiple alternatively spliced protein variants (at least six), which each contain different combinations of protein-interaction-mediating domains. No fewer than 13 different mutant mouse lines have been reported thus far, which disrupt different exons of Shank3. While the majority of lines show deficits in social (nine lines), repetitive (nine lines), or vocalization (four lines) behavior, each line shows a different combination of behavioral and molecular deficits, depending on which Shank3 isoforms are disrupted (reviewed in [24]). For example, in a complete knockout line, *reducing* mGluR5 activity normalized repetitive grooming [25], while in an exon 11 deletion line, *enhancing* mGluR5 activity rescued abnormal grooming [26]. Similarly, at the level of electrophysiology, *reduced* striatal mEPSP amplitude and frequency has been reported in adult Shank3B$^{-/-}$ striatum [27], reduced amplitude but increased frequency in Shank3Δex4–9$^{+/-}$ hippocampus [28], increased mEPSP frequency and amplitude in p14 Shank3B$^{-/-}$ striatum [29], and increased activity in p14 Shank3B$^{-/-}$ cortex [29]. Thus, even models targeting the same gene display different phenotypes dependent on mutation type, age, and brain region. For the majority of ASD genes, only a single model (typically a complete knockout) has been published, and the ages and brain regions targeted differ between labs, complicating attempts at directly comparing pathology between published studies.

This study was designed to make a series of identical, directly comparable molecular measurements in several mouse models of autism, in order to address the question of molecular convergence among models. We compared measurements of synaptic proteins in two brain regions (frontal cortex and hippocampus), in age-and-sex-matched adult (postnatal day 60) animals from six genetic and one environmental model of ASD. We used a novel proteomic technique, Quantitative multiplex co-immunoprecipitation (QMI), that compares the abundance of, and interactions among, a panel of native proteins in mutant animals vs. a matched wildtype littermate control. In QMI, protein complexes are immunoprecipitated onto 5 um polystyrene latex beads and probed with fluorophore-coupled antibodies to quantitatively measure the amount of proteins in shared complexes. The resulting fluorescent signals are read on a flow cytometer, and raw abundance measures are normalized to wildtype controls run on the same plate to cancel out batch effects; only fold-change values compared to control are reported [30].

QMI is a candidate-based approach that targets carefully selected networks of interacting proteins. The high-dimensional data produced is linear over a large dynamic range and is several-fold more sensitive than traditional Western blotting techniques [31]. We used a previously published QMI panel that targets 16 synaptic proteins and measures 240 binary proteins in shared complexes by exposed surface epitopes (PiSCES). This panel consists of ASD-linked proteins that are known to physically interact at the synapse [32]. In each mouse model, we identified a unique combination of disrupted

PiSCES, with occasional overlap of disruptions that were common to multiple models. We then clustered the data by model and brain region to reveal possible higher-level relationships among the seven animal models, and we confirmed a previously unreported molecular deficit in one model that was predicted by our clustering. Our approach has the potential to identify unexpected commonalities among genetic autisms and to suggest novel treatments based on shared molecular pathology.

Methods

Animal models

The specific identity of all mouse strains used is shown in Table 1. Littermate mice were co-housed in groups of 2–5 under standard laboratory conditions. At 60 days of age, mice were deeply anesthetized with isofluorane, decapitated, and brains were removed. We chose day 60 because we wanted to focus on adult animals, since the majority of animal models have been behaviorally tested as adults (see Table 1). We used two males and two females for each genotype to focus our study on robust, non-sex-dependent effects, except FMR1$^{-/y}$ mice and controls, which were all male since FMR1 is an X-linked gene. We used frontal cortex for all models and hippocampus for some models because these two brain regions have been frequently analyzed in electrophysiology and biochemical studies of ASD models (see Table 1). For frontal cortex, the rostral 3 mm of cortex was cut with a razor blade in a metal brain mold, making sure not to include any striatal tissue in the section, and the olfactory bulb was removed; for hippocampus, bilateral hippocampi were removed with curved forceps. Tissue was frozen in liquid nitrogen and stored at − 80 until homogenization. All work was performed under an approved animal protocol at Seattle Children's Research Institute (#15580).

VPA mice were prepared at McMaster University in compliance with standards of the Canadian Council on Animal Care and with approval from the McMaster University Animal Research Ethics Board. CD-1 female mice were mated until a sperm plug was detected (E0). On day 12.5 after conception (E12.5), pregnant mice received a single intraperitoneal (i.p.) injection of 500 mg/kg sodium valproate (VPA; Sigma, Oakville, ON, Canada) dissolved in 0.9% NaCl solution, while controls were injected with only saline. E12.5 was chosen to match previous reports from our group and others (see [32]). Pups were weaned on postnatal day (PD) 21 and subjected to behavioral assays (three-chamber sociability, elevated plus maze, and marble-burying assays for social behavior, anxiety, and repetitive behavior, respectively) on PDs 29–34. Animals were killed by decapitation on PD 35, and brains were rapidly dissected and stored at − 80 °C.

QMI analysis

Tissue was homogenized in 0.32 M Sucrose in HEPES buffer, pH 7.4 with Sigma protease (Cat # P8340) and phosphatase (Cat # P5726) inhibitors (Sigma Aldrich), using 12 strokes of a glass-Teflon homogenizer. Samples were spun at 1000×g for 5 min to pellet membranes, then spun at 10,000×g for 15 min to pellet P2 synaptosomes. Synaptosomes were solubilized on ice in 200 ul lysis buffer (150 mM NaCl, 50 mM Tris (pH 7.4), 1% NP-40, 10 mM NaF, 2 mM sodium orthovanadate + protease/phosphatase inhibitor cocktails [Sigma]) for 15 min, spun at 4 °C at 10,000×g for 15 min to remove insoluble material, and protein concentration was measured by BCA assay (Thermo-Fisher).

QMI beads (Luminex) were prepared as previously described [32], with each bead color-class coupled to a distinct immunoprecipitating antibody, as shown in Table 2. Equal amounts of protein from each matched pair of animals (transgenic vs. wild type littermate or VPA- vs. saline-treated control) were incubated with QMI beads overnight at 4 °C, with constant rotation. Beads from each sample were then distributed into 32 wells of a 96-well plate, approximately 250 beads of each class per well, and each of 16 probe antibodies was added, in duplicate, to individual wells. Beads were then washed with ice-cold Fly-P buffer [50 mM Tris (pH 7.4), 100 mM NaCl, 1% bovine serum albumin, and 0.01% sodium azide], incubated for 30 min with streptavidin-PE (1:200, BioLegend), washed again, and read on a custom refrigerated Bioplex 200 flow cytometer (BioRad), which recorded the bead classification (corresponding to IP'd protein, X) and PE fluorescence (corresponding to the amount of probe antibody target protein, Y) of each bead. An above-background reading for IP:X Probe:Y indicates the occurrence of a protein complex containing both X and Y [33].

Data analysis

Data were exported in .xml files containing all data on a bead-by-bead, well-by-well basis. A custom Javascript was written to generate histograms showing bead distributions for a given bead class in a given well and to extract the median fluorescent intensity of each bead class in each well for export to Excel and R (faculty.washington.edu/seps/program). A custom MatLab script, "Adaptive Non-parametric statistical test with an adjustable alpha Cutoff" (abbreviated ANC), previously described in detail [30], was used to identify interactions that changed significantly in > 70% of experiments; these interactions are referred to as "hits." ANC first uses a K-S test to compare histogram distributions of technical replicates to both discard duplicate wells that are significantly different from each other (presumed manual error) and to adjust the alpha value based on technical error. K-S test results from comparisons between an experimental

Table 1 Animal models used in this study

Strain	Source and background	First citation	Behavioral phenotype	Synaptic proteins	Electrophysiology
Shank3B⁻/⁻	Jax #017688 C57BL/6J	[27]	Abnormal social behavior; excessive grooming leading to self-injury.	Reduced PSD levels of GluR2, NR2A/2B, Homer.	In striatum: reduced mEPSP frequency and amplitude; reduced population spike amplitude.
Shank3Δex4-9+/-	Jax #017890 C57BL/6J	[28]	Less social sniffing, fewer vocalizations in males exposed to females.	Reduced GluR1 immunofluorescent puncta in hippocampus.	In hippocampus: reduced mEPSP amplitude but increased frequency. AMPAR-dependent deficit in population spike amplitude. Impaired LTP, normal LTD.
Ube3a²ˣᵀᴳ	Jax #017482 FVB	[34]	Abnormal social behavior, fewer ultrasonic vocalizations in adult animals, increased repetitive grooming	Reduced ARC levels.	In whisker barrel cortex: reduced mEPSP frequency and amplitude; reduced evoked EPSC amplitude.
Cntnap2⁻/⁻	Jax #017482 C57BL/6J	[46]; in ASD context [64]	Abnormal social behavior, fewer pup ultrasonic vocalizations, increased repetitive grooming		Somatosensory cortex: reduced population synchronization by Ca2+ imaging.
TSC2+/-	Jax #004686 B6129SF2/J	[65]	Abnormal social behavior [63], impaired hippocampal-dependent memory [37]. Abnormal pup vocalizations [66]	Hippocampus: increased mGluR5 [67].	Hippocampus: enhanced LTP [37], reduced LTD in juveniles, abnormal but present LTD in adults [67].
FMR⁻/y	Jax #003025 C57BL/6 J	[68]	Abnormal social behavior, increased repetitive behaviors, impaired memory; reviewed in [69].	Less mGluR5 in forebrain PSD preps; normal levels of other GluRs; normal levels of all receptors in total membrane lysates. [70].	Hippocampus: enhanced, abnormal LTD; LTP reported impaired or normal (reviewed by [69]). Cortex: normal LTP at 2 months, abnormal at 12 months [71].
VPA	Generated by M. Fahnestock, McMaster U. CD-1	[72] (established model); [73] (tested behavior)	Reduced social interaction, increased repetitive/stereotyped behaviors [73], reduced vocalizations [74].	Cortex of 2-week-old rats: increased NR2A/B, [35]; adult rats: reduced PSD95 [52].	Cortical pyramidal neurons: enhanced NMDAR-mediated currents, enhanced LTP [35].

Table 2 QMI targets, autism linkage, and antibody information

Gene name	Protein name	Description	Simons score	Evidence in ASD	IP antibody	Probe antibody
GRM5	mGluR5	Metabotropic glutamate receptor. G-protein coupled receptor activates Erk and PI3K cascades in response to glutamate.	NS	Rare variants identified in ASD patients [61, 75]. Plays a key role in Fragile X [41] and possibly other ASD models.	Millipore 5675 Cat#AB5675	Neuromab N75/3 Cat# 75-115
GRIN1	NMDAR1	NMDA-type glutamate receptor subunits. NMDARs are heterotetramers with high Ca2+ permeability, essential for learning and memory. Subunits confer different functional properties to the receptor.	3	Rare variant in ASD siblings [76]	Thermo 54.1 Cat# 02-0500	Santa Cruz polyclonal C20 Cat# sc-1467
GRIN2A	NMDAR2A		4	Genetic association [77]	Neuromab N327/95 Cat#75-288	Biolegend N327A/38 Cat# 832401
GRIN2B	NMDAR2B		1	Multiple rare variants identified in ASD patients. [4, 78, 79]	Biolegend N59/20 Cat# 832501	Biolegend N59/36 Cat# 818701
GRIA1	GluR1	AMPA-type glutamate receptor subunits. AMPARs are also tetramers. Subunits confer different functional properties to the receptor.	2	Recurrent missense mutations [4, 80]	Biolegend N355/1 Cat# 819801	Millipore polyclonal 1504 Cat# AB1504
GRIA2	GluR2		–	Contained in an ASD-linked deletion [81]	Biolegend L21/32 Cat# 810501	Santa Cruz polyclonal C20 Cat# sc-7610
NLGN3	NL3	Postsynaptic Neuroligin 3 binds presynaptic neurexins to create trans-synaptic adhesion bridges. Cleavage following activity may be involved in cell signaling.	2	Rare mutations; TADA study [82, 83]	Thermo 566209 Cat# MA5-24253	Santa Cruz G2 Cat # sc-271880
HOMER1	Homer1	Postsynaptic scaffold linking Shanks, mGluRs, and many other postsynaptic components. Forms homo-tetramer via N-terminal coiled-coil domain.	4	Rare variants [61]	Lifespan Biosciences AT1F3 Cat# LS-C103482	Santa Cruz D3 Cat# SC-17842
	Homer1A	Activity-dependent isoform of Homer1 that lacks coiled-coil domain and acts as a dominant negative, preventing scaffolding by long Homers.			–	Santa Cruz polyclonal M13 Cat# sc-8922
DLG4	PSD95	Major component of postsynaptic density, scaffolds NMDARs and other components of the PSD via multiple binding domains.	NS	Rare variants and network gene analyses [84–86]	Biolegend K28/74 Cat# 810301	Biolegend K28/43 Cat# 810401
DLG1	SAP97	Scaffold with similar function to PSD95, but different specific binding affinities.	NS	Exome sequencing revealed rare variants [85]	Enzo RPI197.4 Cat# ADI-VAM-PS00	SantaCruz polyclonal H60 Cat# sc-25661
SHANK3	SHANK3	Scaffolding protein that forms a polymeric structure with Homer, and links multiple receptor types to downstream signaling pathways	1S	Recurrent rare de novo mutations and copy number variations (deletions) [87]	NeuroMab N367/62 Cat# 75-344	Enzo Life Sciences RPI197.4 Cat# ADI-VAM-PS00
UBE3A	Ube3A	E3 ubiquitin ligase, phospho-regulated by synaptic activity, that ubiquitinates Arc as well as other neuronal targets; also acts as a transcriptional regulator.	3S	Rare variants and copy number variations (duplications) [88, 89]	Santa Cruz H182 Cat# sc-25509	Santa Cruz E-4 Cat # sc-166689
SYNGAP1	SynGAP1	A RAS GTPase that is heavily expressed at the PSD. Negatively regulates RAS. PSD95 binding may be important in regulating synaptic binding "slots."	1S	Multiple rare variants [90]	Cell Signaling D20C7 Cat# 5539	SantaCruz polyclonal R19 Cat# sc8572
FYN	Fyn Kinase	Associates with PSD95 and NMDARs, phosphorylates the latter. Also binds and is activated by mGluRs.	–	None reported	Santa Cruz Fyn15 Cat# sc-434	BioLegend FYNS9 Cat# B149751
PIK3R1	PI3K	PI3K is a lipid kinase that phosphorylates membrane phospholipids and initiates PI3K/AKT/mTOR signaling. The enzyme consists of a p85 regulatory and p110 catalytic subunit. Our antibodies target p85alpha.	–	PI3K subunits PIK3CG and PIK3R2 (Simons score 4 and 5, respectively) have been linked to autism [91, 92]	Thermo-Fisher U5 Cat# MA1-74183	Millipore AB6 Cat# 05-212

NS Listed in SFARI gene but not scored; – not listed

sample and a matched control are then corrected for multiple comparisons and technical errors to obtain a final p value. "Hits" were interactions with $p < 0.05$. Please see [30] for details. Prior QMI analysis in both T cells [30] and neural tissue [32] found that N of four biological replicates are sufficient to produce a consistent number of significant hits, so an N of at least four matched pairs was used. To eliminate batch effects due to both technical and biological variation, we limit comparisons to ASD model animals and co-housed, littermate controls euthanized on the same day and run on the same assay plate; ANC statistics are therefore based on consistent differences in paired comparisons for $N = 4$ experiments (each run with technical replicates). Workflow and examples of smoothed histograms are shown in Fig. 1.

Data matrices for each matched pair were exported from Java to Excel. For each matrix position, we divided the median fluorescence value (of the two technical replicates) of each ASD model animal by its wildtype littermate control and $\log_2$-transformed the result. Then, $\log_2$ fold change ($\log_2 FC$) matrices from $N = 4$ experiments were averaged to generate a single mean $\log_2 FC$ matrix per genotype/tissue type, shown in Additional file 1: Table S1. ANC significant hits were identified and imported into Cytoscape for visualization. Significant interactions are represented by an edge connecting two protein nodes; the color and width of the edge corresponds to the direction (red = up, blue = down) and magnitude of the change (Fig. 1e, f). Changes in protein abundance (IP probe of same target protein) are represented by loops.

To cluster samples by shared ANC-significant hits, we used the hclust(dist()) and heatmap.2 functions in R. To cluster samples by average fold-change matrices shown in Additional file 1: Table S1, we first performed principal component analysis to reduce noise due to nonspecific background fluctuations using the "PCA" function in the "FactomineR" package for R; then we used the "HCPC" function in the same package to cluster genotypes/tissue types by principal components. To test the robustness of clustering, we used the "pvclust" function in R. All options were used in the default settings.

Western blots were run on cortical tissue using standard protocols. Briefly, cortical P2 fractions were lysed in lysis buffer, protein concentrations were normalized using BCA assays, equal amounts of protein were loaded into each well and run at 110 V. Protein was transferred onto PVDF membranes, blocked with 5% milk in TBS-T, primary antibodies were incubated overnight at 4C, followed by washes, species-specific secondary antibody incubation (anti-mouse or rabbit, 1:10,000, Jackson Immunoresearch), and luminol detection (Pierce Femto reagent). Antibodies used (all 1:1000 dilutions) the following: Ube3a clone E-4 (Santa Cruz), pAKTs473 clone D9E, pAKTt308 clone 244F9, panAKT clone 40D4, pMTOR polyclonal Cat #2971, and pS6 clone D57.2.2 (all from Cell Signaling).

Results

Additional file 1: Table S1 shows the median $\log_2$ fold change values for the complete dataset ($N = 92$ samples from 56 animals; 7 ASD models, with 4 ASD model animals and 4 WT controls per group, except $N = 6$ for Shank3B hippocampus; some animals contributed both cortical and hippocampal tissue). Numbers in bold case

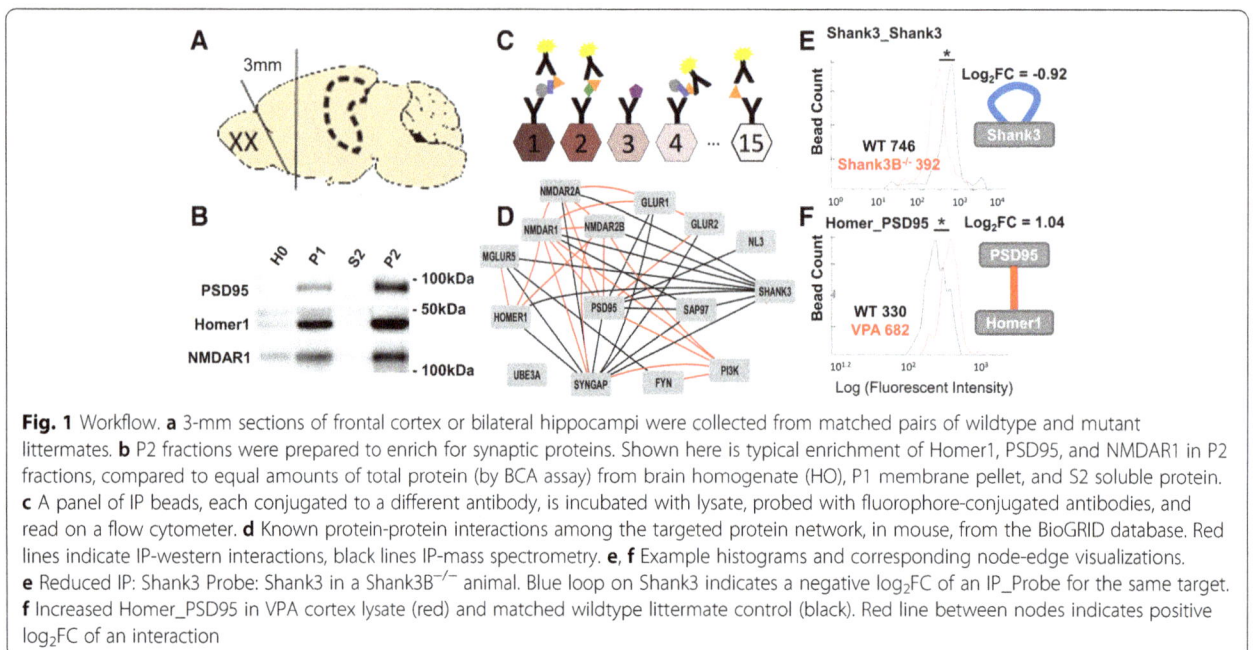

Fig. 1 Workflow. a 3-mm sections of frontal cortex or bilateral hippocampi were collected from matched pairs of wildtype and mutant littermates. b P2 fractions were prepared to enrich for synaptic proteins. Shown here is typical enrichment of Homer1, PSD95, and NMDAR1 in P2 fractions, compared to equal amounts of total protein (by BCA assay) from brain homogenate (HO), P1 membrane pellet, and S2 soluble protein. c A panel of IP beads, each conjugated to a different antibody, is incubated with lysate, probed with fluorophore-conjugated antibodies, and read on a flow cytometer. d Known protein-protein interactions among the targeted protein network, in mouse, from the BioGRID database. Red lines indicate IP-western interactions, black lines IP-mass spectrometry. e, f Example histograms and corresponding node-edge visualizations. e Reduced IP: Shank3 Probe: Shank3 in a Shank3B$^{-/-}$ animal. Blue loop on Shank3 indicates a negative $\log_2 FC$ of an IP_Probe for the same target. f Increased Homer_PSD95 in VPA cortex lysate (red) and matched wildtype littermate control (black). Red line between nodes indicates positive $\log_2 FC$ of an interaction

indicate fold changes > 1.19 or < 0.84 (which corresponds to ± 0.25 in log$_2$ scale), while red highlighting indicates that a value was statistically significant by ANC statistical analysis. Note that while some ANC-significant values are smaller than ± 0.25, indicating a small but high-confidence change, several bolded cells are not ANC-significant due to biological or technical variation and the stringent requirements of our statistical test. Below, we first focus our analysis on only significant ANC hits, then we perform inter-model comparisons using the entire data matrix to attempt to cluster models into biologically relevant groups.

Cortex

Overall, we found 32 statistically significant differences across the 7 mouse models (Additional file 1: Table S1 Sheet 2, and Fig. 2). Of 240 total IP_Probe combinations,

9 proteins (IP probe for the same target) and 18 proteins in shared complexes (PiSCES—IP probe for different proteins) showed differences in abundance across the 7 models. Four PiSCES (Homer1_PSD95, Homer_NMDAR1, SynGAP_PSD95 and NL3_FYN) and three abundance measures (FYN, SynGAP and PSD95) were significantly different in multiple models, while the remaining differences were unique to a single model.

Shank3B$^{-/-}$ animals (Fig. 2a) showed a reduction in Shank3 protein levels and an increased co-association of Homer with PSD95 and NMDAR1. This is counterintuitive, since Homer-PSD interactions are likely mediated by Shank proteins, and may be expected to be reduced in Shank3 animals. These results may reflect changes in Shank1/2 vs. 3 scaffolding, or an increase in these activity-labile interactions [32] may be downstream of

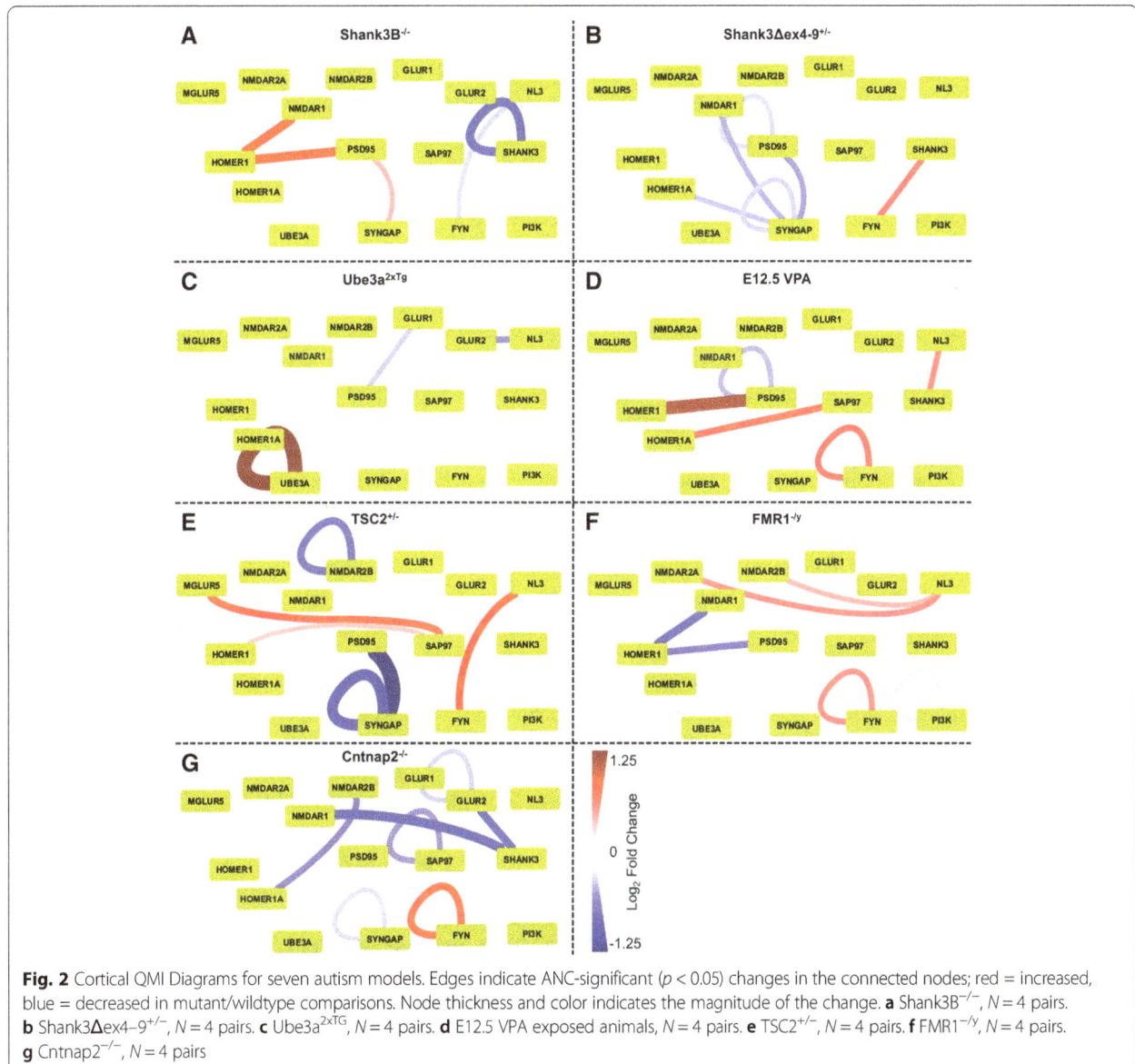

Fig. 2 Cortical QMI Diagrams for seven autism models. Edges indicate ANC-significant (*p* < 0.05) changes in the connected nodes; red = increased, blue = decreased in mutant/wildtype comparisons. Node thickness and color indicates the magnitude of the change. **a** Shank3B$^{-/-}$, *N* = 4 pairs. **b** Shank3Δex4–9$^{+/-}$, *N* = 4 pairs. **c** Ube3a^{2xTG}, *N* = 4 pairs. **d** E12.5 VPA exposed animals, *N* = 4 pairs. **e** TSC2$^{+/-}$, *N* = 4 pairs. **f** FMR1$^{-/y}$, *N* = 4 pairs. **g** Cntnap2$^{-/-}$, *N* = 4 pairs

reduced synaptic activity in mutant animals [27]. Interestingly, these same two interactions were changed, but in the opposite direction, in FMR$^{-/y}$ mice (see below), which have increased basal activity, potentially supporting an activity-dependent mechanism (see discussion). We also observed a small increase in SynGAP_PSD95 (also activity-labile) and a small decrease in FYN_NL3, interactions that were both observed in the opposite direction in the TSC2$^{+/-}$ model.

Shank3Δex4–9$^{+/-}$ animals (Fig. 2b) were tested as heterozygotes because the heterozygotes showed abnormal behavior in the original publication [28] and more accurately represent the human condition, a heterozygous deletion/mutation. Consistent with only moderately reduced Shank3 levels, a modest reduction in Shank3 (log$_2$FC = − 0.227) was not significant by ANC. Remarkably, there was no overlap in significant hits with Shank3B knockouts; in fact, SynGAP_PSD95 was significant in the opposite direction in the two models. Similar to the TSC2$^{+/-}$ animals, Shank3Δex4–9$^{+/-}$ animals showed significant decreases in SynGAP_SynGAP and SynGAP_PSD95, in addition to reductions in SynGAP_Homer1A and SynGAP_NMDAR1 that were unique to this model. Finally, a moderate *increase* in FYN_Shank3 was observed. While published electrophysiology revealed reduced excitatory transmission in both the Shank3B$^{-/-}$ and Shank3Δex4–9$^{+/-}$ animals [27, 28], the experiments were performed in different brain areas (striatum and hippocampus, respectively) and showed small but important differences, such as reduced vs. increased miniature EPSP frequency, respectively. In summary, while QMI data from the Shank3Δex4–9$^{+/-}$ animals highlight reduced SynGAP associations with NMDARs and scaffolds, the Shank3B animals show differences in Homer-PSD-NMDAR complexes but no changes in SynGAP. These data suggest that the molecular deficits in the two animal models may be quite different, consistent with the different isoforms that are affected in the two models [24].

Ube3a^{2xTg} mice (Fig. 2c) showed an expected increase in the amount of Ube3a and reduced co-association between GluR1_PSD95 and NL3_GluR2. Prior work in the cortex of Ube3a animals showed reduced glutamatergic transmission [34] and reduced scaffolding of GluRs is therefore consistent with prior observations.

E12.5 VPA mice (Fig. 2d) are the only non-genetic model analyzed here. Mice were generated by injection of VPA on E12.5, and the efficacy of the treatment was confirmed by behavioral testing (as in [32]) of the adult offspring before dissection and QMI analysis. We observed a large increase in the amount of co-associated Homer_PSD95. In all other models, the amount of Homer_NMDAR1 correlated with Homer_PSD95, and VPA mice were trending towards an increase in this interaction as well (log$_2$FC = 0.48, NS). In addition, levels

of Fyn were increased, PSD95 were decreased, and interactions between SAP97_Homer1A and Shank3_NL3 were increased. Prior reports in VPA-treated rat cortex showed enhanced NMDAR-mediated synaptic currents and enhanced LTP [35], consistent with the observed increase in Homer-NMDAR scaffolding. Decreased levels of PSD95 have also been reported by Western blotting [52].

TSC2$^{+/-}$ mice (Fig. 2e) showed large reductions in the abundance of SynGAP and SynGAP_PSD95. The mTOR activator Rheb (ras homolog enriched in brain), which is directly suppressed by the TSC1/2 complex, is activated by SynGAP following NMDAR stimulation [36], so the reduction of SynGAP may be a homeostatic response to chronically activated Rheb. Reduced levels of NMDAR2B were also observed, along with increased abundance of complexes containing SAP97_mGluR5, Homer1_SAP97, and Fyn_NL3. Taken together, these data indicate reduced NMDAR2B and SynGAP expression, abnormal scaffolding of mGluR5 to Sap97, and abnormal FYN signaling, which could contribute to the altered LTP phenotype reported in the hippocampus of TSC mice [37].

Fragile X mice (Fig. 2f) showed increased abundance of complexes containing NMDAR2A_NL3 and NMDAR2B_NL3. Both NMDA receptors [38] and Neuroligins [39] bind PSD95, which could mediate this observed interaction. FragileX mice also showed reduced complexes with Homer1_PSD95 and Homer1_NMDAR1, demonstrating disrupted Homer-Shank-PSD95-NMDAR complexes, consistent with previous reports [40–42]. These activity-dependent interactions were also significant hits in the Shank3B and E12.5 VPA models, but in the opposite direction, possibly reflecting hyper- vs. hypo-activity of cortical neurons in these models. Finally, reduced levels of PI3K and increased Fyn were detected, consistent with disrupted kinase cascades downstream of mGluR5 in FMR1 mice [43–45].

CNTNAP 2 KO mice (Fig. 2g) showed the greatest number of ANC hits (7) as well as many large but non-significant changes. The abundance of GluR2 was reduced, accompanied by reduced GluR2_Shank3, NMDAR1_Shank3, and NMDAR2B_Homer1A, consistent with reduced scaffolding and expression of glutamate receptors. In addition, the detected levels of Sap97 and SynGAP were reduced, while Fyn was increased, a change also observed in the Fragile X model. While the CNTNAP2 gene product CASPR is known to cluster at the nodes of Ranvier following myelination [46], acute CASPR knockdown acts cell-autonomously to reduce both AMPA and NMDA-mediated EPSPs [47], congruent with reduced NMDAR and AMPAR levels and scaffolding observed here.

Hippocampus

In four models, we also isolated P2 fractions from the hippocampi of the same animals that supplied cortical tissue. We identified 45 statistically significant differences across the 4 mouse models, with the majority of differences, 21, found in the VPA hippocampus (Fig. 3). Nine proteins showed differences in protein abundance (IP probe for the same target), and 32 protein interactions showed differences (IP probe for different targets). However, only three complexes (Homer_mGluR5, Sap97_NMDAR1, and SynGAP_NMDAR2A) and 1 abundance measure (PSD95) were detected in multiple models, while the remainder was unique to a single model. Below, we describe the findings from each model, compared with prior data from the cortex of the same model.

Shank3B$^{-/-}$ hippocampal tissue (Fig. 3a) showed an increase in PSD95 levels and a decrease in FYN levels, neither of which were observed in cortical tissue. A decrease in NMDAR1_mGluR5 likely reflects disrupted scaffolding linking the two receptor types via PSD95/Shank3/Homer linkages [24]. We observed an increase in Homer1_SYNGAP, PSD95_GluR1, and, counter-intuitively, PSD95_Shank3. The latter interaction may reflect elevated expression of an alternative isoform of Shank3 that lacks the PDZ domains in complex with PSD95, possibly mediated via another protein such as Homer. Besides this interaction, no major changes in Shank3 were detected, likely due to the fact that very little Shank3 was detected from Shank3 IPs or probes, consistent with low hippocampal Shank3 expression. We are unable to relate these changes to known electrophysiological abnormalities in these animals, since to our knowledge, hippocampal electrophysiology has not been reported in this model.

Shank3Δex4–9$^{+/-}$ animals (Fig. 3b) showed reduced levels of SynGAP, consistent with cortical tissue from these animals. Interactions involving SynGAP_NMDAR2A were reduced, while SynGAP_GluR2 were increased. Complexes containing NL3_NMDAR2A and _FYN were reduced. Complexes containing PI3K_Sap97, _GluR2, and _SynGAP were all increased. Hippocampal electrophysiology in this model indicated reduced basal AMPA-mediated transmission, and a failure of hippocampal LTP that was correlated with failure to maintain spine expansion following a tetanizing stimulation [28]. Our results indicate that SynGAP, a critical mediator of signal transduction downstream of NMDARs [36, 48], is dysregulated in hippocampal tissue prior to any type of stimulation. Further, changes in FYN and PI3K suggest downstream disruption of signaling cascades.

Ube3a^{2xTG} hippocampus (Fig. 3c) showed the expected increase in Ube3a expression, the only change that was consistent between hippocampus and cortex. A reduction in mGluR5 levels, Homer_mGluR5, and Homer_GlurR2 suggest reduced Homer-mediated scaffolding. Ube3A_Homer interactions were strongly increased, although the significance of this increase is unclear since Ube3a has not been documented to bind directly to or ubiquinate/degrade Homer proteins. The amount of PSD95_Shank3 was increased, as was SAP97_NMDAR1 and SAP97_Shank3. Finally, the amount of Homer1A was increased. These data demonstrate complex changes in scaffolding of AMPA, NMDA, and metabotropic glutamate receptors mediated by both Homer and DLG scaffolds in the Ube3a^{2xTG} animal. Hippocampal electrophysiology has not been reported in these animals, although LTP disruptions due to lack of small conductance potassium channel 2 (SK2) channel regulation have been reported in the Ube3a knockout animal [49].

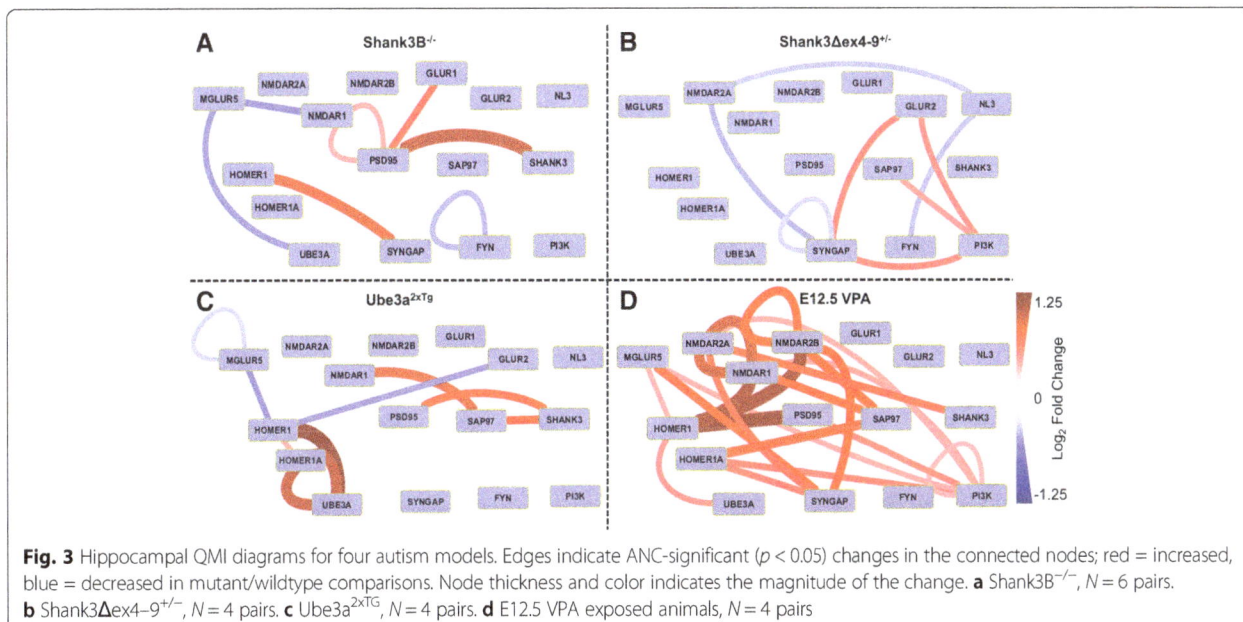

Fig. 3 Hippocampal QMI diagrams for four autism models. Edges indicate ANC-significant (*p* < 0.05) changes in the connected nodes; red = increased, blue = decreased in mutant/wildtype comparisons. Node thickness and color indicates the magnitude of the change. **a** Shank3B$^{-/-}$, *N* = 6 pairs. **b** Shank3Δex4–9$^{+/-}$, *N* = 4 pairs. **c** Ube3a^{2xTG}, *N* = 4 pairs. **d** E12.5 VPA exposed animals, *N* = 4 pairs

VPA hippocampus yielded 21 significant QMI hits, the most of any sample tested, all in the positive direction. PI3K was involved in six significant interactions, with _mGluR5, _NMDAR1, _NMDAR2A, _PSD95, _HOMER1A, and _PI3K. These disruptions in PI3K, which controls AKT/mTOR signaling, is consistent with several reports implicating dysregulated mTOR signaling in the VPA model [32]. The amount of Homer_PSD95, Homer_NMDAR2B, and Homer_NMDAR1 were each increased by almost twofold, reflecting increased NMDAR scaffolding and/or expression. Levels of detected NMDAR1 and NMDAR2B were also increased. These data support prior studies showing increased NMDAR expression in rats following VPA exposure in the cortex [35], although note that a separate study did not find differences in mRNA expression in the cortex or hippocampus [50]. Other notable hits included SynGAP_NMDAR2A and B, SAP97_NMDAR1 and 2B, and Homer_mGLUR5. Comparing these results with VPA cortex, only 2/5 QMI hits in the cortex were shared with the hippocampus, Homer_PSD95 and SAP97_HOMER1A. However, several other interactions that were significant in hippocampus were trending towards significance in cortex; for example, Homer_NMDAR1 and _NMDAR2B were increased by 1.29 and 1.37-fold in the cortex, respectively, but were not significant by ANC criteria (see Additional file 1: Table S1).

Comparisons between models

For the most stringent possible clustering analysis between models, we set all non-ANC-significant measurements to 0 and performed unsupervised clustering using the "complete" method, based on the Euclidian distance matrix of all samples. Because interactions that were significant in a single sample are irrelevant for clustering using this method, we only included the 16 interactions that were significant in two or more samples (Fig. 4). The plot highlights the correlation between certain interactions, such as Homer_PSD95 and Homer_NMDAR1, or SynGAP_PSD95 and SynGAP_SynGAP. However, it is clear from this plot that because there were relatively few interactions that reached ANC significance in multiple models, the clustering is not robust; for example, FragileX and CNTNAP2 mice are shown associated with each other on the basis of a single shared ANC-significant hit, Fyn_Fyn.

To overcome this limitation, we repeated our cluster analysis with all $\log_2FC$ data, reasoning that smaller changes that did not reach the high bar for ANC significance could still be informative for clustering analysis. However, we were concerned about noise contributed by interactions that did not change, but fluctuated randomly around 0, so we first performed principal component analysis (PCA) to focus on factors that contributed the most variation to the dataset. PCA was performed on the mean $\log_2FC$ values of

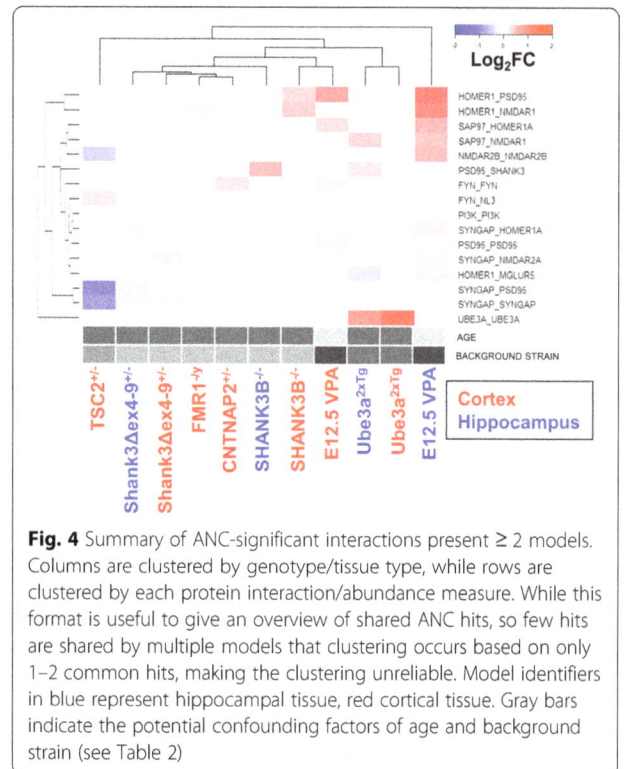

Fig. 4 Summary of ANC-significant interactions present ≥ 2 models. Columns are clustered by genotype/tissue type, while rows are clustered by each protein interaction/abundance measure. While this format is useful to give an overview of shared ANC hits, so few hits are shared by multiple models that clustering occurs based on only 1–2 common hits, making the clustering unreliable. Model identifiers in blue represent hippocampal tissue, red cortical tissue. Gray bars indicate the potential confounding factors of age and background strain (see Table 2)

each interaction for all genotypes/tissue types using default settings. Plotting the data by principal components 1 and 2, which accounted 30.1% and 12.1% of total variation, respectively (Fig. 5a), revealed clear clustering of tissue types within models; in all cases, the hippocampal and cortical tissue shared similar coordinates in PCA space. Both Shank3 models and Fragile X animals were in close proximity in PCA space, and Ube3a^{2xTG} were near VPA animals. To mathematically determine the relationships between models in PCA space, we used a hierarchical clustering on principal component (HCPC) analysis using default settings in the FactoMineR package and cutting the HCPC tree at the recommended level to maximize inertia gain (Fig. 5b). HCPC yielded four clusters: CNTNAP animals were an outgroup (group1). Group 2 contained all Shank3 models, and FMR1 animals. TSC2 animals, alone in group 3, were clustered on a branch adjacent to group 4, which contained cortical and hippocampal tissue from both VPA and Ube3a models. We calculated approximately unbiased p values for the clustering based on multiscale bootstrap resampling. The co-clustering of Shank3B hippocampus with Shank3Δex4–9$^{+/-}$ tissues, and the clustering of VPA tissue with Ube3a cortical tissue reached statistical significance (AU < 0.95); AU values for all other branches are shown in Fig. 5b.

Shared molecular pathology in cluster 4

We noticed from the structure of the clustering that groups 3 and 4 contained two models with known abnormalities in

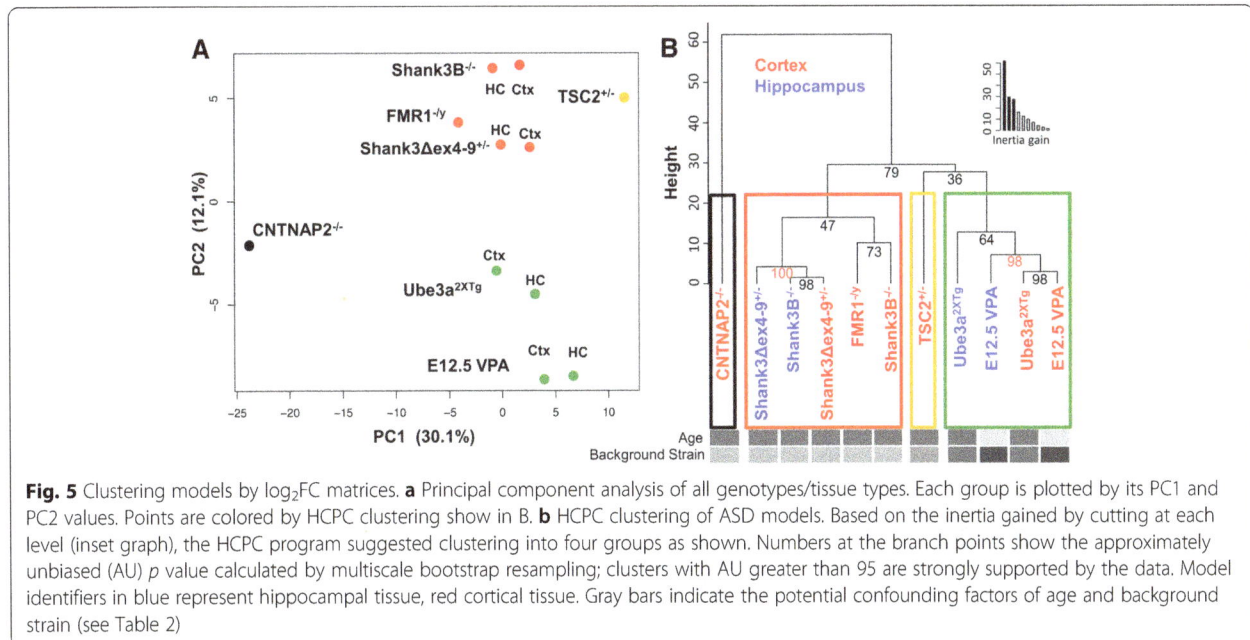

Fig. 5 Clustering models by log2FC matrices. **a** Principal component analysis of all genotypes/tissue types. Each group is plotted by its PC1 and PC2 values. Points are colored by HCPC clustering show in B. **b** HCPC clustering of ASD models. Based on the inertia gained by cutting at each level (inset graph), the HCPC program suggested clustering into four groups as shown. Numbers at the branch points show the approximately unbiased (AU) *p* value calculated by multiscale bootstrap resampling; clusters with AU greater than 95 are strongly supported by the data. Model identifiers in blue represent hippocampal tissue, red cortical tissue. Gray bars indicate the potential confounding factors of age and background strain (see Table 2)

the AKT/mTOR signaling pathway; in fact, mTOR inhibitors have been reported to rescue behavioral deficits in both models [37, 51]. TSC2$^{+/-}$ mice are heterozygous for a critical inhibitor of the mTOR complex and show sustained mTOR activation and abnormalities throughout the pathway [37]. VPA animals also show abnormal AKT signaling, with a recent report showing reduced levels of AKT and mTOR, as well as reduced ratios of phospho-to-total AKT and mTOR in VPA exposed rats [52]. Ube3a^{2xTG} mice clustered closely with VPA mice, but AKT/mTOR has never been implicated in this model. Indeed, mining the factors that differentiated HCPC clusters indicated that PI3K was a significant factor that differentiated group 4, and Ube3a hippocampal issue showed a large, but non-ANC-significant increase in PI3K_PI3K (log2FC = 0.42, NS). We therefore performed phospho-Western blots on cortical samples from an independent cohort of Ube3a^{2xTG} animals

(Fig. 6). AKT phosphorylation was reduced by 41% at p-Ser473, while no difference was observed at p-Thr308. Total AKT levels were similar. Downstream of AKT, mTOR phosphorylation was also similar, as were levels of p~S6. We confirmed previous reports of altered p-AKT levels in cortical tissue from VPA animals and found that p-AKT and total AKT levels were normal in cortical tissue from all other models examined (Additional file 2: Figure S1). These data confirm the predictions of our clustering that Ube3a^{2xTG} mice share a core deficit in the PI3K/AKT/mTOR pathway with the VPA mice that share the same branch of the HCPC cluster tree.

Discussion

The goal of these experiments was to perform a series of identical protein measurements of brain tissue from multiple mouse models of autism, with the aim of cutting

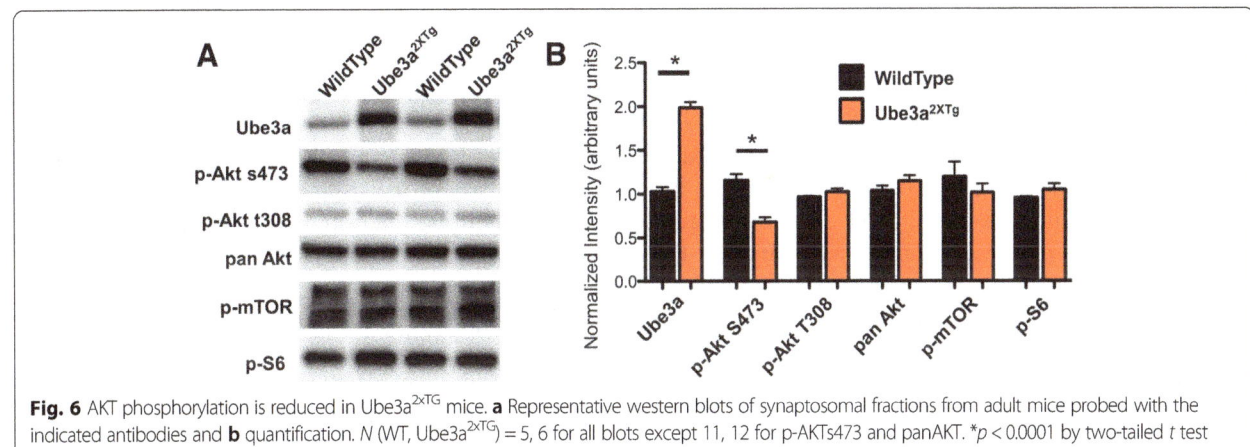

Fig. 6 AKT phosphorylation is reduced in Ube3a^{2xTG} mice. **a** Representative western blots of synaptosomal fractions from adult mice probed with the indicated antibodies and **b** quantification. *N* (WT, Ube3a^{2xTG}) = 5, 6 for all blots except 11, 12 for p-AKTs473 and panAKT. *$p < 0.0001$ by two-tailed *t* test

through the immense heterogeneity of the diagnostic entity and identifying some underlying points of convergence. We did not expect every animal model to show an identical set of protein network disturbances. Rather, we hypothesized that a set of interactions might be disrupted in more than one model; perhaps we would be able to identify subtypes of genetic autisms that share distinct sets of disrupted interactions. Indeed, our stringent ANC criteria identified several interactions that were common to multiple genetic models, but clustering by only ANC-significant interactions was not robust. Bioinformatics analysis using PCA and HCPC clustered the models by both genotype and tissue type indicated generally similar changes in cortical and hippocampal tissue from the same models. For such a clustering approach to be broadly useful, it would need to make testable predictions about pathologic mechanisms. Indeed, analysis of the interactions that contributed to clustering suggested that Ube3a^{2xTG} mice might share a molecular deficit with the other models sharing its branch of the tree, namely disrupted AKT/mTOR signaling. Western blots revealed that AKT signaling was disrupted in Ube3a^{2xTG} and VPA mice, but not other models, confirming clustering predictions. We have therefore successfully identified a set of protein-protein interactions that are disrupted in multiple animal models of autism, clustered models based on high-dimensional QMI data, and used our clusters to make testable predictions about the molecular pathology of closely clustered models.

Proteins or protein interactions that were ANC-significant in multiple models identified here share striking similarity to a set of interactions that we recently reported to be activity-dependent. In response to 5 min of acute stimulation with glutamate, QMI identified significant changes in 26 protein-protein interactions [32]. Homer, Shank and SynGAP were the most connected nodes, each changing its interactions with several other members of the network. Many of these activity-dependent interactions were also identified here as significantly different in ASD models vs. wildtype controls. For example, Homer1_PSD95 and the abundance of the Ras GTPase SYNGAP were each altered in four sample types, and interactions between Homer1_NMDAR1 and SYNGAP_PSD95 were each altered in three sample types. Of the 26 Glutamate-significant interactions, only 15 were included in the QMI panel presented in this paper; but of those 15 interactions, 9 were "hits" in the ASD models (Additional file 1: Table S1, sheet 2). Notably, the directionality of these changes was variable. For example, Homer_PSD95 levels were increased in VPA cortex, but decreased in Fragile X cortex.

Differences in synaptic activity are a defining and unifying characteristic of animal models of autism—virtually, every report of an autism model includes electrophysiological characterization showing altered synaptic transmission. The directionality of change in synaptic activity is also variable between models; for example Ube3a^{2xTG} mice show reduced cortical excitability [32] while Fragile X [53, 54] mice show increased. Viewed through this activity-dependent lens, the bidirectionality of our data makes more sense. Glutamate stimulation results in dissociation of Homer-PSD95 complexes [32]; thus, the reduced amount of this interaction seen in the fragile X model could reflect the hyperactive tonic signaling that has been previously reported [53, 54]. Conversely, in the VPA model, a reduction in intrinsic cortical activity has been reported [55, 56], which would be predicted to cause increased levels of this activity-labile interaction. Future studies could manipulate activity in ASD models and measure the resulting QMI profiles to directly test this hypothesis and disentangle activity-dependent from activity-independent processes.

However, activity-dependent interactions were not uniformly altered within models; for example, while Homer1_PSD95 and Homer1_NMDAR1 were reduced by activity and increased in the VPA model, Syn-GAP_PSD95 was also reduced by activity [32], but unchanged in the VPA model. This could imply an underlying dysregulation in the network response to activity, or a de-coupling of normally correlated molecular processes due to differences in the cell's ability to compensate for some long-term changes better than others. An analogous network-level dysregulation has been observed in transcriptomic analysis of post-mortem autism brain tissue, where individual mRNAs show normal levels of abundance, but the coordinated expression of mRNAs is dysregulated, reflecting disrupted regulatory mechanisms [18]. In the future, it will be informative to design experiments that can de-couple acute, activity-dependent changes from long-term, genotype-dependent changes in PPI networks. The stimulus-dependent dynamics of protein interaction networks encode cellular information, such that different cellular inputs lead to different rearrangements of the interactome, encoding different cellular responses [57]. Understanding how information processing through this synaptic network differs in ASD models could lead to further insights into disease pathogenesis.

To our knowledge, only one other study has attempted to subtype a large number of mouse models of autism [58]. This MRI-based study found great heterogeneity in the relative size of many brain areas in ASD models vs. matched controls, but was able to identify clusters of animal models that shared similar patterns of changes. Three models were analyzed by both the current study and the Ellegood et al. study, FMR1, CNTNAP2, and Shank3B. Both Ellesgood et al. and our study clustered the FMR1 and Shank3B mice as neighbors on the same branch of the dendrogram, suggesting both structural and molecular convergence between the two models.

Indeed, prior work has shown that Shank3 mRNA is posttranscriptionally regulated by FMR1 [59], and that FMR1 mice show deficits in mGluR signaling [25, 26] that is mediated by Homer and Shank-containing scaffolds [42]. More generally, genetic studies [60, 61] have implicated several genes or gene regulatory networks related to mGluR signaling in autism. It is plausible that our "cluster 2" may represent a subtype encompassing Shank3 and Fragile X models, previously and independently identified in the Ellesgood study. However, the models may have co-clustered in both studies by chance.

The PI3K/AKT/mTOR pathway has also been implicated in many diverse models of ASD [14, 52, 62], so it was noteworthy that two models with known disruptions to the mTOR pathway appeared together in clusters 3/4. TSC2 is directly involved in regulating mTORC1 downstream of AKT, and autism-linked mutations in TSC2 cause increased mTOR activation and a de-coupling of mTOR from AKT [63]. Prenatal VPA exposure causes reduced mTOR pathway protein expression and phosphorylation [52], which we confirmed here (Additional file 2: Figure S1). After our clustering results suggested a potential mTOR deficit in Ube3a^{2xTG} animals, we found by phospho-Western blots that Ube3a^{2xTG} animals showed reduced AKT S473 phosphorylation, but normal levels of T308 phosphorylation and normal phosphorylation of other components of the mTOR pathway. Rapamycin treatment has been shown to rescue behavior in both TSC2 and VPA models [51, 63], and future work could explore if correction of AKT phosphorylation in the Ube3a model might similarly correct behavioral deficits.

Limitations

Several limitations of our study should be noted. The background strain was different among several of the models, the age of the VPA mice was different from the other six models, and mice of both sexes were used. Our analysis approach, in which each mutant animal was normalized to a matched littermate control, was designed to cancel out these effects, as well as assay-dependent batch effects, to identify differences caused by each mutation. However, this experimental design prevents us from making wildtype-to-wildtype comparisons (since batch effects cannot be normalized for mice run on different assay plates), so we are unable to unambiguously demonstrate that our clustering was not driven by uncorrected effects stemming from these differences in background, age, or sex. QMI is a candidate-based approach and shares limitations with all antibody-based assays, including potential antibody cross-reactivity and issues of binding epitope access in native protein complexes. The absence of a detected interaction cannot be interpreted as unambiguously indicating that the interaction does not exist in vivo, since occlusion of binding sites could lead to false negative results. We carefully selected and screened all antibodies used in the QMI panel [32], but antibody caveats are unavoidable. We used NP40 detergent after pilot data showed that it produced higher mean matrix MFIs than TritonX100, Digitonin, or Deoxycholate [32]. However, NP40 does not fully solubilize the core postsynaptic density, where several of our protein targets are enriched (discussed in [32]). Since detergents that solubilize the PSD also disrupt protein interactions, detergent selection is necessarily a trade-off, and further studies could more thoroughly quantify differences in synaptic QMI networks due to different detergent conditions. Finally, many of our interactions vary with neuronal activity or by brain region. Small variations in microdissection (e.g., inclusion of small amounts of striatal tissue in cortical samples) or euthanasia protocols (i.e., animal sleep/wake state prior to euthanasia) could have large effects on protein detection (e.g., Shank3, which is highly expressed in striatum, or PSD95_SynGAP, which is activity-dependent). While we were careful to perform our dissections as consistently as possible, at a similar time of day and using metal brain molds to ensure consistent slicing, thinner vibratome slicing followed by a period of controlled slice recovery in ACSF, as for electrophysiology, may be a more optimal experimental strategy to ensure normalization of both activity and location.

Conclusions

In conclusion, we performed a series of identical QMI experiments to measure differences in the abundance of, and binary interactions among, 16 synaptic proteins in 7 mouse models of autism. Employing a mutant-littermate control design, we found a unique combination of disrupted protein interactions in each model and tissue type measured. Many of the disrupted interactions were identified as activity-dependent interactions in a separate study, highlighting the complex relationships between ASD risk genes and activity-dependent homeostatic processes [21]. PCA and cluster analysis of models revealed two identifiable sub-groups, with VPA and TSC2 mice comprising a hypothetical "mTOR" cluster, and Shank3 and FragileX mice comprising a second cluster; the latter co-clustering was consistent with a prior MRI study [58]. The inclusion of Ube3a^{2xTG} mice in the mTOR cluster led to our identification of AKT phosphorylation deficits in this model. Our data highlight the heterogeneity of ASD models, while offering hope that high-dimensional measures of biologically relevant molecular processes may allow differentiation of subtypes of ASD amenable to common treatment strategies. Future work to expand the number of ASD models analyzed and to perform similar QMI experiments in human iPS-derived neurons could offer further insights into the complex relationships among autism risk factors.

Additional files

Additional file 1: Table S1. Sheet 1: Log$_2$ fold change (log$_2$FC) matrices from $N = 4$ experiments were averaged to generate a single mean log$_2$FC matrix per genotype/tissue type. Cells highlighted in red are ANC-significant, numbers in bold case indicate a fold change greater than 0.25 or less than -0.25. Sheet 2: All hits are sorted by the number of times they appeared as ANC-significant. A red-shaded "1" indicates an ANC-significant hit in a particular model. If a hit was also significant following 5 minutes of glutamate stimulation [32], "yes" is entered into the "Glutamate hit" column. (XLSX 46 kb)

Additional file 2: Figure S1. AKT phosphorylation is reduced in VPA mice but normal in all other models examined. Related to Fig. 6 (A) Representative western blots of cortical samples from adult mice probed with the indicated antibodies. (B) Quantification, axes match Fig. 6. $N = 3–10$ individuals per genotype. *$p < 0.001$ by two-tailed t test, Bonferroni-corrected for multiple comparisons. (PDF 194 kb)

Abbreviations
ASD: Autism spectrum disorder; PiSCES: Proteins in shared complexes; QMI: Quantitative multiplex co-immunoprecipitation; VPA: Valproic acid

Acknowledgements
We thank Dr. Raymond Tervo for critical support in the early stages of this work. We also thank Dr. Rachel (Michelle) Reith and Carolyn Smith for providing mouse brain tissue, and all of the investigators who deposited their mouse models at Jax for distribution.

Funding
Funding was provided by R00MH102244 and R01MH113545, A Brain Research Foundation NARSAD Grant #25037, The Dana Foundation at Mayo Clinic (SEPS), the Autism Research Training (ART) program (CN), and Mayo Graduate School, T32AI7425 and T32AI007386 (SN).

Authors' contributions
SS conceived the project. EB, JL, TD, EG, AV, and SS collected the data. SN and NT coded the statistical programs. CN and MF generated the VPA mice. JL, AV, EG, AS, and SS analyzed the data. SS wrote the manuscript. All authors read and approved the final submission.

Competing interests
The authors declare that they have no competing interests.

Author details
[1]Center for Integrative Brain Research, Seattle Children's Research Institute, Seattle, WA, USA. [2]Department of Immunology, Mayo Clinic College of Medicine, Rochester, MN, USA. [3]Present address: Department of Biomedical Engineering, UT Austin, Austin, TX, USA. [4]Present address: Nanostring, Seattle, WA, USA. [5]Present address: Department of Cancer Immunology and Virology, Dana-Farber Cancer Institute, Boston, MA, USA. [6]Present address: Department of Medicine, Harvard Medical School, Boston, MA, USA. [7]Present address: Broad Institute of Harvard and MIT, Cambridge, MA, USA. [8]Department of Psychiatry & Behavioural Neurosciences, McMaster University, Hamilton, ON, Canada. [9]Departments of Molecular Microbiology & Immunology, Surgery and Bioengineering, University of Missouri, Columbia, MO, USA. [10]Department of Pediatrics and Graduate Program in Neuroscience, University of Washington, Seattle, WA, USA.

References
1. Baio J, Wiggins L, Christensen DL, Maenner MJ, Daniels J, Warren Z, Kurzius-Spencer M, Zahorodny W, Robinson Rosenberg C, White T, et al. Prevalence of autism Spectrum disorder among children aged 8 years - autism and developmental disabilities monitoring network, 11 sites, United States, 2014. MMWR Surveill Summ. 2018;67:1–23.
2. O'Roak BJ, Deriziotis P, Lee C, Vives L, Schwartz JJ, Girirajan S, Karakoc E, MacKenzie AP, Ng SB, Baker C, et al. Exome sequencing in sporadic autism spectrum disorders identifies severe de novo mutations. Nat Genet. 2011;43:585–9.
3. Iossifov I, O'Roak BJ, Sanders SJ, Ronemus M, Krumm N, Levy D, Stessman HA, Witherspoon KT, Vives L, Patterson KE, et al. The contribution of de novo coding mutations to autism spectrum disorder. Nature. 2014;515:216–21.
4. De Rubeis S, He X, Goldberg AP, Poultney CS, Samocha K, Cicek AE, Kou Y, Liu L, Fromer M, Walker S, et al. Synaptic, transcriptional and chromatin genes disrupted in autism. Nature. 2014;515:209–15.
5. Patterson PH. Maternal infection and immune involvement in autism. Trends Mol Med. 2011;17:389–94.
6. Edmiston E, Ashwood P, Van de Water J. Autoimmunity, autoantibodies, and autism spectrum disorder. Biol Psychiatry. 2017;81:383–90.
7. Shelton JF, Geraghty EM, Tancredi DJ, Delwiche LD, Schmidt RJ, Ritz B, Hansen RL, Hertz-Picciotto I. Neurodevelopmental disorders and prenatal residential proximity to agricultural pesticides: the CHARGE study. Environ Health Perspect. 2014;122:1103–9.
8. Weiner DJ, Wigdor EM, Ripke S, Walters RK, Kosmicki JA, Grove J, Samocha KE, Goldstein JI, Okbay A, Bybjerg-Grauholm J, et al. Polygenic transmission disequilibrium confirms that common and rare variation act additively to create risk for autism spectrum disorders. Nat Genet. 2017;49:978–85.
9. Grzadzinski R, Huerta M, Lord C. DSM-5 and autism spectrum disorders (ASDs): an opportunity for identifying ASD subtypes. Mol Autism. 2013;4:12.
10. Donovan AP, Basson MA. The neuroanatomy of autism - a developmental perspective. J Anat. 2017;230:4–15.
11. Fernandez M, Mollinedo-Gajate I, Penagarikano O. Neural circuits for social cognition: implications for autism. Neuroscience. 2018;370:148–62.
12. Parikshak NN, Gandal MJ, Geschwind DH. Systems biology and gene networks in neurodevelopmental and neurodegenerative disorders. Nat Rev Genet. 2015;16:441–58.
13. Hormozdiari F, Penn O, Borenstein E, Eichler EE. The discovery of integrated gene networks for autism and related disorders. Genome Res. 2015;25:142–54.
14. Huber KM, Klann E, Costa-Mattioli M, Zukin RS. Dysregulation of mammalian target of rapamycin signaling in mouse models of autism. J Neurosci. 2015; 35:13836–42.
15. Estes ML, McAllister AK. Immune mediators in the brain and peripheral tissues in autism spectrum disorder. Nat Rev Neurosci. 2015;16:469–86.
16. Ashwood P, Krakowiak P, Hertz-Picciotto I, Hansen R, Pessah I, Van de Water J. Elevated plasma cytokines in autism spectrum disorders provide evidence of immune dysfunction and are associated with impaired behavioral outcome. Brain Behav Immun. 2011;25:40–5.
17. Vargas DL, Nascimbene C, Krishnan C, Zimmerman AW, Pardo CA. Neuroglial activation and neuroinflammation in the brain of patients with autism. Ann Neurol. 2005;57:67–81.
18. Voineagu I, Wang X, Johnston P, Lowe JK, Tian Y, Horvath S, Mill J, Cantor RM, Blencowe BJ, Geschwind DH. Transcriptomic analysis of autistic brain reveals convergent molecular pathology. Nature. 2011;474:380–4.
19. Pardo CA, Farmer CA, Thurm A, Shebl FM, Ilieva J, Kalra S, Swedo S. Serum and cerebrospinal fluid immune mediators in children with autistic disorder: a longitudinal study. Mol Autism. 2017;8:1.
20. Zoghbi HY, Bear MF. Synaptic dysfunction in neurodevelopmental disorders associated with autism and intellectual disabilities. Cold Spring Harb Perspect Biol. 2012;4:a009886.
21. Mullins C, Fishell G, Tsien RW. Unifying views of autism spectrum disorders: a consideration of autoregulatory feedback loops. Neuron. 2016;89:1131–56.
22. Bourgeron T. From the genetic architecture to synaptic plasticity in autism spectrum disorder. Nat Rev Neurosci. 2015;16:551–63.

23. Masi A, DeMayo MM, Glozier N, Guastella AJ. An overview of autism spectrum disorder, heterogeneity and treatment options. Neurosci Bull. 2017;33:183–93.

24. Monteiro P, Feng G. SHANK proteins: roles at the synapse and in autism spectrum disorder. Nat Rev Neurosci. 2017;18:147–57.

25. Wang X, Bey AL, Katz BM, Badea A, Kim N, David LK, Duffney LJ, Kumar S, Mague SD, Hulbert SW, et al. Altered mGluR5-Homer scaffolds and corticostriatal connectivity in a Shank3 complete knockout model of autism. Nat Commun. 2016;7:11459.

26. Vicidomini C, Ponzoni L, Lim D, Schmeisser MJ, Reim D, Morello N, Orellana D, Tozzi A, Durante V, Scalmani P, et al. Pharmacological enhancement of mGlu5 receptors rescues behavioral deficits in SHANK3 knock-out mice. Mol Psychiatry. 2017;22:689–702.

27. Peca J, Feliciano C, Ting JT, Wang W, Wells MF, Venkatraman TN, Lascola CD, Fu Z, Feng G. Shank3 mutant mice display autistic-like behaviours and striatal dysfunction. Nature. 2011;472:437–42.

28. Bozdagi O, Sakurai T, Papapetrou D, Wang X, Dickstein DL, Takahashi N, Kajiwara Y, Yang M, Katz AM, Scattoni ML, et al. Haploinsufficiency of the autism-associated Shank3 gene leads to deficits in synaptic function, social interaction, and social communication. Mol Autism. 2010;1:15.

29. Peixoto RT, Wang W, Croney DM, Kozorovitskiy Y, Sabatini BL. Early hyperactivity and precocious maturation of corticostriatal circuits in Shank3B(−/−) mice. Nat Neurosci. 2016;19:716–24.

30. Smith SE, Neier SC, Reed BK, Davis TR, Sinnwell JP, Eckel-Passow JE, Sciallis GF, Wieland CN, Torgerson RR, Gil D, et al. Multiplex matrix network analysis of protein complexes in the human TCR signalosome. Sci Signal. 2016;9:rs7.

31. Smith SE, Bida AT, Davis TR, Sicotte H, Patterson SE, Gil D, Schrum AG. IP-FCM measures physiologic protein-protein interactions modulated by signal transduction and small-molecule drug inhibition. PLoS One. 2012;7:e45722.

32. Nicolini C, Fahnestock M. The valproic acid-induced rodent model of autism. Exp Neurol. 2018;299:217–27.

33. Lautz JD, Brown EA, AAW VS, SEP S. Synaptic activity induces input-specific rearrangements in a targeted synaptic protein interaction network. J Neurochem. 2018; https://doi.org/10.1111/jnc.14466.

34. Smith SE, Zhou YD, Zhang G, Jin Z, Stoppel DC, Anderson MP. Increased gene dosage of Ube3a results in autism traits and decreased glutamate synaptic transmission in mice. Sci Transl Med. 2011;3:103ra197.

35. Rinaldi T, Kulangara K, Antoniello K, Markram H. Elevated NMDA receptor levels and enhanced postsynaptic long-term potentiation induced by prenatal exposure to valproic acid. Proc Natl Acad Sci U S A. 2007;104:13501–6.

36. Wang CC, Held RG, Hall BJ. SynGAP regulates protein synthesis and homeostatic synaptic plasticity in developing cortical networks. PLoS One. 2013;8:e83941.

37. Ehninger D, Han S, Shilyansky C, Zhou Y, Li W, Kwiatkowski DJ, Ramesh V, Silva AJ. Reversal of learning deficits in a Tsc2+/− mouse model of tuberous sclerosis. Nat Med. 2008;14:843–8.

38. Kornau HC, Schenker LT, Kennedy MB, Seeburg PH. Domain interaction between NMDA receptor subunits and the postsynaptic density protein PSD-95. Science. 1995;269:1737–40.

39. Irie M, Hata Y, Takeuchi M, Ichtchenko K, Toyoda A, Hirao K, Takai Y, Rosahl TW, Sudhof TC. Binding of neuroligins to PSD-95. Science. 1997;277:1511–5.

40. Toft AK, Lundbye CJ, Banke TG. Dysregulated NMDA-receptor signaling inhibits long-term depression in a mouse model of fragile X syndrome. J Neurosci. 2016;36:9817–27.

41. Guo W, Ceolin L, Collins KA, Perroy J, Huber KM. Elevated CaMKIIalpha and hyperphosphorylation of Homer mediate circuit dysfunction in a fragile X syndrome mouse model. Cell Rep. 2015;13:2297–311.

42. Ronesi JA, Collins KA, Hays SA, Tsai NP, Guo W, Birnbaum SG, Hu JH, Worley PF, Gibson JR, Huber KM. Disrupted Homer scaffolds mediate abnormal mGluR5 function in a mouse model of fragile X syndrome. Nat Neurosci. 2012;15:431–40. S431

43. Gross C, Chang CW, Kelly SM, Bhattacharya A, McBride SM, Danielson SW, Jiang MQ, Chan CB, Ye K, Gibson JR, et al. Increased expression of the PI3K enhancer PIKE mediates deficits in synaptic plasticity and behavior in fragile X syndrome. Cell Rep. 2015;11:727–36.

44. Gross C, Raj N, Molinaro G, Allen AG, Whyte AJ, Gibson JR, Huber KM, Gourley SL, Bassell GJ. Selective role of the catalytic PI3K subunit p110beta in impaired higher order cognition in fragile X syndrome. Cell Rep. 2015;11:681–8.

45. Hays SA, Huber KM, Gibson JR. Altered neocortical rhythmic activity states in Fmr1 KO mice are due to enhanced mGluR5 signaling and involve changes in excitatory circuitry. J Neurosci. 2011;31:14223–34.

46. Poliak S, Salomon D, Elhanany H, Sabanay H, Kiernan B, Pevny L, Stewart CL, Xu X, Chiu SY, Shrager P, et al. Juxtaparanodal clustering of Shaker-like K+ channels in myelinated axons depends on Caspr2 and TAG-1. J Cell Biol. 2003;162:1149–60.

47. Anderson GR, Galfin T, Xu W, Aoto J, Malenka RC, Sudhof TC. Candidate autism gene screen identifies critical role for cell-adhesion molecule CASPR2 in dendritic arborization and spine development. Proc Natl Acad Sci U S A. 2012;109:18120–5.

48. Krapivinsky G, Medina I, Krapivinsky L, Gapon S, Clapham DE. SynGAP-MUPP1-CaMKII synaptic complexes regulate p38 MAP kinase activity and NMDA receptor-dependent synaptic AMPA receptor potentiation. Neuron. 2004;43:563–74.

49. Sun J, Zhu G, Liu Y, Standley S, Ji A, Tunuguntla R, Wang Y, Claus C, Luo Y, Baudry M, Bi X. UBE3A regulates synaptic plasticity and learning and memory by controlling SK2 channel endocytosis. Cell Rep. 2015;12:449–61.

50. Roullet FI, Wollaston L, Decatanzaro D, Foster JA. Behavioral and molecular changes in the mouse in response to prenatal exposure to the anti-epileptic drug valproic acid. Neuroscience. 2010;170:514–22.

51. Zhang J, Liu LM, Ni JF. Rapamycin modulated brain-derived neurotrophic factor and B-cell lymphoma 2 to mitigate autism spectrum disorder in rats. Neuropsychiatr Dis Treat. 2017;13:835–42.

52. Nicolini C, Ahn Y, Michalski B, Rho JM, Fahnestock M. Decreased mTOR signaling pathway in human idiopathic autism and in rats exposed to valproic acid. Acta Neuropathol Commun. 2015;3:3.

53. Ethridge LE, White SP, Mosconi MW, Wang J, Pedapati EV, Erickson CA, Byerly MJ, Sweeney JA. Neural synchronization deficits linked to cortical hyper-excitability and auditory hypersensitivity in fragile X syndrome. Mol Autism. 2017;8:22.

54. Lovelace JW, Ethell IM, Binder DK, Razak KA. Translation-relevant EEG phenotypes in a mouse model of fragile X syndrome. Neurobiol Dis. 2018;115:39–48.

55. Rinaldi T, Silberberg G, Markram H. Hyperconnectivity of local neocortical microcircuitry induced by prenatal exposure to valproic acid. Cereb Cortex. 2008;18:763–70.

56. Rinaldi T, Perrodin C, Markram H. Hyper-connectivity and hyper-plasticity in the medial prefrontal cortex in the valproic acid animal model of autism. Front Neural Circuits. 2008;2:4.

57. Pawson T. Dynamic control of signaling by modular adaptor proteins. Curr Opin Cell Biol. 2007;19:112–6.

58. Ellegood J, Anagnostou E, Babineau BA, Crawley JN, Lin L, Genestine M, DiCicco-Bloom E, Lai JK, Foster JA, Penagarikano O, et al. Clustering autism: using neuroanatomical differences in 26 mouse models to gain insight into the heterogeneity. Mol Psychiatry. 2015;20:118–25.

59. Darnell JC, Van Driesche SJ, Zhang C, Hung KY, Mele A, Fraser CE, Stone EF, Chen C, Fak JJ, Chi SW, et al. FMRP stalls ribosomal translocation on mRNAs linked to synaptic function and autism. Cell. 2011;146:247–61.

60. Hadley D, Wu ZL, Kao C, Kini A, Mohamed-Hadley A, Thomas K, Vazquez L, Qiu H, Mentch F, Pellegrino R, et al. The impact of the metabotropic glutamate receptor and other gene family interaction networks on autism. Nat Commun. 2014;5:4074.

61. Kelleher RJ 3rd, Geigenmuller U, Hovhannisyan H, Trautman E, Pinard R, Rathmell B, Carpenter R, Margulies D. High-throughput sequencing of mGluR signaling pathway genes reveals enrichment of rare variants in autism. PLoS One. 2012;7:e35003.

62. Zhang J, Zhang JX, Zhang QL. PI3K/AKT/mTOR-mediated autophagy in the development of autism spectrum disorder. Brain Res Bull. 2016;125:152–8.

63. Sato A, Kasai S, Kobayashi T, Takamatsu Y, Hino O, Ikeda K, Mizuguchi M. Rapamycin reverses impaired social interaction in mouse models of tuberous sclerosis complex. Nat Commun. 2012;3:1292.

64. Penagarikano O, Abrahams BS, Herman EI, Winden KD, Gdalyahu A, Dong H, Sonnenblick LI, Gruver R, Almajano J, Bragin A, et al. Absence of CNTNAP2 leads to epilepsy, neuronal migration abnormalities, and core autism-related deficits. Cell. 2011;147:235–46.

65. Onda H, Lueck A, Marks PW, Warren HB, Kwiatkowski DJ. Tsc2(+/−) mice develop tumors in multiple sites that express gelsolin and are influenced by genetic background. J Clin Invest. 1999;104:687–95.

66. Young DM, Schenk AK, Yang SB, Jan YN, Jan LY. Altered ultrasonic vocalizations in a tuberous sclerosis mouse model of autism. Proc Natl Acad Sci U S A. 2010;107:11074–9.

67. Potter WB, Basu T, O'Riordan KJ, Kirchner A, Rutecki P, Burger C, Roopra A. Reduced juvenile long-term depression in tuberous sclerosis complex is mitigated in adults by compensatory recruitment of mGluR5 and Erk signaling. PLoS Biol. 2013;11:e1001627.

68. Consortium TD-BFX. Fmr1 knockout mice: a model to study fragile X mental retardation. Cell. 1994;78:23–33.

69. Kazdoba TM, Leach PT, Silverman JL, Crawley JN. Modeling fragile X syndrome in the Fmr1 knockout mouse. Intractable Rare Dis Res. 2014;3:118–33.

70. Giuffrida R, Musumeci S, D'Antoni S, Bonaccorso CM, Giuffrida-Stella AM, Oostra BA, Catania MV. A reduced number of metabotropic glutamate subtype 5 receptors are associated with constitutive homer proteins in a mouse model of fragile X syndrome. J Neurosci. 2005;25:8908–16.

71. Martin HGS, Lassalle O, Brown JT, Manzoni OJ. Age-dependent long-term potentiation deficits in the prefrontal cortex of the Fmr1 knockout mouse model of fragile X syndrome. Cereb Cortex. 2016;26:2084–92.

72. Rodier PM, Ingram JL, Tisdale B, Nelson S, Romano J. Embryological origin for autism: developmental anomalies of the cranial nerve motor nuclei. J Comp Neurol. 1996;370:247–61.

73. Schneider T, Przewlocki R. Behavioral alterations in rats prenatally exposed to valproic acid: animal model of autism. Neuropsychopharmacology. 2005;30:80–9.

74. Gandal MJ, Edgar JC, Ehrlichman RS, Mehta M, Roberts TP, Siegel SJ. Validating gamma oscillations and delayed auditory responses as translational biomarkers of autism. Biol Psychiatry. 2010;68:1100–6.

75. Iossifov I, Ronemus M, Levy D, Wang Z, Hakker I, Rosenbaum J, Yamrom B, Lee YH, Narzisi G, Leotta A, et al. De novo gene disruptions in children on the autistic spectrum. Neuron. 2012;74:285–99.

76. Rossi M, Chatron N, Labalme A, Ville D, Carneiro M, Edery P, des Portes V, Lemke JR, Sanlaville D, Lesca G. Novel homozygous missense variant of GRIN1 in two sibs with intellectual disability and autistic features without epilepsy. Eur J Hum Genet. 2017;25:376–80.

77. Barnby G, Abbott A, Sykes N, Morris A, Weeks DE, Mott R, Lamb J, Bailey AJ, Monaco AP, International molecular genetics study of autism C. Candidate-gene screening and association analysis at the autism-susceptibility locus on chromosome 16p: evidence of association at GRIN2A and ABAT. Am J Hum Genet. 2005;76:950–66.

78. Platzer K, Yuan H, Schutz H, Winschel A, Chen W, Hu C, Kusumoto H, Heyne HO, Helbig KL, Tang S, et al. GRIN2B encephalopathy: novel findings on phenotype, variant clustering, functional consequences and treatment aspects. J Med Genet. 2017;54:460–70.

79. Iossifov I, Levy D, Allen J, Ye K, Ronemus M, Lee YH, Yamrom B, Wigler M. Low load for disruptive mutations in autism genes and their biased transmission. Proc Natl Acad Sci U S A. 2015;112:E5600–7.

80. Geisheker MR, Heymann G, Wang T, Coe BP, Turner TN, Stessman HAF, Hoekzema K, Kvarnung M, Shaw M, Friend K, et al. Hotspots of missense mutation identify neurodevelopmental disorder genes and functional domains. Nat Neurosci. 2017;20:1043–51.

81. Ramanathan S, Woodroffe A, Flodman PL, Mays LZ, Hanouni M, Modahl CB, Steinberg-Epstein R, Bocian ME, Spence MA, Smith M. A case of autism with an interstitial deletion on 4q leading to hemizygosity for genes encoding for glutamine and glycine neurotransmitter receptor sub-units (AMPA 2, GLRA3, GLRB) and neuropeptide receptors NPY1R, NPY5R. BMC Med Genet. 2004;5:10.

82. Jamain S, Quach H, Betancur C, Rastam M, Colineaux C, Gillberg IC, Soderstrom H, Giros B, Leboyer M, Gillberg C, et al. Mutations of the X-linked genes encoding neuroligins NLGN3 and NLGN4 are associated with autism. Nat Genet. 2003;34:27–9.

83. Sanders SJ, He X, Willsey AJ, Ercan-Sencicek AG, Samocha KE, Cicek AE, Murtha MT, Bal VH, Bishop SL, Dong S, et al. Insights into autism spectrum disorder genomic architecture and biology from 71 risk loci. Neuron. 2015; 87:1215–33.

84. Feyder M, Karlsson RM, Mathur P, Lyman M, Bock R, Momenan R, Munasinghe J, Scattoni ML, Ihne J, Camp M, et al. Association of mouse Dlg4 (PSD-95) gene deletion and human DLG4 gene variation with phenotypes relevant to autism spectrum disorders and Williams' syndrome. Am J Psychiatry. 2010;167:1508–17.

85. Li J, Shi M, Ma Z, Zhao S, Euskirchen G, Ziskin J, Urban A, Hallmayer J, Snyder M. Integrated systems analysis reveals a molecular network underlying autism spectrum disorders. Mol Syst Biol. 2014;10:774.

86. Stessman HA, Xiong B, Coe BP, Wang T, Hoekzema K, Fenckova M, Kvarnung M, Gerdts J, Trinh S, Cosemans N, et al. Targeted sequencing identifies 91 neurodevelopmental-disorder risk genes with autism and developmental-disability biases. Nat Genet. 2017;49:515–26.

87. Durand CM, Betancur C, Boeckers TM, Bockmann J, Chaste P, Fauchereau F, Nygren G, Rastam M, Gillberg IC, Anckarsater H, et al. Mutations in the gene encoding the synaptic scaffolding protein SHANK3 are associated with autism spectrum disorders. Nat Genet. 2007;39:25–7.

88. Nurmi EL, Bradford Y, Chen Y, Hall J, Arnone B, Gardiner MB, Hutcheson HB, Gilbert JR, Pericak-Vance MA, Copeland-Yates SA, et al. Linkage disequilibrium at the Angelman syndrome gene UBE3A in autism families. Genomics. 2001;77:105–13.

89. Glessner JT, Wang K, Cai G, Korvatska O, Kim CE, Wood S, Zhang H, Estes A, Brune CW, Bradfield JP, et al. Autism genome-wide copy number variation reveals ubiquitin and neuronal genes. Nature. 2009;459:569–73.

90. Hamdan FF, Daoud H, Piton A, Gauthier J, Dobrzeniecka S, Krebs MO, Joober R, Lacaille JC, Nadeau A, Milunsky JM, et al. De novo SYNGAP1 mutations in nonsyndromic intellectual disability and autism. Biol Psychiatry. 2011;69:898–901.

91. Riviere JB, Mirzaa GM, O'Roak BJ, Beddaoui M, Alcantara D, Conway RL, St-Onge J, Schwartzentruber JA, Gripp KW, Nikkel SM, et al. De novo germline and postzygotic mutations in AKT3, PIK3R2 and PIK3CA cause a spectrum of related megalencephaly syndromes. Nat Genet. 2012;44:934–40.

92. Serajee FJ, Nabi R, Zhong H, Mahbubul Huq AH. Association of INPP1, PIK3CG, and TSC2 gene variants with autistic disorder: implications for phosphatidylinositol signalling in autism. J Med Genet. 2003;40:e119.

16

Integrated genome-wide Alu methylation and transcriptome profiling analyses reveal novel epigenetic regulatory networks associated with autism spectrum disorder

Thanit Saeliw[1], Chayanin Tangsuwansri[1], Surangrat Thongkorn[1], Weerasak Chonchaiya[2], Kanya Suphapeetiporn[3,4], Apiwat Mutirangura[5], Tewin Tencomnao[6], Valerie W. Hu[7] and Tewarit Sarachana[6]* [iD]

Abstract

Background: Alu elements are a group of repetitive elements that can influence gene expression through CpG residues and transcription factor binding. Altered gene expression and methylation profiles have been reported in various tissues and cell lines from individuals with autism spectrum disorder (ASD). However, the role of Alu elements in ASD remains unclear. We thus investigated whether Alu elements are associated with altered gene expression profiles in ASD.

Methods: We obtained five blood-based gene expression profiles from the Gene Expression Omnibus database and human Alu-inserted gene lists from the TranspoGene database. Differentially expressed genes (DEGs) in ASD were identified from each study and overlapped with the human Alu-inserted genes. The biological functions and networks of Alu-inserted DEGs were then predicted by Ingenuity Pathway Analysis (IPA). A combined bisulfite restriction analysis of lymphoblastoid cell lines (LCLs) derived from 36 ASD and 20 sex- and age-matched unaffected individuals was performed to assess the global DNA methylation levels within Alu elements, and the Alu expression levels were determined by quantitative RT-PCR.

Results: In ASD blood or blood-derived cells, 320 Alu-inserted genes were reproducibly differentially expressed. Biological function and pathway analysis showed that these genes were significantly associated with neurodevelopmental disorders and neurological functions involved in ASD etiology. Interestingly, estrogen receptor and androgen signaling pathways implicated in the sex bias of ASD, as well as IL-6 signaling and neuroinflammation signaling pathways, were also highlighted. Alu methylation was not significantly different between the ASD and sex- and age-matched control groups. However, significantly altered Alu methylation patterns were observed in ASD cases sub-grouped based on Autism Diagnostic Interview-Revised scores compared with matched controls. Quantitative RT-PCR analysis of Alu expression also showed significant differences between ASD subgroups. Interestingly, Alu expression was correlated with methylation status in one phenotypic ASD subgroup.

(Continued on next page)

* Correspondence: tewarit.sa@chula.ac.th
[6]Age-related Inflammation and Degeneration Research Unit, Department of Clinical Chemistry, Faculty of Allied Health Sciences, Chulalongkorn University, 154 Soi Chula 12, Rama 1 Road, Wangmai, Pathumwan, Bangkok 10330, Thailand
Full list of author information is available at the end of the article

(Continued from previous page)

Conclusion: Alu methylation and expression were altered in LCLs from ASD subgroups. Our findings highlight the association of Alu elements with gene dysregulation in ASD blood samples and warrant further investigation. Moreover, the classification of ASD individuals into subgroups based on phenotypes may be beneficial and could provide insights into the still unknown etiology and the underlying mechanisms of ASD.

Keywords: Autism spectrum disorder, Alu elements, Retrotransposon, DNA methylation, Epigenetic regulation, Gene expression profiles, Subgrouping, Lymphoblastoid cell lines, Sex bias, Neuroinflammation,

Background

Autism spectrum disorder (ASD) refers to a group of complex neurodevelopmental disorders that are characterized according to the Diagnostic and Statistical Manual of Mental Disorders, Fifth Edition (DSM-5) criteria by two domains: (i) behavioral impairment, including significant deficits in social interactions and communication, and (ii) restricted interests and repetitive behaviors [1]. Recent data released from the Autism and Developmental Disabilities Monitoring Network have shown a 78% increase in ASD prevalence over the past decade, and approximately 1 in 68 children in the USA have ASD [2]. This increase in ASD prevalence leads to a large economic burden, including costs for healthcare, ASD-related therapy, family-coordinated services, and special education systems [3].

A number of studies have supported the hypothesis that genetic factors are strongly associated with the etiology and susceptibility of ASD. However, abnormalities in genomic DNA are found in only 10–20% of ASD cases accumulatively, partly due to the etiological heterogeneity of ASD, which has a wide variety of different risk factors in addition to genetic factors [4]. A broad variability in clinical phenotypes of ASD individuals are thought to result from complicated interactions between genetic and environmental factors that increase ASD risk [5, 6]. Although the concordance rate among monozygotic (MZ) twins was found to range from 60% to as high as 90%, notable discordance in the ASD diagnosis within monozygotic twin pairs and significant differences in the ASD severity within ASD-concordant monozygotic twin pairs have also been observed [7, 8]. This evidence strongly suggests that environmental factors may play an important role in the etiology and/or the susceptibility of ASD.

DNA methylation is a major epigenetic regulator of gene expression and associated phenotypes. Methylation patterns in genomic DNA are generated during embryogenesis and early fetal development and are altered throughout life in response to endogenous or exogenous environmental signals. Recently, differentially methylated variants (DMVs) at specific CpG sites or differentially methylated regions (DMRs) have been investigated in ASD individuals using various types of tissues, including lymphoblastoid cell lines (LCLs) [9], whole blood [10], and brain tissue samples [11–13]. Nguyen and colleagues

performed a large-scale methylation profiling analysis of LCLs derived from discordantly diagnosed (i.e., ASD and non-ASD) monozygotic twins and sibling pairs [9]. The results revealed differentially methylated genes associated with several biological functions, including gene transcription, nervous system development, and other biological mechanisms implicated in ASD. Moreover, the mRNA expression level of one ASD candidate gene (e.g., retinoic acid-related orphan receptor-alpha gene, *RORA*), which exhibits a differential methylation pattern in ASD, was also decreased in LCLs. Reduced RORA protein levels were also observed in the brain tissues of ASD individuals. This finding suggests that molecular changes in ASD peripheral cells may reflect at least some pathobiological conditions in the brain.

Several studies involving the gene expression profiling of blood or blood-derived cell lines from ASD and non-ASD subjects reported different (but somewhat overlapping) sets of differentially expressed genes (DEGs), most likely due to the heterogeneity within the ASD population. To reduce phenotypic variability and increase statistical power, Hu and Steinberg defined phenotypes within ASD based on cluster analyses of Autism Diagnostic Interview-Revised (ADI-R) scores [14]. Interestingly, gene expression profiling among the LCLs of ASD subgroups also showed differential expression [15]. This result suggested that the sub-classification of ASD patients could help identify subphenotype-specific risk factors in heterogeneous ASD populations. However, most global methylation and gene expression profiling studies have focused on protein-coding regions rather than noncoding regions that include repetitive sequences.

Alu elements are a group of repetitive sequences or mobile genetic elements with copy numbers in excess of one million in the human genome, thus contributing to almost 11% of the human genome [16]. Alu elements belong to a class of retrotransposons termed SINEs (short interspersed elements). Several reports have demonstrated that Alu elements can influence gene expression via insertion into the gene structure and can attract transcription factor binding to regulate gene expression [17]. Alu elements have many CpG residues in their sequences, and these CpG residues are common methylation sites. Methylated CpGs represent approximately

23% of all methylated residues in the human genome [18]. DNA methylation can be altered by exposure to environmental factors that can reduce Alu element methylation in human tissues [19], and there is evidence that Alu methylation plays an important role in cell proliferation and resistance to DNA damage [20]. However, the role of Alu elements and their methylation in ASD remains unclear.

In this study, we therefore aimed to investigate the association between Alu elements and altered gene expression profiles in ASD. First, publicly available gene expression data from previously published ASD transcriptome profiling studies were downloaded from the GEO DataSets database. DEGs from each ASD transcriptome study were identified, and the association between the DEGs from each study and human Alu-inserted genes were determined by Fisher's exact test. Moreover, the DEGs with Alu insertion were identified and subsequently subjected to Ingenuity Pathway Analysis (IPA) to predict the biological functions,

canonical pathways, and gene regulatory networks associated with ASD. A combined bisulfite restriction analysis (COBRA) of Alu was then performed to assess DNA methylation within Alu elements and associated CpGs, which might regulate the expression of Alu elements and Alu-inserted genes. The schematic diagram showing the experimental workflow of this study is illustrated in Fig. 1.

Methods
Data collection
Gene expression profiles of ASD and control individuals were obtained from the NCBI Gene Expression Omnibus database (GEO DataSets: http://www.ncbi.nlm.nih.gov/gds) using the following criteria: the included studies must be ASD studies; the studies must include blood-based gene expression profiles from microarray experiments; and the sample sizes must be greater than or equal to 40 samples. All supplementary information, including series matrix files and related platforms, was

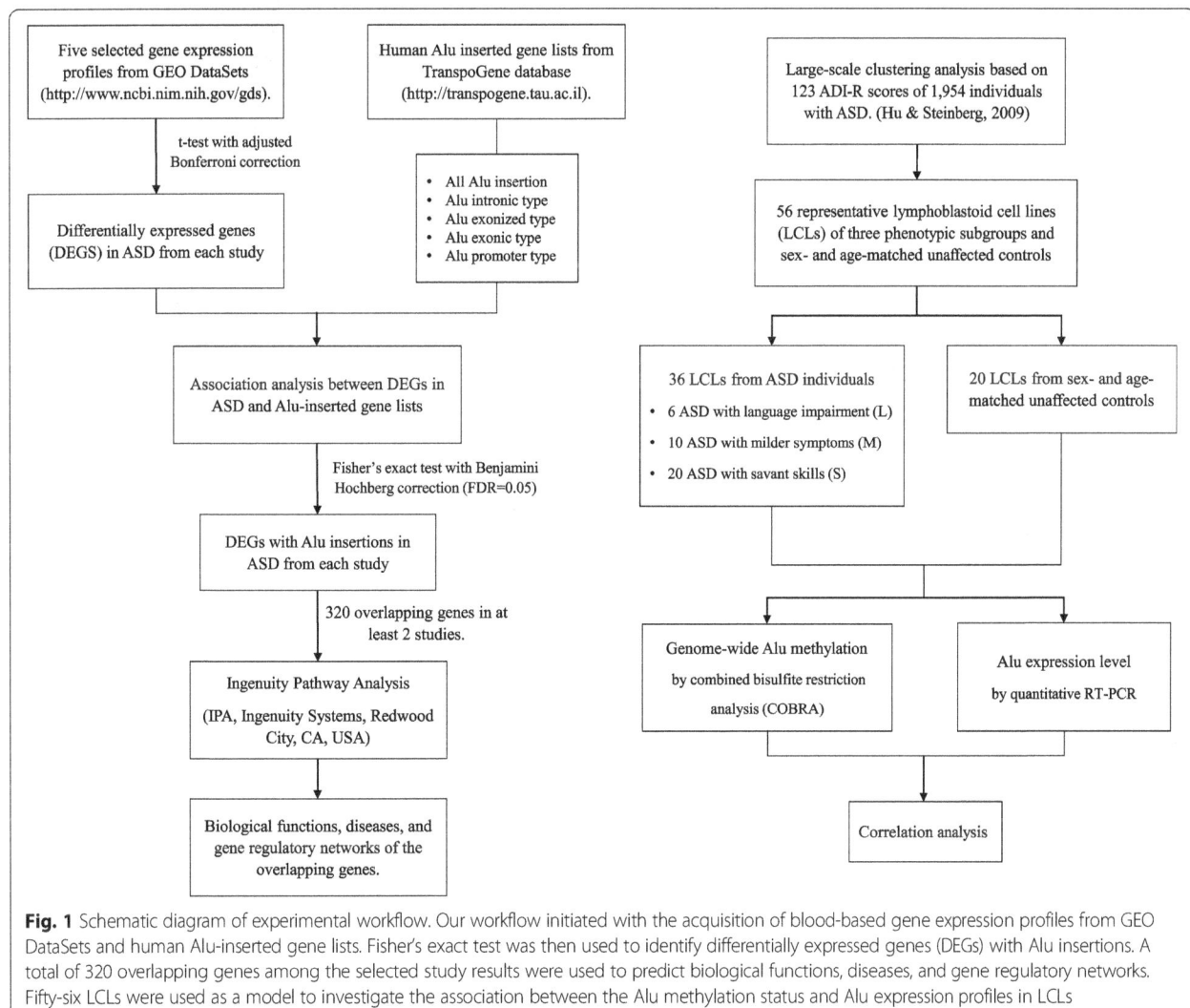

Fig. 1 Schematic diagram of experimental workflow. Our workflow initiated with the acquisition of blood-based gene expression profiles from GEO DataSets and human Alu-inserted gene lists. Fisher's exact test was then used to identify differentially expressed genes (DEGs) with Alu insertions. A total of 320 overlapping genes among the selected study results were used to predict biological functions, diseases, and gene regulatory networks. Fifty-six LCLs were used as a model to investigate the association between the Alu methylation status and Alu expression profiles in LCLs

freely available in GEO DataSets [21, 22]. The details of each study are provided in Table 1.

Alu subfamily-inserted gene lists of Human Genome 18 (UCSC hg18, NCBI build 36.1) were downloaded from the TranspoGene database (http://transpogene.tau.ac.il), which is a publicly available database of transposed elements (TEs) located within protein-coding genes [23]. For the human Alu-inserted genes, a single gene can be inserted by multiple Alu elements with different insertion types. In this study, we obtained all genes with at least one instance of one of the four types of Alu insertions, namely, the exonic, exonized, intronic, and promoter inserts (Table 2). All human Alu subfamily consensus sequences were obtained from Repbase, which is a database of repetitive elements in eukaryotic genomes [24].

Identification of DEGs and association with Alu-inserted genes

The transcriptome profile from each study was analyzed separately by Multiple Experiment Viewer (MEV) [25]. All transcriptome data were filtered using a 70% cutoff, which removes transcripts for which intensity values are missing in > 30% of the samples. The available transcripts were used for identifying DEGs in ASD with two-tailed t tests with adjusted Bonferroni correction. All studies obtained from GEO DataSets employed ASD samples vs. sex- and/or age-matched controls in the analyses. The DEGs and non-DEGs were intersected with the human Alu-inserted gene lists, and the number of intersected genes was classified based on a crosstab 2×2 table into four categories, namely, DEGs with Alu

Table 2 Total number of the Alu-inserted gene lists from TranspoGene database

Insertion type	Alu-inserted genes (n)
All insertion types*	13,534
Exonized type	812
Exonic type	1593
Intronic type	13,245
Promoter type	557

We obtained the lists of human genes with at least one Alu elements from the TranspoGene database. The lists can be categorized into five types of Alu insertions: exonized, exonic, intronic, promoter, and all insertion. Note that multiple Alu elements can be inserted within a single gene with different insertion types. Therefore, the total number of Alu-inserted genes is less than the sum of the exonic, exonized, intronic, and promoter types. These lists of Alu-inserted genes were used for subsequent overlap analyses with differentially expressed genes (DEGs) in ASD
*List of genes with at least one instance of one of the four types of Alu insertions

insertion, DEGs without Alu insertion, non-DEGs with Alu insertion, and non-DEGs without Alu insertion. Fisher's exact test was then used to determine whether the DEG distributions were dependent on the human Alu-inserted gene lists. Moreover, the DEGs were classified as downregulated or upregulated and used for comparison with the human Alu-inserted gene lists. These processes were repeated with each type of human Alu insertion, including intronic, exonized, exonic, and promoter type. A Fisher's exact test P value with Benjamini-Hochberg correction (FDR = 0.05) of less than 0.05 was considered significant.

To identify the reproducibility of the human Alu-inserted genes that were differentially expressed in

Table 1 Details of the gene expression profiles obtained from GEO DataSets

GSE DataSets	Titles	Sample type	Sample information			Number of transcripts		References
			Sample matching	Sample size	Total	Cutoff filter at 70%	Available transcripts with Alu insertion	
GSE15402	Gene expression profiling differentiates autism case-controls and phenotypic variants of autism spectrum disorders	Lymphoblastoid cell lines (LCLs)	Sex (male) and age-matched	87 ASD and 29 controls	116	14,834	6118	Hu VW et al. [15]
GSE18123	Blood gene expression signatures distinguish autism spectrum disorders from controls	Whole blood	Sex (male) and age-matched	170 ASD and 115 controls	285	42,150	8575	Kong SW et al. [32]
GSE25507	Autism and increased paternal age-related changes in global levels of gene expression regulation	Peripheral blood lymphocytes	Sex (male) matched	82 ASD and 64 controls	146	43,735	9437	Alter MD et al. [30]
GSE42133	Disrupted functional networks in autism underlie early brain mal-development and provide accurate classification	Whole blood	Sex (male) matched	91 ASD and 56 controls	147	24,933	7873	Pramparo T et al. [33]
GSE6575	Gene expression in blood of children with autism spectrum disorder	Whole blood	Sex (male) and age-matched	35 ASD and 12 controls	47	43,745	9437	Gregg JP et al. [31]

peripheral blood and cell lines derived from ASD individuals, the significant gene lists from the individual studies were used to create Venn diagrams (http://bioinformatics.psb.ugent.be/webtools/Venn). The DEGs found in at least two studies were selected to identify biological functions and gene regulatory networks that were enriched by Alu elements in ASD.

Identification of biological functions, canonical pathways, and gene regulatory networks associated with Alu elements in ASD

IPA (QIAGEN Inc., https://www.qiagenbioinformatics.com/products/ingenuity-pathway-analysis/) is a powerful bioinformatics tool that is helpful for understanding complex "-omics" data, such as data from microarray experiments. In this study, IPA was used to identify the biological functions, diseases, canonical pathways, and gene regulatory networks of genes that were identified in at least two studies using Fisher's exact tests with Benjamini-Hochberg correction (FDR = 0.05, P value < 0.05).

Experimental models and cell culture

LCLs derived from the peripheral lymphocytes of male individuals were obtained from the Autism Genetic Resource Exchange Repository (AGRE, Los Angeles, CA, USA). Our subjects included LCLs from 36 ASD individuals and 20 sex- and age-matched unaffected controls. These individuals were previously used in large-scale clustering analysis for identification of phenotypic subgroups within ASD based on the Autism Diagnostic Interview-Revised (ADI-R) scores, as previously described in detail [14]. As a result, a total of 1954 individual ASD probands were subdivided into four phenotypic groups based on the scores of the ADI-R questionnaire. Then, we selected representative samples from the groups after excluding ASD individuals with cognitive impairment (Raven's scores < 70), known genetic or chromosomal abnormalities (e.g., Fragile X, Rett syndrome, tuberous sclerosis, chromosome 15q11–q13 duplication), or diagnosed comorbid psychiatric disorders (e.g., bipolar disorder, obsessive compulsive disorder, severe anxiety). Impairment in spoken language was also confirmed based on low standard scores (< 80) on the Peabody Picture Vocabulary Test. Individuals born prematurely (< 35 weeks gestation) were also excluded from this study. These exclusion criteria are expected to reduce the heterogeneity of subjects to study idiopathic autism. Our LCLs represented individuals from three phenotypic groups: severe language impairment (subgroup L), milder symptoms (subgroup M), and savant skills (subgroup S). The demographic information of the LCLs used in this study is shown in Additional file 1. The LCLs were cultured according to the protocol of the Rutgers University Cell and DNA Repository, which maintains the AGRE collection of biological materials from autistic individuals

and their relatives. Briefly, cells were cultured in RPMI 1640 medium supplemented with 15% fetal bovine serum and 1% penicillin/streptomycin. The cultures were split 1: 2 every 3–4 days and harvested for DNA and RNA isolation 3 days after splitting, when the cultures were in the logarithmic growth phase.

Quantitative reverse transcription-PCR analysis

Total RNA was isolated from LCLs of ASD individuals and sex- and age-matched unaffected controls using the GENEzol Reagent (Geneaid, Taiwan) according to the manufacturer's recommended protocol. The RNA concentration was determined using a NanoDrop 1000 spectrophotometer (Thermo Scientific, USA). Quantitative reverse-transcription-PCR (RT-PCR) analysis was used to determine AluS subfamily expression in the LCLs of ASD individuals and controls. First, 5 μg of extracted RNA was treated with DNase enzyme in a 10-μl reaction (RQ1 RNase-Free DNase, Promega), and then, 2 μl of the DNase-treated RNA was reverse-transcribed to complementary DNA (cDNA) using AccuPower® RT PreMix (Bioneer, Korea) and oligo dT$_{18}$ primer in a volume of 20 μl, according to the manufacturer's instructions. The quantitative PCR assay was performed in triplicate using 1 μl of the cDNA in master mix reactions according to the manufacturer's instructions (AccuPower® 2X GreenStar™ qPCR MasterMix, Bioneer, Korea). The amplification cycles consisted of an initial denaturing cycle at 95 °C for 15 min followed by 40 cycles of 45 s at 95 °C for denaturing and 45 s at 60 °C for annealing/extension. Product formation was confirmed by melting curve analysis (55 to 94 °C). The AluS transcript-specific primers were as follows: forward 5′-GTGGCTCACGCCTGTAATC-3′ and reverse 5′-GTAGAGACGGGGTTTCACCA-3′. The number of AluS transcripts was normalized to the housekeeping gene *GAPDH* whose expression was measured using the following primer sequences (forward 5′-ATGTTCGTCATGGGTGTGAA-3′ and reverse 5′-ACAGTCTTCTGGGTGGCAGT-3′), and the AluS expression level was calculated using the $2^{-\Delta\Delta Ct}$ method.

Determination of the Alu methylation levels and patterns in LCLs

Genomic DNA was isolated from LCLs of ASD individuals and sex-/age-matched unaffected controls using the GENEzol Reagent (Geneaid, Taiwan) according to the manufacturer's recommended protocol. The DNA concentration was determined using a NanoDrop 1000 spectrophotometer (Thermo Scientific, USA). COBRA is designed to determine methylation levels and patterns of two CpG loci within AluS subfamilies with the highest number of copies and CpG loci in the human genome (Fig. 2a). Briefly, 1 μg of genomic DNA from each

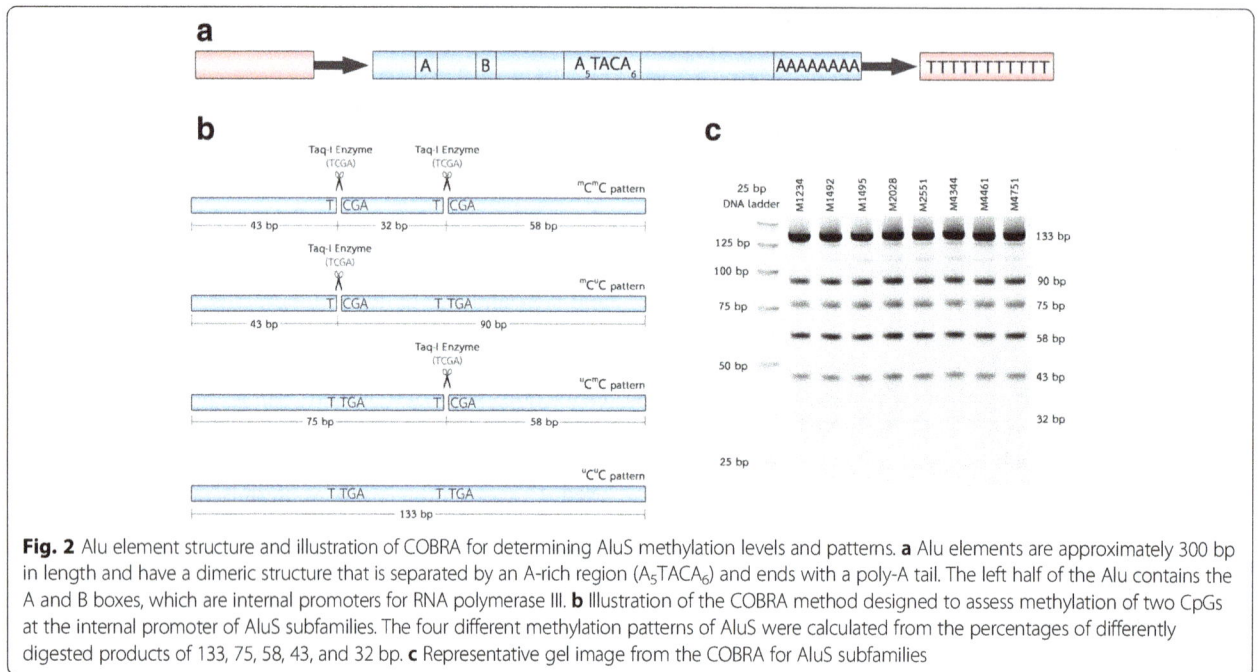

Fig. 2 Alu element structure and illustration of COBRA for determining AluS methylation levels and patterns. **a** Alu elements are approximately 300 bp in length and have a dimeric structure that is separated by an A-rich region (A$_5$TACA$_6$) and ends with a poly-A tail. The left half of the Alu contains the A and B boxes, which are internal promoters for RNA polymerase III. **b** Illustration of the COBRA method designed to assess methylation of two CpGs at the internal promoter of AluS subfamilies. The four different methylation patterns of AluS were calculated from the percentages of differently digested products of 133, 75, 58, 43, and 32 bp. **c** Representative gel image from the COBRA for AluS subfamilies

sample was treated with sodium bisulfite using EZ DNA Methylation-Gold™ Kit (Zymo, Irving, CA, USA). The bisulfite-treated DNA was subjected to 45 cycles of PCR (Hot Start Taq DNA polymerase, QIAGEN, USA) with two specific primers for AluS subfamilies, AluS-F (5′-GGRGRGGTGGTTTARGTTTGTAA-3′) and AluS-R (5′-CTAACTTTTTATATTTTTAATAAAAA-CRAAATTTCACCA-3′), at 53 °C for annealing. Then, the AluS amplicons were digested with TaqI restriction enzyme (Thermo Scientific, USA) in TaqI buffer and incubated at 65 °C overnight. Finally, the digested products were electrophoresed on an 8% non-denaturing polyacrylamide gel, and band intensities were determined for assessment of the AluS methylation levels and patterns as described previously [26].

Upon gel electrophoresis, the digested Alu-amplicons were resolved into six fragments of 133, 90, 75, 58, 43, and 32 bp, which represented different methylation states (Fig. 2b, c), including the $^uC^uC$ methylation state (represented by the 133-bp fragment). The $^mC^uC$ methylation state was represented by the 90-bp fragment. The $^uC^mC$ methylation state was represented by the 75- and 58-bp fragments. The $^mC^mC$ methylation state was represented by the 43- and 32-bp fragments. The calculation for percent AluS methylation was performed as follows. First, the percentage of band intensity was divided by the length (bp) of each DNA fragment: %133/133 = A, %58/58 = B, %75/75 = C, %90/90 = D, %43/43 = E, and %32/32 = F. The percentages of Alu methylation levels and patterns were then calculated using the following formulas: percentage methylated loci (%^mC) = 100 × (E + B)/(2A + E + B + C + D), percentage of

hypermethylated pattern (%$^mC^mC$) = 100 × F/(A + C + D + F), percentage of partially methylated pattern (%$^uC^mC$) = 100 × C/(A + C + D + F), percentage of partially methylated pattern (%$^mC^uC$) = 100 × D/(A + C + D + F), and percentage of partially hypomethylated pattern (%$^uC^uC$) = 100 × A/(A + C + D + F).

Statistical analyses

DEGs were determined using two-tailed t tests with adjusted Bonferroni correction, and adjusted P values less than 0.05 were considered significant. Fisher's exact test with Benjamini-Hochberg (FDR = 0.05) correction was used to investigate the association between the DEG lists and the human Alu-inserted gene lists. P values less than 0.05 were considered significant. Pathway and function analyses were performed with IPA using Fisher's exact test with Benjamini-Hochberg correction for multiple testing (FDR = 0.05); P values less than 0.05 were considered significant. Two-tailed t tests with Benjamini-Hochberg correction (FDR = 0.05) were used to analyze the differences in AluS methylation and expression level; the adjusted P value threshold was 0.05.

Results

Genes containing Alu elements are differentially expressed in ASD blood based on the integration of data from multiple studies

We hypothesized that Alu elements are associated with altered gene expression in the peripheral blood and blood-derived cell lines of ASD individuals and provided CpG sites for DNA methylation within Alu-inserted genes. To test this hypothesis, we obtained five transcriptome profiles from ASD studies available in GEO DataSets and identified a list of DEGs from each study. We then overlapped these DEG lists with the human Alu-inserted genes using Fisher's exact test; the results are shown in Table 3. These results showed that the DEGs in the peripheral blood of ASD individuals were significantly associated with the Alu-inserted gene lists. For the group of all Alu insertion types, the lists of DEGs (up- and downregulated genes) were significantly associated with Alu elements. These lists consist of 388, 869, 1001, and 1492 DEGs from the GSE6575, GSE25507, GSE42133, and GSE18123 studies, respectively. We subsequently identified the up- and downregulated DEGs and assessed their overlap with the "all Alu insertion" gene list type; the results showed a strong association for downregulated genes (adjusted P value < 0.0005). However, the "all Alu insertion" type was only

weakly associated with upregulated genes (adjusted P value = 0.015) in the GSE42133 study and showed a weaker association in the other studies. DEGs were also compared with the other types of Alu insertion gene lists, including the exonic, exonized, intronic, and promoter types. The results are shown in Table 3. These results showed that the DEGs were more strongly associated with the Alu intronic lists than with the other types of Alu insertions. Intronic Alu elements were also strongly associated with the downregulated gene lists. Moreover, because the GSE15402 study has also reduced the heterogeneity of ASD by subgrouping ASD individuals based on their clinical phenotypes using supervised and unsupervised clustering analyses of ADI-R scores, we further investigated whether Alu insertions were associated with DEGs in each ASD subgroup. Interestingly, we found that genes with Alu insertion were significantly

Table 3 Association analyses between the differentially expressed genes (DEGs) in ASD and the human Alu-inserted gene lists

Insertion type	Comparison	GEO datasets	All differentially expressed genes		Upregulated genes		Downregulated genes	
			P value	Genes (n)	P value	Genes (n)	P value	Genes (n)
All insertion	ASD vs. control	GSE15402	0.799	215	0.926	100	0.799	116
		GSE18123	< 0.00005	1492	1.000	255	< 0.00005	1245
		GSE25507	0.012	869	0.256	522	< 0.00005	355
		GSE42133	< 0.00005	1001	0.015	387	< 0.00005	624
		GSE6575	< 0.00005	388	0.955	123	< 0.00005	266
Intronic	ASD vs. control	GSE15402	0.784	212	0.926	99	0.784	114
		GSE18123	< 0.00005	1476	0.970	252	< 0.00005	1231
		GSE25507	0.007	860	0.322	516	< 0.00005	352
		GSE42133	< 0.00005	985	0.012	382	< 0.00005	613
		GSE6575	< 0.00005	382	0.882	119	< 0.00005	264
Exonized	ASD vs. control	GSE15402	1.000	15	0.933	6	0.933	9
		GSE18123	0.009	102	0.926	14	0.003	88
		GSE25507	0.825	45	0.008	17	0.012	28
		GSE42133	0.008	75	0.306	27	0.015	49
		GSE6575	0.006	33	1.000	7	< 0.00005	26
Exonic	ASD vs. control	GSE15402	0.450	19	0.904	10	0.426	9
		GSE18123	0.001	177	0.306	21	< 0.00005	158
		GSE25507	0.426	78	0.136	46	0.662	33
		GSE42133	< 0.00005	148	0.799	43	< 0.00005	106
		GSE6575	0.034	48	0.715	16	0.013	33
Promoter	ASD vs. control	GSE15402	0.933	6	0.436	1	0.799	5
		GSE18123	0.240	37	0.898	8	0.268	29
		GSE25507	0.135	22	0.033	11	0.937	11
		GSE42133	0.831	35	0.447	19	0.255	16
		GSE6575	0.466	16	0.716	3	0.123	13

The list of DEGs from each gene expression profiling study was overlapped with the lists of Alu-inserted genes. Alu-inserted genes were categorized into five types of Alu insertions which included exonized, exonic, intronic, promoter, and combined insertion types. Fisher's exact test with Benjamini-Hochberg correction (FDR = 0.05) was used to determine the association the DEGs and Alu-inserted genes, and P values of less than 0.05 were considered significant. The number of DEGs and adjusted P values are shown associated with DEGs in ASD subgroups but not when all ASD cases were combined (Additional file 2).

We subsequently selected the lists of downregulated genes that were significantly associated with all Alu insertion lists from each study. These lists were used to identify overlapping genes among the selected studies using Venn diagram analysis (Fig. 3). Interestingly, the diagram revealed the reproducibility of Alu-inserted genes that were differentially expressed in ASD whole blood/blood cells. Significant genes that were identified in at least two studies (320 overlapping genes; see Additional file 3) were selected to identify gene regulatory networks, diseases, and biological functions that were associated with Alu elements in ASD.

Biological functions, canonical pathways, and gene regulatory networks of dysregulated genes containing Alu elements are associated with neurological functions and neurodevelopmental disorders

IPA was used to predict the diseases, biological functions, canonical pathways, and gene regulatory networks that were associated with Alu elements in ASD. The results showed that the overlapping genes (320 genes) were significantly associated with neurological diseases and nervous system development and function (adjusted Fisher's exact test, P value < 0.05) (Table 4). Interestingly, 21 overlapping genes were associated with autism or intellectual disability. Eighteen and 20 of the overlapping genes were also associated with mental retardation and cognitive impairment, respectively, which were classified as neurodevelopmental disorders comorbid with ASD. The IPA results also revealed significant canonical

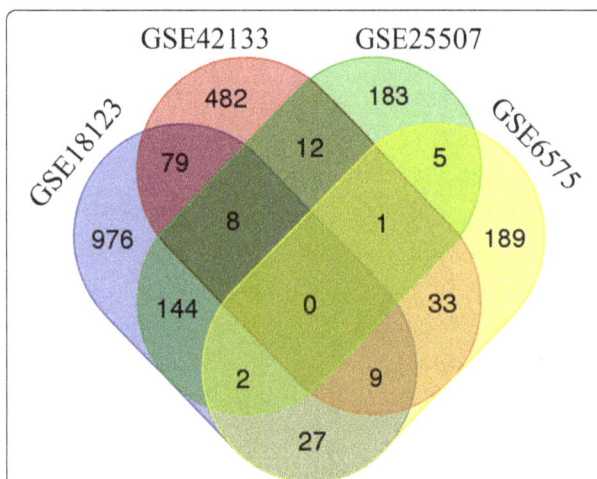

Fig. 3 Venn diagram of genes containing Alu that are differentially expressed in ASD. The significant DEGs with Alu insertions from each study based on Fisher's exact test overlapped. The diagram shows the reproducibility of Alu-inserted genes that were differentially expressed in peripheral blood and blood-derived cell lines from ASD individuals. A total of 320 genes were selected to identify biological functions and gene regulatory networks through an Ingenuity Pathway Analysis (IPA)

pathways associated with the overlapping genes (Table 5), including neurotrophin/TRK signaling, ERK/MAPK signaling, axonal guidance signaling, CREB signaling in neurons, estrogen receptor signaling, androgen signaling, IL-6 signaling, and neuroinflammation signaling, all of which have been associated with ASD.

Gene regulatory networks are sets of genes that interact to control a specific cell function, including cell differentiation, metabolism, cell cycle, and response to environmental cues. A representative gene network associated with neurological disease (Fig. 4) revealed the interaction of overlapping genes with additional molecules from the IPA database involved in estrogen receptor and androgen signaling, axonal guidance signaling, CREB signaling in neurons, and neurotrophin/TRK signaling. This network suggested that some ASD-related biological pathways are associated with Alu-inserted DEGs in the blood of ASD individuals.

AluS methylation levels and patterns in LCLs

To determine the levels of DNA methylation within Alu elements, which contributes to a large proportion of the CpG sites in the human genome, we used LCLs as a model and conducted a COBRA. Specifically, a COBRA of AluS subfamilies was performed to determine the percentages of AluS methylation levels (^{m}C) and patterns ($^{m}C^{m}C$, $^{m}C^{u}C$, $^{u}C^{m}C$, $^{u}C^{u}C$) in LCLs, and the results showed that comparisons of the AluS methylation levels and patterns between the ASD ($n = 36$) and sex- and age-matched unaffected control ($n = 20$) groups were not significantly different (Table 6). The levels and patterns of Alu methylation in individual LCLs are shown in Additional file 4. Due to heterogeneity within ASD individuals, our LCLs were categorized into three subgroups, namely, savant (S), mild (M), and language-impaired (L), based on the ADI-R interview scores according to Hu and Steinberg [14]. In addition, Hu and colleagues reported that the gene expression profiles of LCLs were significantly different among these ASD subgroups [15].

We then compared the AluS methylation levels and patterns between each ASD subgroup and the sex- and age-matched groups. Interestingly, the results showed significant AluS methylation patterns associated with specific ASD subgroups. The percentage of the partially methylated pattern $^{u}C^{m}C$ (20.06% ± 0.92%, adjusted P value = 0.043) was significantly increased in ASD subgroup M (Table 6, Fig. 5). In addition, the percentage of the partially methylated pattern $^{m}C^{u}C$ (20.43% ± 1.17%, adjusted P value = 0.010) was significantly decreased in ASD subgroup S compared with sex- and age-matched controls. There were no significant patterns of AluS methylation in ASD subgroup L. These findings suggested that methylation of Alu elements might play a role in AluS expression and/or transcriptional profile of some ASD subgroups but not all ASD individuals.

Table 4 Diseases and biological functions associated with reproducible DEGs with Alu insertion predicted by the Ingenuity Pathway Analysis (IPA)

Disease or function annotation	Benjamini-Hochberg P value	No. of genes	Gene symbol
Autism or intellectual disability	2.19E–04	21	ABCB1, ADNP, ANKRD11, ARID1A, ATP6V1A, CAMTA1, CASP2, CDC42, CHD4, COL4A3BP, CREBBP, GNB1, OPA1, PTEN, SLC35A3, SMARCA2, SON, TRIO, UBE3A, YY1, ZMYND11
Neuromuscular disease	5.70E–04	34	ABCB1, ADAM10, ALCAM, ANKRD11, ATP2A2, ATP6V1A, ATXN1, CANX, CASP2, CFLAR, GSK3B, HBP1, HMGCR, HSPA5, IFNAR2, IL7R, KIF1B, LDLR, MAP2K4, MBP, MBTPS1, NOTCH2, OSBPL8, PPP3CB, PTPRC, PTPRE, RUNX3, SSX2IP, TLR2, TOMM20, TRIO, USP13, WNK1, XRCC6
Synthesis of reactive oxygen species	7.52E–04	14	CANX, CDC42, CYBB, ETS1, FCER1A, HGF, ITGB1, MAP2K4, MAPK1, PIK3CG, PTEN, SHC1, TLR2, TXNRD1
Disorder of basal ganglia	9.21E–04	29	ABCB1, ANKRD11, ATP2A2, ATP6V1A, ATXN1, CA2, CASP2, CFLAR, GSK3B, HBP1, HMGCR, HSPA5, KIF1B, LDLR, MAP2K4, MBP, MBTPS1, NOTCH2, OSBPL8, PTPRE, RUNX3, SAMHD1, SSX2IP, TOMM20, TRIO, USP13, WNK1, XPR1, XRCC6
Dyskinesia	9.44E–04	23	ABCB1, ANKRD11, ATP2A2, ATP6V1A, ATXN1, CASP2, CFLAR, HBP1, HMGCR, HSPA5, LDLR, MAP2K4, MBTPS1, NOTCH2, OSBPL8, PTPRE, RUNX3, SSX2IP, TOMM20, TRIO, USP13, WNK1, XRCC6
Mental retardation	1.13E–03	18	ADNP, ANKRD11, ARID1A, ATP6V1A, CAMTA1, CASP2, CDC42, CHD4, COL4A3BP, CREBBP, GNB1, OPA1, SLC35A3, SMARCA2, SON, TRIO, YY1, ZMYND11
Brain lesion	1.36E–03	33	ANKRD11, ANXA7, APC, ARCN1, ARID1A, ATP6V1A, CA2, CBL, CREBBP, CTBP2, DICER1, DOCK5, EHD4, HGF, HMGCR, IRS2, LDLR, LYST, NCOA1, NF1, PABPC1, PIK3R1, PRKCSH, PTEN, PTPN11, SAP130, SON, TBK1, TOP1, TRIM33, TRIP11, TRRAP, ZCCHC6
Cognitive impairment	1.44E–03	20	ADNP, ANKRD11, ARID1A, ATP6V1A, CA2, CAMTA1, CASP2, CDC42, CHD4, COL4A3BP, CREBBP, GNB1, HMGCR, OPA1, SLC35A3, SMARCA2, SON, TRIO, YY1, ZMYND11
Dementia	1.62E–03	27	ADAM10, APLP2, ATXN1, CA2, CANX, CASP2, DICER1, GSK3B, HMGCR, HSPA5, LDLR, LIMS1, NFE2L2, OPA1, PIK3R1, PTEN, PTPRE, RUNX3, SLC6A6, SMPD1, SPG21, SRPK2, TBK1, TFCP2, TRIO, UBQLN1, WDR7

Neurological diseases and functions are significantly associated with 320 overlapping genes that were identified in multiple studies. P values calculated by Fisher's exact test with Benjamini-Hochberg correction (FDR = 0.05) and the number of genes for each function are shown

Quantitative reverse transcription-PCR analysis of the AluS expression levels in 56 LCLs

To understand the influence of DNA methylation within AluS elements on AluS expression levels, a quantitative RT-PCR analysis was performed using the LCLs of ASD and sex- and age-matched unaffected control groups. The results showed no significant differences in AluS expression between the ASD and the matched control groups (fold change (FC) = 1.75, adjusted P value 0.316, Table 7), which was similar to the results obtained from the AluS methylation level and pattern analyses. However, comparisons of the AluS expression levels between the ASD phenotypic subgroups and sex- and age-matched control groups revealed that these were significantly different. Specifically, the AluS expression levels were significantly decreased in ASD subgroup L (FC = 0.29, adjusted P value = 0.032) and significantly increased in ASD subgroup S (FC = 3.68, adjusted P value = 0.038). However, in ASD subgroup M, the AluS expression level was not significantly different.

Correlation analysis between AluS methylation levels and AluS expression levels

To demonstrate that AluS methylation regulates the expression of AluS elements, we correlated the DNA methylation and expression levels of AluS subfamilies in the LCLs from ASD individuals and sex- and age-matched controls. The correlation analyses revealed non-linear relationships between DNA methylation and the expression of AluS subfamilies in all groups (ASD + control, Fig. 6). However, when analyzed within the ASD subgroups, we found that the partially methylated pattern $^uC^mC$ showed a moderate positive relationship with AluS expression in ASD subgroup M (coefficient $r = 0.5149$, Fig. 7), whereas other AluS methylation patterns did not correlate with ASD subgroup M. Similarly, DNA methylation and expression of AluS subfamilies were not correlated in ASD subgroups L and S (Additional files 5 and 6). These findings suggested that the partially methylated pattern $^uC^mC$ might regulate the expression of AluS elements in ASD subgroup M.

Discussion

The mechanisms through which human Alu elements are involved in ASD are unclear. In a previous study, Mbarek et al. found a polymorphism of an Alu element in the blood of ASD individuals with more severe clinical symptoms [27]. This allele is located in intron 27b of the neurofibromatosis type 1 (NF1) gene, which is reported to be an ASD risk gene. However, substantially more information was needed to conclude that Alu elements play important roles in ASD. Our findings provide

Table 5 Canonical pathways associated with reproducible DEGs with Alu insertion predicted by the Ingenuity Pathway Analysis (IPA)

Ingenuity canonical pathways	Benjamini-Hochberg P value	Gene symbol
ILK signaling	6.39E−08	PPP2R5E, GSK3B, CDC42, PTEN, IRS2, CREB1, PIK3R4, RHOQ, PIK3R1, MYH9, PIK3CG, PTPN11, MAP2K4, ITGB1, MAPK1, CREBBP, LIMS1, FNBP1, NACA
Neurotrophin/TRK signaling	3.20E−07	CDC42, MAP3K5, IRS2, CREB1, PTPN11, MAP2K4, PIK3R4, MAPK1, CREBBP, PIK3R1, SHC1, PIK3CG
NGF signaling	5.11E−07	CDC42, MAP3K5, IRS2, CREB1, PIK3R4, SMPD1, PIK3R1, PIK3CG, PTPN11, MAP2K4, TRIO, MAPK1, CREBBP, SHC1
Reelin signaling in neurons	1.02E−06	GSK3B, ITGAL, IRS2, FYN, PTPN11, MAP2K4, ITGB1, PIK3R4, PIK3R1, YES1, LYN, PIK3CG
HGF signaling	1.24E−06	CDC42, MAP3K5, IRS2, PIK3R4, ELF2, PIK3R1, PIK3CG, PTPN11, MAP2K4, ITGB1, MAPK1, ETS1, HGF
ERK/MAPK signaling	2.73E−06	PPP2R5E, PAK2, IRS2, CREB1, PIK3R4, ELF2, PRKAG2, PIK3R1, PIK3CG, FYN, PTPN11, ITGB1, MAPK1, CREBBP, ETS1, SHC1
Insulin receptor signaling	5.09E−06	GSK3B, PTEN, IRS2, PIK3R4, PRKAG2, RHOQ, PIK3R1, CBL, PIK3CG, FYN, PTPN11, MAPK1, SHC1
Axonal guidance signaling	2.47E−05	SEMA4D, GSK3B, CDC42, PAK2, IRS2, PIK3R4, PLXNC1, GNB1, PPP3CB, PRKAG2, ADAM10, PIK3R1, RASSF5, PIK3CG, GNAI2, FYN, PPP3R1, PTPN11, ITGB1, MAPK1, PLCL2, SHC1
IL-6 signaling	4.05E−05	ABCB1, MAP4K4, IRS2, PTPN11, MAP2K4, PIK3R4, MAPK1, PIK3R1, SHC1, IL6ST, PIK3CG
Neuroinflammation signaling pathway	4.51E−05	GSK3B, IRS2, CREB1, PIK3R4, PPP3CB, PIK3R1, TBK1, PIK3CG, CFLAR, PPP3R1, PTPN11, MAP2K4, MAPK1, CREBBP, CYBB, TLR2, NFE2L2
Glucocorticoid receptor signaling	4.78E−05	IRS2, CREB1, NCOA1, PIK3R4, SMARCA2, PPP3CB, PRKAG2, PIK3R1, PIK3CG, TAF4, PPP3R1, PTPN11, MAP2K4, HSPA5, MAPK1, CREBBP, ARID1A, SHC1
PI3K/AKT signaling	1.22E−04	PPP2R5E, GSK3B, MAP3K5, PTEN, ITGB1, MAPK1, LIMS1, PIK3R1, SHC1, PIK3CG
CREB signaling in neurons	1.49E−04	IRS2, CREB1, PIK3R4, GNB1, PRKAG2, PIK3R1, PIK3CG, GNAI2, PTPN11, MAPK1, CREBBP, PLCL2, SHC1
Synaptic long-term potentiation	6.29E−03	PPP3R1, CREB1, PPP3CB, MAPK1, CREBBP, PRKAG2, PLCL2
Estrogen receptor signaling	9.05E−03	TAF4, NCOA1, CTBP2, MAPK1, CREBBP, TRRAP, SHC1
Androgen signaling	1.19E−02	GNAI2, NCOA1, GNB1, MAPK1, CREBBP, PRKAG2, SHC1

Canonical pathways are significantly associated with 320 overlapping genes that were identified in multiple studies. P values calculated by Fisher's exact test with Benjamini-Hochberg correction (FDR = 0.05) for each function are shown

preliminary information regarding the association between DEGs and Alu elements in the peripheral blood samples of ASD individuals. It is important to note that Alu elements have the potential to influence gene expression through insertion into the gene structure and through the contribution of gene regulatory elements, such as transcription binding sites and CpG sites [17]. Moreover, Alu elements can act as enhancers, alternate promoters, transcription start sites, and inhibitors of transcription via heterochromatin formation [28, 29].

Several studies have reported altered gene expression profiles in the peripheral blood or blood-derived cell lines of ASD individuals [15, 30–33]. However, no studies have identified an association between DEGs in ASD and Alu elements that could influence gene expression. We first performed multiple gene expression profile comparisons with human Alu-inserted genes in ASD samples using Fisher's exact test. Interestingly, we found that the Alu-inserted genes were associated with DEGs in ASD individuals in four studies (Table 3). These results indicated a strong association of Alu insertion with downregulated genes in ASD, suggesting that Alu

elements could affect gene downregulation. Another interesting question is whether the specific Alu-inserted positions are associated with gene regulation. For this analysis, the Alu-inserted gene list was categorized into four types of Alu insertions: intronic, exonized, exonic, and promoter inserts. Interestingly, we found that intronic Alu insertion was significantly associated with DEGs in ASD individuals. According to a previous study by Tsirigos et al., a genome-wide computational analysis showed that Alu elements selectively retained in the intronic region of inserted genes were associated with specific functions, including the regulation of transcription, RNA processing and splicing, and translation [34]. However, it remains unclear how intronic Alu insertions can influence the expression of genes associated with ASD-related biological functions, and this topic should be investigated further in future research.

We then explored the biological functions associated with 320 DEGs with Alu insertions that overlapped between the selected studies. These overlapping genes were significantly associated with autism or intellectual disability and ASD co-morbid disorders, including

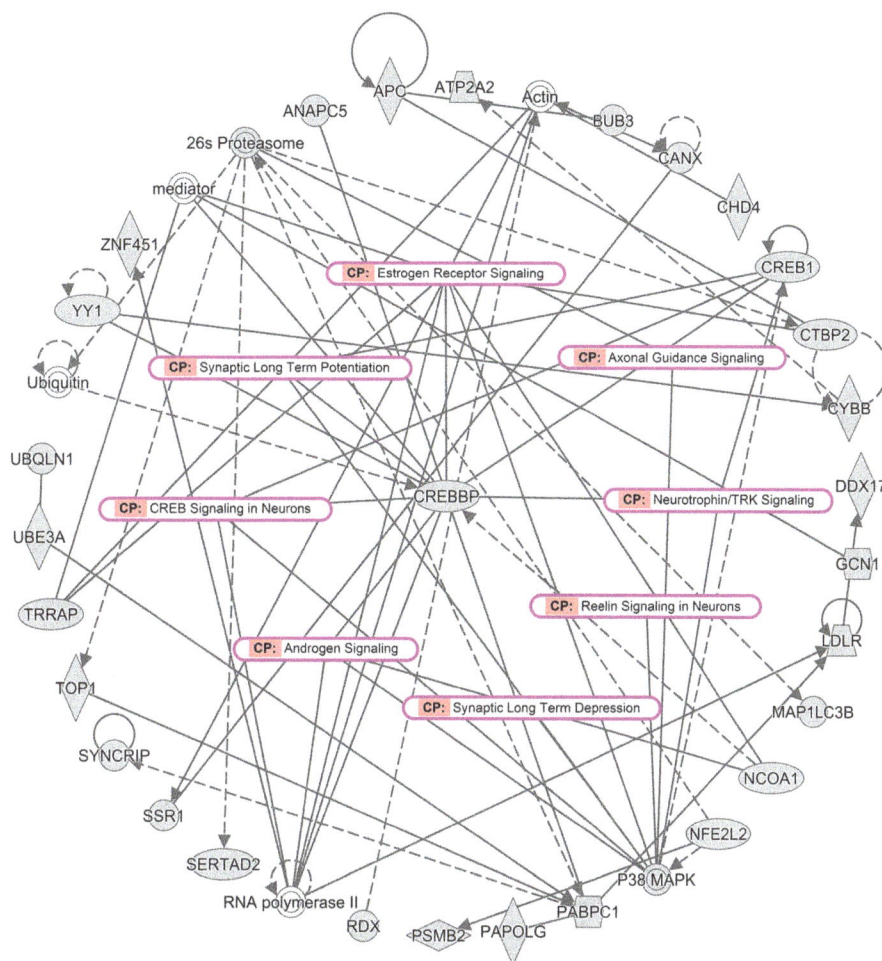

Fig. 4 Predicted gene regulatory network of the overlapping genes associated with neurological disease. This network revealed interactions or relationships among the overlapping molecules (gray background) and with other molecules from the IPA database (white background) that play a role in several mechanisms associated with neurological disease and estrogen receptor and androgen signaling, which is known to be associated with sex bias in ASD (labeled pink)

mental retardation and cognitive impairment. It is noteworthy that sex hormone signaling pathways, including estrogen receptor signaling and androgen signaling pathways, were also associated with DEGs containing Alu elements. ASD is biased towards males with a male-to-female ratio of at least 4:1, and there is accumulating evidence showing that sex hormones and related pathways may play an important role in the sex bias of ASD [35–37]. Recent studies have found that high testosterone exposure during pregnancy significantly correlates with the development of ASD, social development, and language development [38–40]. Moreover, the expression levels of estrogen receptor mRNA and protein were found to be reduced in the brain tissues and serum of ASD individuals [41, 42]. Interestingly, one of the DEGs with Alu insertion related to estrogen receptor and androgen signaling is *NCOA1*, which is a gene encoding the nuclear receptor coactivator 1 protein. This

coregulatory protein has been reported to interact with estrogen receptor and androgen receptor, which oppositely regulate the transcription of the *RORA* gene encoding the retinoic acid-related (RAR) orphan receptor-alpha (RORA) protein [36]. RORA is a hormone-dependent transcription factor that regulates many genes, including *CYP19A1* (aromatase), an enzyme that converts testosterone to estrogen [37, 43–45]. Our previous study also found that RORA binds NCOA1 and regulates the transcription of the *CYP19A1* gene [36]. Thus, it is possible that Alu elements are associated with the sex bias of ASD by disrupting the androgen receptor/estrogen receptor-mediated regulation of *RORA* and *CYP19A1*. Other interesting pathways that are known to be associated with ASD include neurotrophin/TRK signaling [46], ERK/MAPK signaling [47], axonal guidance signaling [48], CREB signaling in neurons [49], IL-6 signaling [50], and neuroinflammation signaling [51].

Table 6 COBRA-derived percentages of AluS methylation and patterns in LCLs from ASD individuals and sex- and age-matched controls

Comparison	Sample groups	Age (mean ± SD)	Percentages of AluS methylation patterns				
			%^{m}C	%^{m}C^{m}C	%^{u}C^{m}C	%^{m}C^{u}C	%^{u}C^{u}C
ASD vs. control (sex- and age-matched)	Control (n = 20)	15 ± 6.97	37.98 ± 1.36	25.70 ± 2.36	18.71 ± 1.15	21.76 ± 1.03	33.83 ± 1.69
	ASD (n = 36)	13.4 ± 4.55	37.86 ± 2.07	25.92 ± 2.69	18.72 ± 1.66	21.22 ± 1.76	34.13 ± 3.00
	P value		0.866	0.866	0.974	0.315	0.845
Subgroup M vs. control (sex- and age-matched)	Control (n = 10)	12.1 ± 3.81	38.07 ± 1.52	25.57 ± 2.31	18.76 ± 0.87	22.06 ± 0.69	33.62 ± 1.85
	ASD subgroup M (n = 10)	12.1 ± 3.73	39.03 ± 1.16	25.17 ± 1.15	20.06 ± 0.92	22.99 ± 0.82	31.77 ± 1.76
	P value		0.293	0.845	*0.043*	0.089	0.168
Subgroup L vs. control (sex- and age-matched)	Control (n = 6)	13.7 ± 1.64	37.84 ± 1.51	24.88 ± 2.94	19.10 ± 1.60	22.25 ± 1.03	33.77 ± 1.84
	ASD subgroup L (n = 6)	13.5 ± 1.97	36.024 ± 1.43	23.37 ± 2.63	19.32 ± 1.69	20.93 ± 2.52	36.38 ± 2.29
	P value		0.168	0.569	0.866	0.502	0.168
Subgroup S vs. control (sex- and age-matched)	Control (n = 20)	15 ± 6.97	37.98 ± 1.36	25.70 ± 2.36	18.71 ± 1.15	21.76 ± 1.03	33.83 ± 1.69
	ASD subgroup S (n = 20)	15 ± 5.41	37.83 ± 2.23	27.06 ± 2.67	17.88 ± 1.44	20.43 ± 1.17	34.64 ± 3.00
	P value		0.866	0.242	0.168	*0.010*	0.502

The percentages of AluS methylation patterns were determined based on four patterns: the hypermethylated pattern (^{m}C^{m}C), two partially methylated patterns (^{m}C^{u}C, ^{u}C^{m}C), and the hypomethylated pattern (^{u}C^{u}C). Comparisons of the methylation status between ASD and sex- and age-matched unaffected control groups and between ASD phenotypic subgroups and the matched unaffected controls were also performed. Statistically significant P values < 0.05 with Benjamini-Hochberg correction (FDR = 0.05) are shown in italics

Although these biological functions and pathways associated with DEGs in ASD with Alu element insertion have been strongly implicated in ASD, we cannot exclude the possibility that all Alu-inserted genes might be enriched for these functions or pathways, regardless of whether they exhibit differential expression in ASD. The full list of Alu-inserted genes could have been used for IPA analysis as a control to address this question. However, IPA does not allow the use of a gene list larger than 8000 genes. This issue should be investigated in future research studies using other pathway analysis programs.

To date, several DMVs at specific CpG sites or DMRs have been identified in many ASD tissue types, including LCLs [9], whole blood [10], and brain [11]. However, these studies did not cover noncoding regions, including repetitive sequences and retrotransposons. DNA methylation is the major epigenetic mechanism that represses retrotransposons in the human genome, particularly Alu elements due to their relatively high CpG density [18, 52, 53]. Kochanek and colleagues found that DNA methylation at CpG sites within an internal promoter (B box) of Alu elements could inhibit their transcriptional activity [54]. In this study, we also assessed the DNA methylation and expression level of AluS subfamilies that contributed the most Alu element copies and CpG sites in the human genome [18]. COBRA of AluS was designed to measure CpG methylation at the internal promoter, including the B box, in LCLs from ASD patients and sex- and age-matched controls. The LCLs were representative samples from three phenotypic groups based on previous multivariate cluster analyses of ADI-R scores of 1954 individuals with ASD. Our

results revealed that the AluS methylation levels and patterns in the LCLs of the combined group of ASD individuals compared with sex- and age-control groups were not significantly different. However, when LCLs were divided into phenotypic subgroups, the AluS methylation patterns in two of the ASD subgroups were significantly different compared with those in the sex- and age-matched controls. In the ASD subgroup with mild symptoms (M), the AluS methylation pattern ^{u}C^{m}C was increased compared with that in the sex- and age-matched controls. Furthermore, the AluS methylation pattern ^{m}C^{u}C was reduced in the ASD subgroup with savant skill (S) compared with the sex- and age-matched controls. Although the abovementioned methylation patterns are statistically significant within a specific ASD subtype, it is also worth noting that other AluS methylation patterns were not much altered in ASD in comparison with control groups. One possible explanation is that AluS elements may be dysregulated only at certain sites in the genome, such as in exonic regions. However, the COBRA analysis used in this study does not measure methylation of AluS at specific genomic locations. Thus, it is likely that signals from significant methylation sites were dampened by noise from a large number of Alu elements located in other non-significant sites in the genome.

We then measured the expression of AluS in the LCLs from the subgroups of ASD and found that AluS was over-expressed in ASD subgroup S and downregulated in the ASD subgroup with severe language impairment (L) relative to their respective sex- and age-matched controls. To investigate whether DNA methylation patterns regulated the expression of Alu elements, we

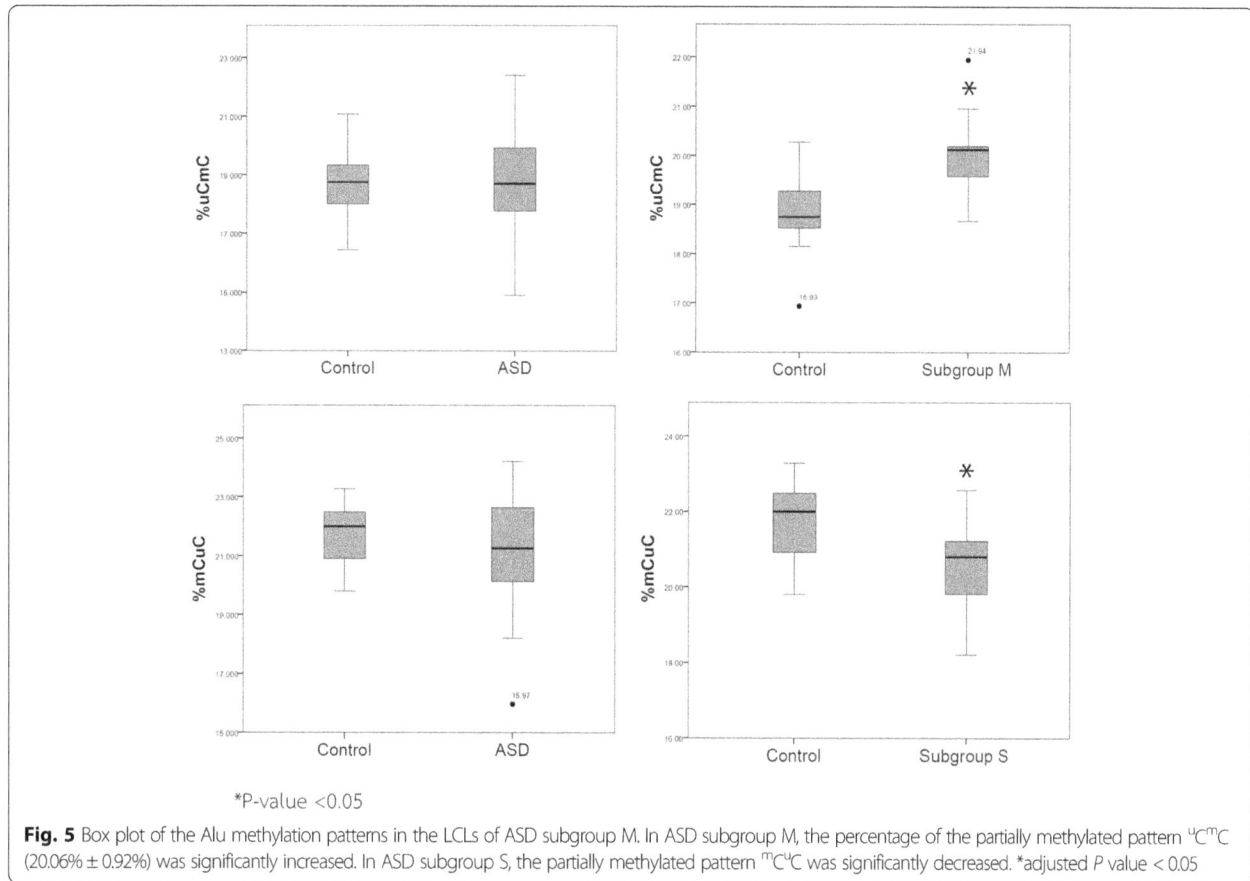

*P-value <0.05

Fig. 5 Box plot of the Alu methylation patterns in the LCLs of ASD subgroup M. In ASD subgroup M, the percentage of the partially methylated pattern $^{u}C^{m}C$ (20.06% ± 0.92%) was significantly increased. In ASD subgroup S, the partially methylated pattern $^{m}C^{u}C$ was significantly decreased. *adjusted P value < 0.05

analyzed the correlations between AluS methylation and expression levels. A positive correlation between AluS methylation and expression was only observed in ASD subgroup M and in sex- and age-matched controls in which the methylation pattern $^{u}C^{m}C$ showed a moderate correlation with AluS expression. It is interesting to note that the methylation pattern $^{u}C^{m}C$ was also significantly increased in subgroup M in the COBRA analysis. These findings suggest that AluS expression may be regulated by the AluS methylation pattern $^{u}C^{m}C$. However, such relationships were not found when all ASD individuals were combined or in other ASD subgroups. In ASD subgroup S, the AluS methylation patterns and

expression levels were not correlated, although the AluS methylation pattern $^{m}C^{u}C$ was significantly reduced, and AluS expression was over-expressed. Moreover, ASD subgroup L showed a significant reduction in AluS expression, but not DNA methylation, indicating that the decrease in AluS expression in ASD subgroup L might result from other epigenetic or gene regulatory mechanisms, such as the disrupted transcription of genes containing an Alu element by altered transcription factor binding at the promoter of the genes but not at the Alu promoter or the other gene regulatory mechanism that have been implicated in LCLs of ASD individuals [55]. These findings suggest that the AluS regulatory mechanism related to methylation might be unique for a specific ASD subpopulation, and there might be other regulatory mechanisms involved in the regulation of AluS methylation and expression, which should be investigated in future research.

The changes of Alu RNAs in LCLs from some ASD subgroups might reflect molecular function because Alu RNAs are involved in transcriptome diversity by contributing recognition sites for RNA editing and alternative splicing within Alu sequences [56]. Altered DNA methylation within Alu elements may have a negative impact on gene regulatory networks, which

Table 7 Quantitative RT-PCR analyses of AluS expression levels in the LCLs of ASD and control groups

Group	Fold change (FC)	$\log_2$ (FC)	P value
ASD vs. control	1.75	0.81	0.316
Subgroup M vs. control	1.05	0.06	0.953
Subgroup L vs. control	0.29	− 1.77	0.032
Subgroup S vs. control	3.68	1.88	0.038

The levels of Alu transcripts were normalized to the housekeeping gene *GAPDH*. The AluS expression levels were calculated using the $2^{-\Delta\Delta Ct}$ method, and differences with a P value < 0.05, as determined by two-tailed *t* tests with Benjamini-Hochberg correction, were considered significant

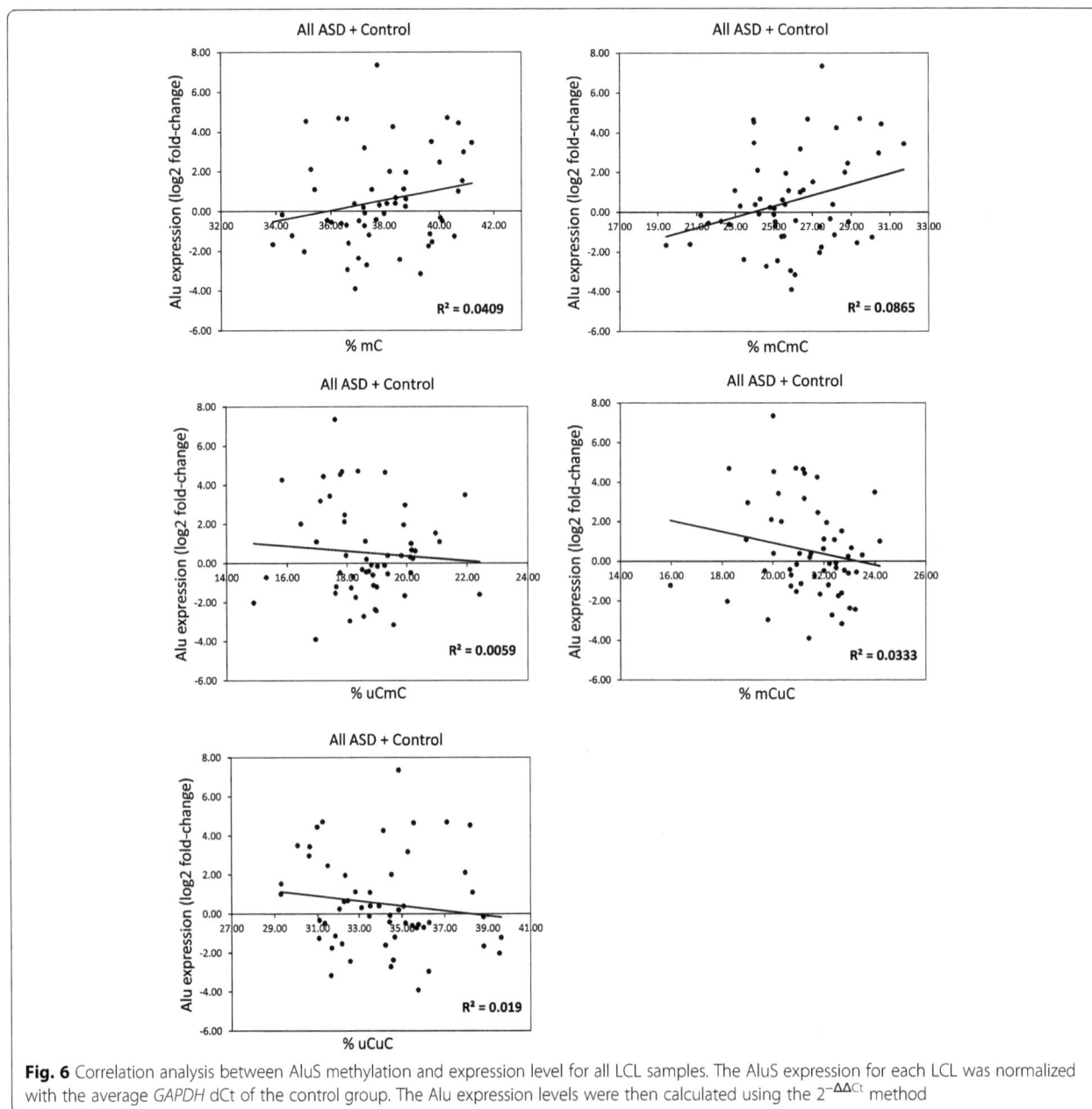

Fig. 6 Correlation analysis between AluS methylation and expression level for all LCL samples. The AluS expression for each LCL was normalized with the average *GAPDH* dCt of the control group. The Alu expression levels were then calculated using the $2^{-\Delta\Delta Ct}$ method

in turn, may affect the biological functions associated with ASD (Fig. 8). The exact mechanisms remain unclear, but it is possible that altered methylation within the Alu promoter, together with other gene regulatory mechanisms, may lead to changes in Alu transcript expression and retrotransposition. Because Alu elements contain transcription factor binding sites within their sequences, these elements could disrupt gene structure and functions by serving as an alternative transcription start site, enhancer, or promoter for cis-/trans-regulation of the target genes once inserted into a new genomic location by the retrotransposition [28, 29, 57–59].

We obtained transcriptomic data from five different studies that used different sample types (e.g., whole blood, leukocytes, and LCLs) as well as different cohorts of subjects with ASD. It remains unclear whether ASD gene expression or methylation signatures will be similar across tissue sources. There might be variations in gene expression and methylation patterns among different sample types and among different cells in the same tissue type. This issue is a potential limitation of this study and should be investigated further in future research. In addition, some of the five selected transcriptome studies did not subgroup ASD individuals before performing DEG analysis and there were no ADI-R scores available

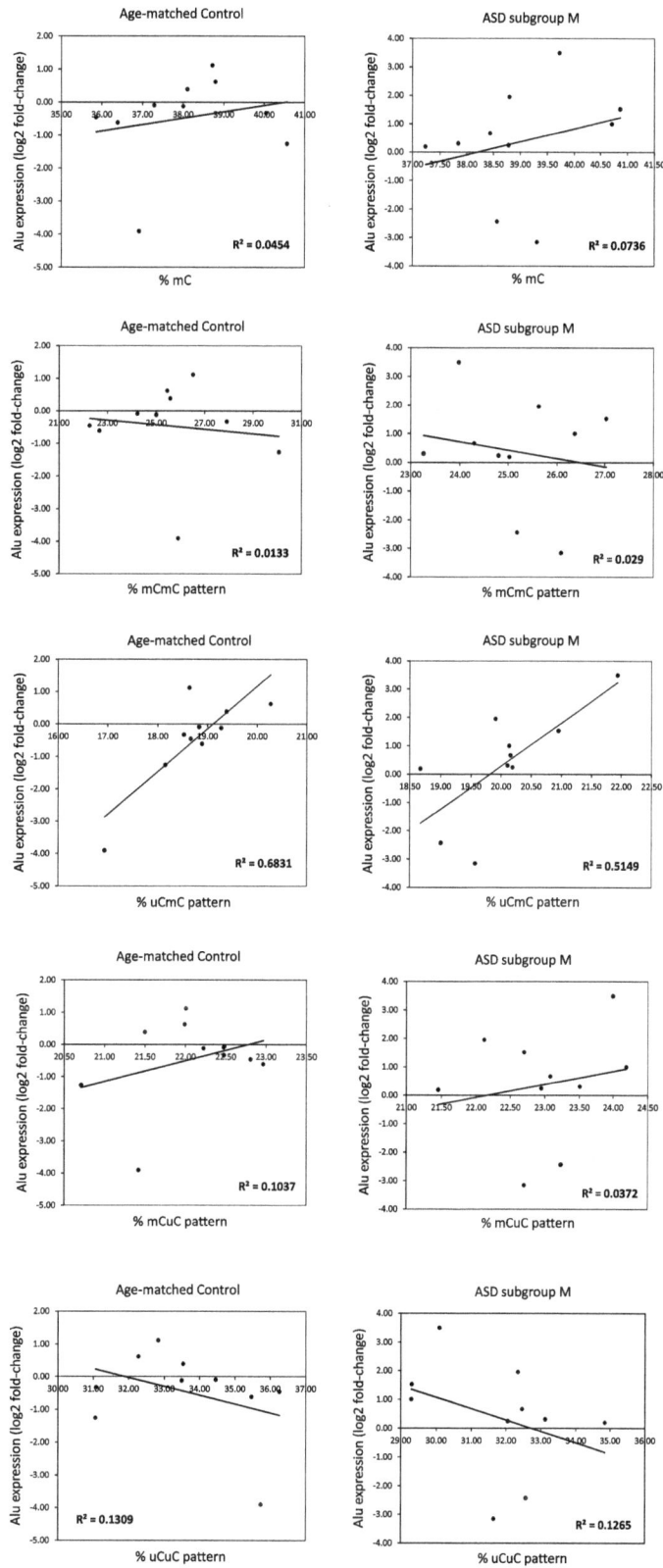

Fig. 7 Correlation analysis between AluS methylation and expression levels in ASD subgroup M and sex- and age-matched controls. The AluS expression of each LCL was normalized to the average *GAPDH* dCt of the control group. The Alu expression levels were then calculated using the $2^{-\Delta\Delta Ct}$ method

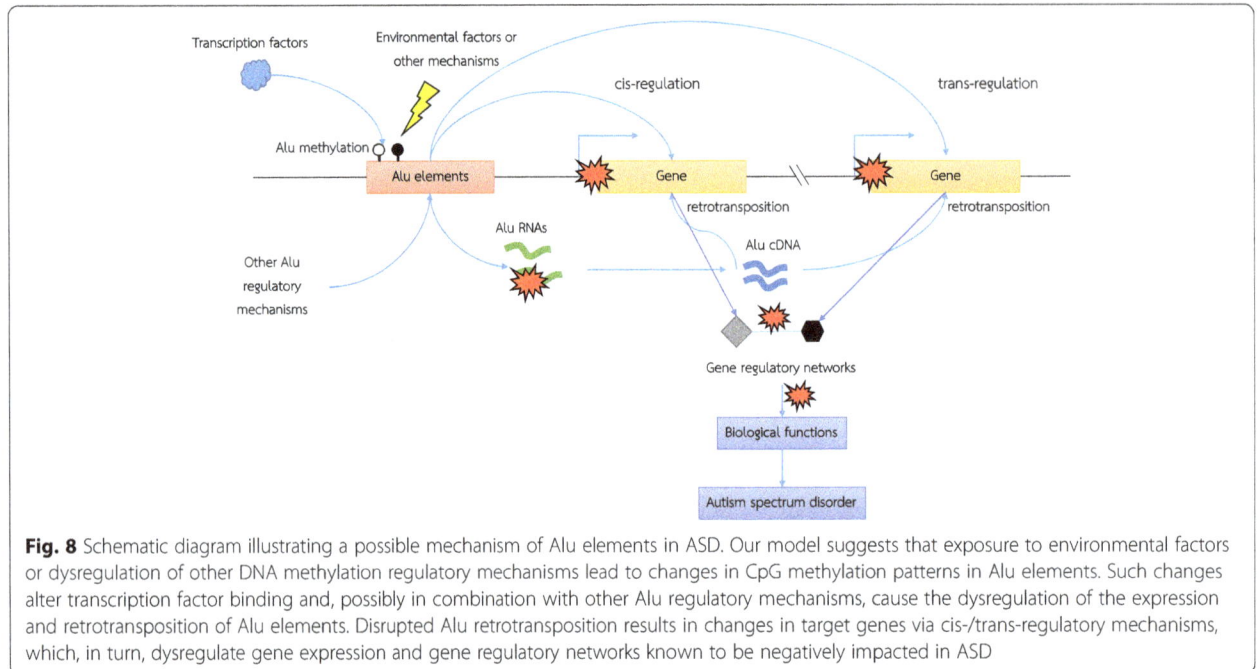

Fig. 8 Schematic diagram illustrating a possible mechanism of Alu elements in ASD. Our model suggests that exposure to environmental factors or dysregulation of other DNA methylation regulatory mechanisms lead to changes in CpG methylation patterns in Alu elements. Such changes alter transcription factor binding and, possibly in combination with other Alu regulatory mechanisms, cause the dysregulation of the expression and retrotransposition of Alu elements. Disrupted Alu retrotransposition results in changes in target genes via cis-/trans-regulatory mechanisms, which, in turn, dysregulate gene expression and gene regulatory networks known to be negatively impacted in ASD

for meta-analysis, whereas others used different criteria and strategies to divide ASD into subgroups. It is therefore difficult to relate our methylation analysis findings to previous analyses of Alu-inserted DEGs in which all ASD individuals were combined or studies using different subgrouping strategies. However, we performed Fisher's exact tests using the microarray data from a previous study (GSE15402) that used the same subgrouping criteria and the same cell model (LCLs) used in this study. Interestingly, we found that genes with Alu element insertion were associated with specific subgroups of ASD rather than with all individuals with ASD. The results of Alu methylation analysis using COBRA and Alu expression analysis using qRT-PCR also showed that the dysregulation of Alu methylation and Alu expression were observed only when ASD cases were divided into subgroups. This finding suggests that the subgrouping of ASD individuals will help reduce heterogeneity and may lead to the discovery of novel mechanisms associated with Alu element in ASD subpopulations. A better understanding of the molecular mechanisms specific for each ASD subgroup might allow the identification of biomarkers and treatment strategies personalized to each subgroup in the future. However, the sample size of this study is relatively small, especially when individuals with ASD were further divided into subgroups. The role of Alu in the context of ASD deserves further studies using a larger cohort. Most importantly, more experiments are needed to verify that Alu elements play important roles in ASD. Brain tissue samples may be used to confirm these findings, and single-cell RNA sequencing might help reduce cell heterogeneity.

Conclusion

Our findings show that the DEGs in males with ASD from several studies with different sample groups are associated with human Alu elements. Differentially expressed genes with Alu insertions were associated with neurodevelopmental disorders and neurological functions involved in the etiology of ASD. In particular, genes involved in estrogen receptor and androgen signaling pathways, which have been reported to be related with sex bias in ASD, were identified as DEGs with Alu insertions. In addition, the global methylation of AluS subfamilies in LCLs was investigated and revealed different AluS methylation patterns within specific ASD phenotypic subgroups. Our findings suggest that the classification of ASD patients into subgroups based on the clinical or behavioral phenotypes of individual patients might help improve our understanding of ASD etiology by reducing the inherent heterogeneity within the ASD population. In addition, this study provides suggestive evidence for an association between Alu elements and ASD.

Additional files

Additional file 1: Demographic information of LCLs used in this study. (DOC 73 kb)

Additional file 2: Association analysis between the DEGs in ASD from GSE15402 and the human Alu-inserted genes lists when ASD individuals were sub-grouped based on ADI-R scores. The comparisons were performed for five types of Alu insertions, including exonized, exonic, intronic, promoter and all types. The Fisher's exact test P value and number of DEGs are shown. (DOC 46 kb)

Additional file 3: List of the overlapping genes. (DOC 118 kb)

Additional file 4: Levels and patterns of Alu methylation in each individual. (DOC 98 kb)

Additional file 5: Correlation analysis between AluS methylation and expression level of ASD subgroup L. (PDF 329 kb)

Additional file 6: Correlation analysis between AluS methylation and expression level of ASD subgroup S. (PDF 333 kb)

Abbreviations

ADI-R: Autism Diagnostic Interview-Revised; ASD: Autism spectrum disorder; COBRA: Combined bisulfite restriction analysis; DEGs: Differentially expressed genes; DMRs: Differentially methylated regions; DMVs: Differentially methylated variants; DSM-5: The Diagnostic and Statistical Manual of Mental Disorders, Fifth Edition; ERK: Extracellular signal-regulated kinases; GEO: Gene Expression Omnibus; IPA: Ingenuity Pathway Analysis; LCLs: Lymphoblastoid cell lines; MAPK: Mitogen-activated protein kinases; RORA: Retinoic acid receptor-related orphan receptor alpha; RPMI: Roswell Park Memorial Institute; RT-PCR: Reverse transcription-polymerase chain reaction; SINEs: Short interspersed elements; TEs: Transposed elements; TRK: Tyrosine kinases

Acknowledgements

TSae, CT, and ST are graduate students in the M.Sc. Program in Clinical Biochemistry and Molecular Medicine, Faculty of Allied Health Sciences, Chulalongkorn University. This work is part of TSae's thesis research to be presented in partial fulfillment of the requirements for the M.Sc. degree. This research was supported by the Ratchadaphiseksomphot Endowment Fund part of the "Research Grant for New Scholar CU Researcher's Project" (GDNS 57-034-37-002) and the Faculty of Allied Health Sciences Research Fund (AHS-CU 58003) to TS. TSae, CT, and ST were financially supported by The 90th Anniversary Chulalongkorn University Fund (Ratchadaphiseksomphot Endowment Fund: TSae-GCUGR1125601055M 53-1; CT-GCUGR1125601058M 53-4; ST-GCUGR1125601056M 53-2). TSae and ST received additional financial support from "The Scholarship from the Graduate School, Chulalongkorn University to commemorate the 72nd anniversary of His Majesty King Bhumibala Aduladeja," while CT received the Research Assistant Scholarship, Chulalongkorn University. WWH is supported by NIEHS grant R21 ES023061. AM is supported by the Thailand Research Fund (DPG5980005). KS is supported by the Thailand Research Fund (BRG5980001). We wish to thank Dr. Charoenchai Puttipanyalears for teaching TSae and CT to conduct the COBRA. We also gratefully acknowledge the resources provided by the Autism Genetic Resource Exchange (AGRE) Consortium* and the participating AGRE families. The Autism Genetic Resource Exchange is a program of Autism Speaks and is supported, in part, by grant 1U24MH081810 from the National Institute of Mental Health to Clara M. Lajonchere (PI). *The AGRE Consortium: Dan Geschwind, M.D., Ph.D., UCLA, Los Angeles, CA; Maja Bucan, Ph.D., University of Pennsylvania, Philadelphia, PA; W.Ted Brown, M.D., Ph.D., F.A.C.M.G., N.Y.S. Institute for Basic Research in Developmental Disabilities, Long Island, NY; Rita M. Cantor, Ph.D., UCLA School of Medicine, Los Angeles, CA; John N. Constantino, M.D., Washington University School of Medicine, St. Louis, MO; T.Conrad Gilliam, Ph.D., University of Chicago, Chicago, IL; Martha Herbert, M.D., Ph.D., Harvard Medical School, Boston, MA; Clara Lajonchere, Ph.D, Cure Autism Now, Los Angeles, CA; David H. Ledbetter, Ph.D., Emory University, Atlanta, GA; Christa Lese-Martin, Ph.D., Emory University, Atlanta, GA; Janet Miller, J.D., Ph.D., Cure Autism Now, Los Angeles, CA; Stanley F. Nelson, M.D., UCLA School of Medicine, Los Angeles, CA; Gerard D. Schellenberg, Ph.D., University of Washington, Seattle, WA; Carol A. Samango-Sprouse, Ed.D., George Washington University, Washington, D.C.; Sarah Spence, M.D., Ph.D., UCLA, Los Angeles, CA; Matthew State, M.D., Ph.D., Yale University, New Haven, CT. Rudolph E. Tanzi, Ph.D., Massachusetts General Hospital, Boston, MA.

Funding

This research was supported by the Ratchadaphiseksomphot Endowment Fund part of the "Research Grant for New Scholar CU Researcher's Project" (GDNS 57-034-37-002) and the Faculty of Allied Health Sciences Research Fund (AHS-CU 58003) to TS. TSae, CT, and ST were financially supported by The 90th Anniversary Chulalongkorn University Fund (Ratchadaphiseksomphot Endowment Fund: TSae-GCUGR1125601055M 53-1; CT-GCUGR1125601058M 53-4; ST-GCUGR1125601056M 53-2). TSae and ST received additional financial support from The Scholarship from the Graduate School, Chulalongkorn University to commemorate the 72nd anniversary of His Majesty King Bhumibala Aduladeja," while CT received the Research Assistant Scholarship, Chulalongkorn University. WWH is supported by NIEHS grant R21 ES023061. AM is supported by the Thailand Research Fund (DPG5980005). KS is supported by the Thailand Research Fund (BRG5980001).

Authors' contributions

TSae performed all the experiments, analyzed the data, and drafted the manuscript under the supervision of TS, AM, TT, WC, and KS. CT assisted TSae in performing COBRA and real-time RT-PCR experiments. ST conducted LCL culture and genomic DNA and RNA extraction. AM and TT provided the enzymes and reagents required for the COBRA analysis. WWH provided all LCLs and the Ingenuity Pathway Analysis program. TS conceived of the study, designed the experiments, and participated in the writing and editing of this manuscript. All the authors read and approved the final manuscript.

Competing interests

The authors declare that they have no competing interests.

Author details

[1]M.Sc. Program in Clinical Biochemistry and Molecular Medicine, Department of Clinical Chemistry, Faculty of Allied Health Sciences, Chulalongkorn University, Bangkok, Thailand. [2]Maximizing Thai Children's Developmental Potential Research Unit, Department of Pediatrics, Faculty of Medicine, Chulalongkorn University and King Chulalongkorn Memorial Hospital, the Thai Red Cross Society, Bangkok, Thailand. [3]Center of Excellence for Medical Genetics, Department of Pediatrics, Faculty of Medicine, Chulalongkorn University, Bangkok, Thailand. [4]Excellence Center for Medical Genetics, King Chulalongkorn Memorial Hospital, Thai Red Cross Society, Bangkok, Thailand. [5]Center of Excellence in Molecular Genetics of Cancer and Human Diseases, Department of Anatomy, Faculty of Medicine, Chulalongkorn University, Bangkok, Thailand. [6]Age-related Inflammation and Degeneration Research Unit, Department of Clinical Chemistry, Faculty of Allied Health Sciences, Chulalongkorn University, 154 Soi Chula 12, Rama 1 Road, Wangmai, Pathumwan, Bangkok 10330, Thailand. [7]Department of Biochemistry and Molecular Medicine, The George Washington University School of Medicine and Health Sciences, The George Washington University, Washington, DC, USA.

References

1. American Psychiatric Association: Diagnostic and Statistical Manual of Mental Disorders. 5th edition. Arlington, VA: 2013.
2. Christensen DL, Baio J, Braun KV, Bilder D, Charles J, Constantino JN, Daniels J, Durkin MS, Fitzgerald RT, Kurzius-Spencer M, et al. Prevalence and characteristics of autism spectrum disorder among children aged 8 years—autism and developmental disabilities monitoring network, 11 sites, United States, 2012. Morbidity Mortal Weekl Repo Surveillance Summ (Washington, DC : 2002). 2016;65(3):1–23.
3. Lavelle TA, Weinstein MC, Newhouse JP, Munir K, Kuhlthau KA, Prosser LA. Economic burden of childhood autism spectrum disorders. Pediatrics. 2014; 133(3):e520–9.
4. Schaefer GB, Mendelsohn NJ. Genetics evaluation for the etiologic diagnosis of autism spectrum disorders. Genet Med. 2008;10(1):4–12.
5. Moosa A, Shu H, Sarachana T, Hu VW. Are endocrine disrupting compounds environmental risk factors for autism spectrum disorder? Horm Behav. 2017. https://doi.org/10.1016/j.yhbeh.2017.10.003.
6. Tordjman S, Somogyi E, Coulon N, Kermarrec S, Cohen D, Bronsard G, Bonnot O, Weismann-Arcache C, Botbol M, Lauth B, et al. Gene x environment interactions in autism spectrum disorders: role of epigenetic mechanisms. Front Psychiatry. 2014;5:53.

7. Bailey A, Le Couteur A, Gottesman I, Bolton P, Simonoff E, Yuzda E, Rutter M. Autism as a strongly genetic disorder: evidence from a British twin study. Psychol Med. 1995;25(1):63–77.

8. Hallmayer J, Cleveland S, Torres A, Phillips J, Cohen B, Torigoe T, Miller J, Fedele A, Collins J, Smith K, et al. Genetic heritability and shared environmental factors among twin pairs with autism. Arch Gen Psychiatry. 2011;68(11):1095–102.

9. Nguyen A, Rauch TA, Pfeifer GP, Hu VW. Global methylation profiling of lymphoblastoid cell lines reveals epigenetic contributions to autism spectrum disorders and a novel autism candidate gene, RORA, whose protein product is reduced in autistic brain. FASEB J. 2010;24(8):3036–51.

10. Wong CC, Meaburn EL, Ronald A, Price TS, Jeffries AR, Schalkwyk LC, Plomin R, Mill J. Methylomic analysis of monozygotic twins discordant for autism spectrum disorder and related behavioural traits. Mol Psychiatry. 2014;19(4):495–503.

11. Ginsberg MR, Rubin RA, Falcone T, Ting AH, Natowicz MR. Brain transcriptional and epigenetic associations with autism. PLoS One. 2012;7(9):e44736.

12. Ladd-Acosta C, Hansen KD, Briem E, Fallin MD, Kaufmann WE, Feinberg AP. Common DNA methylation alterations in multiple brain regions in autism. Mol Psychiatry. 2014;19(8):862–71.

13. Nardone S, Sams DS, Reuveni E, Getselter D, Oron O, Karpuj M, Elliott E. DNA methylation analysis of the autistic brain reveals multiple dysregulated biological pathways. Transl Psychiatry. 2014;4:e433.

14. Hu VW, Steinberg ME. Novel clustering of items from the Autism Diagnostic Interview-Revised to define phenotypes within autism spectrum disorders. Autism Res. 2009;2(2):67–77.

15. Hu VW, Sarachana T, Kim KS, Nguyen A, Kulkarni S, Steinberg ME, Luu T, Lai Y, Lee NH. Gene expression profiling differentiates autism case-controls and phenotypic variants of autism spectrum disorders: evidence for circadian rhythm dysfunction in severe autism. Autism Res. 2009;2(2):78–97.

16. Batzer MA, Deininger PL. Alu repeats and human genomic diversity. Nat Rev Genet. 2002;3(5):370–9.

17. Polak P, Domany E. Alu elements contain many binding sites for transcription factors and may play a role in regulation of developmental processes. BMC Genomics. 2006;7:133.

18. Luo Y, Lu X, Xie H. Dynamic Alu methylation during normal development, aging, and tumorigenesis. Biomed Res Int. 2014;2014:784706.

19. Baccarelli A, Bollati V. Epigenetics and environmental chemicals. Curr Opin Pediatr. 2009;21(2):243–51.

20. Patchsung M, Settayanon S, Pongpanich M, Mutirangura D, Jintarith P, Mutirangura A. Alu siRNA to increase Alu element methylation and prevent DNA damage. Epigenomics. 2018;10(2):175–85.

21. Barrett T, Troup DB, Wilhite SE, Ledoux P, Evangelista C, Kim IF, Tomashevsky M, Marshall KA, Phillippy KH, Sherman PM, et al. NCBI GEO: archive for functional genomics data sets—10 years on. Nucleic Acids Res. 2011;39(Database issue):D1005–10.

22. Edgar R, Domrachev M, Lash AE. Gene Expression Omnibus: NCBI gene expression and hybridization array data repository. Nucleic Acids Res. 2002;30(1):207–10.

23. Levy A, Sela N, Ast G. TranspoGene and microTranspoGene: transposed elements influence on the transcriptome of seven vertebrates and invertebrates. Nucleic Acids Res. 2008;36(Database issue):D47–52.

24. Bao W, Kojima KK, Kohany O. Repbase update, a database of repetitive elements in eukaryotic genomes. Mob DNA. 2015;6:11.

25. Saeed AI, Sharov V, White J, Li J, Liang W, Bhagabati N, Braisted J, Klapa M, Currier T, Thiagarajan M, et al. TM4: a free, open-source system for microarray data management and analysis. BioTechniques. 2003;34(2):374–8.

26. Tiwawech D, Srisuttee R, Rattanatanyong P, Puttipanyalears C, Kitkumthorn N, Mutirangura A. Alu methylation in serum from patients with nasopharyngeal carcinoma. Asian Pac J Cancer Prev. 2014;15(22):9797–800.

27. Mbarek O, Marouillat S, Martineau J, Barthelemy C, Muh JP, Andres C: Association study of the NF1 gene and autistic disorder. Am J Med Genet 1999, 88(6):729-732.

28. Elbarbary RA, Lucas BA, Maquat LE. Retrotransposons as regulators of gene expression. Science (New York, NY). 2016;351(6274):aac7247.

29. Ichiyanagi K. Epigenetic regulation of transcription and possible functions of mammalian short interspersed elements, SINEs. Genes Genet Syst. 2013;88(1):19–29.

30. Alter MD, Kharkar R, Ramsey KE, Craig DW, Melmed RD, Grebe TA, Bay RC, Ober-Reynolds S, Kirwan J, Jones JJ, et al. Autism and increased paternal age related changes in global levels of gene expression regulation. PLoS One. 2011;6(2):e16715.

31. Gregg JP, Lit L, Baron CA, Hertz-Picciotto I, Walker W, Davis RA, Croen LA, Ozonoff S, Hansen R, Pessah IN, et al. Gene expression changes in children with autism. Genomics. 2008;91(1):22–9.

32. Kong SW, Collins CD, Shimizu-Motohashi Y, Holm IA, Campbell MG, Lee IH, Brewster SJ, Hanson E, Harris HK, Lowe KR, et al. Characteristics and predictive value of blood transcriptome signature in males with autism spectrum disorders. PLoS One. 2012;7(12):e49475.

33. Pramparo T, Lombardo MV, Campbell K, Barnes CC, Marinero S, Solso S, Young J, Mayo M, Dale A, Ahrens-Barbeau C, et al. Cell cycle networks link gene expression dysregulation, mutation, and brain maldevelopment in autistic toddlers. Mol Syst Biol. 2015;11(12):841.

34. Tsirigos A, Rigoutsos I. Alu and b1 repeats have been selectively retained in the upstream and intronic regions of genes of specific functional classes. PLoS Comput Biol. 2009;5(12):e1000610.

35. Baron-Cohen S, Auyeung B, Norgaard-Pedersen B, Hougaard DM, Abdallah MW, Melgaard L, Cohen AS, Chakrabarti B, Ruta L, Lombardo MV. Elevated fetal steroidogenic activity in autism. Mol Psychiatry. 2015;20(3):369–76.

36. Sarachana T, Hu VW. Differential recruitment of coregulators to the RORA promoter adds another layer of complexity to gene (dys) regulation by sex hormones in autism. Mol Autism. 2013;4(1):39.

37. Sarachana T, Xu M, Wu RC, Hu VW. Sex hormones in autism: androgens and estrogens differentially and reciprocally regulate RORA, a novel candidate gene for autism. PLoS One. 2011;6(2):e17116.

38. Knickmeyer R, Baron-Cohen S, Raggatt P, Taylor K, Hackett G. Fetal testosterone and empathy. Horm Behav. 2006;49(3):282–92.

39. Tordjman S, Ferrari P, Sulmont V, Duyme M, Roubertoux P. Androgenic activity in autism. Am J Psychiatry. 1997;154(11):1626–7.

40. Whitehouse AJ, Maybery MT, Hart R, Mattes E, Newnham JP, Sloboda DM, Stanley FJ, Hickey M. Fetal androgen exposure and pragmatic language ability of girls in middle childhood: implications for the extreme male-brain theory of autism. Psychoneuroendocrinology. 2010;35(8):1259–64.

41. Crider A, Thakkar R, Ahmed AO, Pillai A. Dysregulation of estrogen receptor beta (ERbeta), aromatase (CYP19A1), and ER co-activators in the middle frontal gyrus of autism spectrum disorder subjects. Mol Autism. 2014;5(1):46.

42. Altun H, Kurutas EB, Sahin N, Sinir H, Findikli E. Decreased levels of G protein-coupled estrogen receptor in children with autism spectrum disorders. Psychiatry Res. 2017;257:67–71.

43. Hu VW, Nguyen A, Kim KS, Steinberg ME, Sarachana T, Scully MA, Soldin SJ, Luu T, Lee NH. Gene expression profiling of lymphoblasts from autistic and nonaffected sib pairs: altered pathways in neuronal development and steroid biosynthesis. PLoS One. 2009;4(6):e5775.

44. Hu VW, Sarachana T, Sherrard RM, Kocher KM. Investigation of sex differences in the expression of RORA and its transcriptional targets in the brain as a potential contributor to the sex bias in autism. Mol Autism. 2015;6:7.

45. Sarachana T, Hu VW. Genome-wide identification of transcriptional targets of RORA reveals direct regulation of multiple genes associated with autism spectrum disorder. Mol Autism. 2013;4(1):14.

46. Correia CT, Coutinho AM, Sequeira AF, Sousa IG, Lourenco Venda L, Almeida JP, Abreu RL, Lobo C, Miguel TS, Conroy J, et al. Increased BDNF levels and NTRK2 gene association suggest a disruption of BDNF/TrkB signaling in autism. Genes Brain Behav. 2010;9(7):841–8.

47. Mukaetova-Ladinska EB, Arnold H, Jaros E, Perry R, Perry E. Depletion of MAP2 expression and laminar cytoarchitectonic changes in dorsolateral prefrontal cortex in adult autistic individuals. Neuropathol Appl Neurobiol. 2004;30(6):615–23.

48. Suda S, Iwata K, Shimmura C, Kameno Y, Anitha A, Thanseem I, Nakamura K, Matsuzaki H, Tsuchiya KJ, Sugihara G, et al. Decreased expression of axon-guidance receptors in the anterior cingulate cortex in autism. Mol Autism. 2011;2(1):14.

49. Ebert DH, Greenberg ME. Activity-dependent neuronal signalling and autism spectrum disorder. Nature. 2013;493(7432):327–37.

50. Wei H, Zou H, Sheikh AM, Malik M, Dobkin C, Brown WT, Li X. IL-6 is increased in the cerebellum of autistic brain and alters neural cell adhesion, migration and synaptic formation. J Neuroinflammation. 2011;8:52.

51. El-Ansary A, Al-Ayadhi L. Neuroinflammation in autism spectrum disorders. J Neuroinflammation. 2012;9:265.

52. Liu WM, Maraia RJ, Rubin CM, Schmid CW. Alu transcripts: cytoplasmic localisation and regulation by DNA methylation. Nucleic Acids Res. 1994;22(6):1087–95.

53. Xing J, Hedges DJ, Han K, Wang H, Cordaux R, Batzer MA. Alu element mutation spectra: molecular clocks and the effect of DNA methylation. J Mol Biol. 2004;344(3):675–82.

54. Kochanek S, Renz D, Doerfler W. Transcriptional silencing of human Alu sequences and inhibition of protein binding in the box B regulatory elements by 5'-CG-3' methylation. FEBS Lett. 1995;360(2):115–20.
55. Sarachana T, Zhou R, Chen G, Manji HK, Hu VW. Investigation of post-transcriptional gene regulatory networks associated with autism spectrum disorders by microRNA expression profiling of lymphoblastoid cell lines. Genome Med. 2010;2(4):23.
56. Sorek R, Ast G, Graur D. Alu-containing exons are alternatively spliced. Genome Res. 2002;12(7):1060–7.
57. Deininger P. Alu elements: know the SINEs. Genome Biol. 2011;12(12):236.
58. Deininger PL, Batzer MA. Alu repeats and human disease. Mol Genet Metab. 1999;67(3):183–93.
59. Hasler J, Strub K. Alu elements as regulators of gene expression. Nucleic Acids Res. 2006;34(19):5491–7.

Permissions

All chapters in this book were first published in MA, by BioMed Central; hereby published with permission under the Creative Commons Attribution License or equivalent. Every chapter published in this book has been scrutinized by our experts. Their significance has been extensively debated. The topics covered herein carry significant findings which will fuel the growth of the discipline. They may even be implemented as practical applications or may be referred to as a beginning point for another development.

The contributors of this book come from diverse backgrounds, making this book a truly international effort. This book will bring forth new frontiers with its revolutionizing research information and detailed analysis of the nascent developments around the world.

We would like to thank all the contributing authors for lending their expertise to make the book truly unique. They have played a crucial role in the development of this book. Without their invaluable contributions this book wouldn't have been possible. They have made vital efforts to compile up to date information on the varied aspects of this subject to make this book a valuable addition to the collection of many professionals and students.

This book was conceptualized with the vision of imparting up-to-date information and advanced data in this field. To ensure the same, a matchless editorial board was set up. Every individual on the board went through rigorous rounds of assessment to prove their worth. After which they invested a large part of their time researching and compiling the most relevant data for our readers.

The editorial board has been involved in producing this book since its inception. They have spent rigorous hours researching and exploring the diverse topics which have resulted in the successful publishing of this book. They have passed on their knowledge of decades through this book. To expedite this challenging task, the publisher supported the team at every step. A small team of assistant editors was also appointed to further simplify the editing procedure and attain best results for the readers.

Apart from the editorial board, the designing team has also invested a significant amount of their time in understanding the subject and creating the most relevant covers. They scrutinized every image to scout for the most suitable representation of the subject and create an appropriate cover for the book.

The publishing team has been an ardent support to the editorial, designing and production team. Their endless efforts to recruit the best for this project, has resulted in the accomplishment of this book. They are a veteran in the field of academics and their pool of knowledge is as vast as their experience in printing. Their expertise and guidance has proved useful at every step. Their uncompromising quality standards have made this book an exceptional effort. Their encouragement from time to time has been an inspiration for everyone.

The publisher and the editorial board hope that this book will prove to be a valuable piece of knowledge for researchers, students, practitioners and scholars across the globe.

List of Contributors

Stavros Stivaros
Academic Unit of Paediatric Radiology, Royal Manchester Children's Hospital, Central Manchester University Hospitals NHS Foundation Trust, Manchester Academic Health Sciences Centre, Manchester, UK
Division of Informatics, Imaging and Data Sciences, School of Health Sciences, Faculty of Biology, Medicine and Health, University of Manchester, Manchester Academic Health Science Centre, Manchester, UK

Stephen Williams
Division of Informatics, Imaging and Data Sciences, School of Health Sciences, Faculty of Biology, Medicine and Health, University of Manchester, Manchester Academic Health Science Centre, Manchester, UK

Shruti Garg and Jonathan Green
Division of Neuroscience and Experimental Psychology, School of Biological Sciences, Faculty of Biology, Medicine and Health, University of Manchester, Manchester Academic Health Science Centre, Manchester University NHS Foundation Trust, Greate Manchester Mental Health NHS Foundation Trust, Room 3.311, Jean McFarlane Building, Oxford Road, Manchester M13 9PL, UK

Maria Tziraki, Karolina Szumanska-Ryt, Laura M Parkes, Hamied A. Haroon and Daniela Montaldi
Division of Neuroscience and Experimental Psychology, School of Biological Sciences, Faculty of Biology, Medicine and Health, University of Manchester, Manchester Academic Health Science Centre, Manchester, UK

Ying Cai and Alcino J. Silva
Departments of Neurobiology, Psychiatry and Biobehavioral Sciences and Psychology, Integrative Center for Learning and Memory, Brain Research Institute, Brain Research Institute, University of California, California, LA 90095, USA

Owen Thomas
Academic Unit of Radiology, Salford Royal Foundation NHS Trust, Manchester Academic Health Sciences Centre, Manchester, UK

Joseph Mellor and John Keane
Computer Science, University of Manchester, Manchester, UK

Andrew A. Morris
Manchester University NHS Foundation Trust, Manchester Academic Health Sciences Centre, Manchester, UK

Carly Jim
Manchester Metropolitan University, Manchester, UK

Nicholas Webb
Department of Paediatric Nephrology, Royal Manchester Children's Hospital, Manchester University NHS Foundation Trust, Academic Health Sciences Centre, Manchester, UK

Francisco X. Castellanos
Hassenfeld Children's Hospital at NYU Langone, Nathan S. Kline Institute for Psychiatric Research, New York, USA

Sue Huson and D. Gareth Evans
Manchester Centre for Genomic Medicine, St Mary's Hospital, Manchester University NHS Foundation Trust, Academic Health Sciences Centre, Manchester, UK

Richard Emsley
Centre for Biostatistics, School of Health Sciences, Faculty of Biology, Medicine and Health, University of Manchester, Manchester, UK

Monica Sonzogni, Ilse Wallaard, Sara Silva Santos, Jenina Kingma, Dorine du Mee, Geeske M. van Woerden and Ype Elgersma
Department of Neuroscience, Erasmus Medical Center, Rotterdam, Netherlands
ENCORE Expertise Center for Neurodevelopmental Disorders, Erasmus Medical Center, Rotterdam, Netherlands

Wing-Chee So, Miranda Kit-Yi Wong, Wan-Yi Lam, Chun-Ho Cheng, Jia-Hao Yang, Ying Huang, Phoebe Ng, Wai-Leung Wong, Chiu-Lok Ho, Kit-Ling Yeung and Cheuk-Chi Lee
Department of Educational Psychology, The Chinese University of Hong Kong, Hong Kong, Special Administrative Region of China

Weiguo Xie, Athena Yao, Min Li, Xiang Gong, Zhigang Chu and Xiaodong Huang
Institute of Rehabilitation Center, Tongren Hospital of Wuhan University, Wuhan 430060, People's Republic of China

Paul Yao
Institute of Rehabilitation Center, Tongren Hospital of Wuhan University, Wuhan 430060, People's Republic of China
Department of Pediatrics, Hainan Maternal and Child Health Hospital, Haikou 570206, People's Republic of China

Xiaohu Ge, Xiaoyan Wang, Haijia Chen and Yifei Wang
SALIAI Stem Cell Institute of Guangdong, Guangzhou SALIAI Stem Cell Science and Technology Co. LTD, Guangzhou 510055, People's Republic of China

Ling Li, Yun Jiao, Meifang Xiao, Wei Xiang and Zhe Lu
Department of Pediatrics, Hainan Maternal and Child Health Hospital, Haikou 570206, People's Republic of China

Hyeong-Min Lee, Ellen P. Clark and M. Bram Kuijer
Department of Cell Biology and Physiology, University of North Carolina School of Medicine, Neuroscience Research Building, Room 5119 115 Mason Farm Rd., Campus Box 7545, Chapel Hill, NC 27599-7545, USA

Benjamin D. Philpot
Department of Cell Biology and Physiology, University of North Carolina School of Medicine, Neuroscience Research Building, Room 5119 115 Mason Farm Rd., Campus Box 7545, Chapel Hill, NC 27599-7545, USA
UNC Neuroscience Center, Carolina Institute for Developmental Disabilities, University of North Carolina School of Medicine, Chapel Hill, NC, USA

Mark Cushman
Department of Medicinal Chemistry and Molecular Pharmacology, Purdue University School of Pharmacy and the Purdue Center for Cancer Research, West Lafayette, IN, USA

Yves Pommier
Developmental Therapeutics Branch and Laboratory of Molecular Pharmacology, Center for Cancer Research, National Cancer Institute, Bethesda, MD, USA

Adrienne Moore, Madeline Wozniak, Andrew Yousef, Cindy Carter Barnes, Debra Cha, Eric Courchesne and Karen Pierce
Autism Center of Excellence, Department of Neurosciences, University of California San Diego, La Jolla, CA, USA

Sophie Carruthers, Emma Kinnaird, Ioannis Bakolis and Rosa A Hoekstra
Institute of Psychiatry, Psychology and Neuroscience, King's College London, London, UK

Alokananda Rudra
Psychology, Ben-Gurion University of the Negev, Beer Sheva, Israel

Paula Smith, Carrie Allison and Simon Baron-Cohen
Autism Research Centre, Department of Psychiatry, University of Cambridge, Cambridge, UK

Bonnie Auyeung
Department of Psychology, School of Philosophy, Psychology and Language Sciences, University of Edinburgh, Edinburgh, UK

Bhismadev Chakrabarti
Centre for Autism, School of Psychology and Clinical Language Sciences, University of Reading, Reading, UK

Akio Wakabayashi
Chiba University, Chiba, Japan

Jesse Barnes
Department of Genetics, Albert Einstein College of Medicine, Bronx, New York, USA

Herbert M. Lachman
Department of Genetics, Albert Einstein College of Medicine, Bronx, New York, USA
Department of Psychiatry and Behavioral Sciences, Albert Einstein College of Medicine, Bronx, New York, USA
Department of Neuroscience, Albert Einstein College of Medicine, Bronx, New York, USA
Department of Medicine, Albert Einstein College of Medicine, Bronx, New York, USA

Franklin Salas and Erika Pedrosa
Department of Psychiatry and Behavioral Sciences, Albert Einstein College of Medicine, Bronx, New York, USA

Ryan Mokhtari
Department of Neuroscience and Physiology, SUNY Upstate Medical University, Syracuse, New York, USA

Hedwig Dolstra
Swammerdam Institute of Life Sciences, University of Amsterdam, Amsterdam, Netherlands

Virginia Carter Leno, Susie Chandler, Pippa White, Isabel Yorke and Andrew Pickles
Institute of Psychiatry, Psychology and Neuroscience, King's College London, 16 De Crespigny Park, London SE5 8AF, UK

Emily Simonoff and Tony Charman
Institute of Psychiatry, Psychology and Neuroscience, King's College London, 16 De Crespigny Park, London SE5 8AF, UK

South London and Maudsley NHS Foundation Trust (SLaM), London, UK

Christine Bole-Feysot, Nicolas Cagnard, Olivier Alibeu and Patrick Nitschke
INSERM UMR 1163, Laboratory of Molecular and pathophysiological bases of cognitive disorders, Imagine Institute, Necker-Enfants Malades Hospital, 24 Boulevard du Montparnasse, 75015 Paris, France

Laurence Colleaux, Lam Son Nguyen and Julien Fregeac
INSERM UMR 1163, Laboratory of Molecular and pathophysiological bases of cognitive disorders, Imagine Institute, Necker-Enfants Malades Hospital, 24 Boulevard du Montparnasse, 75015 Paris, France
Paris Descartes–Sorbonne Paris Cité University, 12 Rue de l'École de Médecine, 75006 Paris, France

Anand Iyer, Jasper Anink and Eleonora Aronica
Department of (Neuro) Pathology, Academic Medical Center, University of Amsterdam, 1105 AZ Amsterdam, The Netherlands

Katherine B. Martin, Jennifer C. Britton, Anibal Gutierrez and Daniel S. Messinger
Department of Psychology, University of Miami, 5665 Ponce de Leon Blvd, Coral Gables, FL 33146, USA

Zakia Hammal
Robotics Institute, Carnegie Mellon University, 5000 Forbes Ave, Pittsburgh, PA 15213, USA

Gang Ren
Center for Computational Science, University of Miami, 1320 S Dixie Hwy, Miami, FL 33146, USA

Jeffrey F. Cohn
Department of Psychology, University of Pittsburgh, 210 S. Bouquet St., Pittsburgh, PA 15260, USA

Justine Cassell
Human Computer Interaction, Carnegie Mellon University, 5000 Forbes Avenue, Pittsburgh, PA 15213, USA

Mitsunori Ogihara
Department of Computer Science, University of Miami, 1365 Memorial Drive, Coral Gables, FL 33146, USA

Denise Haslinger, Regina Waltes, Afsheen Yousaf, Silvia Lindlar, Christine M. Freitag and Andreas G. Chiocchetti
Department of Child and Adolescent Psychiatry, Psychosomatics and Psychotherapy, University Hospital Frankfurt, JW Goethe University Frankfurt, Frankfurt am Main, Germany

Ines Schneider and Simone Fulda
Institute of Experimental Cancer Research in Pediatrics, Frankfurt am Main, Germany

Chai K. Lim and Gilles J. Guillemin
Faculty of Medicine and Health Sciences, Macquarie University, Sydney, New South Wales, Australia

Meng-Miao Tsai and Till Acker
Neuropathology, University of Giessen, Giessen, Germany

Boyan K. Garvalov
Neuropathology, University of Giessen, Giessen, Germany
Department of Microvascular Biology and Pathobiology, European Center for Angioscience (ECAS), Medical Faculty Mannheim, University of Heidelberg, Heidelberg, Germany

Amparo Acker-Palmer
Institute of Cell Biology and Neuroscience and Buchman Institute for Molecular Life Sciences (BMLS), JW Goethe University of Frankfurt, Frankfurt am Main, Germany

Nicolas Krezdorn and Björn Rotter
GenXPro GmbH, Frankfurt am Main, Germany

Marcos Campolongo, Nadia Kazlauskas and Natalí Salgueiro
Universidad de Buenos Aires, Facultad de Ciencias Exactas y Naturales, Departamento de Fisiología, Biología Molecular y Celular, Buenos Aires, Argentina
CONICET-Universidad de Buenos Aires, Instituto de Fisiología, Biología Molecular y Neurociencias (IFIBYNE), Buenos Aires, Argentina

Amaicha Mara Depino
Universidad de Buenos Aires, Facultad de Ciencias Exactas y Naturales, Departamento de Fisiología, Biología Molecular y Celular, Buenos Aires, Argentina
CONICET-Universidad de Buenos Aires, Instituto de Fisiología, Biología Molecular y Neurociencias (IFIBYNE), Buenos Aires, Argentina
UBA-CONICET, Ciudad Universitaria, Int. Guiraldes 2160, Pabellon 2, Ciudad de Buenos Aires, Argentina

German Falasco and Leandro Urrutia
FLENI, Centro de Imágenes Moleculares, Laboratorio de Imágenes Preclínicas, Buenos Aires, Argentina

Christian Höcht
Facultad de Farmacia y Bioquímica, Cátedra de Farmacología, Universidad de Buenos Aires, Buenos Aires, Argentina

Allison Durkin and Jordana Weissman
Seaver Autism Center, Icahn School of Medicine at Mount Sinai, New York, NY 10029, USA

François Muratet, Danielle Halpern, Maria del Pilar Trelles, Silvia De Rubeis, Paige M. Siper and A. Ting Wang
Seaver Autism Center, Icahn School of Medicine at Mount Sinai, New York, NY 10029, USA Department of Psychiatry, Icahn School of Medicine at Mount Sinai, New York, NY 10029, USA

Reymundo Lozano
Seaver Autism Center, Icahn School of Medicine at Mount Sinai, New York, NY 10029, USA Department of Psychiatry, Icahn School of Medicine at Mount Sinai, New York, NY 10029, USA
Department of Pediatrics, Icahn School of Medicine at Mount Sinai, New York, NY 10029, USA
Department of Genetics and Genomic Sciences, Icahn School of Medicine at Mount Sinai, New York, NY 10029, USA

Alexander Kolevzon
Seaver Autism Center, Icahn School of Medicine at Mount Sinai, New York, NY 10029, USA
Department of Psychiatry, Icahn School of Medicine at Mount Sinai, New York, NY 10029, USA
Department of Pediatrics, Icahn School of Medicine at Mount Sinai, New York, NY 10029, USA
Mindich Child Health and Development Institute, Icahn School of Medicine at Mount Sinai, New York, NY 10029, USA

Joseph D. Buxbaum
Seaver Autism Center, Icahn School of Medicine at Mount Sinai, New York, NY 10029, USA. Department of Psychiatry, Icahn School of Medicine at Mount Sinai, New York, NY 10029, USA
Department of Genetics and Genomic Sciences, Icahn School of Medicine at Mount Sinai, New York, NY 10029, USA
Department of Neuroscience, Icahn School of Medicine at Mount Sinai, New York, NY 10029, USA
Friedman Brain Institute, Icahn School of Medicine at Mount Sinai, New York, NY 10029, USA
Mindich Child Health and Development Institute, Icahn School of Medicine at Mount Sinai, New York, NY 10029, USA

Yitzchak Frank
Seaver Autism Center, Icahn School of Medicine at Mount Sinai, New York, NY 10029, USA
Department of Neurology, Icahn School of Medicine at Mount Sinai, New York, NY 10029, USA

J. Lloyd Holder Jr
Division of Neurology and Developmental Neuroscience, Department of Pediatrics, Baylor College of Medicine and Texas Children's Hospital, Houston, TX 77030, USA

Catalina Betancur
Sorbonne Université, INSERM, CNRS, Neuroscience Paris Seine, Institut de Biologie Paris Seine, 75005 Paris, France

Emily A. Brown, Jonathan D. Lautz, Edward P. Gniffke and Noah Tashbook
Center for Integrative Brain Research, Seattle Children's Research Institute, Seattle, WA, USA

Stephen E. P. Smith
Center for Integrative Brain Research, Seattle Children's Research Institute, Seattle, WA, USA
Department of Pediatrics and Graduate Program in Neuroscience, University of Washington, Seattle, WA, USA

Alison A. W. VanSchoiack
Center for Integrative Brain Research, Seattle Children's Research Institute, Seattle, WA, USA
Present address: Nanostring, Seattle, WA, USA

Tessa R. Davis
Department of Immunology, Mayo Clinic College of Medicine, Rochester, MN, USA
Present address: Department of Biomedical Engineering, UT Austin, Austin, TX, USA

Steven C. Neier
Department of Immunology, Mayo Clinic College of Medicine, Rochester, MN, USA
Present address: Department of Cancer Immunology and Virology, Dana-Farber Cancer Institute, Boston, MA, USA
Present address: Department of Medicine, Harvard Medical School, Boston, MA, USA
Present address: Broad Institute of Harvard and MIT, Cambridge, MA, USA

Chiara Nicolini and Margaret Fahnestock
Department of Psychiatry and Behavioural Neurosciences, McMaster niversity, Hamilton, ON, Canada

Adam G. Schrum
Departments of Molecular Microbiology and Immunology, Surgery and Bioengineering, University of Missouri, Columbia, MO, USA

Thanit Saeliw, Chayanin Tangsuwansri and Surangrat Thongkorn
M.Sc. Program in Clinical Biochemistry and Molecular Medicine, Department of Clinical Chemistry, Faculty of Allied Health Sciences, Chulalongkorn University, Bangkok, Thailand

Weerasak Chonchaiya
Maximizing Thai Children's Developmental Potential Research Unit, Department of Pediatrics, Faculty of Medicine, Chulalongkorn University and King Chulalongkorn Memorial Hospital, the Thai Red Cross Society, Bangkok, Thailand

Kanya Suphapeetiporn
Center of Excellence for Medical Genetics, Department of Pediatrics, Faculty of Medicine, Chulalongkorn University, Bangkok, Thailand
Excellence Center for Medical Genetics, King Chulalongkorn Memorial Hospital, Thai Red Cross Society, Bangkok, Thailand

Apiwat Mutirangura
Center of Excellence in Molecular Genetics of Cancer and Human Diseases, Department of Anatomy, Faculty of Medicine, Chulalongkorn University, Bangkok, Thailand

Tewarit Sarachana and Tewin Tencomnao
Age-related Inflammation and Degeneration Research Unit, Department of Clinical Chemistry, Faculty of Allied Health Sciences, Chulalongkorn University, 154 Soi Chula 12, Rama 1 Road, Wangmai, Pathumwan, Bangkok 10330, Thailand

Valerie W. Hu
Department of Biochemistry and Molecular Medicine, The George Washington University School of Medicine and Health Sciences, The George Washington University, Washington, DC, USA

Index

www.ingramcontent.com/pod-product-compliance
Lightning Source LLC
Chambersburg PA
CBHW080514200326
41458CB00012B/4210